KU-026-501

CONTROVERSIES IN THERAPEUTICS

Edited by

LOUIS LASAGNA, M.D.

Professor and Chairman, Department of Pharmacology and Toxicology, University of Rochester School of Medicine and Dentistry, Rochester, New York

1980

W. B. SAUNDERS COMPANY

Philadelphia • London • Toronto

W. B. Saunders Company: West Washington Square
Philadelphia, PA 19105

1 St. Anne's Road
Eastbourne, East Sussex BN21 3UN, England

1 Goldthorne Avenue
Toronto, Ontario M8Z 5T9, Canada

Library of Congress Cataloging in Publication Data

Main entry under title:

Controversies in therapeutics.

1. Chemotherapy. 2. Pharmacy—Social aspects.
I. Lasagna, Louis, 1923- [DNLM: 1. Drug therapy. WB330 C764]
RM263.C68 615'.58 77-86015

Controversies in Therapeutics ISBN 0-7216-5653-6

Last digit is the print number: 9 8 7 6 5 4 3 2 1

Dedication

For David Seegal and Houston Peterson,
who helped me to understand and appreciate controversy.

Where there's a will, there's a won't.

Ambrose Bierce

It is better to debate a question without settling it than to settle a question without debating it.

Joseph Joubert

The gods did not reveal, from the beginning,
All things to us, but in the course of time
Through seeking we may learn and know things better.
But for certain truth, no man has known it,
Nor shall he know it, neither of the gods
Nor yet of all the things of which I speak.
Nor even if by chance he were to utter
The final truth, he would himself not know it:
For all is but a woven web of guesses.

Xenophanes

Contributors

Harold Aaron, M.D. Chairman, Editorial Board, *The Medical Letter.*
Saccharin Should Not Be Banned

W. L. Asher, M.D. Director of Professional Affairs, American Society of Bariatric Physicians; Courtesy Staff, Porter Memorial Hospital, Denver, Colorado.
Drugs Are Useful in Treating Obesity

Daniel L. Azarnoff, M.D. Professor of Medicine and Pharmacology, University of Kansas, College of Health Sciences, Kansas City, Kansas; Attending Physician, University of Kansas Medical Center, Kansas City, Kansas, and Kansas City Veterans Administration Hospital, Kansas City, Missouri.
Monitoring and Control of Physician Prescribing Are Needed

William R. Barclay, M.D. Clinical Professor of Medicine, University of Chicago, Chicago, Illinois; Editor, *Journal of the American Medical Association.*
How Appropriate Is the Proposed Patient Package Labeling?

William T. Beaver, M.D. Associate Professor of Pharmacology and Anesthesia, Georgetown University Schools of Medicine and Dentistry, Washington, D.C.; General Staff, Department of Anesthesia, Georgetown University Hospital, Washington, D.C.
The Medical Costs of Doing Without Opium Derivatives

Burtis B. Breese, M.D. Clinical Professor of Pediatrics, Emeritus, University of Rochester School of Medicine and Dentistry, Rochester, New York.
How Should One Treat Sore Throats?

Robert L. Brent, M.D., Ph.D. Professor and Chairman, Department of Pediatrics; Professor of Anatomy, Professor of Radiology, Jefferson Medical College, Thomas Jefferson University, Philadelphia, Pennsylvania. Chief of Pediatrics, Thomas Jefferson University Hospital, Philadelphia, Pa.
The Prediction of Human Diseases From Laboratory and Animal Tests for Teratogenicity, Carcinogenicity, and Mutagenicity

Rubin Bressler, M.D. Professor and Head, Department of Internal Medicine; Professor of Pharmacology, University of Arizona School of Medicine, Tucson, Arizona.
The Routine Use of Hexachlorophene (HCP) in the Newborn Nursery Should Be Banned

Henry Brill, M.D. Professor of Clinical Psychiatry, School of Medicine, State University of New York at Stony Brook, New York; Consultant in Psychiatry, South Side Hospital, Bay Shore, N.Y., and South Oaks Hospital, Amityville, N.Y.
Should We Do Without Opium Derivatives?

Dale J. Chodos, M.D. Group Research Manager, Medical Affairs, The Upjohn Company, Kalamazoo, Michigan.
Generic Substitution: A Form of Pharmaceutical Russian Roulette?

C. N. Christensen, M.D., Vice President, Lilly Research Laboratories.
Should Trials of Drugs in Children Be Required Before Market Approval for Use in Adults Is Granted?

Leighton E. Cluff, M.D. Adjunct Professor of Medicine, University of Pennsylvania School of Medicine, Philadelphia, Pennsylvania; Vice President, Robert Wood Johnson Foundation, Princeton, New Jersey.
Is Drug Toxicity a Problem of Great Magnitude? Yes!

William H. Crosby, M.D. Adjunct Professor of Medicine, University of California, San Diego, School of Medicine, La Jolla, California; Head, Division of Hematology-Oncology, Scripps Clinic and Research Foundation, La Jolla, Calif.
Should Foods Be Fortified With Iron?

R. John Dobbs, M.B., Ch.B.; D.C.H.; M.R.C.P.(U.K.) Lecturer in Clinical Pharmacology, St. George's Hospital Medical School, London, England; Honorary Senior Medical Registrar, St. George's Hospital, London, England.
Problems With the Use of Drug Blood Levels in Patient Management

Sylvia M. Dobbs, M.B., Ch.B.; MSc.; M.D.(Manchester) Lecturer in Clinical Pharmacology, The Middlesex Hospital Medical School, London, England.
Problems With the Use of Drug Blood Levels in Patient Management

R. Gordon Douglas, Jr., M.D. Professor of Medicine and Microbiology, University of Rochester School of Medicine, Rochester, New York; Head, Infectious Disease Unit, University of Rochester School of Medicine; Senior Attending Physician, Strong Memorial Hospital, Rochester, N.Y.
Amantadine: Should It Be Used as an Antiviral?

Marion J. Finkel, M.D. Associate Director for New Drug Evaluation, Bureau of Drugs, Food and Drug Administration, Rockville, Maryland.
Certain New Drugs Should Be Evaluated in Children Before Marketing

Lawrence Fleckenstein, Pharm.D. Assistant Clinical Professor, Pharmacy, University of California, San Francisco, School of Medicine, San Francisco, California; Director, Drug Information Service, Alta Bates Hospital, Berkeley, Calif.
Patient Package Inserts Will Benefit Consumers

John P. Fox, M.D., Ph.D. Professor of Epidemiology, School of Public Health and Community Medicine, University of Washington, Seattle, Washington.
Which Is Better in Preventing Flu Epidemics–Amantadine or Vaccine?

Edward D. Frohlich, M.D. Vice President, Education and Research, Alton Ochsner Medical Foundation; Director, Division of Hypertensive Diseases, Ochsner Clinic, New Orleans, Louisiana.
Are Beta Blockers Too Dangerous for General Clinical Use?

John Fry, M.D. Family Physician, Beckenham, Kent, England.
Should One Treat All Mild Hypertension? No.

Vincent A. Fulginiti, M.D. Professor and Head, Departmernt of Pediatrics, University of Arizona School of Medicine, Tucson, Arizona.
The Routine Use of Hexachlorophene (HCP) in the Newborn Nursery Should Be Banned

George D. Giraud, B.Sc. (Pharm.) Canadian Heart Foundation Medical Scientist Fellow; University of Calgary Faculty of Medicine, Calgary, Alberta, Canada.
Fixed Ratio Drug Combinations–Sense and Nonsense

Louis Gluck, M.D. Professor of Pediatrics and Reproductive Medicine, University

of California, San Diego, School of Medicine, La Jolla, California; Head, Division of Neonatal/Perinatal Medicine, University Hospital-UCSD Medical Center, San Diego, Calif.
Hexachlorophene: A Useful and Lifesaving Drug

Merwyn R. Greenlick, Ph.D. Adjunct Professor of Sociology, Portland State University; Associate Clinical Professor of Preventive Medicine and Public Health, University of Oregon Medical School, Director, Health Services Research Center, Kaiser Foundation Hospitals.
What Should Be the Standard Approach to Diagnosis and Treatment of Common, Acute Respiratory Infections and Streptococcal Sore Throats in Outpatients?

Birgir Gudjonsson, M.D. Assistant Professor of Medicine, Yale University School of Medicine, New Haven, Connecticut; Attending Gastroenterologist, Yale-New Haven Hospital, New Haven, Conn.
What Is the Best Antacid?

Robert Herschler, B.S. Consultant on Dimethyl Sulfoxide, Medical Research Foundation of Oregon.
The Case of Dimethyl Sulfoxide

Leo E. Hollister, M.D. Professor of Medicine and Psychiatry, Stanford University School of Medicine, Stanford, California; Veterans Administration Hospital, Palo Alto, Calif.
Are Drugs Useful for Treating Senile Dementia?

Richard A. Horvitz, M.D. Clinical Pathologist, Butterworth Hospital, Grand Rapids, Michigan.
Generic Substitution: A Way to Cut Medical Costs

Arnold V. Hurtado, M.D. Associate Clinical Professor of Medicine, University of Oregon Medical School, Portland, Oregon; Medical Director, Sunnyside Medical Center, Portland, Oregon.
What Should Be the Standard Approach to Diagnosis and Treatment of Common, Acute Respiratory Infections and Streptococcal Sore Throats in Outpatients?

Peter Barton Hutt, A.B., LL.B., LL.M. Partner, Covington and Burling, Washington, D.C.; Former Chief Counsel, Food and Drug Administration, Washington, D.C.
The Legal Requirement That Drugs Be Proved Safe and Effective Before Their Use

Stanley W. Jacob, M.D. Associate Professor of Surgery, University of Oregon Health Sciences Center-Medical School, Portland, Oregon.
The Case of Dimethyl Sulfoxide

Judith K. Jones, M.D., Ph.D. Director, Division of Drug Experience, Food and Drug Administration, Washington, D.C.
Do Over-The-Counter Drugs Act Mainly as Placebos? Yes.

William B. Kannel, M.D. Professor of Medicine, Boston University Medical School, Boston, Massachusetts; Consultant, Framingham Union Hospital; Attending Physician, University Hospital, Boston, Evans Memorial.
Should All Mild Hypertension Be Treated? Yes.

Fred E. Karch, M.D. Assistant Professor of Pharmacology, Toxicology and Medicine, University of Rochester School of Medicine and Dentistry, Rochester, New York; Associate Physician, Strong Memorial Hospital, Rochester, N. Y.
Is Drug Toxicity a Problem of Great Magnitude? Probably Not.

Nathan Kase, M.D. Professor of Obstetrics and Gynecology, Yale University School of Medicine, New Haven, Connecticut; Attending Physician, Yale-New Haven Hospital, New Haven, Conn.
A Statement in Favor of Estrogen Replacement Therapy

Irving I. Kessler, M.D., Ph.D. Professor and Chairman, Department of Epidemiology and Preventive Medicine, University of Maryland School of Medicine.
Saccharin Should Not Be Banned

Ambrose J. King, M.B.B.S., F.R.C.S. Consulting Venereologist, The London Hospital, London, England.
All Venereal Disease Contacts Need Not Be Treated

Philip R. Lee, M.D. Professor of Social Medicine, Health Policy Program, University of California, San Francisco School of Medicine, San Francisco, California.
America Is an Overmedicated Society

Samuel Livingston, M.D. Associate Professor Emeritus of Pediatrics, The Johns Hopkins University School of Medicine, Baltimore, Maryland; Director Emeritus and Physician-in-Charge Emeritus, The Johns Hopkins Hospital Epilepsy Clinic, Baltimore, Md.
Clinical Reponse Is More Important Than Measurement of Blood Levels in Managing Epileptic Patients

Keith L. MacCannell, M.D., Ph.D. Professor of Pharmacology and Therapeutics and Professor of Internal Medicine, University of Calgary Faculty of Medicine, Calgary, Alberta, Canada.
Fixed Ratio Drug Combinations – Sense and Nonsense

John M. Mazzullo, M.D. Assistant Professor of Medicine, Harvard Medical School, Boston, Massachusetts; Assistant Physician, Beth Israel Hospital, Boston, Mass.
Generic Substitution and Grandma's Secret Recipe

John P. Morgan, M.D. Associate Professor, School for Biomedical Education, City College of New York, New York, New York; Associate Professor of Medicine and Pharmacology, Mt. Sinai Hospital School of Medicine, New York, N.Y.
The Politics of Medication

Ralph W. Moss, Ph.D. Editor, *Second Opinion.*
In Defense of Laetrile

J. Fraser Mustard, M.D., Ph.D. Professor of Pathology, McMaster University, Hamilton, Ontario, Canada.
Are Aspirin and Sulfinpyrazone Useful in the Prevention of Myocardial Infarction, Strokes, or Venous Thromboembolism?

Marian A. Packham, Ph.D. Professor of Biochemistry, University of Toronto, Toronto, Ontario, Canada.
Myocardial Infarction

Carl C. Peck, M.D. Assistant Clinical Professor of Medicine, University of California, San Francisco School of Medicine, San Francisco, California; Associate Professor of Medicine and Pharmacology, Uniformed Services University of the Health Sciences, Bethesda, Maryland; Consultant in Clinical Pharmacology, Letterman Army Medical Center and Moffitt Hospital, San Francisco, Calif.
Should We Improve Patient Compliance With Therapeutic Regimens, and if so, How?

Joseph M. Pisani, M.D. Clinical Associate Professor of Medicine, George Washington University School of Medicine, Washington, D.C.; Medical Staff, George

Washington University Hospital, Washington, D.C.

Are Most Over-The-Counter Medicines Really Placebos? Definitely Not.

Thaddeus E. Prout, M.D. Associate Professor of Medicine, The Johns Hopkins University School of Medicine, Baltimore, Maryland; Chief of Medicine, The Greater Baltimore Medical Center, Baltimore, Md.

The Myth of the Usefulness of Amphetamines in the Long-Term Management of Obesity

Irving Pruce, B.S., R.Ph. Director of Research, The Samuel Livingston Epilepsy Diagnostic and Treatment Center, Baltimore, Maryland.

Clinical Response Is More Important Than Measurement of Blood Levels in Managing Epileptic Patients

Ellen D. Rie, Ph.D. Adjunct Assistant Professor of Psychology, Case Western Reserve University, Cleveland, Ohio.

Problems in the Use of Stimulant Drugs for Hyperkinesis

Herbert E. Rie, Ph.D. Professor and Chairman, Department of Psychology, Case Western Reserve University, Cleveland, Ohio.

Problems in the Use of Stimulant Drugs for Hyperkinesis

Albert B. Sabin, M.D. Distinguished Research Professor of Biomedicine, Medical University of South Carolina, College of Medicine, Charleston, South Carolina.

Amantadine and Influenza: Evaluation of Conflicting Reports

David L. Sackett, M.D. Professor of Clinical Epidemiology and Biostatistics and Professor of Medicine, McMaster University, Hamilton, Ontario, Canada. Attending Physician, McMaster University Medical Center.

Is There a Patient Compliance Problem? If so, What Do We Do About It?

David S. Salsburg, Ph.D. Pfizer Central Research, Groton, Connecticut.

Are Carcinogenicity Tests Useful?

James H. Sammons, M.D. Executive Vice President, American Medical Association.

New Controls on Physician Prescribing Are Not Needed

Lewis B. Sheiner, M.D. Associate Professor of Medicine and Laboratory Medicine, University of California, San Francisco School of Medicine, San Francisco, California.

Intelligent Use of Drug Blood Level Data Is Helpful in Managing Patients

Ira Shoulson, M.D. Assistant Professor of Neurology, Medicine and Pharmacology, University of Rochester School of Medicine and Dentistry, Rochester, New York; Attending Neurologist and Physician, Strong Memorial Hospital, Rochester, N.Y.

Rational Pharmacotherapy in Dementia: Hazards of "Vasodilator Therapy"

Harold S. Solomon, M.D. Assistant Professor of Medicine, Harvard Medical School, The Peter Bent Brigham Hospital, Boston, Massachusetts; Director, Hypertension Clinic, Peter Bent Brigham Division of the Affiliated Hospital Center, Inc.

How to Improve Patient Compliance

Howard M. Spiro, M.D. Professor of Medicine, Yale University School of Medicine, New Haven, Connecticut; Attending Gastroenterologist, Yale-New Haven Hospital, New Haven, Conn.

What Is the Best Antacid?

Richard K. Tompkins, M.D. Associate Professor of Health Services and Medicine, University of Washington, Seattle, Washington; Director, U.S. Public Health Service Hospital, Seattle, Wash.

A Management Strategy for Sore Throat Based on Cost-Effectiveness Analysis

M. Verstraete, M.D., Ph.D. Professor, University of Leuven, Belgium; Director, Center for Thrombosis and Vascular Research, University of Leuven, Belgium.
Can Drugs, by Suppressing Some Platelet Functions, Prevent Postoperative Deep Vein Thrombosis and Coronary Heart Disease

Philip D. Walson, M.D. Associate Professor of Pediatrics and Assistant Professor of Pharmacology, University of Arizona School of Medicine, Tucson, Arizona.
The Routine Use of Hexachlorophene (HCP) in the Newborn Nursery Should Be Banned

Murray Weiner, M.D. Clinical Professor of Medicine, University of Cincinnati College of Medicine, Cincinnati, Ohio; Vice President, Research and Scientific Affairs, Merrell Research Center.
Should the Public Have the Legal Right to Use Unproven Remedies? Yes.

Michael Weintraub, M.D. Associate Professor of Pharmacology and Medicine, University of Rochester School of Medicine and Dentistry, Rochester, New York.
Fixed Ratio Combinations – Pro Position

Paul H. Wender, M.D. Professor of Psychiatry, University of Utah College of Medicine, Salt Lake City, Utah; Attending Psychiatrist, University Hospital, University of Utah College of Medicine, Salt Lake City, Utah.
The Role of Stimulant Medication in the Treatment of the Hyperactive Child

Richard R. Willcox, M.D., F.R.C.P. Honorary Consulting Venereologist, St. Mary's Hospital, London, England; Consultant Venereologist, King Edward VII Hospital, Windsor, England; Member, World Health Organization Expert Panel on Venereal Infections and Treponematoses.
Should Venereal Disease Contacts Be Treated? A Qualified Yes.

Harry K. Ziel, M.D. Assistant Clinical Professor of Obstetrics and Gynecology, University of Southern California School of Medicine, Los Angeles, California; Clinical Associate, Department of Nursing, California State University, Los Angeles, Calif; Attending Obstetrician and Gynecologist, Kaiser Foundation Hospital, Los Angeles, Calif.
The Negative Side of Long-Term Postmenopausal Estrogen Therapy

Preface

A perverse characteristic of the human race is its preference for spurious simplicity as opposed to truthful complexity. Doctors are not immune to this virus, and indeed they are often inoculated with large quantities of it in their medical education by well meaning pedagogues who try to ease student anxieties by "not making the practice of medicine too complicated." Nor is this teaching principle devoid of merit—it often seems easier to build upon a solid bedrock of general (and generally valid) principles than to start with a foundation shot full of caveats and exceptions.

But sooner or later departures from the party line must be incorporated into one's medical thought if the magnificent richness of patient complaints, syndromes, and therapies is to be adequately encompassed. A wise physician once said that doctors have to learn to live with ambiguity. They need not (and indeed cannot) resign themselves to diagnostic or therapeutic paralysis, but it is surely better in the long run to acknowledge the fact that one does not know for certain what is the "right" thing to do, even as one makes the best judgment possible at any given time.

This book tries to convey the disagreements that characterize some of society's most pressing therapeutic questions. A good course in therapeutics could certainly be organized around the opposing positions taken by men of good will and expertise in the pages that follow.

Some readers may recall the delightful (but now defunct) television program called "Omnibus," hosted by the urbane and witty Alastair Cooke. One such program featured a playlet by William Saroyan about an old lady and a necktie salesman. These parts were played—if memory serves correctly—by Helen Hayes and Burgess Meredith. At one point the lady asks the salesman whether he wouldn't think it splendid to die for something in which he truly believed. "No," he replied, "I might be wrong."

As I get older, I find myself thinking more and more like the necktie salesman and less and less like the old lady. Not that I have lost my passion for vigorous stands, but rather that I more readily appreciate how easy it is to make a reasonable case for the other fellow's position. I am reminded of the prodigious ambivalence of the famous southern politician when asked for his stand on alcohol:

> If you mean that most fiendish, corrupt and hell-soaked institution that ever crawled out of the eternal pit; that open sore of the land; the scourge that transforms the loving husband and father to a heartless wretch to steal the shoes from his starving babe's feet; the devil's own, that robs your innocent daughter of her virtue and transforms her into a wanton harlot; then I'm against it! But if you mean that pleasant refreshment of mankind that promotes good comradeship to dedicate man to the values of fellowship, equality and euphoria; providing a warm and quiet retreat where man and women may explore the pleasures of friendship away from the nagging cares of creditor, spouse and clergyman; where one can lift the burdens of caste and status and grasp the dim image of his own individuality; then I'm for it.*

Louis Lasagna, M.D.

* Palmer, G.C.: The truth about alcohol. der Sitzmarker 24:6, 1974.

Acknowledgments

I am most grateful to Marie D. Low, Medical Editor of the W.B. Saunders Company, whose idea it was to put this volume together, and to her associate Jill Goldman, who worked so hard over the final processing of the many contributions.

In my own office, I am indebted to Kris Wemett, who helped during the painful early months when the line-up of authors was being decided, and who, along with Linda Donovan, prodded recalcitrant authors to get in their promised contributions. Typing of manuscripts, quotations, and commentary was ably provided by Ruth Kimmerer, and most of the correspondence was handled by Holley Swanson.

I hope all these friends are pleased with the book, but they are blameless for any of its faults.

Louis Lasagna

Contents

SECTION I – BASIC ISSUES

SECTION II – SPECIFIC PROBLEMS

SECTION I

Basic Issues

1

Are We an Overmedicated Society?

As to disease, make a habit of two things—to help, or at least to do no harm.

Hippocrates, *Epidemics*

Even in medicine, though it is easy to know what honey, wine and hellebore, cautery and surgery are, to know how and to whom and when to apply them so as to effect a cure is no less an undertaking than to be a physician.

Aristotle, *Nichomachean Ethics*

It is a great mistake to suppose that Nature always stands in need of the assistance of Art . . . nor do I think it below me to acknowledge that, when no manifest indication pointed out to me what was to be done, I have consulted the safety of my patient and my own reputation effectually by doing nothing at all.

Thomas Sydenham

Nothing kills like doing nothing.

Danish proverb

Introduction

Few topics in medicine elicit such passions in the hearts of physicians as the question "Are we an overmedicated society?" Some, like Dr. Lee, are convinced that we resort too often to medicines and that physicians are active partners with many patients in indulging in an all too common tendency "to seek a pill for every ill."

Lee finds the great increase in prescriptions and drug sales in the last quarter century disquieting, and he singles out in particular the inappropriate use of antibiotics, psychotropic drugs, analgesics, and hormones.

Morgan, in contrast, finds the expenditures by our society on medicines to be small in comparison with what we spend on tobacco, alcohol, telephones, and automobile tires. He asks whether the increasing drug use may not simply reflect the market availability of more drugs and the better care of the ill. Unlike Lee, Morgan finds little of concern in the usage of minor tranquilizers and antibiotics, and he reminds us that hypertensive patients are still seriously undertreated.

Perhaps the important message in Dr. Morgan's contribution lies in his urging that we analyze *why* the segments of our society think as they do about drug use—regardless of their final opinion.

LOUIS LASAGNA, M.D.

America Is an Overmedicated Society

Philip R. Lee, M.D.
University of California, San Francisco

The discussion of whether America is an overmedicated society must begin with the definition of *overmedication*. Overmedication exists when drug use is either unjustified or inappropriate. Use is unjustified when there is no proper indication for the drug or when the drug is ineffective. Use is inappropriate when more effective or less hazardous drugs are available, when a drug is used in excessive amounts or for an excessive length of time, when a fixed combination drug is used and only one of the components is indicated, or when a costly drug is prescribed and a less costly one of equal effectiveness is available.

What is the evidence of overmedication? It begins with data that demonstrate the remarkable increase both in sales of prescription drugs and in volume of prescriptions during the past 30 years. It includes the changing patterns of prescription drug use during that period, the data on the extent of prescription and over-the-counter (OTC) drug use in population samples in the United States, and an international comparative study that revealed the highest volume of prescription and OTC drug use per person in North America as compared with those in Europe and Latin America. But the case for overmedication, especially with respect to prescription drugs, must be built on more than a recitation of gross statistics. It must rest on evidence gleaned from a careful examination of prescribing practices for certain classes of drugs and for specific drugs within those classes.

Growth in Prescription Drug Sales

The growth in American drug industry sales during the past two decades reflects the remarkable amount of drug use in this country, as witnessed by the more than sixfold increase in sales over the past 23 years. In 1954, drug firms headquartered in the U.S. reported domestic sales of approximately \$1.3 billion; by 1965, sales had risen to \$2.8 billion; and in 1977, the figure stood at an estimated \$8.7 billion (Pharmaceutical Manufacturers Association, 1977). These sales are for finished human dosage form pharmaceuticals only. Increased sales have been particularly dramatic for antibiotics, psychotropic drugs, analgesics, and hormones. The figures reflect the increasing number of prescriptions dispensed annually during this period.

Growth in Volume of Prescriptions

It is estimated that over 70 million Americans regularly use prescription or OTC drugs. Since 1950, the average number of prescriptions dispensed by community pharmacies, discount stores, and physicians has risen from 2.4 per person each year to 6.9 in 1976, almost a threefold increase in 25 years. The per capita increase is also reflected in the total number of prescriptions dispensed in community pharmacies—from 363 million in 1950 to an estimated 1.518 billion in 1974. The number has dropped slightly since then to 1.473 billion in 1976 (National Prescription Audit, IMS America, Ltd., 1977), which still represents a fourfold increase in 26 years.

The number of outpatient prescriptions filled in hospitals reached 237 million annually, and the number of inpatient prescriptions was almost 1 billion annually in 1974. The total number of prescriptions dispensed by all vendors—community pharmacies, other retail outlets, and hospital pharmacies—to outpatients and inpatients reached 2.704 billion in 1974, the latest year for which complete data exist. If this total is used as a base, per capita use of prescription drugs now stands at 12.7 prescriptions per year.

For ambulatory patients—this includes 75 percent of the U.S. population who make at least one physician visit during the year, or a total of about one billion visits annually—the number of new and refill prescriptions issued by physicians averages 1.7 per visit. Almost 67 percent of all office visits to a physician result in the prescription or the use of a drug for therapeutic or preventive purposes. A drug is prescribed in 44 percent of all visits, an injection is given in 13.8 percent, and an immunization or desensitization is a feature of 4.5 percent (National Center for Health Statistics, 1977).

For short-term hospital inpatients—this includes the 11 percent of the population who are hospitalized at least once a year—it appears that one prescription is dispensed for every day of hospitalization, or about eight for a typical hospital stay.

Although these gross statistics are not proof of overmedication, they demonstrate that physicians are prescribing drugs far more often to inpatients and outpatients than they did 10 or 25 years ago. The problem is not limited to the use of prescription drugs.

Drug Use in United States Population Samples

How many people in the United States take prescription drugs? How many take OTC drugs? How does drug use in the United States compare with that in Canada, Europe, and Latin America?

A sample of U.S. households in 1972 showed that 95 percent of all households procured at least one drug during a 30-week period (Knapp and Knapp, 1972). The average number of drugs purchased was 13.7; the average number of drugs in the house was 22.5—17.2 OTCs and 5.3 prescription drugs. This same study showed that prescription drugs were used in about 33 percent of episodes of illness or injury and OTC drugs in over 70 percent. Over 90 percent of illness episodes were treated with some medication.

Another household sample, this one conducted in the Baltimore, Maryland area in 1968-1969 (Rabin and Bush, 1975) as part of a WHO collaborative study, showed that 56 percent of the population had used one or more medicines in the two days before the survey interviews. Pain relievers, vitamins, and cough and cold medicines were the most frequently used drugs. Of the people taking prescription drugs, 40 percent were also using OTC drugs for self-medication. People in ill health took more drugs than people who described themselves as healthy. However, people who said they were healthy still took drugs; over 40 percent said they used prescription or OTC drugs.

The WHO/International Collaborative Study of Medical Care Utilization found that "the volume of prescribed and nonprescribed medicine use and rates per person were highest by far in the North American Study areas" (White et al., 1977). The mean for the 12 study areas was 910 medicines per 1000 population within a two-day period. The volume of different medicines used ranged from lows of 391 and 424 per 1000 population in Banat (Serbia) and Rijeka (Croatia) to highs of 1202 and 1047 in northwestern Vermont and in Baltimore, Maryland. The U.S. sites were also highest for people using prescription drugs, with rates more than double those at the lowest site (Table 1–1). As one might expect, the extent of prescription drug use was controlled principally by physicians.

Factors Influencing Drug Use

How is it possible to explain the rapid increase in the use of prescription drugs during the past 30 years? How can we explain the high rates in the United States and Canada, compared with rates in Europe and Latin America?

Some might justify the rate increase seen in the United States on the basis of the new drugs introduced during this period, many of which are very effective. Certainly this is a factor. Population growth, the increased number of aged, and the increased use of medical and hospital services (especially since the imple-

Table 1-1. *Rates and Standard Errors (SE) per 1000 Population for Persons Using Services and Volume of Services Used*

Site	Volume of Different Medicines Used		Persons Using Prescribed Medicines		Persons Using Nonprescribed Medicines	
	Rate	± SE	Rate	± SE	Rate	± SE
Grande Prairie, Canada	920	17	273	6	355	7
Saskatchewan, Canada	1046	22	300	8	384	9
Fraser, Canada	900	15	262	6	369	7
Jersey, Canada	922	17	269	6	354	7
Northwestern Vermont, USA	1202	26	344	9	399	10
Baltimore, USA	1047	21	328	7	337	8
Buenos Aires, Argentina	814	19	304	7	184	6
Liverpool, England	816	33	247	12	317	14
Helsinki, Finland	948	18	280	6	295	7
Lodz, Poland	724	24	194	6	130	5
Banat, Yugoslavia	391	11	160	5	97	4
Rijeka, Yugoslavia	424	16	183	7	101	6

From White, K.L., Anderson, D.O., Kalimo, E., Kleczkowski, B.M., Purola, T., and Vukmanovic, C.: *Health Services: Concepts, and Information for National Planning and Management.* Geneva, World Health Organization, 1977.

mentation of Medicare and Medicaid) have all contributed, but I do not believe that they solely account for the high figures.

Ample evidence exists to show that many other factors, in addition to morbidity, play a role in the use of prescription and OTC drugs. Age, sex, race, marital status, social status, education, place of residence, and family size have all been found to influence drug use (Rabin and Bush, 1974). Health and illness behavior, access to health care services, type and scope of health insurance coverage, physician prescribing habits, physician specialty, and practice organization (e.g., group or solo practice) are other important determinants. The influence of drug promotion by the pharmaceutical firms cannot be ignored, nor can the regulatory role of the Food and Drug Administration (FDA) be overlooked.

Symbolism is also important in prescribing. Pellegrino has offered a perceptive analysis of the symbolic meaning of drugs and prescribing for both patients and physicians. He observed that for many physicians, "it is prescribing which makes a clinical situation legitimately medical. In its absence, he may regard the patient's problem as a personal or social matter outside the domain of medicine entirely" (Pellegrino, 1976). As patients bring more and more psychosocial problems to the physician, there is need for both physician and patient to have these problems considered as legitimate medical issues.

Why Are Drugs Prescribed?

Ambulatory care data for the United States suggest that a patient's appearance in a physician's office, rather than the patient's specific problem or complaint, may be the chief indication for the use of a prescription, injection, or immunization. Drugs are prescribed or used for therapeutic or preventive purposes in approximately 67 percent of all visits to office-based physicians. Among general and family practitioners, this figure is even higher; in 80 percent of all visits, a prescription or OTC drug is administered or recommended, or an injection, immunization, or desensitization is given (The National Ambulatory Medical Care Survey, 1977). Among all office-based physicians, prescription or OTC drugs are recommended in over 70 percent of cases for half the leading 20 symptomatic complaints. For only a few complaints are drugs recommended less than 50 percent of the time. Indeed, there appear to be no instances, either among symptomatic or nonsymptomatic visits—pregnancy exams, general medical exams, gynecologic exams, well baby exams—in which a drug is not used or recommended (except visits for required medical exams).

Short-term hospital utilization data for this country show a 50 percent increase in the number of discharges during the last two decades. This huge increase in the number of people being treated in hospitals has also contributed to the increase in drug use. Patients are probably sicker and have more complex problems, and there are more drugs available now to treat them. However, this hardly explains the widespread use of antibiotics for prophylaxis or the extensive use of sedatives and tranquilizers for symptomatic care.

It is not surprising that multiple episodes of acute and chronic illness and a variety of symptomatic complaints result in the use of vast amounts of prescription and OTC drugs. The question is: is the use of certain drugs justified or appropriate?

The Use of Specific Therapeutic Classes of Drugs

To demonstrate that American patients are overmedicated, it is necessary to go beyond an examination of gross statistics on drug use and to look closely at prescribing patterns for specific therapeutic classes of drugs and for specific drugs within those classes. Although evidence of overmedication might be marshaled for certain drugs in almost every major class, I will cite as examples antiinfectives, psychotherapeutics, analgesics, and hormones, since they are among the most frequently prescribed types of therapeutic drugs.

Antiinfectives

In 1976, systemic antiinfectives ranked number one in terms of all prescriptions, both new and refill, dispensed by retail pharmacies (National Prescription Audit, IMS America, Ltd., 1977). These drugs accounted for 14.1 percent of all prescriptions. Year in and year out, antibiotics represent from 15 to 20 percent of all drugs prescribed in hospitals (Simmons and Stolley, 1974). Broad- and medium-spectrum antibiotics represent about 67 percent of the U.S. market for antiinfectives; penicillin products account for a little less than 33 percent; and others make up the small fraction of the remaining sales.

Inappropriate and unjustified use of antibiotics continues each year. Studies and reports spanning more than a decade reveal misuse of antibiotics in community, university, and Veterans Administration hospitals (Castle et al., 1977; Jones et al., 1977; Counts, 1977; Chodak and Plaut, 1977; Kass, 1976; May et al., 1974; Kunin et al., 1973; Gibbs et al., 1973; Roberts and Visconti, 1972; Adler et al., 1971; Scheckler and Bennett, 1970; Muller, 1965; Smith et al., 1966). In a number of hospitals either antimicrobial therapy was not indicated at all or an inappropriate drug or dosage had been used in from 30 to 60 percent of treated patients. In another study in 20 community hospitals, for only 41 percent of the patients treated with antibiotics was there an unambiguous statement in the patient's chart linking the initiation of treatment with a particular antimicrobial agent to a specific diagnosis, operation, or nonoperative procedure.

The prophylactic use of antibiotics in patients undergoing surgery often represents unjustified or inappropriate use of antiinfectives. In a study of antimicrobial use in community hospitals, Kass found that 30 percent of all antimicrobial courses were administered prophylactically in patients undergoing surgery or nonoperative procedures. Courses given for longer than four days accounted for 78 percent of all prophylactic dosage. Merely reducing the use to two days would have eliminated 20 percent of all hospital antibiotic use. There is no evidence to suggest that prolonging prophylactic use of antibiotics beyond 48 hours has any value (Kass, 1976).

After a careful review of 131 published studies, only 24 of which were well designed enough to permit valid judgments to be made, Chodak and Plaut concluded that antibiotic prophylaxis was of value in hysterectomy, cesarean section, total hip replacement, and microsurgical craniotomies. They found no prophylactic value for laparotomies or inguinal hernia repair. They found antibiotics to be used often for prophylaxis without evidence of value and concluded, "Current practices of antibiotic prophylaxis in surgery too often result from custom, unsupported belief or dependence on poorly designed clinical trials" (Chodak and Plaut, 1977).

Cephalosporins are particularly popular with surgeons in many hospitals. Dramatic reductions in the excessive use of cephalosporins were achieved in a Veterans Administration hospital by requiring consultation prior to use (Kunin et al., 1973) and in a community hospital through effective utilization review (Zeman et al., 1974). A recent attempt to reduce inappropriate use at the University of California, San Francisco hospitals through an educational campaign did not prove successful.

The potential significance of controlling the excessive use of antibiotics in hospitals is great. Hospital use of antibiotics accounts for about 40 percent of all antibiotic use and about 50 percent of the dollar value of annual antibiotic sales. Not only would the risk of adverse drug reactions and the development of antibiotic resistant infections be reduced but cost savings would be substantial. It has been estimated that reducing prophylactic antibiotics in surgical patients to 48 hours might result in a savings of $200 million annually in hospital costs (Kass, 1976).

Inappropriate and unjustified use of antiinfectives is not confined to the hospital. The use of antibiotics for ambulatory patients, particularly those with viral upper respiratory infection, is excessive. In the classic study by Dingle and his associates of 25,155 illnesses in Cleveland, Ohio families over a 10-year period, 62.7 percent of all illnesses were found to be acute respiratory illnesses (Dingle et al., 1964); 95 percent were classified as "common cold, rhinitis, pharyngitis, bronchitis and other acute respiratory illness of undifferentiated types." None of these was bacterial in origin. Streptococcal tonsillitis and pharyngitis constituted only 2.7 percent of all acute respiratory illnesses; the remainder included primary atypical pneumonia, pneomococcal pneumonia, and a variety of bacterial and viral infections. If the Cleveland studies are at all representative, the current practice of prescribing antibiotics for 50 to 60 percent of patients who consult physicians with colds and other common respiratory infections cannot be justified. It has been repeatedly demonstrated that antibiotics do not shorten the course of viral upper respiratory infections, nor do they prevent complications or shorten the course of illness.

The use of injectable antibiotics among New Mexico Medicaid patients treated in physicians' offices was found to be excessive on the basis of peer judgment. Dramatic declines in the use of these drugs followed one-to-one physician counseling, combined later with the denial of payment for such injections by the state Medicaid program. In a two-year period, it was estimated that 45,000 unnecessary injections were prevented (Brook and Williams, 1976).

Based on the limited number of diseases for which tetracyclines are the treatment of choice, it is particularly difficult to understand or justify their widespread use. Tetracyclines are prescribed more often than broad-spectrum penicillins (e.g., ampicillin), penicillin V and VK, and erythromycin (National Prescription Audit, IMS America, Ltds., 1977). The most obvious unjustified use of tetracycline is in children under eight years of age. Despite repeated advice to physicians on its dangers, this practice continues (Ray et al., 1977).

The problem is not new. Current practices in the use of antibiotics recall the dismal performance of physicians in the use of chloramphenicol over a 20-year period (Silverman and Lee, 1974). Unfortunately, the practice of excessive prescribing of chloramphenicol by a small percentage of physicians persists.

Use of fixed combination antibiotic products—often combining an antibiotic, an antihistamine, and a decongestant—was a popular practice for many years. The FDA removed these products from the market in the early 1970s because they were judged to be ineffective. In addition to prescribing these fixed combination products for colds, cough, and related upper respiratory symptoms, prescribing antibiotics in fixed combinations was also a popular practice. Again, it required the FDA's removal of these drug products from the market to terminate use of these irrational mixtures.

Psychotropic Drugs

Psychotropic drugs, perhaps more than any other class of drugs, are at the center of controversy in the debate about what constitutes appropriate drug therapy. Evidence of both unjustified and inappropriate use of psychotropic drugs, particularly during the past 20 years, exists. Psychotropic drug prescriptions filled in U.S. drug stores more than doubled between 1958 and 1976, growing from 42.7 million to an estimated 90 million prescriptions. The total number of prescriptions for psychotropic drugs reached 193 million in 1976 (National Prescription Audit, IMS America, Ltd., 1977; Balter and Levine, 1969). The peak was reached a few years earlier, in 1973, when the total number reached 223 million. The decline between 1973 and 1976 was due primarily to decreasing numbers of prescriptions for stimulants, hypnotics, and sedatives.

Several studies in the past decade have identified some of the characteristics of patients who use psychotropic drugs and the physicians who prescribe them. General practitioners, surgeons, and internists prescribe 70 percent of all psychotropic drugs. Indeed, the top 25 percent of prescribers account for as much as 50 percent of all prescriptions for psychotropic drugs (Balter and Levine, 1969). Females, particularly those of middle age, come to physicians most often, and they receive a disproportionate number of prescriptions for psychotropic drugs. Females aged 40 to 59 are the highest consumers of psychotropic drugs. The highest proportion of emotional disorders are thought to occur in women of this age group, and women are perceived by physicians as frequently presenting such symptoms as fatigue, tension, anxiety, and lassitude. Minor tranquilizers are frequently prescribed for problems of this type. The result: 67 percent of all psychotropic drugs are prescribed for females, and stimulants and antidepressants are used overwhelmingly by females—accounting for 82 percent and 74 percent of use respectively.

Advertising plays a role in the use of these drugs. Not only are psychotropic drugs promoted as being effective, but their use for a wide range of vague complaints and for the normal trials and tribulations of daily life also is encouraged (Stolley, 1976; Lennard et al., 1970). Recently, minor tranquilizers have been promoted to produce "a less demanding and complaining patient" (Waldron, 1977).

MINOR TRANQUILIZERS. Minor tranquilizers, including diazepam (Valium), chlordiazepoxide (Librium), and meprobamate, are among the most popular prescription drugs. Their use has increased rapidly, particularly after the introduction of chlordiazepoxide in 1960 and diazepam in 1963. In 1973, 100 million prescriptions were dispensed for minor tranquilizers, accounting for the sale of approximately five billion tablets. During that year, one out of every ten Americans 18 years of age or older was reported to have taken diazepam at one time or another.

About 30 percent of prescriptions for minor tranquilizers are for anxiety or insomnia; the remaining 70 percent are for a wide variety of problems including muscloskeletal disorders, circulatory disorders, gastrointestinal complaints, asthma, menopausal symptoms, and postoperative care (Blackwell, 1973; Rickels, 1977). Although the efficacy of diazepam for anxiety varies from one study to the next, it often appears to be an effective drug for short-term use (Blackwell, 1973; Kline, 1974; Waldron, 1977). There is much less evidence supporting long-term use for anxiety. Analyzing data from the medical literature of the early 1960s to 1973, Cooperstock found "little to support the use of psychotropic drugs as an adjunct in the maintenance therapy of common physical illness" (Cooperstock, 1973). Similar observations have been made for the use of benzodiazepines for such disorders as hypertension, angina pectoris, peptic ulcer, and asthma (Greenblatt and Shader, 1977). Often, it seems that physicians prescribe minor tranquilizers for hospitalized patients in anticipation that the patients will suffer anxiety or other emotional problems (Rickels, 1977). The reasons given for prescribing such drugs are often vague (Raft et al., 1975).

In January, 1978, the FDA took steps to alert physicians that there is no evidence that diazepam or other minor tranquilizers are effective for long-term use. The new label on these drugs will incorporate the following instruction: "The physician should periodically reassess the usefulness of the drug for the individual patient."

Several developments lie behind this new warning. First, evidence of the adverse effects of the benzodiazepines has been mounting. Physiologic dependence on these drugs has been demonstrated, not only for patients taking large doses over long periods, but also for adults taking therapeutic doses for 20 or more weeks (Zisook and DeVaul, 1977). Adverse effects have been reported, particularly paradoxic psychologic reactions such as hostility and rage. The risk of suicide, formerly thought to be virtually nonexistent, is also a factor.

MAJOR TRANQUILIZERS. Major tranquilizers constituted only 1.3 percent of all new prescriptions filled in retail pharmacies in 1976 (National Prescription Audit, IMS America, Ltd., 1977). However, these drugs are often prescribed by general practitioners and family physicians, and there is evidence of their inappropriate use in general and psychiatric hospitals (Hesbacker et al., 1976; Schroeder et al., 1977; Laska et al., 1973). These drugs are used in excessive dosage, often with little regard for the diagnosis (Altman et al., 1972). They may be prescribed with other psychotropic drugs and, in some general hospitals, with other major tranquilizers (Davidson et al., 1975), thus increasing the risk of adverse drug reactions.

STIMULANTS. The most serious misuse of prescribed stimulants, particularly amphetamines, is in the treatment of obesity. There are 12 drug entities approved for the treatment of obesity. All of them, except mazindol, are related in chemical structure, all are central nervous system stimulants, and all are scheduled under the Controlled Substance Act of 1970.

In addition to determining appropriate control schedules for anorectic drugs, the FDA undertook a variety of other actions between 1971 and 1976 designed to limit the misuse of anorectics (U.S. Congress, 1976). The result of these actions was that the number of amphetamine prescriptions per year dropped from over 20 million in 1970 to about 5.5 million in 1973. They have remained at that level.

The FDA began the slow process of removing all combination drug products containing amphetamines from the market in 1973. By late 1976, several drugs were still under review but the majority had been eliminated. The FDA also rescinded approval of the use of methamphetamine preparations for a number of conditions for which NSA/NRC panels had found them ineffective.

Despite the fact that there is some evidence supporting the short-term (8 to 12 week) use of prescription anorectics in achieving weight loss and that some physicians prescribing these drugs certainly consider them effective (Lasagna, 1973), I agree with the view that these drugs are used excessively and with minimal effectiveness (Edison, 1977). This view is supported by the Canadian government, which withdrew the approval of amphetamine and related compounds for the treatment of obesity several years ago. Recently, the FDA initiated an action to prohibit the labeling of amphetamines for the treatment of obesity and to limit approved labeling solely to the treatment of narcolepsy and minimal brain dysfunction. Banning amphetamines as a weight reduction aid might eliminate up to 88 percent of their present legal use.

One interesting instance of doctors combating misuse of amphetamines took place in Jacksonville, Florida. The county medical society leadership, convinced that amphetamines were overprescribed locally (more than one million such prescriptions in a four-month period in 1977), jointly sponsored a plan that reduced amphetamine prescriptions by 81 percent and reduced pharmacy robberies and street traffic in the drugs as well. There was a verbal campaign to inform physicians about problems relating to stimulants. Pharmacists volunteered to remove all amphetamine stocks from their stores, and they instituted a delay in filling these prescriptions for two days. The program gave them an opportunity to track down false prescriptions, and it gave notice to physicians that people were concerned about overprescribing amphetamines. The society's president reported that physicians welcomed the restrictions, and that they were interested in applying their experience to other dangerous drugs (American Medical News, 1978).

Sedatives and hypnotics. Sedatives and hypnotics continue to be used excessively. Hypnotics are used by almost 3 percent of the population. These drugs carry a high abuse potential, and the consequences of their abuse are staggering: 5000 deaths a year are associated with sleeping pills, and barbiturate users make about 25,000 trips to hospital emergency rooms every year because of drug-related problems (DuPont, 1977).

Hypnotic prescriptions rose from less than 30 million new and refill prescriptions in the 1960s to 42.1 million prescriptions in 1971 (U.S. Department of Health, Education, and Welfare, 1977). Since that time, the number of prescriptions has decreased to 27.3 million. The change in barbiturate hypnotic prescriptions has been dramatic—from 20.4 million in 1971 to 5.5 million in 1976. Prescriptions for all the nonbarbiturate hyponotics, except flurazepam (Dalmane), also declined during this period.

For all barbiturate sedatives, there has also been a marked decline in prescriptions in recent years. This followed the increased use of diazepam for daytime sedation and flurazepam for insomnia, as well as the classification of the barbiturates as scheduled drugs under the Controlled Substances Act of 1970.

How is it possible to justify the use of barbiturates in the amounts prescribed in the 1960s and early 1970s? Certainly their use for insomnia cannot be condoned. A recent study by the National Institute of Drug Abuse reported that physicians' prescribing of hypnotics and sedatives for insomnia was not consistent with their pharmacologic effects or clinical effectiveness (U.S. Department of Health, Education, and Welfare, 1977). Not only do these drugs not relieve insomnia but they may aggravate it.

In my view, there is no question that psychotherapeutic drugs—major tranquilizers, minor tranquilizers (especially the benzodiazepines), stimulants, and hypnotics—are used inappropriately or without justification in the United States.

The opinion that psychotropic drugs are overused is not shared by some thoughtful students of drug use. Based on their studies in the United States as well as in Europe, Parry, Balter, and associates concluded that "There is no evidence that the American people are overmedicated with respect to psychotherapeutic drugs" (Parry et al., 1973). This view is shared by a number of leaders in the field (Hollister, 1975; Kline, 1974; Gardner, 1974). I believe that the evidence supports the contrary view, which is shared by many physicians and scientists (Greenblatt and Shader, 1974; Lennard et al., 1970; Muller, 1972) as well as by the general public. In a national survey of psychotropic drug use, 60 percent of those surveyed agreed that "many doctors prescribed tranquilizers more than they should" (Manheimer et al., 1973).

Whether one agrees that psychotropic drugs often are prescribed inappropriately or without justification, certainly we can agree that patients would be well served if physicians followed Katz's recommendation:

> . . . every time a physician reaches for his prescription pad, he (should) ask himself if he is prescribing a sedative or tranquilizer because he has a roomful of patients waiting and is in a hurry to get to the next patient, whose illness he considers more serious, or whether he has carefully considered all the evidence, has found that sympathy, understanding, suggestion and reassurance are not sufficient, and has decided to prescribe a sedative or tranquilizer for positive reasons rather than as an easy way out (Katz, 1972).

Analgesics

Aspirin, one of the most frequently used OTC drugs, is found in hundreds of analgesic preparations as well as in cough and cold mixtures. The FDA panel on analgesics reviewed the evidence on safety and effectiveness of these drugs and recommended a series of actions designed to limit the misuse of analgesics. The FDA is requiring labeling changes for many analgesics that contain aspirin. Claims that the drugs are effective for treatment of arthritis, rheumatism, bursitis, and gout will be eliminated. The problem identified by the analgesic panel was not so much related to the commonly used ingredients as to labeling and promotional claims regarding specific conditions, and promotion that might well result in overuse or misuse under these conditions.

Among OTC drugs, aspirin is the leading cause of adverse drug reactions leading to hospitalization, and it is usually found among the top ten on any list of drugs causing adverse reactions serious enough to result in hospitalization. Aspirin is not only a major culprit in drug-induced illness, but is also a major cause of childhood poisoning. It has been estimated that 20 percent of the three million accidental poisonings in children under the age of five each year are due to aspirin (Graedon, 1977).

The panel reviewing analgesics also recommended that phenacetin be made available by prescription only because of the dangers of kidney damage associated with prolonged use. Acetaminophen is another widely used analgesic, which may be found in over 250 different OTC drug products. Most people using acetaminophen are unaware of its potential toxicity—particularly hepatoxicity—and its presence in multiple drug products.

Propoxyphene in its various proprietary forms is among the most commonly prescribed drugs in America. It is often used inappropriately when other equally effective or less costly drugs are available. Propoxyphene is often used to bridge the gap between aspirin and narcotics, but a number of studies indicate that it is no more effective than aspirin and aspirin with codeine in the relief of pain (American Medical Association Department of Drugs, 1977). Reports of propoxyphene abuse have led to a warning in the *Journal of the American Medical Association (JAMA)* about misprescribing analgesics (Lewis, 1974). Recently, a national study of the increasing number of deaths due to propoxyphene illustrated another real danger of this drug (Finkle et al., 1977). The report noted that the number of propoxyphene deaths has been increasing each year at a faster rate than that for total drug deaths.

Why is it that propoxyphene in its various forms continues to be one of the most frequently prescribed drugs? The skillful promotion by the Eli Lilly and Co. apparently has been a key factor in the continued inappropriate prescribing of this drug.

Hormones

Although many hormones are prescribed inappropriately or without justification, the use of estrogens for menopausal symptoms presents a major hazard because of their widespread use. The most frequently used oral estrogens are conjugated estrogens and diethylstilbestrol. In addition, about 1.5 million prescriptions are written for vaginal estrogens each year (National Prescription Audit, IMS America, Ltd., 1977). On the basis of national sales figures, it has been estimated that almost 13 percent of women aged 45 to 64 take oral estrogens (Markush and Turner, 1971). Other estimates range from 8 to 15 percent (Boston Collaborative Drug Surveillance Program, 1974; Pfeffer, 1977), with many women in the seventh and eighth decades continuing to use estrogens. In 1977, the FDA estimated that three million women take estrogens for menopausal symptoms.

How much of this use is justified in view of the risks associated with prolonged estrogen therapy? Risks include hypertension (Pfeffer and Vanden Noort, 1976), ovarian cancer (Hoover et al., 1977), endometrial cancer (Mack et al., 1976; Ziel and Finkel, 1975; Smith et al., 1975), venous thromboembolism, gallbladder disease (Boston Collaborative Drug Surveillance Program, 1974), and glucose intolerance (Ajabor et al., 1972). Most important is the increased risk of endometrial and ovarian cancers. In three recent studies, the risk of endometrial cancer was found to increase by 4.5, 7.6, and 8 times when estrogens were used (Mack et al., 1976; Ziel and Finkel, 1975; Smith et al., 1975). Since the frequency of endometrial cancer in all postmenopausal women who have uteruses is about one in 1000 per year, these studies indicate that the frequency may be high as four to eight in 1000 per year for estrogen users. The risk of endometrial cancer in postmenopausal women using estrogens is greater than the usual combined risk of cervical, breast, and endometrial cancer. The risk of ovarian cancer has recently been documented by Hoover et al., who followed almost 1000 women who had taken oral Premarin for at least six months (Hoover et al., 1977). In this group, the risk of ovarian cancer was two or three times greater than expected. Risk increased with the strength of the Premarin tablet taken but not with the duration of use or the total dose. The excess risk of cancer in this group, however, was chiefly in women who had also used diethylstilbestrol.

The most frequent reasons for the use of estrogens in postmenopausal women are atrophic vaginitis, replacement therapy, osteoporosis, hot flashes and anxiety, depression, fatigue, and headache (Pfeffer, 1977). Do these symptoms justify the present patterns of use, considering the risks in menopausal and postmenopausal women? Certainly, osteoporosis is an appropriate indication, but is the same true of anxiety, depression, fatigue, and headache?

As a result of the risk of endometrial cancer, in July, 1977, the FDA began requiring pharmacists and physicians who dispense estrogens to provide users with a special brochure that emphasizes the risks of long-term use. The FDA had earlier tightened restrictions on drug labeling and instructions. These regulations will very likely result in a sharp decline in the use of estrogens for menopausal and postmenopausal symptoms.

Conclusion

Based on the limited data available on (1) the growing use of prescription drugs in this country, (2) drug use in the United States compared with that in other countries, and (3) the use of prescription antiinfectives, psychotropic drugs, and estrogens, as well as prescription and OTC analgesics, I believe a strong case can be made that America is an overmedicated society.

Although there is evidence that some chronically ill patients are undermedicated, that some hospitalized patients suffering severe pain are given inadequate relief, and that many patients with depression are undertreated or not treated at all, this does not balance the inappropriate and unjustified use of drugs. The question of overmedication cannot be answered by adding up the patients who are overmedicated and subtracting the number of those who are undermedicated. To provide a definite answer, more complete data are needed on patterns of drug use, drug prescribing, and drug safety and effectiveness. Certainly, there will be little agreement on the question until more adequate and definite data are available.

References

Adler, J.L., Burke, J.P., and Finland, M.: Infection and antibiotic usage at Boston City Hospital, January 1970. Arch. Intern. Med. 127:460, 1971.

Ajabor, L.N., Tsai, C.C., Vela, P., et al.: Effect of exogenous estrogen on carbohydrate metabolism in postmenopausal women. Am. J. Obstet. Gynecol. 113:383–387, 1972.

Altman, H., Evenson, R.C., Sietten, I.V., and Cho, D.W.: Patterns of psychotropic drug prescription in four midwestern state hospitals. Curr. Ther. Res. 14:667, 1972.

American Medical Association Department of Drugs: *AMA Drug Evaluations*, 3rd edition. Littleton, Massachusetts, Publishing Sciences Group, Inc., 1977.

American Medical News: MDs curb amphetamine prescribing. March 27, 1978, p. 11.

Balter, M.B., and Levine, J.: The nature and extent of psychotropic drug usage in the United States. Psychopharmacol. Bull. 5:3, 1969.

Blackwell, B.: Psychotropic drugs in use today, JAMA 225:1637, 1973.

Boston Collaborative Drug Surveillance Program: Surgically confirmed gallbladder disease, venous thromboembolism and breast tumors in relation to postmenopausal estrogen therapy. N. Engl. J. Med. 290:15, 1974.

Brook, R.H., and Williams, K.N.: Effect of medical care review on the use of injections. Ann. Int. Med. 85:509, 1976.

Castle, M., Wilfert, C.M., Cate, T.R., and Ostemout, S.: Antibiotic use at Duke University Medical Center. JAMA 237:2819, 1977.

Chodak, G.W., and Plaut, M.E.: Use of systemic antibiotics for prophylaxis in surgery. Arch. Surg. 112:326, 1977.

Cooperstock, R.: Some factors involved in the increased prescribing of psychotropic drugs. Prepared for Symposium on Social Aspects of the Medical Use of Psychotropic Drugs, October 22–25, 1973.

Counts, G.W.: Review and control of antimicrobial usage in hospitalized patients. JAMA 238:2170, 1977.

Davidson, J.R.T., Raft, D., Lewis, F., and Gebhardt, M.: Psychotropic drugs on general medical and surgical wards of a teaching hospital. Arch. Gen. Psychiatry 32:507, 1975.

DeNuzzo, R.V.: Annual prescription survey by the Albany College of Pharmacy. Medical Marketing and Media, April 1977, p. 32.

Dingle, J.H., Badger, G.F., and Jordan, W.S., Jr.: *Illness in the Home.* Cleveland, The Press of Western Reserve University, 1964.

Dupont, R.: Quoted in sleeping pill study citing death, abuse. San Francisco Chronicle, December 7, 1977.

Edison, G.R.: Amphetamines: a dangerous illusion. In U.S. Senate Committee on Small Business, Subcommittee on Monopoly, Competitive Problems in the Drug Industry, Part 31, Safety and Efficacy of Antiobesity Drugs, November 9, 10, 11, 18, and 19, 1976. Washington, D.C., U.S. Government Printing Office, 1977.

Finkle, B.S., McCloskey, K.L., Kiplinger, G.F., and Bennett, I.F.: A national assessment of propoxyphene in postmortem medicolegal investigation, 1972–1975. J. Forensic Sci. 1977.

Gardner, E.A.: Implications of psychoactive drug therapy. N. Engl. J. Med. 290:800, 1974.

Gibbs, C.W., Jr., Gibson, J.T., and Newton, D.S.: Drug utilization review of actual versus preferred pediatric antibiotic therapy. Am. J. Hosp. Pharm. 30:892, 1973.

Graedon, J.: *The People's Pharmacy.* New York, Avon Books, 1977.

Greenblatt, D.J., and Shader, R.I.: *Benzodiazepines in Clinical Practice.* New York, Raven Press, 1974.

Greenblatt, D.J., and Shader, R.I.: Nonprescription psychotropic drugs. J. Fam. Pract. 5:492, 1977.

Hesbacher, P., Rickels, K., Rial, W.Y., Segal, A., and Zamostien, B.B.: Psychotropic drug prescription in family practice. Compr. Psychiatry 17:607, 1976.

Hollister, L.E.: Drugs for emotional disorders. JAMA 234:942, 1975.

Hoover, R., Gray, L.A., Sr., and Fraumeni, J.F., Jr.: Stilbestrol (diethylstilbestrol) and the risk of ovarian cancer. Lancet 533, September 10, 1977.

Jones, S.R., Barks, J., Bratton, T., McRee, E., Pannell, J., Yanchick, V.A., Browne, R., and Smith, J.W.: The effect of an educational program upon hospital antibiotic use. Am. J. Med. Sci. 273:79, 1977.

Kass, E.H.: Quality assurance and the use of antimicrobial drugs in general hospitals: an introduction. Unpublished, 1976.

Kass, E.H.: Lecture, Harvard Medical School, 1976.

Katz, R.L.: Drug therapy: sedatives and tranquilizers. N. Engl. J. Med. 286:757, 1972.

Kline, N.S.: Antidepressant medications: a more effective use by general practitioners, family physicians, internists, and others. JAMA 227:1158, 1974.

Knapp, D.A., and Knapp, D.E.: Decision making and self-medication. Am. J. Hosp. Pharm. 29:1004, 1972.

Kunin, C.M., Tupasi, T., and Craig, W.A.: Use of antibiotics: a brief exposition of the problem and some tentative solutions. Ann. Intern. Med. 79:555, 1973.
Lasagna, L.: Attitudes toward appetite suppressants: a survey of U.S. physicians. JAMA 225:44, 1973.
Laska, E., Varga, E., Wanderling, J., Simpson, G., Logemann, G.W., and Shah, B.K.: Patterns of psychotropic drug use for schizophrenia. Dis. Nerv. Syst. 34:294, 1973.
Lennard, H.L., Epstein, L.J., Bernstein, A., and Ransom, D.C.: Hazards implicit in prescribing psychoactive drugs. Science 169:438, 1970.
Lewis, J.R.: Misprescribing analgesics. JAMA 228:1155, 1974.
Mack, T.M., Pike, M.C., Henderson, B.E., et al.: Estrogens and endometrial cancer in a retirement community. N. Engl. J. Med. 294:1262, 1976.
Manheimer, D.I., Davidson, S.T., Balter, M.B., Mellinger, G.D., Cisin, I.H., and Parry, H.J.: Popular attitudes and beliefs about tranquilizers. Am. J. Psychiatry 130:11, 1973.
Markush, R.E., and Turner, S.L.: Epidemiology of exogenous estrogens. HSMHA Health Reports 86:74, 1971.
May, F.E., Stewart, R.B., and Cluff, L.E.: Drug use in the hospital: evaluation of determinants. Clin. Pharmacol. Ther. 16:834, 1974.
Muller, C.: Medical review of prescribing. J. Chron. Dis. 18:689, 1965.
Muller, C.: The overmedicated society: forces in the marketplace for medical care. Science 176:488, 1972.
National Prescription Audit: IMS America, Ltd., Ambler, Pennsylvania, 1977.
1976: The top 200 drugs. Pharm. Times, April 1977, p. 37.
Parry, H.J., Balter, M.B., Mellinger, G.D., Cisin, I.H., and Manheimer, D.I.: National patterns of psychotherapeutic drug use. Arch. Gen. Psychiatry 28:769, 1973.
Pellegrino, E.D.: Prescribing and drug ingestion: symbols and substances. Paper delivered at the American Association for the Advancement of Science, Annual Meeting, February, 1976.
Pfeffer, R.I.: Estrogen use in postmenopausal women. Am. J. Epidemiol. 105:21, 1977.
Pfeffer, R.I., and Vanden Noort, S.: Estrogen use and stroke risk in postmenopausal women. Am. J. Epidemiol. 103:445, 1976.
Pharmaceutical Manufacturers Association: Annual Survey Report, 1976–1977. Washington, D.C., December 1977.
Rabin, D.L., and Bush, P.J.: The use of medicines: historical trends and international comparison. Int. J. Health Serv. 4:61, 1974.
Rabin, D.L., and Bush, P.J.: Who's using medicines? J. Community Health 1:106, 1975.
Raft, D., Davidson, J., Toomey, T.C., Spencer, R.F., and Lewis, B.F.: Inpatient and outpatient patterns of psychotropic drug prescribing by nonpsychiatrist physicians. Am. J. Psychiatry 132:1309, 1975.
Ray, W.A., Federspiel, C.F., and Schaffner, W.: The mal-prescribing of liquid tetracycline preparations. Am. J. Public Health 67:762, 1977.
Rickels, K.: Valium: a discussion of current issues. Psychosomatics 18:1, 1977.
Roberts, A.W., and Visconti, J.A.: The rational and irrational use of systemic antimicrobial drugs. Am. J. Hosp. Pharm. 29:828, 1972.
Scheckler, W.E., and Bennett, J.V.: Antibiotic usage in seven community hospitals. JAMA 213:264, 1970.
Schroeder, N.H., Caffey, E.M., and Lorei, T.W.: Antipsychotic drug use: physician prescribing practices in relation to current recommendations. Dis. Nerv. Syst. 114, February 1977.
Silverman, M., and Lee, P.R.: *Pills, Profits, and Politics*. Berkeley, University of California Press, 1974.
Simmons, H.E., and Stolley, P.D.: This is medical progress? Trends and consequences of antibiotic use in the United States. JAMA 227:1023, 1974.
Smith, D.C., Prentice, R., Thompson, D.J., et al.: Association of exogenous estrogen and endometrial carcinoma. N. Engl. J. Med. 293:1164, 1975.
Smith, J.W., Seidl, L.G., and Cluff, L.E.: Studies on the epidemiology of adverse drug reactions v. clinical factors influencing susceptibility. Ann. Int. Med. 65:629, 1966.
Stolley, P.D.: Evaluating drugs and determining the drug needs of developed and developing countries. J. Community Health 2:113, 1976.
U.S. Congress, Senate, Committee on Small Business, Subcommittee on Monopoly: Competitive Problems in the Drug Industry. Part 31, Safety and Efficacy of Anti-obesity Drugs, November 9, 10, 11, 18 and 19, 1976. Washington, D.C., U.S. Government Printing Office, 1977.
U.S. Department of Health, Education, and Welfare, Public Health Service, Alcohol, Drug Abuse, and Mental Health Administration, National Institute on Drug Abuse: Sedative-hypnotic drugs: risks and benefits. Edited by Cooper, J.R., August 1977.
U.S. Department of Health, Education, and Welfare, Public Health Service, Health Resources Adminstration, National Center for Health Statistics: The national ambulatory medical care survey, 1975 summary, series 13. No. 33, 1977.

Waldron, I.: Increased prescribing of Valium, Librium, and other drugs—an example of the influence of economic and social factors on the practice of medicine. Int. J. Health Serv. 7:37, 1977.

White, K.L., Anderson, D.O., Kalimo, E., Kleczowski, B.M., Purola, T., and Vukmanovic, C.: *Health Services: Concepts and Information for National Planning and Management.* Geneva, World Health Organization, 1977.

Zeman, B.T., Pike, M., and Samet, C.: The antibiotic utilization committee. Hospitals 48:73, 1974.

Ziel, H.K., and Finkel, W.D.: Increased risk of endometrial cancer among users of conjugated estrogens. N. Engl. J. Med. 293:1167, 1975.

Zisook, S., and DeVaul, R.A.: Adverse behavioral effects of benzodiazepines. J. Fam. Pract. 5:963, 1977.

The Politics of Medication

John P. Morgan, M.D.
City University of New York

The skill demanded for writing a chapter in a point-counterpoint book is often that of writing well what is counter-intuitive. Of all the issues in *Controversy in Internal Medicine* (1966), the one I best recall was that the treatment of essential hypertension with drug therapy was of unproven merit (Goldring and Chassis, 1966). I do not remember the quality of the authors' arguments or data but do easily recall the verve with which they attacked the popularly held view that patients with essential hypertension needed aggressive therapy with the drugs commonly used at the time.

One of the reasons for the success of books dealing with controversies in medicine or science surely has to do with the opportunity they provide to read the scientific or clinical writer turned polemicist. Many people correctly suspect that within each ostensibly rational scientist, there hides a hostile seller of personal viewpoint who itches to slash away with pen if not sword.

Masters of the counter-intuitive phrase or essay abound, but they are usually found writing a column (sometimes complete with their picture) in a political journal or newspaper. Whenever I feel that I have arrived at some personal truth regarding a political or social issue, I know that I will also find a confidently stated viewpoint in the words of a William Safire or William Buckley or George Will or Gary Wills, showing that things are not really as they seem. Not merely may I find an alternative viewpoint but sometimes an interpretation of fact that is so opposite from mine that I can only sit in wonder or occasionally fume in fury.

I find it appropriate to cite political writers because many topics in this volume—and this question in particular—have political dimensions. Surely there will be some who argue the correctness and probity of clinical trials and ion flux interpretations, but the controversies of clinical pharmacology are often the controversies of the social context of drug use; they must therefore be viewed within ethical, economic, and moral frameworks along with the relatively simple scientific ones.

In addition to its political origins, there is at least one other citeable characteristic of the counter-intuitive exercise. We usually know where to look for a certain viewpoint. This evolves from the truism that what one does seems to determine what one thinks. Those in the employ of pharmaceutical firms seldom seem to think that this is an overmedicated society; those in the employ of the FDA or various consumerist liberal groups seldom seem to consider any other position. That leaves the somewhat tattered army of academics between two poles. We, at least those of us in clinical pharmacology, are increasingly supported by industrial funds. The budgetary crisis of recent years has led us to this bed. Few, if any, investigators have compromised the data of clinical trials to conform to industry's wishes. Whether any of us have compromised public utterances or writings must be left to critical readers.

The Prevailing View

The prevailing view of widely distributed cultural groups—including patients, physicians, and editors of popular magazines—is that we are an overmedicated society. In the recent past, I have been asked by high school groups, alcoholism counselors, and freelance writers from *Time Inc.* and *Gentlemen's Quarterly* to comment on overmedication in American society. Everyone seems to know that we are an overmedicated society, and one imagines editors of publications small and large, common and arcane, swallowing benzodiazepines while rushing to meet a deadline with an article on the overmedicated society.

Apparent drug use and the total cost of prescription drugs have expanded notably in the last few decades. This growth and the elastic criteria for drug intervention in humans have produced the view that our society is overmedicated. I have heard surprisingly little comment about society being undermedicated at one time. Since no one maintains that a time of "correct medication" intervened, we must have passed from "under" to "over" without interim "properness." This situation is analogous to a critical assessment of the sexual revolution by someone who claimed that we have progressed from Victorianism to license without an intervening era of proper sensuality.

Is Overmedication Seen in the Cost of Drugs?

The National Prescription Audit (NPA) (IMS America, 1978) is conducted by monitoring selected retail pharmacies. A survey of these data is published annually.

For 1977, 1.42 billion prescriptions were filled by retail druggists at an approximate cost of $5.98 each. This yields a dollar volume for retail sales at $8.5 billion. The per capita cost in America must then approximate $32. Adding in the value of hospital drugs, which increases the total economic sales of the prescription industry to $10.5 to 11.0 billion, probably inflates the per capita cost to approximately $35 to $40. Even though we know that this is not distributed evenly (elderly and seriously ill individuals pay more), this figure is surprising only in its slightness. Americans pay more in dollar volume of sales for tobacco, alcohol, telephone service, and automobile tires, not to mention automobiles.

The claim of overmedication, then, should not be tied to an enormous cost of drugs. Indeed, it cannot even be correlated with a rapidly rising cost of drugs. For years, there has been substantial argument about a consumer price index prepared by the Bureau of Labor, which indicated that the cost of drugs as part of consumer expenditures has actually declined. This survey was regularly criticized because it underrepresented newer and costlier drugs. Firestone has recently submitted convincing data showing that a "comprehensive retail price index" tabulating drug costs between 1960 and 1969 indicates that prescription drug prices at retailer and manufacturer levels actually declined in that decade. The increase of the total drug bill then relates to greater usage, and the increase in average prescription price is secondary to the increased size of the prescription package. Firestone's data would then confirm that more drugs are being used, but they are being bought at a steady or even reduced price (Firestone, 1970). In fact, the recent NPA data even indicate that the absolute number of total prescriptions (new plus refill) has actually declined in the past three years (IMS America, Ltd., 1978).

The mere increase in the total volume of drugs would not in itself justify a claim of overmedication, even for the sharpest critics. The possibility exists that we have generated better treatment for previously untreatable or poorly treated diseases. For example, there has been a dramatic increase in the amount of treatment of arthritics with the newer nonsteroidal antiinflammatory drugs. This may indicate that arthritics were undertreated with previously available drugs. It may also indicate that the newer drugs are better. The aggressive promotion of these agents has surely contributed to their growing use, but how should we regard that? If arthritics are helped and the national economy has gained millions of dollars from their return to work, should we be grateful to the merchandisers and ad men? Or should we cite them again as a cause of overmedication—because antiarthritic drug sales have increased in volume from 36.9 million prescriptions in 1974 to 48.7 million in 1977?

Another response to the overmedication accusation is to point out that the accusation is too broad. If physicians are overanxious to prescribe certain drugs, should we assume that they overmedicate all patients or illnesses? In fact, the evidence shows the opposite to be true. Some studies have referred to the apparent undertreatment of hypertension in America as a national disgrace. Hospitalized patients in the United States are seriously undermedicated for treatment of severe pain (Marks and Sachar, 1973). An indirect commentary on this is provided by the fact that our most effective oral narcotic analgesic, methadone, is scarcely used any longer because of official pressure and unofficial fear (Morgan and Penovich, 1977).

The Cultural Context of Drug Use

One reason we stumble over questions of "appropriate" drug utility is our lack of understanding of the cultural context of drug use. We do not comprehend the wide use of drugs by patients and physicians. We do not know much about the reasons for drug use that differ from our usual "clinical" motives. This is not as surprising as it may appear initially. The era of scientific therapeutics and the emergence of a pharmaceutical science dealing in arcana instead of plant simples is a short 40 years. For centuries, humans engaged in the taking and giving of drug substances for a complex set of reasons, some of which we understand. However, little of that knowledge applies to the same issues in a technological era in which drugs exert profound biologic effects.

We are asked to define a "proper" level of medication in a society when we do not understand the social utility of powerful chemicals. What is the impact on an individual's worklife and sexual function when his blood pressure is lowered? Is he happier? Does he work more effectively? Will he take drugs to lower his blood pressure when he notes very little change in feeling? Why should he take drugs if they make him drowsy? I have jumped to the social utility or dysfunction of drug use. A recent study pointed out that the mere act of *diagnosing* hypertension alters an individual's work habits, regardless of whether he is symptomatic or taking drugs at all (Haynes et al., 1978).

All the questions I have posed for hypertension exist for arthritis or ileitis or leishmaniasis or neurocirculatory asthenia. We operate from the tiny or even puny viewpoint of clinical reasoning. It is presumptuous—even preposterous—to define appropriateness solely from a clinical viewpoint. Even if that narrow view were desirable as a starting point, we cannot even accomplish that with certainty. Patients take medications and physicians prescribe them for reasons we can hardly guess. Patients are made worse and made better by medications in ways that we can hardly guess. Until we make more progress in defining the social utility of drugs and the social utility of health and well-being, it behooves us to be a bit more humble about appropriateness. Linn has demonstrated that physicians find it generally appropriate to give a sedative/tranquilizer to students who are too nervous to study for an exam, but they generally deem inappropriate the giving of a stimulant to a tired student to help him study (Linn, 1971). Can anyone doubt that that decision principally reflects a social phenomenon? What diagnostic skill and clinical reasoning go into such a decision?

Valium

What is the rationale for the accusation of *overmedication*? Muller's article, which utilizes the phrase in her title, describes the usual basis neatly (Muller, 1972). Most complaints and critical articles focus on the expanding use of pyschotropic agents, particularly benzodiazepine tranquilizers. Admittedly, critics also cite an insouciant use of antibiotics, and earlier articles have criticized anorexiant prescribing and the easy use of cough and cold preparations, but these criticisms are relatively quiet compared with the volume of criticism about the use of Valium and its congeners.

Barry Blackwell's paper entitled *Psychotropic Drugs in Use Today* effectively frames the discussion (Blackwell, 1973). Blackwell had originally subtitled a preprint of the paper "The Age of Valium." Surely, the unimaginative editor at the Journal of the American Medical Association (JAMA) should have his or her blue pencil removed, because Blackwell's original phrase not only is apt but might well become a phrase with the staying power of "The Dark Ages," "The Restoration," or "Ten Days That Shook the World." He details the growth of psychotropic drug prescribing during the last decade and shows that the principal growth has been due to benzodiazepines, principally Valium. Other psychotropic agents are surely important, but he notes that there has been relatively little increase or an actual decline in the use of most others, including phenothiazines, antidepressants, sedative-hypnotics, and psychostimulants. Blackwell points out that the annual *increase* in Valium sales during the decade examined was greater that the *average yearly sales* of tricyclic antidepressants. This incredible growth rate means that today, Valium is the most commonly prescribed drug in the world. It is prescribed by 97 percent of all internists and family practitioners. The worldwide market for benzodiazepines probably went over the billion dollar mark in the mid 1970s.

I have not yet seen data that clearly document the impact of moving Valium to schedule IV, but the principal practical impact of that rescheduling has been to limit refills to a six-month period after issuance of the prescription. Since 1974, the ratio of refills to new benzodiazepine prescriptions has fallen, and that decrease in Valium refills is the most likely explanation for the previously mentioned fact that after years of steady increase in prescription volume, the total volume of written prescriptions in America has fallen for the past three years (IMS America, Ltd., 1978).

The enormous growth in Valium (and other benzodiazepine) use can be viewed positively. There is some reason to believe that these drugs are more effective as antianxiety drugs than the previously available psychotropic agents. They are surely less hazardous in terms of fatal overdose and physical dependence liability than the previously utilized sedatives such as chloral hydrate, barbiturates, and meprobamate. The increase in the use of flurazepam as a hypnotic can be viewed in a similarly positive light, as this drug steadily displaces agents that can successfully be used for suicide. These advantages have been emphasized by some, principally those who work in the drug industry. Much more obvious, however, is the strident criticism of the expansion of benzodiazepine use. Indeed, even physicians who use these drugs frequently seem to suffer from some guilt and join in the criticism. The objections are often not clearly focused. Some cite the biologic hazards of the agents. The literature contains some cases of physical dependence (usually in alcoholics), and these cases are often cited. More often, the criticism seems to have a moral character, even if it is only implicit. These writers clearly do not like the widespread use of these agents and apparently feel that such use is undermining some moral structure of the culture. A 1973 editorial in the Lancet was entitled "Benzodiazepines: Use, Overuse, Misuse, Abuse?" (Anonymous, 1973). A survey of a few other titles supports this viewpoint: "Housewife Drug Abuse" (Brahen, 1973), "Mood-Modifying Drugs Prescribed in a Canadian City: Hidden Problems" (Cooperstock and Sims, 1971), and (my favorite) "Is It Right to Perform a Pharmacological Leucotomy on a Large Section of Contemporary Society?" (Parish, 1973). In the last article, Parish suggests that contrary to treating any 'illness,' physicians are relying far too heavily on drug-induced symptomatic relief and are suppressing the emotional lives of their patients. Lennard has gone further with this style of analysis. Not only does he believe that the prescribing of psychoactive drugs is overmedication, but he sees a relationship between the "legitimate" use of psychotropic drugs and drug abuse (Lennard, Epstein, et al., 1970).

Another Viewpoint

Literature critically assessing the use of psychotropic agents in our culture recently has been supplemented by literature that agrees that their use has increased but states that such use is indicated in terms of psychiatric morbidity. Some authors believe that if any malprescribing exists, it is characterized by too little use, not too much (Balter and Levine, 1969; Balter and Levine, 1971; Balter, Levine, and Manheimer, 1974). Balter and Levine, in association with others, have surveyed and judged American and international psychotropic drug use. Their conclusions, released in a 1969 publication, have not changed: "The data available to us . . . do not indicate that a large proportion of Americans are becoming chronic or dependent users of psychotropic drugs . . ." They believe that Americans are conservative in their use of drugs that relieve psychic distress: "Further evidence of the conservative behavior of the American public can be found in the fact that 67% of these persons classified as high on both psychic distress and life crises did not use any psychotherapeutic drug in the year preceding the interview."

One reason for closely examining the Valium issue is that it clearly displays the dilemma of a social induction of drug use. Earlier, I discussed our paucity of knowledge about the social utility of drugs or even the social utility of health and well-being. In general, authors on both sides of the psychotropic appropriateness issue cite the same findings and data. They differ in their interpretation of the social utility or moral framework of the drug-human-cultural interaction. Both camps are made up principally of physician-warriors who use what we could call the *clinical ruse.* They try to anchor their interpretations of appropriateness (on nonappropriateness) to proper diagnosis and to the clinical model. Critics of current prescribing habits feel that the drugs are given to those with problems of everyday life and that such sufferers could do better with spiritual coaching (psychotherapy) and their own social resources. Balter and Levine feel that there is much untreated psychiatric illness that, if subjected to careful diagnostic precision, would lead to a justification for the use of more psychotropic agents. The point missed here by both sides is that diagnosis and conventional medical thought have essentially nothing to do with the usual use of benzodiazepines, except to serve occasionally as a post hoc justification for their use. Blackwell's survey of diagnoses justifying Valium use illustrated that the uses are essentially limitless. One study of psychiatric diagnoses showed little correlation between a benzodiazepine prescription and whether a particular diagnosis of neurosis or depression was made (Ballinger, 1972). When I think of diagnostic justification for the use of Valium, I always recall a young lawyer who asked me for a prescription for the drug. He had noted that a small dose taken before a courtroom appearance stilled his shaking hands and quavering voice. His life seemed otherwise notably free from anxiety and psychic distress. Of course, I wrote the prescription for him. The drug is probably often used for such social facilitation, and the appending of clinical diagnostic terms is meaningless regardless of whether such terms are slated for removal from The American Psychiatric Association Diagnostic Handbook.

One can search long to find a spirited defense of Valium use. My friend, a teacher and practitioner of family practice, does so with verve. He states that the prescription for Valium saves enormous amounts of time, gives his patients what they need, and is much more effective in treating anxiety than the usually encouraged counseling.

Antibiotic Use

Another heavily criticized aspect of prescribing is the use of antibiotics. It is likely that no other area of drug development has meant as much to patients as the development of effective antimicrobials. Such development does not exceed public health measures in the battle against severe infectious disease, but nonetheless, the development of penicillins, cephalosporins, and aminoglycosides does pharmaceutical science proud.

Concern over the misuse and overprescribing of antibiotics has grown with their use. Profligate use contributes to morbidity in the form of needless drug toxicity, superinfections, induction of resistance, and possible shifts in nosocomial bacterial populations. Critics have said that (1) American physicians often prescribe antibiotics without any attempt to culture for bacterial identification, (2) antibiotics are commonly given for viral illnesses, and (3) patient pressure for antibiotics is a factor in their use. Further, the common use of antibiotics for prophylaxis against infection seldom is based on proven efficacy. A review and extremely discouraging overview of these problems was presented by Simmons and Stolley in 1974. They pointed out, in addition to problems already mentioned, that antibiotic use continues to expand and has exceeded the growth of the population. These authors call for moderate controls of antibiotic use, particularly in-hospital reviews. Such muscle exerted by the infectious disease division and the pharmacy and therapeutics committees at teaching hospitals is becoming increasingly apparent.

Here begins the counter-intuitive section—written with some commitment, although not with single-mindedness. Some benefits may relate to the willing (even easy) use of antibiotics. There has been a dramatic decrease in some infections and infectious complications. Overall mortality and case-fatality rates have clearly declined for pneumococcal pneumonia, meningococcal meningitis, subacute bacterial endocarditis, rheumatic fever, and syphilis. Now, a ruptured appendix is seldom fatal. One writer, in response to the Simmons and Stolley article, attributed the relatively high occurrence of otitis media and its complications in American Indian and Alaskan Eskimo populations to the underuse of medication (Chang, 1974). As for Stolley and Simmons, most of their data on emergence of resistance and increasing rates of bacteremia originate from in-hospital reports. Even if outpatient prescribing is more casual than we like, is there any evidence that it is to be tied to the serious complications that have emerged from in-hospital use? Further, is the increased incidence of gram-negative septicemia solely related to overuse of antibiotics? There are other factors that warrant consideration. More elderly patients are now seen in the hospital population, and they might be more susceptible to gram-negative infection. There are more patients with serious underlying diseases, more undergoing heroic surgical procedures, and more simultaneously receiving steroids and immunosuppressive drugs than before. Surely, more gram-negative illness is now diagnosed, particularly in patients with serious illness, because we often look for it with blood cultures.

The counter-intuitive blow has been struck, and it may even have some merit.

Hypertension

Although other areas of prescribing might be examined, I conclude this exercise with one that is not so controversial. Physicians underprescribe for the treatment of hypertension. Of the 25 to 30 million American hypertensives, approximately half are undiagnosed, only half of those diagnosed are receiving any therapy, and the usual estimate is that half of these are treated adequately. In the light of studies showing positive effects from drug intervention, this becomes a tragedy of enormous magnitude. Indeed, it signals to our "overmedicated society" the failure of our system to deliver drug therapy adequately to those who need it.

Conclusion

This volume contains considerations of a variety of prescribing dilemmas. The issue of overmedication looms large and is, to some, analogous to environmental pollution as an unwelcome cohort of the technological revolution. Technology has given us powerful drugs that can both help and harm greatly. That knowledge, like the evidence of particle-filled skies and DDT levels in peregrine falcons, causes great ambivalence about the benefits of technology. Indeed, one could classify some strident critics of American drug use as pharmacologic Luddites who, with a bit more power, might smash all the bubbling retorts and tablet punches and return us to the era of herbal medicine. These words surely do not mean that I think all is well. It would be foolish to ignore the criticism of antibiotic profligacy and the careless expenditure of such valuable resources as drugs. However, reflex criticism of "overmedication" may be extremely harmful. The widely held societal belief that physicians create armies of drooling narcotic addicts by treating pain, and ceaseless seekers of barbiturates by treating insomnia, is undocumented and incorrect. A strange specter of national shame seems to surround drug utilization for sickness. The distrust of pharmaceutical technology seems to be rooted in a Calvinistic twitching that implies that if we were truly strong, we would not need these drugs to get by. In fact, problems that may equal overmedication include noncompliance and individual undermedication. Physicians and patients seem to conspire together to give a little bit of drug and often a little bit of the wrong drug. I prefer therapeutic aggressiveness coupled with a sure conservatism regarding ritual use of small drug in small amounts.

In summary, there is still much wrong with American prescribing habits. Some of what is wrong relates to our inability to view and to analyze the social context of drug use without recourse to the clinical ruse. Other problems include timidity, underprescribing, a costly Puritanical approach to needed therapy, and, in some instances (and only some), overprescribing.

References

Anonymous: Benzodiazepines: use, overuse, misuse, abuse? Lancet 1:1101, 1973.

Ballinger, B.R.: Drug dependence in psychiatric admissions. Br. J. Addict. 67:215, 1972.

Balter, M.B., and Levine, J.: The nature and extent of psychotropic drug usage in the United States. Psychopharm. Bull. 5:3, 1969.

Balter, M.B., and Levine, J.: Character and extent of psychotherapeutic drug usage in the United States, Excerpta Medica International Congress Series no. 274, Psychiatry (Part I), Proceedings of the V World Congress of Psychiatry, Mexico, D.F., Excerpta Medica, Amsterdam, p. 80, 1971.

Balter, M.B., Levine, J., and Manheimer, D.I.: Drug use as determined by interviews. N. Engl. J. Med. 290:1491, 1974.

Blackwell, B.: Psychotropic drugs in use today. The role of diazepam in medical practice. JAMA 225:1637, 1973.

Brahen, L.S.: Housewife drug abuse. J. Drug Educ. 3:13, 1973.

Chang, T.W.: Trends of antibiotic use in The United States (Letter). JAMA 228:1099, 1974.

Cooperstock, R., and Sims, M.: Mood modifying drugs prescribed in a Canadian city: hidden problems. Am. J. Public Health 61:1007, 1971.

Firestone, J.M.: Trends in prescription drug prices. Washington, American Enterprise Institute, 1970.

Goldring, W., and Chassis, H.: Anti-hypertensive drug therapy: an appraisal. In Ingelfinger, F., *Controversy in Internal Medicine*, Philadelphia, W.B. Saunders Company, 1966.

Haynes, R.B., Sackett, D.L., Taylor, D.W., Gibson, E.B., and Johnson, A.L.: Absenteeism from work after the detection and labeling of hypertensives. N. Engl. J. Med. 299:74, 1978.

IMS America Ltd. National Prescription Audit: General information report, 16th edition. Ambler, Pennsylvania, 1978.

Lennard, H.S., Epstein, L.J., Bernstein, A., and Ransom, D.C.: Hazards implicit in prescribing psychoactive drugs. Science 169:438, 1970.

Linn, L.S.: Physician characteristics and attitudes toward legitimate use of psychotherapeutic drugs. J. Health Soc. Behav. 12:132, 1971.

Marks, R.M., and Sachar, E.J.: Undertreatment of medical impatients with narcotic analgesics. Ann. Int. Med. 78:173, 1973.

Morgan, J.P., and Penovich, P.: Methadone: still an analgesic. Drug Therapy. Hospital Edition 1:18, 1977.

Muller, C.: The overmedicated society: forces in the market place for medical care. Science 176:488, 1972.

Parish, P.A.: Is it right to perform a pharmacological leucotomy on a large section of contemporary society? Drugs and Society 7:11, 1972.

Simmons, H.E., and Stolley, P.D.: This is medical progress? Trends and consequences of antibiotic use in The United States. JAMA 227:1023, 1974.

2

Are Most OTC Drugs Really Placebos?

Do Over-the-Counter Drugs Act Mainly as Placebos? Yes.
Judith K. Jones, M.D., Ph.D.

Are Most Over-the-Counter Medicines Really Placebos? Definitely Not.
Joseph M. Pisani, M.D.

It requires a good deal of faith for a man to be cured by his own placebos.

John L. McClenahan

But let us hence, my sovereign, to provide
A salve for any sore that may betide.

William Shakespeare, *Henry VI, Part III*

Introduction

Over-the-counter drugs (OTCs) are widely used and widely criticized. Critics of OTCs believe that their use is largely a tribute to the effective blandishments of Madison Avenue hyperbole, the hypnotic power of television, and man's desire to take medicine.

Jones argues that the popularity of OTCs is largely due to the circumstances of their use rather than to any of their pharmacologic effects. She stresses the self-limited nature of many ailments, the expectations that accompany the use of OTCs, and the impact of prior favorable experiences with such remedies.

Granting that at least a few OTCs are truly active for pharmacologic reasons, Jones questions the bioavailability of some of the complicated combinations and formulations on the market and the efficacy of some of the older, more exotic ingredients.

Pisani argues to the contrary and stresses the importance and desirability of intelligent self-medication. He points out that the purposeful formulation of combination OTCs and their "track record" may render OTCs more predictable than drug combinations put together at the behest of a physician or a patient. The generally low dosage of ingredients, chosen so as to insure safety, also tends to make difficult the demonstration of efficacy in modern, randomized controlled trials. Pisani reiterates a point made by others: if OTC products are different from prescription drugs, as dictated by law, should they be judged and evaluated by the same standards?

One particular point is not discussed by either contributor. If some people insist on taking medicines, how is one going to obtain for them the benefit of the placebo effect? Even if all OTCs were simply elegant placebos (and they assuredly are not), how could one capture their "placebo power" without at least the presence of allegedly active ingredients, advertising, labeling, etc.? Would the FDA allow the marketing of lactose or saline placebos that were labeled as "good for pain" or "unclogs your nasal passages"? The answer is obviously *no*. So—do we encourage stoicism and the more frequent biting of bullets? Or do we take a more relaxed regulatory view of OTCs?

LOUIS LASAGNA, M.D.

Do Over-the-Counter Drugs Act Mainly as Placebos? Yes.

Judith K. Jones, M.D., Ph.D.
Food and Drug Administration, Rockville, MD*

Over-the-counter drugs (OTCs) act mainly as placebos, despite the fact that some of them contain ingredients that have clearly defined pharmacologic effects. First, it is generally proposed that even for currently available OTC drugs with some known actions, the predominant effect is likely to be that of a placebo. Second, it is contended that the remainder of OTCs, for which specific actions are still to be determined, behave primarily as placebos, making assessment of their true value difficult.

My views are based on two important facts: (1) with some notable exceptions, scientific evidence as to the clinical effectiveness of most OTCs is lacking and (2) the nature of most of the ailments or symptoms treated with OTCs and the context in which OTCs are used are often conducive to a positive placebo effect. Further, most of the symptoms treated are generally responsive to placebo therapy.

Before elaborating, let's consider the scope of over-the-counter products and the context of their use, as compared with those of prescription drugs.

The Spectrum of OTC Products

The range of OTC products is so broad that when the Food and Drug Administration (FDA) began its review of all OTC products available in the United States, it required more than 20 review panels to look at the hundreds of ingredients of over 200,000 products. The number of *active* ingredients, however, was considerably smaller.

Effective or not, OTC compounds are widely utilized. To indicate the breadth of the OTC market, the different pharmacologic categories and products are listed in Table 2–1. Since categories were defined by usage, there is some overlap of products. This distinction may be relevant to the examination of placebo effect, because in one situation the drug may have a pharmacologic action, whereas in another it can have a placebo action. It is important to know at this juncture that the spectrum of ingredients in over-the-counter drugs is constantly changing, especially as the various FDA panels conduct reviews of the safety and effectiveness of these compounds. Therefore, this factor may be subject to future change.

Disorders and Symptoms Treated with OTCs

It is apparent from considering the categories of OTC products that most are directed at and used for relatively mild, self-limited symptoms and ailments. In most cases, the symptom, such as mild pain, itching, anxiety, or gastrointestinal discomfort, is highly subjective and variable in its course. In fact, the assumed therapeutic goals of symptomatic relief are often achieved solely by the passage of time.

* The views expressed by the author are her own and should not be interpreted as those of the Food and Drug Administration.

Table 2-1. *The Categories of OTC Products Reviewed by the Food and Drug Administration OTC Panels*

Antacids and Antiflatulents	Antiperspirants
Antimicrobials	Laxatives and Antidiarrheals
Sedatives and Sleep Aids	Dentifrices and Dental Products
Analgesics	Sunburn Treatments and Preventives
Cold, Cough, Allergy, Bronchodilator, and Antihistaminic Drugs	Contraceptives
Mouthwashes	Stimulants
Antiinfectives	Hemorrhoidals
Hematinics	Dandruff Preparations
Vitamins and Minerals	Menstrual and Vaginal Products
Antiemetics and Emetics	
Ophthalmics	

Modified after Edwards, 1972.

Context of OTC Product Use

"Autotherapy"

The use of OTCs differs from the use of prescription drugs in one major respect. In many cases of OTC use, therapist and patient are one and the same. This is not always the case for children and other dependents, where the medicine distributor (usually the mother) may be the "therapist." Other potential "therapists" for OTC drug use include neighbors and pharmacists. It is also likely that persuasive actor or cartoon selling of OTCs on television and in other media plays the role of therapist. Thus, OTCs are given (or recommended) by "autotherapists" or "pseudotherapists." The latter are so called because they are generally not thought to be credible medical or even paramedical therapists by society, though this in no way necessarily relates to their effectiveness.

Acceptance of Self-Limited, Easily Treated Disease

Historically, it is very difficult to differentiate OTCs from such home remedies as chamomile tea and lemon and sugar for a cough. Older books are replete with herbal remedies that can be compiled at home from garden items or from components obtained through the pharmacist. (The pharmacist and the medicine man vied for the market of what are now OTCs.) It is difficult to ascertain whether the context of the use of home remedies varied greatly from that of OTCs today, although now there appears to be a general acceptance of minor, self-limited complaints or symptoms that can be relieved by simple home remedies or over-the-counter products. This can often lead to expectation of relief, whether due to drugs or to the passage of time.

Casual or Deliberate Use

Use of OTCs varies, depending on the frequency of the occurrence of symptoms. Some OTCs may be kept at home and used when needed, such as aspirin or acetaminophen for headaches or other minor pain. It can be presumed that certain of these OTCs are considered as "staples" and are kept in the home just as naturally as bread and milk are kept. Thus, an expectation of need exists, as does the implication of presumed and potential effectiveness.

Another category of OTCs includes those that are bought only after the need arises, since the need is neither predictable nor frequent. Antidiarrheal and cough or cold OTCs are part of this category. Seeking out, purchasing, and using these types of OTCs may be quite deliberate and may help to determine expectations of relief.

Motivations for Use

It can be reasonably postulated that use of OTCs before or instead of medical therapy may imply (1) expectation that the OTC will probably work, (2) hope that the use of an OTC will make a symptom disappear and prevent the need for medical therapy, and (3) expectation that use of an OTC will avoid the need for interruption of daily activities.

If any of these expectations is borne out, there is in fact an identifiable reward for a specific action. Since use of these products requires some monetary investment, a positive outcome is likewise reinforcement of good judgment.

OTC Users May Be Different

Of interest in this regard is a study by Balter (Cooper, 1973) that suggests that the user of OTC sedative-hypnotics is not usually the one taking prescription sedative-hypnotic formulations. This could indicate (1) that the users are satisfied, (2) that the users have benign medical problems, or (3) that we are dealing with two entirely separate population groups.

Evidence of Effectiveness of OTC Drugs

In the initial review of 422 OTC products by the National Academy of Science/National Research Council in the late 1960s, only one fourth of the OTCs were judged to be effective, based on data available at that time (Edwards, 1973).

There is a paucity of data relating to the use, pharmacologic effects, and safety of OTC preparations. However, with the advent of FDA-mandated reviews of OTC drugs in 1972, some information from the studies has begun to appear, including a few discussions relating to the placebo question (Cooper, 1973). In general, there are no definitive studies that discuss the overall controversy, but a few reports do throw light on this question.

A Few OTCs are Effective Pharmacologically

Both older and more recent studies do confirm the effectiveness of certain OTC products when compared with placebos. These involve the demonstrated effectiveness of aspirin and acetaminophen in relieving simple pain (Beecher, 1957; Beaver, 1965, 1966; Moertel et al., 1972), the antihistaminic actions of certain antihistamines (Douglas, 1975), and the cough-suppressant effects of dextromethorphan and diphenhydramine (Federal Register, 1976), to name a few. However, with the exception of these few ingredients at adequate dosages, evidence of the pharmacologic effectiveness of most OTC products is scant.

Many OTCs Shown to Be No Better than Placebos

Some investigations of over-the-counter drugs show them to be no better than placebos, such as some studies of aspirin and acetaminophen (Beaver, 1965, 1966), the sleep preparation Compoz (Rickels and Hesbacher, 1973), antacids (Sturdevant et al., 1977), and expectorants (Hirsch et al., 1973; Federal Register, 1976).

Most OTCs Never Compared with Placebos

Most OTC products have not been studied or compared with placebos, despite the fact that placebos have been shown to have significant effects on many symptoms. The question of how much of the therapeutic effect is attributable to the drug must also be raised. For example, many studies of antiasthma drugs compare two separate drugs or combinations of drugs without placebo controls, even though certain asthmatics have very clear-cut placebo responses to saline injections or saline aerosols (Godfrey and Silverman, 1973).

Suboptimal Dosage in OTCs

Other reasons for doubt about the supposed benefit of OTCs relate to the vast lack of information about them as they are currently formulated and used. For example, many known pharmacologically active ingredients are present in suboptimal doses in OTCs (A.Ph.A. Project Staff, 1977). The lower limit of effectiveness of these ingredients is often not known, but the action can be presumed to be minimal.

The small amounts of antihistamines in analgesic and sleep and cold preparations serve as examples.

Mutiple Combinations of Similar Drugs—Are They Additive?

Further, many OTCs contain combinations of two or more drugs of the same class in suboptimal doses based on the presumption that they are additive, although there is little information to substantiate this.

Combination Products—Interactive or Bioavailable?

Since very few studies have been performed to evaluate the overall effects of combination OTCs as compared with placebos, these OTCs often raise other questions relating to the potential for any pharmacologic action. For example, attention must be given to (1) whether the multiple combination products have interactions that *decrease* their effect and (2) whether there is bioavailability of the presumed active ingredient. Although requirements to show bioavailability exist primarily for certain prescription drugs, this question is of particular concern with regard to enteric-coated drugs (e.g., certain forms of aspirin), time-release preparations, and topical formulations, despite the fact that they may contain active drugs at adequate doses.

Many OTC Products Have Unknown Effects

Another area of obscurity relates to the OTC products whose pharmacologic effects are essentially unknown, since the formulations are usually carryovers from much earlier times. Such ingredients include passion flower extract (until recently in Compoz); various "essential" oils such as tolu oil, balsam of Peru, and eucalyptus oil; and buchu and hydrangea extracts (in menstrual products).

Problems in Methodology for Assessing Effectiveness

Finally, although it is possible that in the future many of the unknowns will be eliminated and many OTCs will be studied in well designed clinical trials, it is likely that evidence for true pharmacologic effectiveness will still be moot. This is owing to the difficulty of designing methods to assess the relief of such evanescent and weakly defined symptoms as itch, nasal congestion, expectoration, and premenstrual distress. This is not even to mention the statistical problems in analyzing drugs that are just slightly more effective than placebos.

Thus, although a few over-the-counter drugs such as aspirin, acetaminophen, antihistamines, and cough suppressants have been shown to have clinical effectiveness as a result of their drug action, evidence is sparse for the great majority of OTC products at present.

OTCs Act Mainly as Placebos

Nature of the Placebo Response

The concept of the placebo has varied. The term itself means *I will please*, but it is used in many contexts. From the standpoint of drug studies, a *true placebo* is an agent that has no known pharmacologic effects. From the perspective of drug testing, the term usually implies that the inactive placebo is identical in appearance, taste, and smell to the drug being tested. More appropriate to the question at hand, the *placebo effect* or *response* has been defined as *any change in a patient's symptoms that is the result of a therapeutic intent and not the specific physical/chemical nature of the medical procedure* (Byerly, 1976). The discussion of OTCs acting as placebos will revolve around *placebo effect* or *response*, since at least some OTCs are not pharmacologically inert.

Scientific study of the placebo response has greatly expanded, beginning with the careful study of Lasagna and his colleagues (Lasagna et al., 1954). This study raised many questions about the placebo reactor and the nature of the placebo response.

Determinants of the Placebo Response

In general, Rickels (1968) has related the placebo response (or nonspecific factors in drug responses) to four factors:

1. The patient's unique personality, medical and drug intake history, expectations, attitudes, and social setting
2. The physician's personality, attitudes and expectations
3. The treatment milieu or sites of therapeutic interaction

4. The nontreatment milieu of home and work.

All these factors have been shown at times to have an effect on placebo response in various settings (Rickels, 1968; Shapiro and Morris, 1978). However, in the case of placebo responses to OTC products, the physician plays only an indirect role (in fact, one motivation for using OTC drugs may be to *avoid* the physician), and the therapeutic milieu blends with the nontherapeutic. However, there may be an analogous role to the physician in the person of the aforementioned autotherapist or pseudotherapist.

A recent, very comprehensive review (Shapiro and Morris, 1978) of the placebo response suggested that very few generalizations could be made about this extremely complex phenomenon. The response is not consistently a function of sex, age, IQ, socioeconomic group, race or personality type, although these variables have been shown to be positive or negative factors in individual studies. On the other hand, a placebo response has been shown to relate to therapeutic environment, expectations, and degree and type of symptoms. It has also shown a strong association with personality characteristics (Shapiro and Morris, 1978). Factors that could potentially affect placebo response include suggestibility, persuasion, reinforcements, hope, and previous experience.

The rate of response to placebos for angina, postoperative pain, cough, and mood was long contended by Beecher (Beecher, 1968) to average 35 percent, within a range of 15 percent to 58 percent. More recent reviews suggest that, depending on the conditions of the study and what is studied, the range of placebo response is in fact from 0 percent to 100 percent (Shapiro and Morris, 1978).

Possible Mechanisms of Placebo Response

Various studies have been proposed to explain the mechanism of those factors that can influence placebo response. *Conditioning* has been offered as an explanation for placebo response when there is a preceding response to a similar stimulus (Morris and O'Neal, 1974). For example, if aspirin relieves a headache repeatedly, a placebo or drug called aspirin may be likely to relieve a similar headache. This kind of response has been elicited in animals for some drugs but not for others (Byerly, 1976). In a broad sense, placebo reaction due to a variety of responses in the past has been considered to be a function of the type of conditioning (Bourne, 1978). *Expectations* of the patient, conditioned by media advertising, labeling of the drug, and level of anticipation, may also be regarded as conditioning factors.

Attribution theory (Morris and O'Neal, 1974; Shapiro and Morris, 1978) suggests that the placebo response occurs when individuals attribute their response to a drug when it is actually due to some other factor(s), such as natural resolution of the symptom. This may be especially common in the use of OTC drugs, because many symptoms treated therewith resolve spontaneously.

Another proposed factor is *response bias*, or the effect of influences in the extrinsic milieu such as positive feedback from other people. This mechanism is more likely to apply to the prescribed or experimental drug setting but might occasionally apply to the OTC drug setting, especially when there is a pseudotherapist. For example, an observer's voiced perception that a drug has had certain effects could produce a biased response that is reflected in repeated use or judgment of effectiveness.

Why the Response to OTCs Is Mostly a Placebo Response

Given the lack of scientific proof (and often of pharmacologic rationale) and the context of OTC drug use, there are still logical reasons why most OTC products, often containing ingredients of unproven effectiveness, are very popular and useful. This appears to be true, despite the fact that relief of symptoms is achieved basically through the placebo effect.

Likelihood of placebo effect on subjective symptoms. Since most symptoms for which OTCs are used, such as mild pain, mild anxiety, or cough, are known to be relieved by placebo in 20 percent to 50 percent of cases (Beecher, 1968), there is a good likelihood of a positive patient response whether the OTC is active or not. Other studies likewise contend that these symptoms are the ones most commonly relieved by placebos; therefore, a placebo response would be suggested when any treatment was taken (Campbell and Rosenbaum, 1967; Bourne, 1978). In this setting, an effective drug is difficult to differentiate from a true placebo if it is only slightly more effective.

Positive outcome is rewarded. The context of OTC product use is amenable to placebo response for these reasons:

1. The user or autotherapist will have his judgment and expectations rewarded by a positive placebo response

2. A positive response will avoid need for further medical attention and interruption of daily routine

3. The repetitive user, as autotherapist, is more likely to be a *self-selected* positive responder, and his previous positive response (pharmacologic or placebo) predisposes him to a further positive placebo response (Shapiro and Morris, 1978.)

Misattribution. The benign, often transient nature of the symptoms treated with OTCs is a very likely factor in misattribution. That is, relief of symptoms is mistakenly perceived as being due to the product, and expectation of its continued effect predetermines a further placebo effect.

Incidental effects may suggest that the drug is working. Since some OTCs do have ingredients that produce reactions not necessarily related to proposed therapeutic effectiveness (such as lethargy in the case of antihistamines or stinging in the case of phenol in various solutions or astringents), occurrence of these reactions may be interpreted as indications that the product is "working." In fact, studies exist that either support or refute this type of phenomenon (Kast and Loesch, 1961; Rickels, 1968; Shapiro and Morris, 1978).

The "therapist." Finally, the pseudotherapist (mothers, pharmacists, and the media) must be considered a possible influence on both positive and negative placebo responses, since in other settings the therapist can have a powerful effect on the placebo response (Bourne, 1978; Shapiro and Morris, 1978). For example, mothers and pharmacists desiring positive drug therapy may elicit positive responses secondary to a response bias. The graphic, often colorful media advertising is powerful in promoting sales, and it may also be powerful in eliciting and reinforcing a placebo effect of OTCs used repeatedly (Buckalew, 1972).

Conclusion

All these factors tend to support the contention that with some exceptions, whatever is in the OTC product, for a variety of reasons unrelated to the pharmacology of the drug, a beneficial effect will more than likely be due to a placebo response and will be seen in a substantial number of people who use OTC drugs.

However, this essay is written during a time of change. As the conclusions of the FDA OTC Review evolve, many OTC products are changing in formulation and are being tested more carefully. Although the conditions for high placebo reaction will likely remain and even be enhanced by expectation of greater effect, the proportionate number of truly pharmacologically effective drugs available for OTC use may well also increase.

References

A.Ph.A. Project Staff: *Handbook of Non-Prescription Drugs*, 5th edition. Washington, D.C., American Pharmaceutical Association, 1977.

Beaver, W.T.: Mild analgesics: a review of their pharmacology. Am. J. Med. Sci. 250:577–604, 1965; 251:576, 1966.

Beecher, H.K.: The measurement of pain. Prototype for the quantitative study of subjective responses. Pharmacol. Rev. 9:59, 1957.

Beecher, H.K.: Placebo effects of situations, attitudes, and drugs: a quantitative study of suggestibility. In Rickels, K., editor, *Non-Specific Factors in Drug Therapy*, Springfield, Ill., Charles C Thomas, Publisher, 1968.

Bourne, H.: Rational use of placebos. In Melmon, K.L., and Morrelli, H., editors, *Clinical Pharmacology*, Macmillan Inc., 1978.

Buckalew, L.: An analysis of experimental components in placebo effects. Psychol. Rec. 22:113, 1972.

Byerly, H.: Explaining and exploiting placebo effects. Perspect. Biol. Med. Spring 1976:423.

Campbell, J.H., and Rosenbaum, C.T.: Placebo effect in symptom relief in psychotherapy. Arch. Gen. Psychiatry 16:364, 1967.

Cooper, J.D.: *The Efficacy of Self-Medication*. Washington, D.C., The Interdisciplinary Communication Associates, Inc., 1973.

Douglas, W.W.: Histamine and antihistamine; 5-OH-tryptamine and antagonists. In Goodman, L.S., and Gilman, A., eds., *The Pharmacologic Basis of Therapeutics*, 5th edition, Macmillan, Inc., 1975.

Edwards, C.E.: Closing the gap, OTC drugs. FDA Papers, February 1972.

Federal Register: Over-the-counter drugs. Establishment of a monograph for OTC cough, cold, allergy, bronchodilator and antiasthmatic products. Vol. 41, September 1976.

Godfrey, S., and Silverman, M.: Demonstration of placebo response in asthma by means of exercise testing. J. Psychosom. Res. 17:293, 1973.

Hirsch, S.R., Viernes, P.F., and Cory, R.G.: The expectorant effect of glyceryl guaiacolate in patients with chronic bronchitis. A controlled in vitro and in vivo study. Chest 63:9, 1973.

Kast, E.C., and Loesch, J.: Influence of the doctor-patient relationship on drug action. Ill. Med. J. 119:390, 1961.

Lasagna, L., Mosteller, F., VonFelsinger, J., and Beecher, H.: A study of the placebo response. Am. J. Med. 16:779, 1954.

Moertel, C.G., Ahmann, D.L., Taylor, W.F., and Schwartau, N.: A comparative evaluation of marketed analgesic drugs. N. Engl. J. Med. 286:813, 1972.

Morris, L.A., and O'Neal, E.: Drug name familiarity and the placebo effect. J. Clin. Psychol. 30:280, 1974.

Rickels, K.: Non-Specific factors of drug therapy in neurotic patients. In Rickels, K., editor, *Non-Specific Factors in Drug Therapy*, Springfield, Ill., Charles C Thomas, Publisher, 1968.

Rickels, K., and Hesbacher, P.T.: Over-the-counter daytime sedatives. JAMA 223:29, 1973.

Shapiro, A.K., and Morris, L.I.: The placebo effect in medical and psychological therapy. In Bergin, A., and Garfield, S., editors, *Handbook of Psychotherapy and Behavior Change, An Empirical Analysis*, John Wiley & Sons, Inc., 1978.

Sturdevant, R.A.L., Isenberg, J.I., Secrist, D., and Ansfield, J.: Antacid and placebo produce similar pain relief in duodenal ulcer patients. Gastroenterology 72:1, 1977.

Are Most Over-the-Counter Medicines Really Placebos? Definitely Not.

Joseph M. Pisani, M.D.
Proprietary Association, Washington, D.C.

After two years as an executive in the Food and Drug Administration (FDA), I spent over ten years as a scientific representative of a national trade association representing the manufacturers of nonprescription or over-the-counter (OTC) medicines. The knowledge thus obtained of the pharmaceutical industry and its regulation was furthered during five of these years via service as an Industry Liaison Representative (ILR) on four of the FDA advisory panels engaged in the review and evaluation of the various categories of OTC medicines. The opinions expressed in this article are conclusions that I have drawn through personal experience with a regulatory agency and with a regulated industry as a physician, an administrator, and a consumer.

Terminology

As a preface to discussing over-the-counter drugs (OTCs), some common words and phrases should be elaborated upon so as to provide insight into their usage. The term *medicine* usually conveys the concept of a substance or a preparation to treat disease—a tool of the physician who has decided upon its use and directed or guided its administration. On the other hand, the public's impression of the word *drug* is usually either that of a substance taken for nonmedical reasons or of a powerful preparation (e.g., a narcotic with a strong potential for physical or psychologic dependence) administered by a physician or nurse to alleviate severe suffering. In either case, the "drugged" person is conceptualized somewhat unfavorably. *Medicine* and *drug* are, nevertheless, often used interchangeably. This probably led to the use of the word *pharmaceutical*, which is more sophisticated and usually refers to a medicinal drug.

In most instances, I favor the term *medicine* because it more clearly depicts the salutary effects of such chemical preparations, and I reserve the word *drug* for the aforementioned situations. This approach stresses the positive aspects of medicinal agents when used appropriately, rather than the negative attitudes toward drug use, bordering on therapeutic nihilism, that have been advanced by industry critics. At the same time, this approach may be considered somewhat idealistic, since the law that applies in many cases is the U.S. Food, Drug, and Cosmetic Act (FDC Act). This law contains no definition or reference to *medicine*, but does have a rather technical definition of the word *drug* that reads, in part: "the term 'drug' means . . . (B) articles intended for use in the diagnosis, cure, mitigation, treatment or prevention of disease in man or other animals . . ." (Section 201,g,1). There are other legal-regulatory aspects that would also seem to favor focusing on the term *drug* rather than on *medicine*. Also, the difficulty of attempting to alter widespread traditional use of the word *drug*, especially in scientific circles, is fully appreciated.

Nonprescription Versus Prescription Medicines

By law and regulation, drugs (or medicines) are of two classes: (1) those sold by prescription, with licensed practitioners giving the directions for use, and (2) those sold over-the-counter, without prescription, in which case the product labeling gives the directions for use. According to the 1951 Durham-Humphrey Amendment to the FDC Act, a drug *must* be sold OTC if (1) it is safe per se; (2) adequate directions and indications for use, readily discernible to the average person can be written; and (3) a licensed practitioner's services are not necessary for its administration. As the legislative history of the FDC Act and the 1951 Amendment clearly shows, the intent of Congress was not to prohibit self-medication but rather to insure its safety and effectiveness by making available only those drugs for which adequate directions for self-use could be written.

Passage of the Durham-Humphrey Amendment underscored the important differences between two classes of medicines, with an especially basic distinction being in purpose. Nonprescription medicines are generally used for the temporary relief of mild, often self-limiting symptoms or the treatment of relatively minor ailments and indispositions. These conditions are common and easily self-diagnosed; the intervention of the licensed practitioner is unnecessary. On the other hand, prescription medicines are primarily intended to treat more serious conditions or disease states. They are inappropriate for unsupervised use because of greater potency, a generally narrower margin between benefit and risk, and a higher incidence of side effects. Also, the diseases involved are not self-limiting and necessitate professional diagnosis and management.

From these basic distinctions flow numerous other differences in the ways prescription and nonprescription medicines are developed, manufactured, labeled, promoted, sold, used, and regulated. A discussion of the FDA's regulatory approach to OTCs and its implications for their development and marketing is informative.

The Food and Drug Administration

A commentary in the Journal of the American Medical Association (JAMA) analyzed the dictum *Primum non nocere* (first, do no harm) as to its negative impact on the utilization of therapeutic agents for serious disease (Gifford, 1977). In discussing the current overemphasis on potential risks in benefit-risk considerations, it was observed that "the doctrine also pervades and, I fear, unduly influences the FDA .... since their primary objective is to protect the public from unsafe drugs, foods and cosmetics, and to fulfill that role as it pertains to drugs, it is only natural that they should place emphasis on the risk denominator of the benefit-risk ratio."

During the past decade, other scientists have raised similar questions as to whether the FDA's primary mission is to protect against unsafe products and whether overprotectiveness may not operate to the detriment of the public. These issues stimulated a Special Communication in JAMA to physicians from the FDA Commissioner (Kennedy, 1978). Besides marshaling data to demonstrate that if a "drug lag" exists, it is not indigenous to the U.S., and supporting the view that the chief reason for the decline in the rate of introduction of important new drugs is an "appararent exhaustion of certain basic knowledge on which the industry's earlier breakthroughs were based," the message contains other notable concepts:

> The FDA's responsibility to the public health is often thought of primarily as a matter of guaranteeing safety, but consumers are poorly served when they are denied access to safe products that are effective in the relief of pain or the cure of disease. We must view our role as regulators of technology transfer comprehensively and be just as conscious of the costs of foregone innovation as we are of other kinds of costs.

In discussing FDA and Department of Health, Education and Welfare (DHEW) changes in the FDA Act, being prepared for submission to Congress, Commissioner Kennedy stated:

> The provisions will be aimed at . . . greater flexibility in the clinical testing and marketing of new drug products where they represent significant or urgently sought therapeutic breakthroughs and where efficacy tests are difficult to do . . . and at enhanced ability to keep the use of particular marketed drugs under strict controls . . .

The FDA and OTC Product Regulation

The preceding discussion of the FDA's regulatory approach may seem to involve chiefly prescription medicines. Actually, the doctrine of *Primum non nocere* has more fundamental and greater applicability to OTCs, via the

FDA's implementation of the Durham-Humphrey Amendment, especially as to their *labeling* and *development or formulation.* This is understandable, since nonprescription medicines have different indications than prescription medicines and are to be used directly by the layman without professional supervision. The FDA has traditionally focused on insuring the safe use of such products.

Not only is comprehensive, understandable labeling required by law and regulation, but over the years, much attention—by both government and industry—has been given to avoiding the use of terms on labels that may (1) connote treatment or cure of a disease state, particularly when the latter involves self-diagnosis beyond a nonprofessional's capabilities; (2) encourage chronicity of use rather than occasional, temporary use; or (3) imply permanent relief. Beside adequate indications and directions for use, cautions or warnings appropriate to the various OTC medicine categories are also mandated. Included in these requirements are general admonitions designed to prevent various forms of misuse of OTCs, including overuse and accidental ingestion. For example, advice such as "Keep out of the reach of children," "Do not exceed the recommended dosage," and "If symptoms persist beyond (x) days, or become aggravated, consult your physician" have become common. In addition, industry's voluntary compliance efforts include campaigns encouraging consumers to "Read the Label" in order to insure appropriate OTC usage, "flagging" of labels to call attention to significant labeling changes, and generally supporting safety measures in packaging.

The FDA's evaluation of OTCs has even greater significance in relation to the development and formulation of such medicines. In contrast to prescription medicines, which are often single entity preparations directed at a particular disease state, a sizable majority of OTCs are combinations of active ingredients directed at a given symptom complex and premeasured, blended, and balanced for the dosage level and schedule appropriate for the majority of the target population. Owing to pretesting and experience with such mixtures, there is no need to be concerned that the various ingredients may interact or that their various dosages may not be in proper balance. The dosage is relatively low and the safety margin is wide, since these principles have always been a major focus of the FDA.

Starting in the mid-1950s, as a consequence of the Durham-Humphrey Amendment, a series of prescription-exemption regulations, popularly known as "switch-over regs," were initiated by the FDA. They provide specific potency, dosage ceilings, and labeling requirements for certain commonly used preparations that allow them to be marketed on an OTC basis and to be exempt from prescription drug requirements. These regulations were periodically updated, and there are currently 26 of them in effect.

Various ingredients are covered by "switch-over regs," such as analgesics (acetaminophen and sodium gentisate), antifungals (diamthazole and tolnaftate), anticholinergics (dicyclomine and diphemanil), dentifrice–caries preventatives (sodium fluoride and sodium monoflurophosphate), an antitussive (dextromethorphan), a number of antihistamines (e.g., meclizine and chlorcyclizine), and decongestants (tuaminoheptane and methoxyphenomine). In addition, consultations between the industry and the FDA often resulted in similar guidelines concerning potencies and dosages for certain other preparations not formally covered in these regulations.

Several important considerations arose from such regulatory determinations:

1. Delineation of important differences between OTCs and prescription medicines and the impact of potency limitations imposed by the "switch-over regs" and other FDA controls on OTC ingredients do not imply the absence of effectiveness of such OTC products for their intended use, but rather highlight the difficulty of demonstrating efficacy via double-blind, randomized, well controlled clinical investigations.

2. Not infrequently, the potency and dosage ceilings arrived at were "guesstimates," with the figures being selected primarily on the basis of a wide margin of safety and less on the grounds of demonstrated effectiveness by modern biometric techniques that began to be used in the 1930s and 1940s.

3. Subsequent to the 1962 Kefauver-Harris Amendments to the FDC Act calling for New Drug Applications (NDA's) approved between 1938 and 1962 (primarily precleared for safety) to be reviewed for demonstration of effectiveness, the agency became more concerned about OTCs. The FDA's experience with the Drug Efficacy Study (DES) of the National Academy of Sciences-National Research Council (NAS-NRC) from 1966 to 1969 and their own Drug Efficacy Study Implementation (DESI) Program (1969 to present) convinced

the agency that a massive review of the OTC field should be undertaken under their own auspices rather than on a contract basis (more about this later).

4. In the late 1960s, the FDA began efforts to tighten the regulatory drawstrings by becoming more cognizant of the aforementioned modern biometric techniques. In May, 1970, the FDA indicated that "substantial evidence" (of effectiveness) meant evidence consisting of adequate and well controlled investigations as detailed in then Section 130.12 (a) (5) (ii) of the Code of Federal Regulations (CFR) 21 (currently C.F.R. 21 Section 314.111). The FDA identified the well controlled, double-blind, randomized, statistically evaluated clinical trial as the primary basis for assessment of effectiveness. At the time, it was indicated that this criterion had been used also as the standard for effectiveness in the DES of 1966 to 1969, but this was not confirmed in the final report submitted to the FDA by the NAS-NRC (DES Report, 1969).

Next came the issuance of the FDA's policy on fixed combinations of prescription drugs in October 1971, followed by the OTC Review Procedural Regulations of May 1972 that included an apparently more reasonable approach to standards for OTC drug combinations.

Meanwhile, in 1970 to 1971, leading FDA spokesmen began announcing that one standard would be applied to all drugs both old and new. Although the primary intent of this was to phase out uncontrolled clinical observations as contributory to the proof of effectiveness for prescription drugs, OTC medicines were squeezed by this regulatory belt-tightening maneuver in an illogical fashion.

As has been noted (Pisani, 1974; Lasagna, 1976) it is anomalous for the FDA to limit the potency of OTC ingredients and then turn around and expect the same type of modern biometric evidence to be as readily available as for the more potent prescription medicines, particularly when experience with, and usage of, many of the OTC ingredients antedate the advent of the randomized, controlled clinical trial that per se may not be appropriate as a standard for effectiveness of OTCs.

Where does all this seem to lead? Have I swung around to equating most OTCs with "placebos"? Definitely not! Let's look more closely at the term and other factors that point in the opposite direction.

"Placebos"

Is this an appropriate term to use in relation to OTCs? Not according to the dictionary definition (Webster, 1961). The derivation is from Latin, meaning *I shall please* and it usually refers to *an inert medicament or preparation given for its psychogical effect, especially to satisfy the patient or act as a control in an experimental series.*

The references to *I* and to *satisfy the patient* are explicit allusions to the necessary ingredients of physician *and* patient in placebo reactions. The reference to acting as a control in an experimental series also implies the controlled clinical trials used for the efficacy evaluation of prescription medicines. Interestingly enough, the dictionary definition is incomplete, as it refers just to psychologic effect. While there have been numerous articles in the literature discussing the psychologic effects of placebos, their physiologic and "toxic" effects have also been reported. At least one investigator has shown that placebos can cause the adrenals to fire, and in severely anxious patients, to mimic the effects of ACTH in normal subjects (Cleghorn et al., 1950). Beecher (1955) discussed studies from the literature wherein placebos not only relieved pain arising from physiologic causes but also caused gross physical change. The consistency of the placebo effect as reported in this article (35.2 percent ± 2.2 percent) is remarkable in view of the number and diversity of the studies.

Although there have been numerous studies of OTCs involving placebos, the appropriateness of the type of data ordinarily collected in evaluating medication has been questioned (Feinstein, 1972). The same authority (Feinstein, 1973) also questioned the propriety of clinical studies involving placebos in evaluating OTCs, since they are consumed directly by the individual without the doctor's participation—which, in itself, may produce substantial effects.

What are the alternatives? The problem was discussed in depth some years ago at an interdiciplinary conference sponsored by the Smithsonian Institution (Cooper, 1974), during which the importance of the "track record" or experience with marketed drugs was highlighted, as well as the concept of the need for some means of assessment of consumer symptom relief for new OTCs short of the formal, randomized, blinded clinical trial.

In the latter regard, I had earlier reported

on a suggestion that sociometric measures of consumer satisfaction be employed in evaluating OTCs on normal, healthy people—representing the majority of OTC users—under the natural everyday conditions in which they live, rather than under the artificial conditions of a pharmacologic experiment or the negative selection represented by a hospital or clinic population (Pisani, 1974).

Let's assume agreement that most OTCs are not really "placebos," and rephrase the original question: i.e., "Are most OTC medicines composed of inert ingredients that really do little for the consumer?" My reply is still "Definitely not." Beside many of the points previously discussed, there are yet others that should be cited in support of this view.

CONSIDERATIONS ARISING FROM THE FDA's OTC REVIEW

Summary of the OTC Review

As mentioned earlier, in 1970 to 1971, the FDA began planning for one of the most massive projects in its history: the review of what was originally estimated to be 27 categories of OTCs, involving more than 100,000 products, by 17 advisory panels. After more than a year of planning, the project began early in 1972, and will take a decade or more to complete.

The FDA divided all ingredients of OTCs into therapeutic categories, assigning these and their subcategories to the 17 advisory review panels. Some of the divisions are Internal Analgesics (antipyretic and antirheumatics); Cough and Cold Remedies (allergy, bronchodilator, and antiasthmatic products); Laxatives (antidiarrheals and antiemetics); and Sedatives and Stimulants. Overall, it is now estimated that there will be over 100 categories and subcategories for which OTC monographs will be prepared.

Each of the panels consists of seven voting members, including physicians, dentists, pharmacists, toxicologists, and other specialists, plus liaison representatives from industry and consumer groups who participate in panel discussions but do not have a vote.

Panel deliberations include a review of an FDA literature search on the ingredients being evaluated, together with an invitation for anyone (manufacturers, consumers, physicians, etc.) to submit information. By 1978, 16,000 volumes of data had been submitted, chiefly by manufacturers regarding their products.

Customarily, each panel then holds two or three day meetings at intervals of about six to eight weeks over a period that has varied from one to several years. Each panel is charged with preparing a report that contains recommendations classifying all conditions (ingredients, labeling, etc.) into one of three categories:

I—Those that the panel considers generally recognized as "safe and effective."

II—Those that the panel considers *not* generally recognized as "safe and effective."

III—Those for which, in the panel's opinion, there is insufficient evidence to decide general recognition of safety and effectiveness.

In its Final Report, submitted as recommendations to the FDA, the panel must include reasons for their classifications of the various conditions and must specify what further studies are needed (and by when) to advance Category III conditions to Category I status.

After the panel's report is submitted to the FDA, it becomes publicly available, with 90 to 120 days allowed for comments by any interested party. Subsequently, the FDA evaluates the panel's report and the comments and issues a Tentative Final Monograph, which includes the FDA's views on the report and comments. An additional 30-day period is provided for anyone who wishes to file objections on any issue or to request an oral hearing before the FDA Commissioner. After this time, the FDA issues a Final Monograph for the particular OTC category (or categories). It includes the list of ingredients, formulations, and labeling that the FDA Commissioner decides are in Category I and serves as a kind of "recipe book" for OTC medicine manufacturers. Any product not conforming to the Final Monograph within a time period determined by FDA is liable to regulatory action.

OTC Review Classification of Ingredients

It is estimated that about 500 of the 1100 submitted ingredients have been reviewed to date. Since only the Antacid and Antiflatulent categories have reached the Final Monograph stage, and several review panels have not completed their work or submitted reports, it may be some time before any attempt can be made at an overall assessment of the effectiveness of the many OTC ingredients. Even when the OTC Review is completed, it may be difficult to make such an analysis because the various ingredients may be placed in any one of the three categories by different panels, as a number of them will be under review by more than one panel for different indications. Further, ingredients may be placed in any one of the three categories by a given panel for reasons that may not be directly related to their pharmacologic effectiveness or lack of activity—that is, the classification may be related to another condition pertaining to labeling or formulation.

Nevertheless, certain observations may be made:

1. OTC review panels have seldom placed ingredients in Category II on the sole basis of lack of effectiveness. More commonly, such recommendations are related to a panel's opinion that there is a significiant question as to the safety of a preparation or concern about potential for misuse. Occasionally, this view is supplemented by some doubt as to effectiveness.

2. There are many Category III recommendations for which panels believe that further evidence would enable reclassification into Category I, and no question of safety would be involved.

3. Since the OTC Review started in 1972, there have been three instances in which the FDA felt that substantial questions of safety existed regarding ingredients under review by the panels to a degree that merited removal from the market without following the routine OTC procedures adopted in May 1972. These were as follows:

> ***Hexachlorophene.*** Although the panel considering antimicrobials thought this to be an effective antimicrobial agent, it recommended that hexachlorophene was unsafe for general OTC use, except as part of a preservative system if used in a concentration no greater than 0.1 percent. Because of concern regarding its potential toxicity, especially on damaged skin and the skin of premature infants, and the potential for multiple use on the body, the FDA took action to make hexachlorophene available as an antimicrobial agent only on a prescription basis, and it did so before the Tentative Final Monograph stage was reached in this category.
>
> ***Tribromsalan, dibromsalan, and tetrachlorosalicylanilide.*** Here again, the panel considered tribromsalan to have antimicrobial activity and to have effective deodorant activity. However, the panel was concerned over reports of severe and crippling photosensitivity in some individuals using products with this ingredient. Because of the risk involved, even for just a few individuals, the panel recommended removal of tribromsalan from the market. Further, although data on the other two antimicrobial ingredients were not submitted for review, the panel believed that there was clear evidence that these agents were even more potent photosensitizers than trimbromsalan, and therefore it recommended that all three be banned from use in drugs and cosmetics. Again, the FDA implemented the panel's recommendations without waiting for the usual review procedure phases to be completed.
>
> ***Chloroform.*** While reviewing chloroform as a preservative, the FDA banned it as an OTC ingredient because of studies reporting it to be carcinogenic in mice and rats. Again, the FDA moved ahead without following the usual OTC review procedures because of concern regarding potential toxicity in humans.

4. In its final report, the OTC review panel on Cough, Cold, Allergy, Bronchodilator, and Antiasthmatic Products included recommendations that some 14 ingredients (antihistamines, bronchodilators, and nasal decongestants), then wholly or partially limited to prescription use, be made available for OTC use. In accepting the panel report in September 1976, the FDA also tentatively (1) agreed with panel recommendations for 10 of the ingredients, allowing them to be switched over to nonprescription use; (2) disagreed with the panel about three of the other ingredients for switchover; and (3) postponed action on the fourth. In addition, a few other OTC review panels that have not yet completed their work are considering several other prescription ingredients for recommendation for switchover to OTC use.

It thus appears evident that most OTC medicines are definitely not just "placebos" or products that are pharmacologically inert.

Conclusion

I am convinced that nonprescription (or OTC) medicines should definitely not be considered "just placebos" or "just inert" substances.

The appropriateness of measuring drug effects in well controlled, clinical settings such as the hospital, outpatient clinic, or doctor's office should be reassessed with respect to the evaluation of OTC medicines. Alternative methods of measuring symptomatic relief in the major target population for OTCs—i.e., the average healthy person—under common conditions of use should be sought.

Finally, important differences between prescription and nonprescription medicines and the regulatory constraints placed on both have been discussed in order to highlight the fact that they are different classes of drugs, as per Congressional mandate, and thus they call for different evaluative standards. Last summer, when the FDA Commissioner asked for comments from interested parties on the May 1977 Final Report of the DHEW Review Panel on New Drug Regulation a letter was sent by the trade association representing most large volume, nonprescription medicine manufacturers that also discussed these matters (Cope, 1977). Similar efforts were made at an FDA hearing (November 1977) on a preliminary draft of a proposed Administration Bill to amend the current FDC Act that was referred to earlier in this paper in relation to the FDA Commissioner's recent communication to physicians in response to criticism about a "drug lag" in the U.S. The Commissioner's communication stated, in part, that the bill contemplated ". . . greater flexibility in the clinical testing and marketing of new drug products where they represent significant or urgently sought therapeutic breakthroughs and where efficacy tests are difficult to do. . . ."

While the appeal and importance of "significant or urgently sought therapeutic breakthroughs" for serious disease states are supported by most everyone, the importance of nurturing appropriate self-medication should not be overlooked, particularly in the current era of rising health care costs. If people assume more responsibility for their own good health via constructive preventive medicine measures and habits regarding immunization, diet, and exercise, and they supplement this with responsible self-medication as needed, the burdens on the overall health care system should be lightened through a decreased incidence of chronic and serious disease and the freeing of health professionals to care for such conditions when they do arise.

References

Beecher, H.K.: The powerful placebo. JAMA 159:1602–1606, 1955.

Cleghorn, R.A., et al.: In Proceedings of the First Clinical ACTH Conference. New York, Blakiston (McGraw Hill) 561–65, 1950.

Cooper, J., ed.: The efficacy of self-medication. The Interdisciplinary Communication Associates Inc. of The Smithsonian Institution, Vol. 4, 121–137, 1974.

Cope, J.D.: Letter to FDA Commissioner Kennedy, August 2, 1977.

Drug Efficacy Study Final Report: National Academy of Sciences, 8–9, 1969.

Feinstein, A.: The need for humanized science in evaluating medication. Lancet 774:421–423, 1972.

Feinstein, A.: The efficacy of self-medication. The Interdisciplinary Communication Associates Inc. of the Smithsonian Institution, Vol. 4:141–170, 1973.

Gifford, R.W.: "Primum non nocere." JAMA 238:598–90, 1977.

Kennedy, D.: A calm look at 'drug lag'. JAMA 239:423–26, 1978.

Lasagna, L.: Drug discovery and introduction: regulation and over regulation. Clin. Pharmacol. Ther. 20:507–511, 1976.

Pisani, J.: The PA views OTC—what's in store for OTCs in the future. Wisc. Phar. Ext. Bull. 17:2, 1974.

Webster's Third New International Dictionary (unabridged). G. & C. Merriam Co., 1961.

3

Is Drug Toxicity a Problem of Great Magnitude?

What you should put first in all the practice of our art is how to make the patient well; and if he can be made well in many ways, one should choose the least troublesome.

Hippocrates, *On Joints*

Medicine sometimes removes, sometimes bestows safety. . . .

Ovid, *Tristia*

I do not like to cure trouble by trouble; I hate remedies that are more nuisance than the disease.

Montaigne, *Essays*

Introduction

Science reporters tell us that the public is more concerned about the hazards associated with drug use than with other aspects of pharmacotherapeutics. As Karch points out, the media are not a negligible factor in the evolution of public concern. Is the situation as bad as the public thinks?

Cluff argues that drug toxicity is a problem of great magnitude. He acknowledges that serious drug reactions are rare, but he judges the published literature to indicate that drug-related hospital admissions and hospital-associated drug reactions afflict a considerable number of patients. Cluff also argues that discounting the importance of the problem will hinder efforts to understand and to prevent toxicity.

It is undoubtedly true that the chances of a drug reaction of some sort increase as the number of drugs taken concomitantly (or even sequentially) rises. This is due in part to the greater exposure thus achieved and in part to the possibility of drug-drug interactions. It certainly behooves physicians to advise patients to take drugs only when a good reason exists for so doing.

Cluff also makes a useful point by reminding the reader that fears about drug toxicity and its costs are likely to lead to more and more regulations and controls, and to increased litigation by patients against either doctors or pharmaceutical firms. One result of such fears is the increasing tendency to allow new drugs to be marketed only after long periods of pre-marketing study.

Karch, on the other hand, looking at the same data as Cluff, does not find the picture as gloomy. He is properly skeptical about the extrapolation of individual hospital studies to the national scene and of the ability of doctors (and even experts) to conclude correctly that a drug is at fault.

Karch reminds us that the Food and Drug Administration (FDA) never approves a drug unless it appears that its potential benefits exceed its potential risks. Like Cluff, he believes that there has been a tendency to forget that serious drug toxicity is often seen in critically ill patients in whom drugs are employed as a last-ditch effort to save the patient.

It is both interesting and depressing to see how little attempt has been made to identify *preventable* drug toxicity. Our drugs are, and will continue to be, imperfect tools for controlling disease or ameliorating symptoms. Preventable drug toxicity is to be decried; Karch and Cluff agree on this. Drug toxicity that can neither be predicted nor forestalled is quite another matter.

LOUIS LASAGNA, M.D.

Is Drug Toxicity a Problem of Great Magnitude? Yes!

Leighton E. Cluff, M.D.
University of Florida College of Medicine, Gainesville

Those who experience adverse reactions to drugs consider the reactions to be very important, particularly when the result is serious illness, hospitalization, chronic disability, or death. The child who develops aplastic anemia following administration of chloramphenicol, the elderly woman who cannot walk because of vestibular impairment after receiving streptomycin, the man who cannot work because of exfoliative dermatitis attributable to any of a number of drugs—these patients may not influence national health statistics, but they do have problems of considerable magnitude.

National health statistics do not reflect the magnitude of the problem of drug-induced diseases. A death certificate may indicate that a person died of renal failure, but it may not state that the disease was caused by a drug. Hospital admission or discharge diagnoses often do not indicate when a disease was caused by a drug (Cluff, Thornton, and Seidl, 1964). Physicians are currently not required to report observed cases of drug-induced diseases to a centralized registry. Many diseases or manifestations of illness caused by drugs may also have other causes. Proving that a disease is due to a particular drug can be very difficult. National statistics, therefore, do not provide the information needed to assess the importance to public health of drug toxicity or adverse reactions to drugs. Such data might be useful, but no satisfactory method has yet been developed in the United States to assemble meaningful statistics on drug toxicity.

The rate of *serious* adverse reactions to individual drugs that are given or taken in standard dosages and for medically acceptable reasons is usually quite low. Therefore, one physician will observe such reactions infrequently, rarely, or never in the patients he treats. For example, if aplastic anemia occurs only once in 30,000 patients who have been given chloramphenicol, the probability of a physician observing one such occurrence in the patients he treats during his professional career is small. Some types of drug intoxication, such as nonfatal cardiac arrhythmia due to digitalis, are common, but they may be accepted by physicians as unavoidable consequences of effective drug use, even though they may herald serious problems. Nausea, vomiting, and diarrhea, which have no perceived or actual deleterious influence upon a patient's treatment, also may be interpreted by physicians as inconsequential, even though they often are distressing to affected patients. The significance or importance of drug toxicity as perceived by the physician, therefore, is affected by the probability of its occurring in his patients and by his interpretation of its severity or acceptability.

Data obtained from epidemiologic investigations (conducted mostly in University teaching hospitals) concerning adverse reactions to drugs may not accurately assess the national importance of these clinical problems, but they have demonstrated that such reactions, in these settings at least, are common and important (Gardner and Cluff, 1970; Stewart, Cluff, and Philp, 1977).

Data that identify and characterize the occurrence of drug toxicity may appear to have little value when the problem seems to be unpredictable and not easily preventable. Unfortunately, this is true even of drugs used appropriately for prophylactic or therapeutic purposes. Definition, characterization, and investigation of drug-induced diseases, however, are necessary prerequisites to obtaining the knowledge needed for their control. It behooves us to investigate the mechanisms responsible for adverse drug reactions rather than to question the significance of these reactions. Controversy about the degree of importance of drug-induced diseases can discourage or divert attention from those efforts required to understand and to prevent them. The problem of drug-induced diseases is here, it will not go away, and it may get worse. It should not be ignored or underestimated by questioning its importance.

Unquestionably, drugs that have been developed, particularly those of the past 50 years, have added measurably to the prevention, treatment, and control of disease. In many ways, regulations to insure the safety and claims of efficacy of drugs that have been introduced were established in response to evidence of unacceptable drug toxicity.

Prior to 1927, before the FDA became an independent regulatory agency, dangerous drugs were sold legally in the U.S. because testing for safety was not required. Lethal effects of diethylene glycol, used to dissolve sulfanilamide, were observed in the 1930's after the drug was marketed without having been tested for toxicity in animals. This led Congress to enact a law requiring demonstration of proof of drug safety before marketing. During the subsequent 25 years, 14,000 new drug applications were received by the FDA for certification as to strength, quality, and purity. More stringent requirements for demonstrating the safety of drugs have been legislated and implemented in recent years. The occurrence of congenital anomalies in offspring of pregnant women who had taken thalidomide, coupled with growing national concern about pharmaceutical manufacturers' profits, the costs of drugs, and "me-too" drug development, led to the drug amendments of 1962. These made it necessary for manufacturers to establish evidence of drug effectiveness as well as drug safety. Approval of marketed drugs could be withheld or withdrawn if their safety or efficacy was questionable. Implementation of these regulations has resulted in controversy, but it has improved the safety of drugs and has controlled fraudulent claims of drug efficacy.

Despite regulations that exist or may be established in the future, adverse reactions to drugs will occur as long as it is not possible to predict or to prevent them. It is necessary, then, to balance the therapeutic, diagnostic, or prophylactic importance of a drug against the drug's toxicity. This requires tradeoffs, but such tradeoffs cannot be made rationally without knowing the probability of harm to weigh against the probability of benefit. These probabilities cannot be determined solely from controlled clinical trials of drugs in selected patients; they must be estimated in practical settings that involve many unselected patients with different types of clinical problems, who are treated with many different drugs and managed by many different physicians. The complexity of the studies necessary to determine probabilities of both beneficial and harmful effects of drugs under these circumstances affects the reliability of the data obtained and their interpretation. This further fuels the controversy as to the importance of drug-induced disease. Data obtained in "purer" settings, however, are also subject to controversy, because they may not be applicable to "real life" situations. Drugs are developed for use in real situations, not only for controlled clinical trials; therefore, it is in this setting that adverse reactions must be studied and controlled.

Considerable epidemiologic data from many different sources on drug-induced diseases have been gathered over the past 15 or more years (Gardner and Cluff, 1970; Stewart, Cluff, and Philp, 1977). These data demonstrate the overall significance of drug toxicity and provide information on the probability of adverse reactions to individual drugs. There is a need to continue monitoring these problems and to investigate the occurrence and probability of adverse reactions to additional drugs as they are introduced and used. The great need today, however, is to use data derived from previous and ongoing epidemiologic studies to unravel the reasons for their occurrence and to institute methods to control them. As unrealistic as it may seem now, the goal should be to eliminate or to reduce as far as possible the incidence of death, disability, and illness attributable to those agents given to improve health.

Epidemiologic Evidence

Drug Utilization

Drug toxicity is related to drug utilization;

drug-induced disease does not occur unless drugs are given and taken. As the number of people receiving a particular drug increases, the number who may be harmed also increases. The larger the number of different drugs taken by an individual, the more likely it is that an adverse reaction to at least one of these drugs will occur. Excessive use and misuse of drugs thus contribute to the incidence of drug toxicity. Proper use of drugs is essential, therefore, to insure that adverse reactions are not attributable to inappropriate drug use.

One study showed that on the average, 9.5 drugs were given to adult medical patients in a teaching hospital; pediatric patients in the same hospital received an average of 4.5 drugs during hospitalization (Stewart, Cluff, and Philp, 1977). In another study (Jick et al., 1970), it was found that an average of 8.4 drugs was administered to patients in six hospitals. These findings may not be applicable to all hospitals in the U.S. and patients in community, non-teaching hospitals might receive fewer drugs, but the evidence indicates that hospitalized patients everywhere do receive many different drugs. In addition, numerous diagnostic and therapeutic agents have not been included in some studies on drug utilization. For example, phenylephrine used as a mydriatic, a local anesthetic used prior to ocular tonometry or biopsy, radiopaque diagnostic agents, preoperative medications, and p.r.n. analgesics or sedatives may not be recorded. Therefore, the average number of drugs administered to hospitalized patients may be larger than that which is reported.

Latiolais and Berry (1969) reported that ambulant patients attending a university hospital clinic were taking an average of 2.3 prescribed medications, and that 55 percent of patients were also taking nonprescription, over-the-counter (OTC) drugs. Bleyer, Au, Lange, and Raisz (1970) reported that women in the third trimester of pregnancy had taken an average of 8.7 drugs during this period. They found that an average of 6.9 drugs was taken without the physician's knowledge, hence only 20 percent of the drugs taken were prescribed by the physician.

Stewart and Cluff (1971) similarly found that patients attending a general medical clinic at a university hospital had used an average of 3.2 prescription and 2.9 nonprescription preparations, or an average of 9.5 different medicinal chemicals in the 30 days prior to their visit. Almost half the patients were using drugs prescribed by more than one physician, and these patients were taking drugs that could interact much more frequently than were patients receiving prescriptions from only one physician.

Several investigations have shown a direct relationship between the number of drugs taken by patients and the rate of adverse drug reactions. In one study (Smith, Seidl, and Cluff, 1966), it was found that less than 5 percent of patients receiving fewer than 6 drugs during hospitalization developed an adverse reaction. If the number of different drugs administered exceeded 16, the probability of a reaction occurring increased to over 40 percent. Patients receiving many different drugs are sicker than those receiving fewer drugs, as measured by mortality, duration of hospitalization, and renal failure rates. The combination of multiple drug treatment and renal, cardiovascular, or hepatic failure compounds the problem of detection but increases the frequency of adverse drug reactions (Cluff, Thornton, and Seidl, 1964; Smith, Seidl, and Cluff, 1966).

Many times, physicians are unaware of the medications taken by their patients, except for the ones they have prescribed personally. Patients often do not know the name or the purpose of drugs prescribed for them by their physicians, and they also may have prescriptions filled by different pharmacies. It is no wonder, therefore, that patients often do not take their medications as recommended and take drugs that may interact adversely. Inability or failure of patients to take medications correctly and as prescribed by their physicians may not always result in drug-induced disease, but can result in ineffective control of the illness for which drugs are given. This too might be interpreted as an example of an untoward drug effect.

Retrospective assessment of whether physicians have prescribed drugs to patients appropriately and with supportable reasons may be unfair. Nevertheless, such studies have concluded that drugs are frequently used inappropriately. Antibiotics are administered to approximately 30 percent of hospitalized patients (Caldwell and Cluff, 1974; Stewart, Cluff, and Philp, 1977); analysis has suggested that between 30 and 60 percent of these patients have no clear evidence of infection (Simmons and Stolley, 1974; Stewart, Cluff, and Philp, 1977). Furthermore, many other drugs are unquestionably given unnecessarily.

Because an excessive amount of drugs is consumed, the prevalence of drug toxicity is increased. The magnitude of the problem of drug toxicity, therefore, can in part be related to the unwise, indiscriminate, and unnecessary use of drugs. The syndrome of drug-induced disease is controllable by more discriminating and rational drug use. New information about the problem of drug toxicity is not needed to target efforts at this method of prevention.

Methods have been developed for drug monitoring, and their implementation could contribute to improving drug utilization. Drug monitoring has become a requirement for responsible drug use (Stewart, Cluff, and Philp, 1977). The concept of Drug Utilization Review (DUR) was introduced in the final report of the Secretary of the Health, Education and Welfare's (HEW) Task Force on Prescription Drugs in 1968. It was directed towards review, analysis, and interpretation of drug usage in a health delivery system, whether this be a hospital, group practice, clinic, community, or regional set-up. It included peer review, identification of cases of inappropriate drug utilization, feedback of information, and institution of corrective measures. Some states (e.g., New Jersey) have required pharmacists to maintain drug profiles on patients to whom they dispense drugs. Such information can assist physicians, pharmacists, and patients to prevent adverse drug interactions, and it can provide a foundation for more rational drug use.

Adverse Drug Reactions

Application of the principles of epidemiology to the study of drug toxicity has only begun recently, although adverse reactions to drugs have been noted for as long as drugs have been used. The etiologic relationship of many drugs to particular diseases or clinical problems has often been accepted without calculation of probability or rate of occurrence. Yet, only with such information can the risk of drug toxicity be reasonably estimated in planning patient management. Adverse reactions that are uncommon or not dramatic have been difficult to relate to specific drugs, and relating the numerator data to a meaningful denominator has been necessary to identify probable relationships that may then be quantified and documented. Such studies during the past 15 years have disclosed a very high rate of morbidity due to drug-induced disease and have pointed the way for specific investigation of those factors responsible for their occurrence.

It was reported that 2 to 5 percent of patients admitted to the adult and pediatric medical services of those hospitals studied (Caranasos, Stewart and Cluff, 1974; McKenzie, Marshall, and Netzloff, 1976) are hospitalized with drug-induced diseases; 5 to 30 percent of patients experience untoward reactions to drugs during hospitalization (Gardner and Cluff, 1970). An undetermined number of patients visit physicians' offices because of drug-induced illnesses.

These data may not be used reliably to estimate the prevalence of adverse drug reactions in this country, but it must be concluded that drug-induced illnesses are common. Whether or not less than 1 percent or more than 5 percent of the population is affected, it represents a large number of individuals.

Clinical manifestations of drug toxicity are protean and often are not easily distinguishable from the manifestations of diseases not caused by drugs. Adverse reactions to drugs may be serious and cause death, they may be moderately severe and result in transient or permanent dysfunction, or they may be mild and cause no significant illness (Cluff, Caranasos, and Stewart, 1975). Whether 10, 25, or 30 percent of reactions are serious or moderately severe, the number of patients affected is large.

Most drug-induced diseases are attributable to pharmacologic rather than immunologic mechanisms. When their pharmacologic effects are known (e.g., hypoglycemia following administration of insulin), adverse reactions are usually readily identified and related to the drug. Reactions not recognized or known to be caused by a drug's pharmacologic action, or those not attributable to allergies or other mechanisms, often are not as easily related to a specific drug.

Adverse reactions to drugs may be of little consequence, or they may require extensive medical care. Nausea, vomiting, diarrhea, and dizziness are common manifestations of drug toxicity, but associating them with a specific drug is difficult because they are common symptoms of many illnesses that are not drug related. Seemingly insignificant adverse drug reactions, however, may be premonitory signs of more serious disease and should not be overlooked. For example, the occurrence of pruritus may seem unimportant, but it can precede the development of exfoliative dermatitis. Nausea and vomiting can indicate drug-induced gastritis preceding gastric hemorrhage.

Drug-induced disease may be acute or chronic, may occur during brief or prolonged use of a drug, and also may be recognized only after discontinuance of a drug. Increasingly, it has also been recognized that interaction of two or more drugs is responsible for untoward effects that neither drug alone will produce (Cluff and Petrie, 1974). Unquestionably, predisposition of some people to adverse reactions is attributable to genetic factors, existence of other diseases, organ dysfunction, food intake, age, and many other factors that must be identified. Familiarity with the drugs, circumstances, and predispositions associated with the occurrence of drug-induced diseases is necessary if these problems are to be recognized, prevented, and controlled.

Very few methods are available that confirm or prove the causal relationship between a drug and a disease. Circumstantial evidence of a temporal relationship between administration or discontinuance of a drug and the onset or cessation of illness in an individual may be the only clue to a possible causal relationship. Epidemiologic evidence under these circumstances provides the only reliable means to identify and to quantify this relationship. One may be critical of the variability of such evidence, but in epidemiologic studies the number of illnesses that may be inaccurately attributed to drugs is probably offset by the number of drug-induced illnesses that are unidentified. The statistical magnitude of such evidence, therefore, is probably close to actuality. Undoubtedly, improvements in epidemiologic methods are needed to refine the data so as to define the problem of drug toxicity more clearly, but it seems unlikely that the problem will be made any less important by such refinements, although they may provide better evidence.

Contrasted with the relatively small number of individuals who must be treated to assess drug efficacy, large numbers of individuals receiving a drug must be studied before statistically valid conclusions can be made about adverse reactions. This also indicates why controlled clinical trials may be used to study drug efficacy, but they are of less value in studying drug toxicity. Comparative but noncontrolled studies are the best that can be used for investigation of drug-induced disease in large populations receiving regular medical care.

Much has been made of the frequency of death attributable to drug-induced illnesses. Recent studies (Caranasos, May, Stewart, and Cluff, 1976) have shown, however, that most of these deaths involve patients with ordinarily fatal diseases such as leukemia or other neoplasias who are given drugs to delay the terminal event. Although a crude analysis of drug-induced deaths may suggest that they are unacceptably common, a refined analysis does not support such an interpretation. This does not mean that death caused by drugs is acceptable, but it does place this problem in proper perspective: if death is caused by a drug given unnecessarily to a person whose life is not threatened by an illness for which the drug was given, this is a catastrophe to be avoided. If death is caused by a drug that is given in an attempt to arrest or to delay progression of a fatal disease, however, this should not necessarily be interpreted as an avoidable catastrophe.

Implications

Drug regulation and legislation, medical care costs, litigation, quality of medical care, drug development, drug research, and professional and public attitudes are influenced by the magnitude of the problem of drug toxicity. The implications of drug-induced disease, therefore, extend beyond the individuals who are affected and beyond the drug that is responsible in a particular instance.

A demonstration in 1877 by the British Medical Association that proved that chloroform sensitized the myocardium and predisposed patients to potentially fatal cardiac arrhythmia played a major role in leading to regulation and curtailment of the use of this drug as an anesthetic. Proof that the jaundice occurring in patients given neoarsphenamine was not attributable to drug toxicity but to infectious hepatitis served to protect this important antisyphilitic drug from market restraint after World War I. Forty-five years following the introduction of aminopyrine, the drug was recognized as being responsible for agranulocytosis, and it was eliminated from OTC use. In the past several years, it has been necessary to impose controls on or to eliminate a significant number of drugs because of unacceptable toxicity.

As drugs became increasingly important and effective in control of disease, with the introduction of insulin, sulfonamides, and antibiotics, their beneficial effects markedly outweighed their untoward effects. Furthermore, penicillin has such little toxicity and is so extraordinarily effective that its safety and usefulness have influenced attitudes towards other drugs as well. The occurrence of phocomelia in the offspring of mothers who had taken thalidomide, however, reawakened concern about drug toxicity, and new legislation was introduced that has increasingly regulated the safety and claims of efficacy of drugs.

New problems with drug toxicity continue to appear, attributable both to old and new drugs. Certainly, these problems will perpetuate ongoing debate and may precipitate new concerns about safety that will lead to modification of present legislation or to new legislation and regulation of drugs.

Proportionately, drugs account for only about 10 percent of health care costs, but this exceeds $10 billion each year. With increasing public concern about the cost of health care, drugs have become a focus of attention and evidence of drug toxicity compounds concern. When many patients are hospitalized because of drug-induced disease, and when many patients seem to require prolonged hospitalization becasue of illnesses induced by drugs, the impact of drug toxicity upon health care costs cannot be hidden.

In our present litigious society, it is not surprising that drug toxicity has resulted in an increasing number of claims of malpractice against physicans and that pharmaceutical manufacturers have correspondingly experienced increasing litigation because of drug-induced illnesses. As long as society expects full protection against injury, it can be anticipated that litigation over liability for drug toxicity will increase.

There are no drugs that cannot and will not in some instances cause harm. Personal and public familiarity with this fact, disclosure of such information to individual patients, active rather than passive participation of patients in medical decisions, and recognition that varying degrees of risk are a *sine qua non* of medical care are necessary if litigation over drug toxicity is to diminish. Such litigation will not cease merely by stipulating that drug toxicity is of no great importance.

The availability of an increasing array of drugs capable of alleviating much discomfort and misery, as well as the availability of drugs that for the most part are safe and effective, have made drugs an indispensable component of medical care. A sense that drugs must be available to relieve every physical and emotional problem has developed. This has not been accompanied by the healthy fear of drugs that is necessary if they are to be used with discrimination and care.

Extensive regulations, arising in large part because of concern about drug toxicity and which must be met today before new drugs can be developed and marketed, have had important implications in terms of the cost and feasibility of drug research. In the long run this could profoundly affect the availability of important new drugs in the future, further illustrating that drug toxicity indirectly has been and still is a problem of considerable magnitude.

Conclusion

Unquestionably, drug-induced disease or drug toxicity is of great concern to affected patients. But there are more far-reaching implications that have made this an important problem that must be accepted and recognized. A concentrated effort must be undertaken to improve drug utilization as a means of reducing the problem. This will include more effective provision of needed information to prescribers, dispensers, and consumers of drugs. Investigation of the causes and mechanisms of drug-induced diseases must be encouraged. Monitoring of drug utilization and adverse drug reactions must be encouraged. Short of this, continued controversy will prevail, regulations will increase, and litigation will become more common. Physicians, hospital staff, nurses, pharmacists, pharmaceutical companies, governmental agencies, academicians, scientists, and the public have responsibilities to examine and to contribute to the control of drug-induced disease. For drugs to be used to their best advantage, concerted attention must be given to reducing or eliminating their potentially harmful effects so as to avoid compromising their usefulness.

References

Bleyer, W.A., Au, W., Lange, W.A., and Raisz, L.G.: Studies on the detection of adverse drug reactions in the newborn. I, Fetal exposure to maternal medication. JAMA 213:2046, 1970.

Caldwell, J.R., and Cluff, L.E.: Adverse reactions to antimicrobial agents. JAMA 230:77, 1974.

Caranasos, G.J., May, F.E., Stewart, R.B., and Cluff, L.E.: Drug associated deaths in medical inpatients. Arch. Int. Med. 136:872, 1976.

Caranasos, G.J., Stewart, R.B., and Cluff, L.E.: Drug induced illnesses leading to hospitalization. JAMA 228:713, 1974.

Cluff, L.E., Caranasos, G.J., and Stewart, R.B.: *Clinical Problems with Drugs*. Philadelphia, W.B. Saunders Co., 1975.

Cluff, L.E., and Petrie, J.C.: *Clinical Effects of Interaction between Drugs*. New York, American Elsevier Pub. Co. (Excerpta Medica), 1974.

Cluff, L.E., Thornton, G.F., and Seidl, L.G.: Studies on the epidemiology of adverse drug reactions. I, Methods of JAMA: 976, 1964.

Gardner, P., and Cluff, L.E.: The epidemiology of adverse drug reactions. Johns Hopkins Med. J. 126:77, 1970.

Jick, H., Miettiner, O.S., Shapiro, S., Lewis, G.P., Siskins, V., and Sloane, D.: Comprehensive drug surveillance. JAMA 213:1455, 1970.

Latiolais, C.H., and Berry, L.C.: Misuse of prescription medications by outpatients. Drug Intell. Clin. Pharm. 3:270, 1969.

McKenzie, M.W., Marshall, G.L., and Netzloff, M.L.: Adverse reactions leading to hospitalization in pediatric medicine patients. J. Pediatr. 89:487, 1976.

Simmons, H.E., and Stolley, P.D.: Trends and consequences of antibiotic use in the United States. JAMA 227:1023, 1974.

Smith, J.W., Seidl, L.G., and Cluff, L.E.: Studies on the epidemiology of adverse drug reactions. V, Clinical factors influencing susceptibility. Ann. Int. Med. 65:629, 1966.

Stewart, R.B., and Cluff, L.E.: Studies on the epidemiology of adverse drug reactions. VI, Utilization and interactions of prescription and non-prescription drugs in out-patients. Johns Hopkins Med. J. 129:319, 1971.

Stewart, R.B., Cluff, L.E., and Philp, J.R.: Drug monitoring: a requirement for responsible drug use. Baltimore, Williams and Wilkins Co., 1977.

Is Drug Toxicity a Problem of Great Magnitude? Probably Not.

Fred E. Karch, M.D.
University of Rochester, Rochester, New York

Trying to answer this question is to play what Dr. John Ballin, Director of the AMA Department of Drugs, has called "the ADR numbers game" (Ballin, 1974, 1975). The players, a mixture of legislators, consumer advocates, academic physicians, and pharmaceutical industry representatives, have played the game at congressional hearings, in medical literature, and most noticeably in the press, where headlines have proclaimed "Prescriptions Killing Thousands" (Rensberger, 1976) and "Pharmaceuticals Said to Kill 100 Daily" (New York Times, 1973). Despite this notoriety, the game's final score has been widely disputed. Why?

One explanation for the controversy surrounding the magnitude of the drug toxicity problem is that, as in any game, you have to play by the rules. Yet in the "ADR numbers game," nobody agrees on the rules! Each player seems to have his own, and the final score depends on what rules were used. The issue is even more confusing when you realize that occasionally, the players don't make known what rules they are using.

The first step, then, is to try to establish some "rules," that is, to define the question in clear terms so that we can use appropriate methods to arrive at a conclusion.

When is Drug Toxicity a Problem?

To assess the magnitude of the drug toxicity problem, we must first decide when toxicity should be considered a problem. The simplest approach would be to consider all drug toxicity, including the most trivial and seemingly innocuous reactions, to be a problem, especially for the patient experiencing the drug's ill effects. If we accept this argument, the controversy is easily resolved. Since every available drug is capable of producing toxicity, and since drug use is enormous, the drug toxicity problem must be great. But this approach takes the issue out of context.

In this simplistic and idealistic approach, the only ways to decrease the magnitude of the drug toxicity problem are to develop drugs that have no toxicity or to diminish drug use. Unfortunately, identification of effective drugs that have no toxicity has eluded medical science for centuries. To diminish drug use significantly would be to deny the substantial therapeutic benefits of drugs (Figure 3–1). Thus, this approach does not deal adequately with the real problem.

If we agree that we want to make drugs available and we accept that in the real world, all useful drugs also do harm, the question becomes: when is this harm a problem? For example, is transient asymptomatic hepatitis during isoniazid therapy a problem? Since the long-term consequences of this are unknown, the fact that the patient is asymptomatic is no assurance that the toxicity is not a problem. On the other hand, if it is a problem, at what point does it become so? Is it a problem if the patient's SGOT rises one unit above the upper limit of "normal," or if the SGOT rises but stays within the "normal range"? In what circumstances should the inherent toxicity of a drug be deemed a problem?

Usually this question has been approached by examining the relationship between a drug's toxicity and its therapeutic benefit. This logic

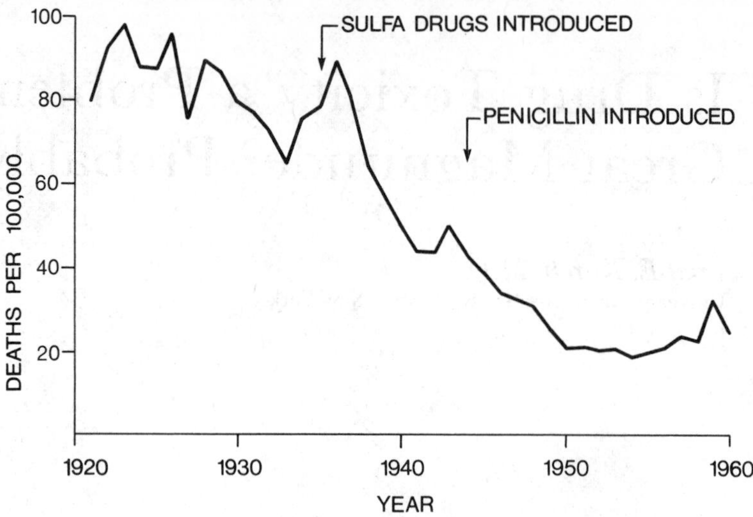

Figure 3-1. Annual death rate from bronchopneumonia and lobar pneumonia in the United States from 1920 to 1960. (Source: Grove, R.D. and Hetzel, A.M.: *Vital Statistics Rates in the United States, 1940-1960.* Washington, D.C.: National Center for health Statistics, 1968.)

weighs potential benefit and toxicity in the overall context of the illness being treated and the availability of other therapy. Serious toxicity during treatment of a mild, self-limiting illness would be a problem, whereas trivial toxicity during the treatment of a life-threatening illness would not be a problem. Thus, drug toxicity is a problem when the severity or frequency of the possible toxicity exceeds the potential therapeutic benefit.

Although this approach seems straightforward, it is not. The difficulty arises in deciding when potential risk exceeds potential benefit. In extreme cases, the decision is easy. However, it becomes much more difficult with most other cases. Risk and benefit cannot be weighed on an objective scale; the balance is a subjective, judgmental determination, and each person has his or her own criteria for acceptable risk (Table 3-1). Although some people have argued that

Table 3-1. *Distribution of Respondents as to Probability of Success Required to Accept an Operation with Outcomes of Either Death or Full Relief of Permanent Bed Confinement* (*N*=279)

Probability of Success	Number	Percent
0.00–0.09	54	19.3
0.10–0.19	46	16.4
0.20–0.29	43	15.4
0.30–0.39	13	4.6
0.40–0.49	12	4.3
0.50–0.59	57	20.4
0.60–0.69	12	4.3
0.70–0.79	16	5.7
0.80–0.89	14	5.1
0.90–0.99	11	3.9
1.00	1	0.2
<0.50	168	60.0
>0.50	111	40.0

Reprinted with permission from *Health Status Indexes*, edited by Robert L. Berg. Copyright 1973 by the Hospital Research and Educational Trust, 840 North Lake Shore Drive, Chicago, Illinois 60611.

the decision on acceptable risk should be made by the individual patient (e.g., in the recent legal battle over the availability of Laetrile—see Chapter 24), the decision on the acceptability of a drug is usually made by a governmental agency, such as the United States Food and Drug Administration (FDA). In the United States no drug is approved for marketing unless the balance between potential toxicity and potential therapeutic benefit is acceptable within the total context of the illness being treated. Thus, FDA approval is presumably evidence that the drug's overall potential benefit exceeds its overall potential toxicity.

Applying the toxicity versus benefit criteria to drugs marketed in the U.S., therefore, means that the toxicity resulting from these drugs should not be considered a problem, but rather the acceptable price of therapeutic advances. However, there are several circumstances in which this reasoning fails. The nature of premarketing studies of drugs limits the amount of information available on drug toxicity. The full spectrum of drug toxicity and the severity of the reactions may not be known until the drug has been in general use for several years. Thus, the initial decision of the FDA may have been wrong, and toxicity might actually be a problem of some magnitude.

Even if the FDA evaluation is correct, their analysis of a drug is usually based on only a few therapeutic indications when the drug has been used according to specific criteria within a limited dose range. But after the drug is marketed, physicians may prescribe the drug to treat illnesses for which the toxicity versus benefit relationship may not have been established (experimental use), or even for cases in which the relationship was deemed unacceptable. They may prescribe the drug in circumstances for which its use is contraindicated, or they may prescribe it in excessive or inadequate dosages. Further, patients may inadvertently misuse the drug, upsetting the balance between toxicity and benefit so that toxicity does become a problem. Thus, although FDA approval of a drug for general marketing usually indicates an acceptable risk versus benefit relationship, several factors may distort this relationship in clinical practice.

Toxicity from experimental drug use is difficult to classify because the toxicity versus benefit criteria cannot be evaluated. One reason why these drugs and their usages are experimental is precisely that their benefits and toxicities have not been fully established and hence, their potential cannot be accurately weighed. Toxicity from experimental drugs should therefore be considered a problem, but it should not be lumped together with problems arising from the routine therapeutic use of drugs. Doing so would confuse the interpretation of the data and detract from our understanding of drug toxicity in general clinical practice.

Another often ignored circumstance in which drug toxicity is a problem is when the fear of toxicity prevents adequate treatment. If the therapeutic benefit of a drug is inappropriately denied through a misperception of potential toxicity, toxicity should also be considered a problem.

These, then, are the "rules" I will use. Drug toxicity will be evaluated on the basis of the potential toxicity versus the potential benefit relationship. Since this evaluation is difficult and highly individual, I will rely on FDA approval of a drug as evidence of an acceptable risk-benefit balance, except when (1) the FDA evaluation is incorrect—as evidenced by subsequent withdrawal of FDA approval, (2) the drug is used experimentally, (3) the drug is prescribed for an inappropriate indication, (4) the drug is prescribed in an excessive or inadequate dosage, or (5) the patient inadvertently misuses the drug. Drug toxicity will also be considered a problem when there is evidence that effective treatment is inappropriately withheld due to the fear of drug toxicity.

Because the focus of this discussion is on toxicity during the general therapeutic use of drugs, data on intentional poisonings, experimental drug use, and toxicity from "recreational" drug use will be excluded.

Examining the Data

Pitfalls in the Use of Available Data

Populations studied. In order to determine the magnitude of the drug toxicity problem, quantitative data must be collected on the general population. Unfortunately, reliable data are not available, and we must depend on that obtained from relatively small samples of the population. If these samples are representative, the data can be easily extrapolated to the general population. If, however, the sample groups are not representative, bias is introduced into the data and the results cannot be fairly applied to the general population.

Most of the quantitative data on drug toxicity have been gathered from studies of hospitalized patients on acute-care internal medicine wards, most often at university hospitals. Are these patients a representative sample of the general population? Clearly, they are not – acute-care internal medicine wards are not comparable to other hospital wards. Drugs used, illnesses being treated, patients' ages, and ways that drugs are used there are different. An internal medicine ward is not the same as an obstetric ward. Further, a university hospital is not comparable to a community general hospital. University hospitals are usually referral centers for patients with complicated medical problems or for patients who require the specialized facilities available at an academic facility (e.g., neonatal intensive care unit). Experimental drugs are often studied at university hospitals, and marketed drugs are occasionally used in experimental ways. Moreover, no hospital-based sample should be considered representative of the general population. The fact that these patients are ill enough to require hospitalization means that they are a biased sample of the general population, and extrapolation from hospitalized patients to the general population will reflect this bias.

Data gathering. Study techniques based on spontaneous reporting of drug toxicity by physicians may serve an important role in the qualitative assessment of drug toxicity, but they are inadequate for quantitative studies. Many factors influence spontaneous reporting schemes (Koch-Weser et al., 1969) and the data are not reliable for quantitative analysis (Karch and Lasagna, 1975; Bennett and Lipman, 1977).

Identifying drug toxicity. Meaningful use of drug toxicity data depends on the accurate identification of clinical drug toxicity, and this is the most troublesome aspect of drug toxicity reports. Evaluation of each specific clinical case "depends on the vagaries of clinical judgment of an array of unstandardized physicians" (Feinstein, 1974). How dependable are those judgments?

The record shows that these judgments are not very reliable. Physicians have reported drug toxicity in patients who had *never* taken the suspect drug or took it only *after* the onset of the alleged toxic reaction (Irey, 1976; Burley and Binns, 1976). Tacit acceptance of physicians' unevaluated judgments may lead to erroneous conclusions.

Expert evaluation of the clinical data, however, may not be completely reliable either. The problem is that each case must be evaluated with limited clinical information. Cases are frequently complicated by underlying illnesses and the concomitant use of several drugs. Further, patients frequently develop symptoms commonly attributed to drugs even when no drugs have been taken (Green, 1964; Reidenberg and Lowenthal, 1968; Kupfer and Detre, 1971; Ciccolunghi and Chaudri, 1975; Joubert et al., 1977). It is usually difficult and occasionally impossible to distinguish these spontaneous events from actual drug toxicity. The impact of these factors makes the clinical evaluation of drug toxicity difficult, and even clinical pharmacologists often have difficulty identifying drug toxicity reliably (Karch et. al., 1976; Koch-Weser et al., 1977).

Inconsistent results. One of the remarkable features of the available data on drug toxicity is the variability of the results. Deviations might be expected between groups due to differences in population samples, in data-gathering techniques, and in methods of identifying drug toxicity, but the variation noted

Table 3-2. *Variability in the Reported Incidence of Drug-Related Deaths*

	Incidence of Fatal Drug Reactions (%)	Δ* (%)	p*†
Johns Hopkins Hospital			
Seidl et al. (1966)	1.54		
Smith et al. (1966)	0.22	−86	<0.01
Boston Collaborative Group			
Shapiro et al. (1971)	0.44		
Miller (1973)	0.29	−34	<0.05
Porter and Jick (1977a)	0.09	−80	<0.0001

* Comparison with initial report from each group.
† Calculated from the X^2 distribution.

in serial reports from individual monitoring programs is also large. This phenomenon is illustrated by the data on drug-induced mortality (Table 3–2). One group has explained that this variability results from important differences in the patients studied (Porter and Jick, 1977b). Thus, the quantitative results from even these large-scale studies of drug toxicity are significantly influenced by patient selection bias, and data from these studies are inadequate for extrapolation to the general population.

Data Selection

Despite the limitations imposed by the deficiencies in the available quantitative data on drug toxicity, we can at least look at the reports to get some idea of the magnitude of the drug toxicity problem. Because we want quantitative data that reasonably reflect the current situation, the analysis will be limited to large-scale epidemiologic studies published since 1976. To apply the criteria established earlier for identifying drug toxicity problems, the reports have to describe sufficient clinical details of the individual cases. Since large scale epidemiologic studies usually only report the clinical details of fatal drug reaction cases, this analysis will be limited to drug-related mortality.

It must be emphasized that the available studies do not represent the general population, and that the data *cannot* be extrapolated to the general population. The authors of several of these studies have cautioned that "extrapolation from the available data to a national incidence of drug-associated deaths is not possible" (Caranasos et al., 1976).

Drug-Related Deaths

Several studies of drug-related deaths have been reported since 1976 (Caranasos et al., 1976; McKenney and Harrison, 1976; Armstrong et al., 1976; McKenzie et al., 1976; Porter and Jick, 1977a). These have been hospital-based studies, and most of the data is from university teaching hospitals. The combined data from these studies involve a total of 47,938 patients from three wards—internal medicine (71 percent), surgical (21 percent), and pediatric (8 percent). The proportion of patients dying from possible drug-related toxicity was 0.12 percent for the medical patients, 0.11 percent for the pediatric patients, and 0.02 percent for the surgical patients.

Drug withdrawn by FDA. No death reported in these studies was associated with the use of a drug that had been initially approved by the FDA for general marketing but subsequently withdrawn from the market.

Drug prescribed for an inappropriate indication. No case described in these reports seems to have resulted from an inappropriate prescription. In one surgical patient, the condition was incorrectly diagnosed, but based on the clinical information available at the time, the therapy used was appropriate for the presumptive diagnosis.

Drug prescribed in an inappropriate dosage. Data on drug dosage are not presented for most of the cases in these reports, so it is not possible to evaluate this factor adequately. However, the clinical information included in the reports *suggests* inappropriate dosages in several cases. Five patients developed fatal pulmonary edema while receiving intravenous fluids, and one patient developed fatal hyperkalemia while receiving potassium chloride therapy. All these patients were severely ill prior to the onset of the drug toxicity. The problem in evaluating these cases is that we do not know if the dose prescribed was inappropriate or if some event (e.g., acute myocardial infarction leading to acute cardiac failure and pulmonary edema or a malfunctioning intravenous fluid administration set leading to excessive fluid infusion) suddenly made the agent toxic. All the cases of fluid and electrolyte toxicity came from just one of these reports (Porter and Jick, 1977a), and it is not clear why similar events did not occur in the other centers. (Conceivably, other centers might not have considered fluid and electrolyte problems as related to "drug toxicity.")

Five patients treated with digitalis for congestive heart failure developed fatal cardiac arrhythmias that may have been due to inappropriate dosage, but the digitalis dosage was not reported. Certainly, congestive heart failure, the indication for digitalis therapy in all these cases, is also a cause of cardiac arrhythmias, and it is often difficult to determine if the arrhythmia is due to the disease or to the drug. But even if the fatal arrhythmias were drug-related, we still do not know if the prescribed dose of digitalis was therapeutically inappropriate:

> A patient who appears to be dying of advanced congestive heart failure and who is not responding to conventional doses of a digitalis preparation may be given larger doses of this drug in a desperate

attempt that is recognized as heroic. Signs of digitalis intoxication may supervene . . . but the use of additional digitalis in this instance was a well considered and warranted intervention (Ingelfinger, 1976).

Although clinical details of the five cases are not described, the authors commented that these deaths were not preventable. Since deaths due to inappropriately prescribed dosages of digitalis certainly could be prevented, it appears that none of these digitalis-related cases resulted from an inappropriately prescribed dosage of medication.

Although some of the reported cases may have resulted from the prescription of inappropriate dosages, the case reports do not provide sufficient data on this question. The best we can say is that the reports *suggest* that prescribed excessive dosages may have been responsible for up to six of the fatal cases, that is, from 0 to 0.01 percent of the patients reported in these studies. All these cases were associated with the use of either intravenous fluids or potassium chloride, and all were reported by one group.

Misuse of drugs by patients. Here again, the reports do not provide sufficient clinical information to determine if inadvertent misuse of drugs was responsible for the toxicity. Since these were hospital-based studies, patient misuse of medication would have occurred prior to hospitalization; patients rarely administer medications to themselves in a hospital. One of the studies specifically excluded toxicity related to drugs taken prior to hospitalization (Porter and Jick, 1977a), but Caranasos et al. (1976) noted that 62.5 percent of the patients who died of drug-related toxicity had developed the toxicity prior to hospitalization. The role of inadvertent misuse of drugs by patients is not discussed, and the brief case descriptions neither suggest nor rule out this factor.

Effective therapy withheld due to fear of toxicity. Since these studies focused only on drugs as a cause of toxicity, deaths due to withholding treatment were not reported. Few studies have examined this problem (Marks and Sachar, 1973; Symmers, 1973), and more data are needed to assess the impact of this factor on patient care.

Summary

Five large scale reports of drug-associated deaths published since 1976, involving almost 50,000 hospitalized patients on acute-care internal medicine, surgical, and pediatric wards, have been reviewed (Caranasos et al., 1976; McKenney and Harrison, 1976; Armstrong et al., 1976; McKenzie et al., 1976; Porter and Jick, 1977a). Using the potential toxicity versus potential benefit balance to define acceptable risk, drug toxicity was considered to be a problem when the risk was unacceptable. Applying the aforementioned criteria for unacceptable risk, such drug toxicity may have been responsible for up to six fatal cases; that is, from 0 to 0.01 percent of the monitored patients in these studies.

Inadvertent misuse of drugs by patients and the withholding of effective drugs due to fear of toxicity may have contributed to some fatal cases, but data are not available to assess the magnitude of these problems.

Conclusion

On the basis of this analysis of recent, large-scale, quantitative, epidemiologic studies, the magnitude of the drug toxicity problem seems small. The studies involved severely ill hospitalized patients on internal medicine, pediatric, and surgical wards, presumably the group of patients at greatest risk for drug toxicity. The frequency of drug toxicity deaths was less than 1 per 10,000 monitored patients. All these fatal cases involved the use of either intravenous fluids or potassium chloride, and all these patients were severely ill at the time the drug toxicity developed. Thus, the problem of severe drug toxicity seems small in terms of both the number of patients and the number of drugs involved.

These results, however, do not mean that drug toxicity is a trivial problem. Since most of the data were obtained from university hospitals, we cannot know if the data accurately represent the experience of community general hospitals or, more important, of the general population. The limitations in the available data prevent extrapolation of the findings, and we simply do not know whether drug toxicity is a minor or a major problem in the general population. But even if the drug toxicity problem is small, we should still encourage efforts to reduce it further. New drugs with an even better toxicity versus benefit balance should be developed. Although the risk of toxicity from a drug may be acceptable given the available alternatives, serious drug toxicity is never acceptable if it might be prevented. Physicians must exercise utmost care in the use of drugs in order to maximize therapeutic benefits and to minimize the potential toxicity.

References

Armstrong, B., Dinan, B., and Jick, H.: Fatal drug reactions in patients admitted to surgical services. Am. J. Surg. 132:643, 1976.

Ballin, J.C.: The ADR numbers game. JAMA 229:1097, 1974.

Ballin, J.C.: The ADR numbers game revisited. JAMA 234:1257, 1975.

Bennett, B.S., and Lipman, A.G.: Comparative study of prospective surveillance and voluntary reporting in determining the incidence of adverse drug reactions. Am. J. Hosp. Pharm. 34:931, 1977.

Berg, R.L.: Establishing the values of various conditions of life for a health status index. In Berg, R.L.: *Health Status Index.* Chicago, Hospital Research and Educational Trust, 1973.

Burley, D.M., and Binns, T.B.: Erroneous adverse reaction reports. Lancet 1:1193, 1976.

Caranasos, G.J., May, F.E., Stewart, R.B., and Cluff, L.E.: Drug-associated deaths of medical inpatients. Arch. Int. Med. 136:872, 1976.

Ciccolunghi, S.N., and Chaudri, H.A.: A methodological study of some factors influencing the reporting of symptoms. J. Clin. Pharmacol. 15:496, 1975.

Feinstein, A.R.: Clinical biostatistics. XXVIII, The biostatistical problems of pharmaceutical surveillance. Clin. Pharmacol. Ther. 16:110, 1974.

Green, D.M.: Pre-existing conditions, placebo reactions, and "side-effects." Ann. Int. Med. 60:255, 1964.

Grove, R.D., and Hetzel, A.M.: *Vital Statistics Rates in the United States 1940–1960.* Washington, D.C., National Center for Health Statistics, 1968.

Ingelfinger, F.J.: Counting adverse drug reactions that count. N. Engl. J. Med. 294:1003, 1976.

Irey, N. S.: Tissue reactions to drugs. Am. J. Pathol. 82:617, 1976.

Joubert, P.H., Jansen van Rijssen, F.W., and Venter, J.P.: Drug side-effects assessed in a naturalistic setting. S. Afr. Med. J. 52:34, 1977.

Karch, F.E., and Lasagna, L.: Adverse drug reactions—a critical review. JAMA 234:1236, 1975.

Karch, F.E., Smith, C.L., Kerzner, B., Mazzullo, J., Weintraub, M., and Lasagna, L.: Adverse drug reactions—a matter of opinion. Clin. Pharmacol. Ther. 19:489, 1976.

Koch-Weser, J., Sidel, V.W., Sweet, R.H., Kanarek, P., and Eaton, A.E.: Factors determining physician reporting of adverse drug reactions. N. Engl. J. Med. 280:20, 1969.

Koch-Weser, J., Sellers, E.M., and Zacest, R.: The ambiguity of adverse drug reactions. Eur. J. Clin. Pharmacol. 11:75, 1977.

Kupfer, D.J., and Detre, T.P.: Once more—on the extraordinary side effects of drugs. Clin. Pharmacol. Ther. 12:575, 1971.

Marks, R.M., and Sachar, E.J.: Undertreatment of medical inpatients with narcotic analgesics. Ann. Int. Med. 78:173, 1973.

McKenney, J.M., and Harrison, W.L.: Drug-related hospital admissions. Am. J. Hosp. Pharm. 33:792, 1976.

McKenzie, M.W., Marchall, G.L., Netzloff, M.L., and Cluff, L.E.: Adverse drug reactions leading to hospitalization in children. J. Pediatr. 89:487, 1976.

Miller, R.R.: Drug surveillance utilizing epidemiologic methods—a report from the Boston Collaborative Drug Surveillance Program. Am. J. Hosp. Pharm. 30:584, 1973.

New York Times: Pharmaceuticals said to kill 100 daily. December 13, 1973, p. 6.

Porter, J., and Jick, H.: Drug-related deaths among medical inpatients. JAMA 237:879, 1977a.

Porter, J., and Jick, H.: Drug-related deaths. JAMA 237:2470, 1977b.

Reidenberg, M.M., and Lowenthal, D.T.: Adverse nondrug reactions. N. Engl. J. Med. 279:678, 1968.

Rensberger, B.: Bad prescriptions kill thousands a year. New York Times, January 28, 1976, pp. 1, 17.

Seidl, L.G., Thornton, G., Smith, J.W., and Cluff, L.E.: Studies on the epidemiology of adverse drug reactions. III, Reactions in patients on a general medical service. Bull. Johns Hopkins Hosp. 119:299, 1966.

Shapiro, S., Slone, D., Lewis, G.P., and Jick, H.: Fatal drug reactions among medical inpatients. JAMA 216:467, 1971.

Smith, J.W., Seidl, L.G., and Cluff, L.E.: Studies on the epidemiology of adverse drug reactions. V, Clinical factors influencing susceptibility. Ann. Int. Med. 65:629, 1966.

Symmers, W. St.C.: Amphotericin pharmacophobia. Br. Med. J. 4:460, 1973.

4

Is Generic Substitution Desirable?

The problem is to induce people to pay twenty-five cents for the liver-encouraging, silent-perambulating, family pills, which cost three cents.

John Shaw Billings

The old saying . . . that the exception proves the rule, is as destitute of truth as it is of meaning. Such an exception can prove one thing . . . that the rule is not fully understood, or completely ascertained.

Elish Bartlett, *Philosophy of Medical Science*

Seek simplicity and distrust it.

Alfred North Whitehead, *The Concept of Nature*

Introduction

Generic substitution is much in the headlines these days. To some, it is "an idea whose time has come"; to others, it is a philosophy both dangerous and naïve, with the potential for jeopardizing the welfare of the sick in return for putative economic savings that may in fact be illusory.

Horvitz dismisses as inconsequential any concerns over chemical or biologic equivalence. He admits to some past problems, but stresses their rarity and the recent decline in their rate of occurrence. He has faith in the FDA's policing of the marketplace. Furthermore, Horvitz argues that imprecision in dosing isn't so important in many areas of medicine and for many drugs. The prospect of saving as much as the $450 million a year he estimates could be involved is obviously attractive to consumers and third-party payers. Because the pharmacy profession is moving away from percentage markups and toward professional fee pricing, Horvitz sees no reason for druggists not to pass on the savings to the consumer. He foresees a growing trend toward the use of generic drugs, either voluntarily or via state substitution laws.

Chodos is not convinced by either the theory or the facts cited by generic drug enthusiasts. He acknowledges that some generic manufacturers do a commendable job, but points out that some fail miserably, and he questions the ability of the FDA to supervise all drug production. In view of the findings in past surveys of troubles that were not generally appreciated, the obvious question must be raised. Are the problems of which we are aware today really the bulk of the trouble that exists, or are we seeing only the tip of the iceberg? The past helps only in one respect: we can be certain that the extent of bioinequivalency is greater than we know at any given moment. How *much* greater is at best an educated guess.

There are many reasons why badly formulated drugs that perform poorly in patients might not be so identified, and Chodos describes some of them. He also argues that the potential savings to the public from generic substitution will never be great, in view of the relatively small contribution of drug costs to the national health care bill.

Mazzullo seconds Chodos on a number of these points. He describes the dangers of relying on simple (and possibly simple-minded) *in vitro* tests on the one hand, and the problems of doing *in vivo* tests on the other. There is good reason for remembering that the most important determinant of drug prices is neither the doctor nor the pharmaceutical firm, but the pharmacist. Every survey I have ever read that investigated the cost of prescriptions has found that enormous price differences are usually encountered when one takes the same prescription to ten different drugstores in any city. This is true whether one has a brand-name prescription, a generically written prescription, or a "substitution permitted" one. Given the available possibilities, a patient may find that occasionally a brand-name prescription may actually cost less than one written any other way! If the consumer or doctor is confused by all this, it's not surprising.

Mazzullo could also have cited another reason for prescribing drugs by brand name. He once wrote a fascinating article entitled "The Nonpharmacologic Basis of Therapeutics." (A later article touched on the same topic, and called the phenomenon "chromoconfusion." See reference listing.) Mazzullo had seen many patients so confused by the need to take different medicines that all looked alike that they made errors in taking their medication. He suggested an ingeniously simple solution: whenever possible, prescribe medicines that *don't* look alike. Instead of three different white tablets, all about the same size and shape as aspirins, how about prescribing a red one, a blue one, or one with a distinctive shape? To do this, however, requires not only a knowledge of the alternatives, but a willingness to prescribe a given brand, or at least a given manufacturer. At the moment, such prescribing would favor brand versions, although there is nothing to prevent generic manufacturers from being imaginative and devising their own distinctive shapes and sizes. (Now, they often try to make their tablets and capsules so much like the innovator's brand that there have been some suits against them for infringement of trademark.) The snag in this idea is that there would have to be advertising costs to communicate the generic manufacturer's specially colored version to the doctor, so that he would know how to order it. This would inevitably raise the costs of the generic version and negate the principal reason for its existence!

LOUIS LASAGNA, M.D.

Biron, P., and Carignan, R.: Chromoconfusion: a new type of pill-pill interaction in cardiology. Can. Med. Assoc. J. 110:1346, 1974.

Mazzullo, J. M.: The nonpharmacologic basis of therapeutics. Clin. Pharmacol. Ther. 13:157, 1972.

Generic Substitution: A Safe Way to Cut Medical Costs

Richard Horvitz, M.D.
Butterworth Hospital, Grand Rapids, Michigan

To prescribe drugs generically or by brand name—this has been one of the most debated questions of modern therapeutic practice. Is there any truth to the statements of brand-name advocates that prescribing by brand will assure that the patient will receive a quality drug of proven effectiveness, and that any savings possibly offered by generic prescribing are not worth the risk of receiving an inferior product? Probably not. The risk that a generically prescribed drug product will be ineffective is almost nonexistent in nearly all cases, and the cost savings available to the patient, and the potential for savings, are large.

The basic concern over generic prescribing is whether generic drugs are equivalent to the brand-name products. How much of a concern is this? What do we mean, furthermore, by *equivalent*? There are a number of aspects of equivalence, which will be discussed. But let us keep the whole issue of equivalency in perspective by considering two important questions. How much difference is there between different products of the same drug? How much of this difference, if any, is likely to be therapeutically significant?

Equivalency

Let us immediately dismiss one myth about generic prescribing—namely, that generic prescriptions are filled with products of small "generic" firms of questionable reputation. Most generic prescriptions in fact are filled with products of large drug companies, firms that are among the best-known in the industry and major promoters of brand-name drugs. Smith-Kline, Lederle, Parke, Davis & Co., Squibb, and Upjohn are among the major suppliers of the generic market. Even the smaller firms often do not produce their own drugs, but purchase them from the larger manufacturers and distribute them under their own labels. For example, there are more than 60 companies marketing ampicillin products, but only 11 companies are licensed by the Food and Drug Administration (FDA) to manufacture this drug. The difference between generic and brand-name prescribing is not in the quality of the drugs dispensed, but in their marketing structure, as will be discussed in the latter part of this article. Most of the generic drugs on the market are products of major and highly reputable manufacturers, and it is reasonable to assume that they are of high quality.

Chemical equivalence. This is the first aspect of equivalency to be examined. Equivalent generic drug products must contain the same amount of active ingredient in an adequately pure form as their brand-name counterparts. In virtually all cases, one can confidently consider this to be upheld. Standards of purity, potency, and content uniformity have long been established by such pharmaceutical compendia as the *United States Pharmacopoeia* (USP) and the *National Formulary* (NF). All drug manufacturers, brand-name and generic alike, are required to meet these criteria. Standards of good manufacturing practice and quality control are established and enforced by the FDA. For some drugs, such as antibiotics, lot-by-lot testing of potency is required. In the early days of generic drug usage, some products of small firms did not meet these standards and this gave all generic drugs a bad name, but today, the general state of pharmaceutical manufacturing appears high. Chemical equivalence can be virtually eliminated as an area of concern.

Biologic equivalence. The greatest area of controversy about generic drugs has been over the question of biologic equivalence. Equivalent generic drug products must not only contain the same amount of active ingredient as their brand-name counterparts, they must also make it available in such a way that it produces equivalent drug levels in the body and equivalent therapeutic effects.

The events that occur between taking a solid drug in tablet or capsule form and the appearance of the drug in active form in the patient's bloodstream are complex. The tablet or capsule must first disintegrate in the gastrointestinal tract. The active drug is released and must then dissolve in the stomach or intestinal fluid before it can be absorbed. Many factors can alter these events. Variations in tablet composition, particle size, crystal form, and inert ingredients (excipients) used in drug formulations can have marked effects. The study of bioavailability, the rate and extent to which a drug is absorbed into the body, has become an area of great interest over the past decade.

Bioavailability

The basic approach to the study of bioavailability has been to measure drug levels in the blood at various intervals after a standard dose of a drug product is given. If the products are biologically equivalent, they should yield similar patterns of blood levels. Other measurements of drug absorption, such as urinary drug excretion, have been used in some studies. Drug absorption has also been correlated with *in vitro* pharmaceutical tests, such as disintegration time (time required for a tablet or capsule to break apart in a test solution) or dissolution rate (time required for the active drug to go into solution). Hundreds of studies, involving dozens of different drugs, have been performed in recent years, and a number of excellent reviews on this subject have been published (Koch-Weser, 1974; Skelly, 1976).

Variations in bioavailability among different products of many drugs have been reported. There have been a few cases where bioavailability problems have been severe enough that clinically ineffective therapy might have been given. Serious deficiencies in bioavailability of several oxytetracycline products were reported a number of years ago. More recently, large differences in bioavailability among various digoxin products have become an issue of concern. But when there have been serious bioavailability problems, corrective action has been undertaken rapidly. The unsatisfactory oxytetracycline products were recalled, and a follow-up report noted that all products remaining on the market produced adequate blood levels (Ballin, 1971). Further studies on the digoxin problem led to the establishment of a correlation between bioavailability and dissolution rate (Lindenbaum et al., 1973), and the FDA took action to require that all digoxin products meet a dissolution standard. With all the awareness and publicity over the issue of bioavailability, one would surely expect that if there were other serious problems, they would be as widely reported in the medical literature as the oxytetracycline and digoxin problems were. In the last five years, no new problems of this magnitude have been reported. This fact alone would suggest that such serious problems are no longer present.

Present status of bioavailability data. Variable differences have been reported for a number of commonly prescribed drugs, but studies of other drugs have shown all products tested to have similar availability. Over the past three years, the American Pharmaceutical Association has published a series of monographs (at least 20 so far) that review published studies and bioavailability data supplied by manufacturers of individual drugs (American Pharmaceutical Association, 1975–1977). The vast majority of the data presented suggests that equivalence is more often the rule than is inequivalence. For several major drugs, including ampicillin, tetracycline, sulfisoxazole, penicillin V, prednisone, hydrochlorothiazide, quinidine, and warfarin, the data supporting equivalence appear overwhelming. For most other drugs, the differences seem relatively minor. In my earlier extensive reviews on this subject (Horvitz, 1973; Horvitz, 1975b), I reached largely the same conclusion. Most of the reported differences add up to less than the therapeutic variability that can be expected from other causes.

This is not to imply that bioavailability can be dismissed as a concern in the choice of drug products. It is only to say that the problem is less severe than many of the advocates of brand-name prescribing make it out to be. I will have more to say about putting the problem in perspective later. Meanwhile, two important trends strongly support the conclusion that whatever problem bioavailability presents now, it will become less and less troublesome in the future.

Trends towards equivalence. The first of these trends is that of drug manufacturers, pharmacists, and regulatory authorities becoming more and more aware of the problem of bioavailability. With this increased awareness, it can be expected that products will be improved and bioavailability problems will decrease. It is in everybody's best interest for all drug products to be optimally bioavailable. Drug companies realize this, and they are making the effort to insure that their products will be effectively absorbed. They are also providing data supporting this fact to pharmacists and others involved in the selection of drug products.

Pharmacists are also very much aware of the issue of bioavailability. Pharmacists are professionals with years of training in drugs and their characteristics, and they are well trained for the selection of effective drug products. Most of the studies on bioavailability have appeared in the pharmacy literature, even before articles on this subject began appearing in the medical literature.

Compendial and regulatory agencies have taken an active role in the problem of bioavailability. Standards of dissolution or other characteristics related to bioavailability have been established for several drugs. Lot-by-lot testing is now required for certain critical drugs. Since 1975, the FDA has required manufacturers introducing new products of a previously marketed drug to document that these are biologically equivalent to the original product. It is to the advantage of manufacturers to do so. Pharmacists are looking for products with documented bioavailability, and products without such support are less competitive on the market. With awareness of the bioavailability problem on all levels, the chance of an ineffective product reaching the patient seems more and more remote.

The second factor involves the enormous methodologic advances in the analysis of drug levels in blood and other biologic samples. A decade ago, when problems of bioavailability were first noticed, analytic methods for most drugs were crude. Antibiotics could be tested by microbiologic assays, but these required long periods for bacterial growth and were only approximately accurate at best. The few analytic methods available for other drugs were mostly colorimetric or spectrophotometric chemical methods that were laborious, relatively imprecise and non-specific, and marginally sensitive for the assay of blood levels. Today much of this has changed. New techniques—gas chromatography, high-performance liquid chromatography, mass fragmentography, radioimmunoassay, and others—have been applied to the assay of drugs in biologic samples. These techniques have been extensively developed during the 1970's and applied to a wide variety of drugs. Sensitivity and specificity have been vastly improved, and assays that used to take hours to complete can now be performed in minutes. Drugs that were previously difficult or impossible to analyze can now be assayed routinely. It was the development of highly sensitive radioimmunoassay methods that made the analysis of serum digoxin levels and the discovery of the bioavailability problems with this drug possible. Many other drugs have been studied with these new methods, and experience with bioavailability studies has become widespread. The necessary equipment and technical expertise are widely available in drug company and other laboratories. Criteria for study design and methodology in the area of bioavailability are now well established. The science of pharmaceutical formulation and the development of effectively absorbed drug products have advanced rapidly in recent years. Many of the problems of bioavailability have already been solved, and the technology to solve those remaining exists today.

Even if differences in bioavailability are still present, the question of their clinical significance still remains. The pattern of clinical use, and the degree to which therapeutic levels are critical, are different for different drugs. (Horvitz, 1973). For an important drug with a narrow range between therapeutic and toxic levels, bioavailability is a justifiable concern. But for drugs with wide ranges of effective levels, or for situations in which indications are less critical and therapy largely empirical, moderate differences in availability are probably of little therapeutic concern. It is well known that blood levels and therapeutic effect produced by a given dose of a drug vary among individuals. These variations are far greater than most of the reported differences in bioavailability.

Table 4-1. *The Top 50 Prescription Drugs*

1. Valium	26. Phenobarbital°
2. Ampicillin°	27. Erythromycin°
3. Lasix	28. Benadryl
4. Tetracycline°	29. Fiorinal
5. Aldomet	30. Aldoril
6. HydroDiuril	31. Lomotil
7. Premarin	32. Ilosone
8. Librium	33. Dilantin
9. Dimetapp	34. Diuril
10. Lanoxin	35. Librax
11. Tylenol/Codeine	36. Butazolidin Alka
12. Empirin Compound/Codeine	37. Prednisone°
13. Actifed	38. Mellaril
14. Motrin	39. Antivert
15. Darvon Compound-65	40. Ser-Ap-Es
16. Dyazide	41. Penicillin V°
17. V-Cillin-K	42. Ortho-Novum
18. Darvocet-N	43. Hygroton
19. Dalmane	44. Thyroid°
20. Inderal	45. Percodan
21. Ovral	46. Achromycin
22. Indocin	47. Triavil
23. Donnatal	48. Aldactazide
24. Keflex	49. Diabinese
25. Elavil	50. Mycolog

° Generically prescribed

From National Prescription Audit, IMS America, Ltd. as reported in *Pharmacy Times,* April 1977.

Table 4-2. *The Top 50 Drugs Classified by Indication and Generic Availability*

	Antibiotics	Tranquilizers	Symptomatic	Physiologic
GENERIC	Ampicillin Tetracycline Erythromycin Penicillin V	Phenobarbital		Prednisone Thyroid
MULTIPLE PRODUCTS	V-Cillin-K Ilosone Achromycin	Librium Elavil	Tylenol/Codeine Empirin Compound/Codeine Darvon Compound-65 Darvocet-N Benadryl	HydroDiuril Premarin Lanoxin Dilantin Diuril
SINGLE SOURCE	Keflex	Valium Dalmane Mellaril	Lomotil Antivert	Lasix Aldomet Motrin Inderal Indocin Butazolidin Alka Hygroton Diabinese
COMBINATION	Mycolog	Triavil	Dimetapp Actifed Donnatal Fiorinal Librax Percodan	Dyazide Ovral Aldoril Ser-Ap-Es Ortho-Novum Aldactazide

Bioavailability and Common Drugs

Let us examine how the question of bioavailability applies to some of the most commonly prescribed drugs. Table 4–1 lists the 50 drugs most commonly prescribed in the United States during 1976 (Pharmacy Times, 1977). These 50 drugs alone account for almost 40 percent of the 1.5 billion prescriptions written annually, or some 600 million prescriptions per year. In Table 4–2, these drugs are subdivided as to their therapeutic use and the availability of generic equivalents. Seven of the top 50 are drugs prescribed generically. Fifteen of these are drugs for which there are multiple products on the market (including some of the common combination analgesics for which generic equivalents of the same composition are widely available). Of the remaining drugs, there are 14 that are still under patent or otherwise available from only one manufacturer, and 14 combination products available as only one brand and generally prescribed as such. Nine of the 50 most prescribed drugs are antibiotics. Antibiotics generally have wide margins between therapeutic and toxic levels, and are used at dosages designed to produce blood levels well above those needed to inhibit the organisms they are being used to treat. Seven of the top 50 drugs are minor or major tranquilizers. Such drugs acting on the central nervous system are used in individualized doses, and there is little correlation established between blood levels and therapeutic effect for most of these drugs. Another 13 drugs are medications used to treat pain, nasal congestion, or other purely symptomatic states for which therapy is largely empirical at best. Only 21 of these are drugs whose primary effect is upon the cardiovascular, endocrine, or other major physiologic systems of the body. Even among these drugs, there are some whose therapeutic use is largely symptomatic, and some for which bioequivalence has now been reasonably well established. There are few drugs for which there is any clear indication for prescribing a specific brand because of concern over bioavailability problems endangering the achievement of an effective therapeutic level. Certainly no antibiotics need be prescribed by brand name, neither do most of the other drugs on this list for which multiple products are available. For most such drugs, brand-name prescribing is likely to assure the patient of little except an unnecessarily high price for his prescription.

Generic Savings

There is ample evidence that generic prescribing saves patients money, at least for certain drugs. Generic prescribing will obviously not lead to any savings if only one product is available or appropriate, which is true for a large number of prescriptions. But with drugs for which alternative products are available, potential for savings clearly exists. Only about 10 percent of all prescriptions, largely those for antibiotics, are now being written generically (Pharmacy Times, 1977). From Table 4–2 and the foregoing discussion, it is obvious that many more prescriptions can be written generically. One can conservatively estimate that 20 percent of all prescriptions are for brand-name drugs for which generic equivalents are available at lower cost. The actual figure may be much higher; one estimate is that nearly 50 percent of all prescriptions are for drugs for which multiple products are available (Goldberg et al., 1977). Even using the conservative figure and estimating an average saving of $1.50 per prescription, one can project an annual saving in prescription costs to consumers of $450 million. A saving of this amount is certainly not something to be ignored. Actual savings may even be far greater.

Savings on generic drugs are possible because of the basically different market structures for brand-name and generic drugs. When a prescription is written for a brand-name drug, the pharmacist is generally obligated (except where the repeal of antisubstitution laws allows him to do otherwise) to fill the prescription with the specific brand. The price the pharmacist must charge the patient is determined largely by the manufacturer's price to the pharmacist. The market for brand-name drugs is essentially monopolized, and anyone with only a minimal knowledge of economics knows that monopoly prices are high. Brand-name prescription drugs, furthermore, represent one of the few markets in our economy in which the person selecting the product to be purchased is not the person purchasing the product. The price factor is essentially absent as a criterion for product selection. Brand-name marketing further supports the artificially high prices. The barrage of blandishments from journal advertisements, direct mailings, salesmen, and the like is too well known to all of us. Pharmaceutical advertising to physicians is an enormous business, valued at nearly $1 billion a year. Little of this benefits patient care, and none of it supports lower drug prices for consumers. Enormous promotion costs constitute a totally unnecessary portion of the health care bill that patients who need medication, and have no choice in the matter, should not have to pay.

Generic drugs are sold under an entirely different economic system because they are marketed primarily to pharmacists. Drug quality and reputation of the manufacturer play important roles in product selection, but so does price. The pharmacist must select a product not only of dependable quality but at a reasonable price. There is plenty of opportunity for him to do so. Generic marketing of drugs, at least for such high-volume items as antibiotics, has become a highly competitive business. Many major drug firms have entered this market, often with the same products also marketed under their own brand-names. Some firms, such as SmithKline and Lederle, have marketed separate product lines for the generic market.

Once the pharmacist has selected an economically priced product, there is plenty of incentive for him to pass the savings along to the consumer. The retail prescription market is quite competitive. More and more pharmacists are changing from mark-up pricing to a professional fee pricing system (cost of the drug plus a fixed fee for filling the prescription), which removes the temptation not to pass savings along. The cost of a generic drug is a truer reflection of the costs of manufacturing, distribution, and dispensing than that of a brand-name drug. The artificial costs of monopoly and marketing are eliminated, and the consumer can only benefit.

Does generic prescribing save the consumer money? Numerous surveys have been done on this subject, by both health professionals and various consumer groups, and I need not review all the literature here. In virtually every study, substantial savings were encountered. The savings were not uniform; prices for both brand-name and generic prescriptions vary widely from one pharmacy to another, and not all pharmacists filled generic prescriptions for a lower price. But enough did so that on the average, the consumer saved money. In most studies, the overall saving amounted to about $1.50 to $2.00 per prescription, but in some cases it was more. Most of the studies, however, surveyed only one or a few drugs (generally the common antibiotics such as tetracycline or ampicillin). One recent study examined a wider range of drugs (Horvitz, 1975a). The number of pharmacies offering savings for each drug and the average of the saving are presented in Table 4–3. For the common antibiotics, most pharmacies offered savings. Every pharmacy surveyed filled generic ampicillin prescriptions at a lower price than those for the major brand. With other drugs, however, savings were obtained less frequently (this study, however, was performed in 1973, and savings may now be more widely available). For several drugs, only one or two pharmacies stocked generic products, but those that did gave large savings. The message of this study is clear: for drugs often prescribed generically, savings are widely available, but for other drugs, they may not be. Pharmacists have little incentive to stock lower-cost generic equivalents if there is no demand for them; manufacturers have no reason to offer economical generic products if there is no market for them. Incentive for generic savings must come from the physician.

Motivating forces for wider use of generic prescribing are already coming from a number of directions. Consumers are starting to become aware of the potential for financial savings—the consumer movement is an increasingly strong force in our society, and prescription prices was one of the first issues it acted upon. More and more patients will be asking that their drugs be prescribed generically, and pharmacists are even starting to encourage patients to do so. Quite a number of pharmacies, including several of the major chains, are beginning advertising campaigns encouraging the use of generic prescribing. They are explaining the potential for savings with generic drugs, encouraging customers to ask their physicians for generic prescriptions, and offering to fill these at lower prices. The consumer clearly benefits from this strategy (as does the pharmacist, who, instead of dispensing an expensive brand that is often priced as a loss leader in the competitive retail market, is able to dispense a product with a lower wholesale cost and a greater profit margin). Third-party and government payers interested in reducing health care costs are also exerting pressure by beginning to limit their reimbursements to generic drug price levels. There is strong pressure in the federal government to enlarge the MAC (maximum allowable cost) program, in which prices for prescription drugs for which multiple products are available would be limited to the lowest wholesale cost at which the drug is generally available plus a pharmacist's dispensing fee. The FDA is considering the issue of bioavailability and is plan-

Table 4-3. *Generic Savings for 12 Drugs*

Drug	Pharmacies Offering Generic Savings°	Average Savings†
Ampicillin (Polycillin)	12/12	$1.44
Erythromycin (Erythrocin)	6/10	2.16
Penicillin V (Pen-Vee-K)	2/11	0.90
Propoxyphene (Darvon)	5/12	1.66
Chlorpheniramine (Chlor-Trimeton)	0/11	no savings
Phenytoin (Dilantin)	0/10	no generics
Dioctyl sodium sulfosuccinate (Colace)	8/10	2.49
Papaverine (Pavabid)	1/9	3.70
Pentaerythritol tetranitrate (Peritrate)	3/12	2.83
Conjugated estrogens (Premarin)	2/12	2.35
Sulfisoxazole (Gantrisin)	1/11	0.90
Methenamine mandelate (Mandelamine)	0/10	no generics

° First number is number of pharmacies filling generic prescription with alternative product at lower cost than for prescription for indicated brand. Second number is number of pharmacies surveyed.

† Average of savings in pharmacies where generic prescription was filled with alternative at lower cost than prescription for indicated brand.

Modified from Horvitz, R.A., Morgan, J.P., and Fleckenstein, L.: Savings from generic prescriptions: a study of 33 pharmacies in Rochester, New York. Ann. Intern. Med. 82:601–607, 1975.

ning to establish a formulary of products for which adequate documentation of equivalency has been established. This plan has already been implemented for several drugs, and more will be included in the future. Medicare and Medicaid will reimburse only up to the MAC limit, and similar limitations can be expected from private insurers and other third-party payers. With the increasing concern over the costs of health care, the inflated costs of brand-name drugs will come under increasing scrutiny.

Another advantage of generic prescribing and the resulting lower prescription prices is the potential for improving patient compliance. Patients are often concerned about the cost of medication, especially since it is an out-of-pocket expense of which they are acutely aware. If money is tight, they may try to economize by taking fewer doses than indicated, or by taking the medication for a shorter time than prescribed (perhaps saving the rest of the prescription for another similar illness for which the medicine may or may not be appropriate). The result is often suboptimal therapy. No medication is going to be fully effective if not taken in the proper dose for the proper period. This is especially true for antibiotics, and price differences between brand-name and generic products of this type may be large. The issue of patient compliance is becoming an area of increasing concern, and generic prescribing, because of its economical aspect, may well help to make therapy more effective.

Conclusion

The practice of generic prescribing is becoming popular and will continue to expand in the future, as will the opportunities for generic savings. More and more generic drugs are becoming available; patents on many commonly used drugs have expired, and several more will do so over the next few years. A patent has a duration of only 17 years from the date of initial discovery and patent (not from the date of marketing, which may be some years later).

Drugs that spearheaded the therapeutic revolutions of the 1950's and 1960's are becoming the generic workhorses of the 1970's and 1980's, and the rate of drug innovation is decreasing. With the growing difficulties and costs of pharmaceutical research, few new drugs are being introduced. More and more of medicine is being practiced with established drugs, and these are the drugs for which generic savings are becoming available. This trend will soon affect the profitability of the drug companies, and the investment community is becoming worried about this (Reynolds Securities Information Report, 1977). Increased use of drug substitution, establishment of MAC and other cost containment programs, promotion of generic drug use by large chain pharmacies, increased marketing of low-price generic product lines—all these forces are cutting into the earning potential of the major drug firms. These and the other factors discussed in this article are acting to change the drug market from an innovative and highly profitable system of brand-name products to a commodity system of competitively priced products. This may not benefit the drug companies and their stockholders, but it certainly does benefit the far larger numbers of patients, citizens, and taxpayers concerned with the high cost of health care.

The issue of brand-name versus generic prescribing has long been one of the great controversies in medicine, but the answer now seems clear as questions over drug quality seem satisfactorily resolved. Most of the drug products on the market are now adequately equivalent, if equivalence is really a significant therapeutic concern in most circumstances. Worries over bioavailability appear exaggerated, and the incentive and technology exist to solve any remaining problems. Savings in prescription costs to the patient are incontrovertible, and savings will be even greater in the future. Health care costs are an increasingly important concern for the individual and for society, and the excessive price of brand-name prescribing is an extravagance we can no longer afford. Generic prescribing is an idea whose time has come.

References

American Pharmaceutical Association: Bioavailability monographs. J. Am. Pharm. Assoc. NS15:43–46, 1975 (digoxin); NS15:409–412, 1975 (nitrofurantoin); NS15:461–463, 1975 (oxytetracycline); NS15:529–532, 1975 (prednisone); NS15:591–594, 1975 (ampicillin); NS15:647–650, 1975 (phenytoin); NS15:709–712, 1975 (tetracycline); NS16:47–50, 1976 (hydrochlorothiazide); NS16:143–146, 1976 (prednisolone); NS16:203–206, 1976 (erythromycin); NS16:271–274, 1976 (warfarin); NS16:365–368, 1976 (phenylbutazone); NS16:415–418, 1976 (quinidine sulfate); NS16:467–470, 1976 (digitoxin); NS16:617–620, 1976 (sulfisoxazole); NS17:107–112, 1977 (aspirin); NS17:173–176, 1977 (meprobamate); NS17:243–246, 1977 (penicillin V potassium); NS17:303–306, 1977 (sustained-release papaverine hydrochloride); NS17:377–380, 1977 (ferrous sulfate).

Ballin, J.C.: Effectiveness of oxytetracyclines. JAMA 215:2095, 1971.

Goldberg, T., Aldridge G.W., DeVito C.A., et al.: Impact of drug substitution legislation; a report of the first year's experience. J. Am. Pharm. Assoc. NS17:216–226, 1977.

Horvitz, R.A.: Bioavailability and generic prescribing; a rational approach. Drug Therapy Vol. 3 (No. 9):22–35, 1973.

Horvitz, R.A., Morgan, J.P., and Fleckenstein, L.: Savings from generic prescriptions; a study of 33 pharmacies in Rochester, New York. Ann. Intern. Med. 82:601–607, 1975a.

Horvitz, R.A.: More on bioavailability and generics. Drug Therapy Vol. 5 (No. 9):125–130, 1975b.

Koch-Weser, J.: Bioavailability of drugs. N. Engl. J. Med. 291:233–237, 503–506, 1974.

Lindenbaum, J., Butler, V.P., Murphy, J.E., and Creswell, R.M.: Correlation of digoxin tablet dissolution rate with bioavailability. Lancet 1:1215–1217, 1973.

Pharmacy Times: 1976: the top 200 drugs. April 1977, pp. 37–44.

Reynolds Securities Information Report: Multi-source drugs; an acceleration in the use of lower-cost substitutes? New York, Reynolds Securities, Research Department, May 1977.

Skelly, J.P.: Bioavailability and bioequivalence. J. Clin. Pharmacol. 16:539–545, 1976.

Generic Substitution: A Form of Pharmaceutical Russian Roulette?

Dale J. Chodos, M.D.
Upjohn Company, Kalamazoo, Michigan

The controversy surrounding the concept of generic drug substitution is different from many medical controversies because of its pervasive nature. It involves almost all physicians and surely every pharmacist. It has been debated in nearly every state legislative body (it has even stimulated bipartisan controversy), in the halls of Congress, and in a variety of state and federal legislative subcommittees. Generic drug substitution has been discussed by the federal executive staff, probably even in the Oval Office, and has been a popular shibboleth for both consumer advocates and the press. Since almost everybody requires drug therapy at some time in his life, inconsistency in the quality, safety, or efficacy of drugs can have enormous consequences. It is small wonder that emotions run high and tempers are hot over this issue.

Despite the notoriety of the issue, arguments presented in this debate seem more emotional than factual. In fact, it is difficult to find much substantial information concerning generic substitution in either medical or lay literature. Particularly disturbing is the fact that the arguments offered are chiefly economic, with little concern expressed for the effect of generic prescribing on the health of the patient, whose general welfare should be paramount.

What are Generic Drugs?

It is surprising to find that confusion still exists concerning the definition and classification of generic drugs. For this discussion, a generic drug will be defined as a *pharmaceutical product manufactured by any company not involved in the development of the drug.* The term *generic* should also include products of manufacturers licensed by the "innovator" to manufacture and market a product still under patent protection. Any drug available from more than one manufacturer will be referred to as a *multi-source drug*. The innovator's product is often called the *standard product*, since most of the efficacy, safety, and pharmacology studies reported in the literature and submitted to the FDA were performed with that drug entity. Assignment of a tradename (trademark) to a duplicator's generic product does nothing to distinguish that product from other generic products; therefore, any comparison of drugs based solely on tradenames is meaningless.

Kinds of Generic Manufacturers

Multi-source drugs are manufactured by various kinds of drug companies, ranging from large, well-established companies with a cadre of experienced, sophisticated experts in their research, manufacturing, and control units to small companies with no research staff and small, inexperienced manufacturing and control staffs. As a result, it is not uncommon to find a range in quality that reflects the experience, expertise, and capability of the manufacturers. The innovator has had years of experience in working with the drug he developed. As sole manufacturer during the patent-protected years, he has produced innumerable lots of the drug and has manufactured it frequently, if not continuously, during each year. As a result, the innovator has learned how to avoid many problems encountered during the manufacturing process. Duplicating companies, regardless of size or experience, will produce smaller quantities of the drug more irregularly and probably will never attain the experience of the innovator. Like any manufacturer's product therefore, drugs can vary in quality, depending upon the expertise of their manufacturer.

What is Generic Substitution?

Generic substitution, as defined by new legislation in many states, allows or mandates a pharmacist to substitute another (usually cheaper) formulation of a drug for the specific drug formulation stipulated by the physician on a prescription or other drug order. Because of differences in legislation from state to state, the practice of generic substitution can vary markedly. Some states, for example, require the physician to state, in his own handwriting, "DAW" (Dispense As Written) or a similar statement if he wants to assure that the patient receives the exact medication prescribed. In some states, two signature spaces are provided: one to permit substitution, the other to forbid it. A few states even require a written statement of "medical justification" for a physician to interdict substitution.

With generic substitution, a patient theoretically could receive a different manufacturer's product any time a prescription is refilled, regardless of whether or not it is done at the same pharmacy.

Are Generic Drugs Alike?

Essential to the question of the desirability of generic substitution is the possibility that different therapeutic effects can result from changing from one multi-source drug to another. A plethora of articles can be found describing substantial differences in absorption among different formulations of the same drug. Unfortunately, these articles rarely appear in journals that physicians commonly read. Furthermore, only a few good review articles summarizing these findings exist, and these, too, are seldom found in medical literature. Most of these studies compare the bioavailability of multi-source drugs.

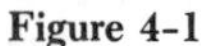

Figure 4-1.

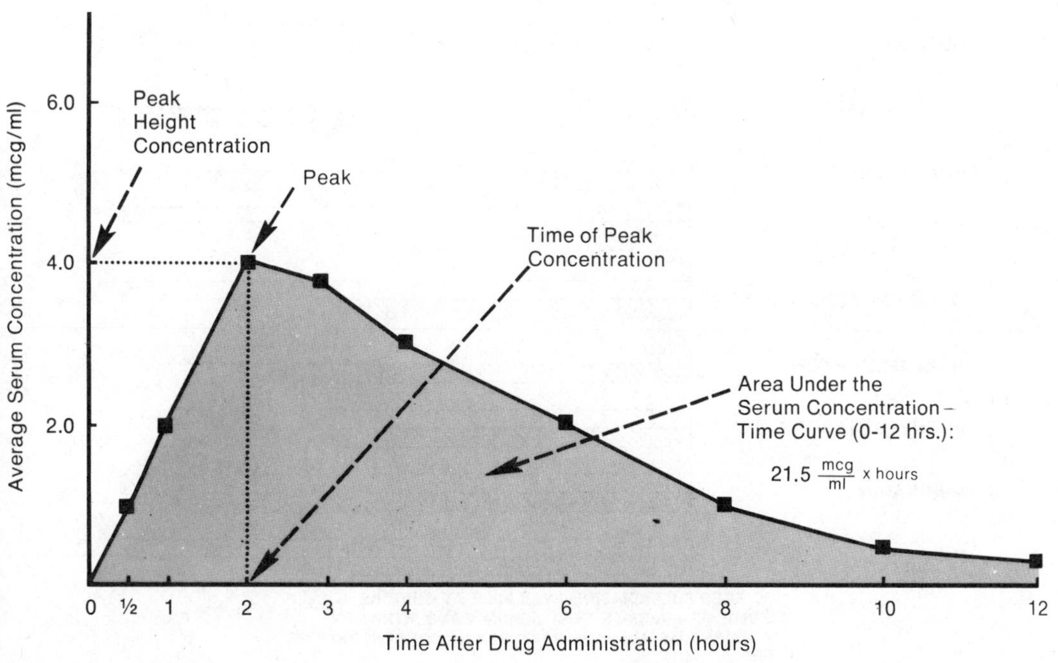

Bioavailability

Bioavailability is commonly defined as *the measurement of the rate and extent of absorption of a drug.* It is usually evaluated by measuring the amount of a drug or its metabolites in sequentially obtained blood or urine specimens. Comparisons of two formulations of the same drug can be made by measuring both rate (speed) and extent of absorption. Rate of absorption can be inferred by measuring the maximum or peak concentration of a drug in the blood and the time at which that maximum concentration occurred. Extent of absorption, or total amount of drug absorbed, is estimated by measuring, mathematically, the *a*rea *u*nder a drug blood level time *c*urve (AUC) (Figure 4-1).

If the rate and extent of absorption are similar for two or more formulations, they are judged *bioequivalent.* From each formulation, the same amount of drug will be delivered at the same

Figure 4-2. Personal file. Reproduced by Upjohn Co.

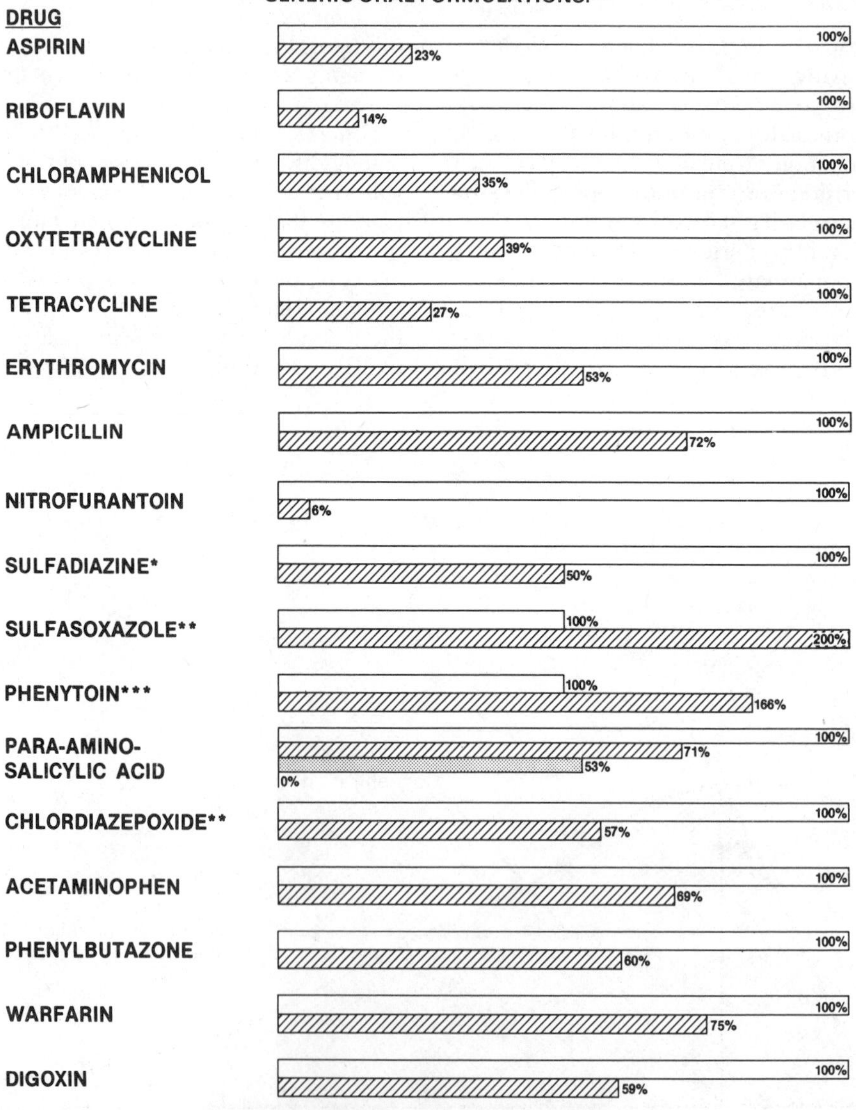

time to the site of pharmacologic activity and, consequently, the formulations will be equivalent in safety and efficacy (therapeutically equivalent). If there are substantial differences among different formulations in either the rate or extent of absorption of the drug, the potential for a difference in clinical effect must be seriously entertained. The difference in bioavailability between two formulations that is necessary to deem them unequal in absorption *(bioinequivalent)* theoretically can vary with each drug, depending upon its pharmacologic dose response. Unfortunately, we have little pharmacologic or therapeutic dose-response information for most drugs. Relatively arbitrary differences in bioavailability parameters of 20 to 25 percent are, therefore, commonly quoted as the lower limits of acceptable variability.

Surveys of bioinequivalent drugs. One of the first surveys highlighted 12 multi-source marketed products with substantial differences in bioavailability (Wagner, 1971). A second review, based on 370 articles, identified five additional drugs with documentable differences in bioavailability (Chodos and DiSanto, 1973). Figure 4–2 illustrates the differences in bioavailability for each of these 17 drugs. The second review also identified 56 additional drugs for which differences in bioavailability or in clinical or pharmacologic effect were documented or strongly suggested, either among different formulations of the same drug or among different salts or esters (pro-drugs) of that drug, when administered orally, parenterally, or topically in man or animals. A third review (Table 4–4) identified 34 multi-source marketed products for which significant aberrations in bioavailability were identified (Koch-Weser, 1974).

A recent review of over 2000 articles evaluating bioavailability suggests that at least 45 different marketed oral multi-source drugs can be identified for which sophisticated testing has revealed significant differences in bioavailability. At least 100 additional drugs can be identified for which either differences among pro-drugs, or among similar formulations of the same drug were documented or strongly suggested when these formulations were administered to man or to animals either orally, parenterally, or topically (Chodos, 1978).

Any drug can be formulated deliberately in such a way that its absorption would differ from that of another formulation. Spontaneously occurring formulation differences have been described with many drugs, and there is little doubt that such differences could occur whenever any drug is manufactured.

Causes of generic inequivalence. Inequivalence among different formulations of the same drug should not be unexpected, since there are a number of factors that may cause differences in absorption of the active ingredient of a drug. Some of these factors are bulk drug characteristics (crystal size and habitus, surface area, polymorphism, etc.); (2) excipients (materials other than the active ingredient in dosage forms—wetting agents, fillers, sweetening agents, dyes, lubricants, etc.); (3) coatings (enteric, film, and sugar); (4) manufacturing variables (filling pressures for capsules, compression pressures for tablets, solvents, drying techniques, pH's, etc.); (5) drug form (different salts or esters); and (6) dosage form (solutions, suspensions, capsules, tablets, sustained release preparations, etc.).

When bioinequivalence is demonstrated, the actual cause is usually not identified. It is probable that there are other unknown mechanisms

Table 4–4. *Drugs for Which Bioinequivalence Between Different Products Has Been Demonstrated*

Acetaminophen	Griseofulvin	Phenylbutazone
Aminophylline	Hydrochlorothiazide	Prednisone
Ampicillin	Methaqualone	Riboflavin
Aspirin	Nalidixic Acid	Salicylamide
Chloramphenicol	Nitrofurantoin	Spironolactone
Chlordiazepoxide	Oxytetracycline	Sulfadiazine
Dextroamphetamine	Para-aminosalicylic Acid	Sulfisoxazole
Diazoxide	Penicillin G	Tetracycline
Digoxin	Penicillin V	Theophylline
Diphenylhydantoin	Pentobarbital	Tolbutamide
Erythromycin	Phenacetin	Triamterene
		Warfarin

From Koch-Weser, J.: N. Engl. Med. 291:233–237, 503–506, 1974.

responsible for inequivalence, in addition to those just mentioned. Often, a combination of two or more of these factors could occur simultaneously, further compounding the problem.

Prevalence of Inequivalent Formulations. Few definitive data are available with which to evaluate the prevalence of bioinequivalent multi-source formulations. A general overview of the literature might suggest that these phenomena are not uncommon, since the preponderance of the literature describes studies documenting or suggesting such differences.

The only substantive information concerning the incidence of bioinequivalence among generic drugs was reported by the Health Protection Branch in Canada (the equivalent of the U.S. FDA). It was found that as many as one of 10 consecutively studied formulations of 229 multi-source drugs was considered bioinequivalent (Ruedy et al., 1977).

Clinical Significance of Bioinequivalence. Bioinequivalence becomes critical to the patient only if the clinical effect of a drug is altered. It has been postulated that if bioavailability differences between duplicator and innovator drugs were important clinically, physicians would have recognized the existence of ineffective or toxic generic products long ago. But it must be recognized that it is difficult for a physician to isolate the cause of therapeutic failure or adverse effect in a patient. Therapeutic misadventure can be related to a number of different factors, including individual patient variability in drug absorption or pharmacologic effect; variability in disease manifestation; drug interactions (recognized and unrecognized); effects of food, age, or environmental factors or drug absorption; placebo reactions; and patient compliance. Physicians have been trained to react to inefficacy or to the occurrence of adverse effects either by altering the dose of the medication or by changing to another drug or even, perhaps, by reevaluating the original diagnosis.

A dramatic example of the failure of physicians to recognize important bioinequivalence phenomena occurred with multi-source digoxin products. Only after a bioavailability study documented a serious inequivalence in absorption was the extent of the clinical problem recognized (Manninen et al., 1971). In retrospect, decreasing the dose of digoxin by 50 percent by substituting a more poorly absorbed formulation must have resulted in frequent therapeutic failure. Increasing the dose by approximately 100 percent by substituting the better-absorbed drug must have created situations of serious toxicity as well.

Another example of clinically significant bioinequivalence that went unrecognized by physicians is found in a report stating that an erythromycin liquid formulation was so poorly absorbed that it failed to treat successfully beta hemolytic streptococcal infections (Howie and Ploussard, 1972). The product had been used by physicians, apparently without complaint, for over 17 years. Once the problem was recognized, the drug was immediately removed from the market by the manufacturer.

Only one review dealing with differences in clinical effects caused by different multi-source drugs has been published (Azarnoff and Huffman, 1976). In that review, 21 drugs that demonstrate substantive differences in clinical effect among multi-source products were identified (Table 4–5). A cursory review of the literature adds at least 13 more drugs to that list: amphotericin B, aspirin, cortisone acetate, erythromycin ethyl carbonate, fluphenazine, isopropylantipyrine, methicillin, molindone, nitroglycerin, pipiazine, prednisone, pyrvinium, sodium salicylate, and tetracaine (Chodos, 1979).

It is true that not every drug for which a bioinequivalence problem has been identified has also had a difference in clinical effect uncovered. However, the array of examples of clinical or pharmacologic differences observed with multisource drugs strongly suggests that

Table 4–5. *Clinical Differences Found among Multi-Source Drug Products*

Tetracycline	Prednisone	Tolbutamide
Oxytetracycline	USP Thyroid Tablets	Phenacetin
Chloramphenicol	Hydrochlorothiazide-Triamterene	Aspirin
Sulfadiazine	Spironolactone	Fluocinolone Acetonide
Griseofulvin	Potassium Chloride	Digoxin
PAS	Phenytoin	Dicumarol
Nitrofurantoin	Indomethacin	
L-dopa		

From Azarnoff, D.L., and Huffmann, D.H.: Ann. Rev. Pharmaceutical Toxicology, Vol. 16, 1976.

such differences, if carefully looked for, could occur with any drug.

Clinical Effects of Drug Substitution

Finally, in attempting to evaluate the potential clinical effect of generic substitution, we must examine the concept of substitution itself. Consider a patient who had been taking an innovator's product and has switched to a generic product absorbed with 50 percent less efficiency. Symptoms may recur and the patient would have to return to the physician to seek relief. The physician, unaware of the substitution, has several options. He can (1) consider increasing the dose of the product and then evaluate the result, (2) change to a more potent medication that could be associated with more serious adverse effects (3) decide that non-drug therapy such as surgery might be indicated or (4) hospitalize the patient to reevaluate either the diagnosis or the treatment. Consider again the first option of increasing (probably doubling in this example) the dose until substantial relief is obtained. When the prescription for the higher dose is filled, it is conceivable that a more completely absorbed product could be substituted. The patient, in effect, could then receive the equivalent of twice the dose of the more completely absorbed product. Since many adverse effects of drugs are dose-related, chances for toxicity could be substantial.

It is apparent that generic substitution has the potential for causing toxicity; for forcing an unnecessary modification of therapy, including the use of more potent and more potentially dangerous drugs; for subjecting a patient needlessly to additional painful or inconvenient investigational procedures, perhaps requiring extensive hospitalization; or perhaps, for prematurely considering surgery or other painful or inconvenient non-medical therapies. Any of these results could increase the cost of therapy substantially. Although it is impossible to measure these kinds of additional costs, they must be considered in any estimation of cost savings attributable to generic substitution.

Other Effects of Generic Substitution

Differences among generically manufactured drugs are not limited solely to differences in clinical effect resulting from bioinequivalence. Other aspects of drugs and drug manufacturers can serve to differentiate multi-source drugs. For example, quality control specifications have been shown to be more extensive, more restrictive, and less variable for some manufacturers' products than for others. Differences in taste, smell, color, consistency, and shape among multi-source products can be important in assuring enhanced compliance in ingesting medication, particularly for pediatric preparations. Provision of unit-dose or calendar-dose packaging by one manufacturer could enhance compliance with his product. Differences in packaging safety, both in terms of safety for children as well as convenience for the elderly and infirm, can distinguish between products. Development of clinical information highlighting new or more appropriate uses of one formulation of a drug might make that product more desirable. Provision of informational services by one company and not another might be a factor in product selection. Provision of a variety of 24-hour services might enhance the desirability of one manufacturer's formulation. The immediate recall capability of a company with a large field force would allow one company to assure that any potentially dangerous product can be removed from the pharmacist's shelf almost immediately. Finally, inspection of pharmacists' stock for outdated merchandise and replacement with fresh drugs by field representatives can serve to distinguish one multi-source product from another.

What Protection is Available to Assure the Quality, Safety, and Efficacy of Generic Drugs?

The FDA has established certain standards of approval for generic counterparts of existing drugs.

FDA Generic Drug Approval Process

Three basic categories of generic drugs can be described based on current regulatory practices.

Generic counterparts of innovator drugs that were marketed before 1938 (the so-called "Grandfather" drugs) do not require FDA approval. Consequently, unless they are registered voluntarily, no standards for safety, efficacy, or quality are imposed on these products.

Generic drugs that are duplicates of products approved by the FDA between 1938 and 1962 require submission of an Abbreviated New Drug Application (ANDA) to the FDA for approval. This submission form provides information concerning the formulation of ingredients for the product, a description of the manufacturing process, a description of the various control procedures that will be used, and, rarely at present, documentation of bioequivalence to an innovator's product. (This ANDA process has been challenged recently by the so-called "Lannett Case," in which a generic manufacturer has, thus far, legally overturned the FDA's authority to mandate approval for this category of drug.)

The ANDA process does not apply to duplicates of drugs approved by the FDA after 1962. Apparently, duplicating companies must submit "full" NDAs that contain efficacy and safety data in order to obtain FDA approval. The extent of the information required by the FDA for a "full" NDA is not known.

Finally, it is recognized that a number of smaller manufacturers have been marketing generic products without notifying the FDA as required. Products from these manufacturers, therefore, would not even be subject to existing standards for quality, safety, and efficacy. (The FDA has confirmed the availability of such unapproved drug products recently by publishing an official list of drugs deemed "therapeutically equivalent" only because they were the subject of an approved NDA or ANDA. Publishing such a list seems tantamount to admitting that there are drugs now marketed without an approved NDA or ANDA. Otherwise, obviously, there would be no use for such a list.)

The FDA has recently published Bioavailability-Bioequivalency Regulations that require the innovator company to develop certain *in vitro* or *in vivo* procedures that would serve as standards for bioavailability and quality testing (Gardner, 1977). These regulations, in effect, will force the innovator to develop methods that will enable generic manufacturers to obtain FDA approval for their generic products much more readily and rapidly in the future.

In these regulations, the FDA has listed 110 FDA-approved drugs with which, because of either known or suspected problems, inequivalent absorption of different formulations of the drug could occur. The FDA has stated its intent to write specific regulations for each generic drug or class of drugs included in the problem list that will provide for either specific bioavailability or *in vitro* standards for these drug entities.

These regulations further suggest, and experience with the regulations published to date indicates, that the FDA frequently will substitute dissolution rate testing for bioavailability testing when approving those 110 potentially troublesome generic products. The dissolution rate assay is an *in vitro* test that measures the time required for dissolution of the parent drug from its final dosage form (tablet, capsule, etc.). The popularity of dissolution rate testing is based on the theoretical concept that the speed with which a drug dissolves is related to its rate and extent of absorption. Although it is undoubtedly a reasonable theory, there are many other factors (known and unknown) unrelated to the dissolution rate of the parent drug that can affect bioavailability. Whereas the dissolution rate is useful as a quality control tool and as a harbinger of potential bioavailability problems, the finding of a significantly prolonged dissolution rate can not be relied upon to document bioinequivalence; neither will the finding of an "acceptable" dissolution rate guarantee bioequivalence and therapeutic equivalence.

The FDA states that there is no need to correlate, statistically, dissolution rate testing with human bioavailability testing or therapeutic equivalence. Inasmuch as there are a number of examples showing a lack of correlation between the dissolution rate and bioavailability, the FDA attitude that proof of the correlation is not necessary because it is too complex seems both puzzling and unscientific.

There is little doubt that a more extensive use of the dissolution rate test would decrease to some extent the rate of occurrence of bioinequivalent formulations. There is no way of knowing, however, how valuable this test would be in substantially reducing the prevalence of inequivalent formulations.

FDA Regulation of Marketed Generic Drugs

The FDA has set up several procedures for monitoring the manufacturing of most multisource products. The Good Manufacturing Practices Regulations determine standards for manufacturing processes. The Quality Assurance Lab evaluates a sampling of randomly selected lots of generic drugs for meeting compendial *(in vitro)* specifications.The Certification Process, utilized exclusively for insulin, antibiotics, and biologicals (serums, vaccines, etc.), requires FDA batch testing and approval of each manufactured lot. Manufacturing plant inspections are undertaken by FDA, which is supposed to inspect each manufacturer's plant every two years, and field inspectors are charged with monitoring the marketplace for violations of FDA Regulations.

The ability of any of these various monitoring schemes to assure the quality, safety, and efficacy of generic products has not been adequately documented. The Quality Assurance Lab and the Certification Process evaluate certain *in vitro* tests described in the recognized drug compendia, the *United States Pharmacopeia* (USP) and the *National Formulary* (NF). These tests are important and helpful in assuring the quality of generic drugs by evaluating them for purity (freedom from contamination), potency (assurance of chemical equivalence with an innovator's product), and chemical stability over time. They were not designed, however, to evaluate the safety and efficacy of drugs, and consequently can not be relied upon to identify bioinequivalent and potentially therapeutically inequivalent products.

Bioavailability comparison is the most sophisticated and practical parameter for predicting therapeutic equivalence. As previously indicated, such studies will be used somewhat more frequently in the future by the FDA in an attempt to insure the safety and efficacy of marketed generic products. Unfortunately, these studies also may have serious drawbacks. Although we can be sure that identically absorbed drugs will be therapeutically equivalent, small differences in absorption may be difficult to evaluate since pharmacologic response may not necessarily parallel changes in blood drug level exactly. It is possible that a small difference in rate or extent of absorption could cause a more marked difference in clinical effect.

A recent study has demonstrated that when two multisource products found to show a small difference in bioavailability when tested in ambulatory normal volunteers were restudied in bedridden subjects, substantial differences in bioavailability were uncovered (Adir and Barr, 1977). Since food and a number of other factors, in addition to ambulation, are also known to affect the bioavailability of drugs, it is not unreasonable to assume that these factors might also exaggerate otherwise small, supposedly inconsequential, bioavailability differences that have been found in studies of other drugs performed in normal volunteers.

If two formulations of a drug were found bioequivalent immediately after manufacture, it is also possible that the bioavailability of one of the formulations might change with increasing shelf life whereas the bioavailability of the other formulation might not.

Lot-to-lot variability in drug absorption is another potential source of therapeutic inequivalence. There is reasonable evidence to suggest that important differences in bioavailability can occur among different lots of the same formulation produced by one manufactuer. However, lot-to-lot variability and variability due to instability have not been studied extensively. Therefore, the prevalence of bioinequivalence resulting from such phenomena is uncertain. There is no provision in present FDA regulations for lot-to-lot or stability bioavailability sampling, although *in vitro* tests including dissolution rates are recommended for that purpose.

Governmental Influences on Generic Substitution and Drug Costs

Any decision by the physician for or against generic substitution will be profoundly influenced by recent and future governmental actions at both state and federal levels.

State and federal antisubstitution laws. State antisubstitution laws, in effect in all states until recently, prevented pharmacists from substituting medications prescribed by a physician. These laws now have either been rescinded or substantially modified in over half the states in the country. The new laws generally allow or require pharmacists to substitute any generic drug unless specifically prohibited in writing by the prescriber.

A similar piece of federal legislation aimed at repealing all state antisubstitution laws has appeared before Congress. The FTC has recently published a model substitution law, requesting its adoption in all states.

MAC legislation. "MAC" (Maximum Allowable Cost) legislation has established a system of price fixing for multi-source pharmaceuticals paid for by the government (VA hospitals, military institutions, Medicaid, Medicare, etc.) This legislation sets maximum prices to be paid by the government based on the lowest priced generic product that is nationally and consistently available.

An Advisory Board was also charged with the evaluation of evidence for bioinequivalence and the rejection of products that have potential problems. The Board was often reassured by the FDA, however, that no equivalence problems existed for the drugs proposed. On a number of occasions, the Board's advice was disregarded by the FDA. Recently the Board was dissolved by the agency.

Cost savings of generic drug substitution. The primary purpose of federal and state regulation and legislation relating to generic drugs is to save money, a laudable goal. The concept of cost containment is critical to those legislators hoping for passage of National Health Insurance legislation. Since pharmaceutical products are perhaps the easiest segment of the health care system to regulate, they have been subjected to intense governmental scrutiny.

It is important, therefore, to put pharmaceutical costs into some sort of perspective. The cost of medication (prescription and OTC) is estimated to be only about 8 percent of the total United States health care bill. Even the most exuberant planner can predict generic substitution savings of no greater than 10 percent. Thus, we are discussing a concept that can save, at most, less than 1 percent of our current health care expenditures.

The actual savings or additional costs that might accrue from generic substitution, however, are exceedingly difficult to estimate. Certain generic drug substitution plans have been presented that claim to have demonstrated significant and substantial savings. Other plans have proved to be miserable failures in their attempts to save money. The difficulty of measuring the administration costs of such a system also must be considered. Further, it is impossible to determine the potential cost of an increased rate of either therapeutic failure or drug toxicity that could result from the dispensing of generic formulations that are potentially therapeutically inequivalent. Figures for cost savings resulting from generic prescribing or mandated drug substitution can be, at best, only vague estimates that would be subject to considerable controversy.

What is the Impact of Generic Inequivalence?

The phamaceutical industry. Generic substitution undoubtedly will seriously affect the profitability base for the innovating segment of the pharmaceutical industry. A reduction in industry profitability should be of concern to all, since it would result in a significant reduction in the funding of research by industry and, consequently, in a further reduction in the number and quality of new therapeutic breakthroughs that have been typical of pharmaceutical industry performance in past years.

The patient. The combination of the repeal of state antisubstitution legislation and the institution of federal MAC legislation now forces certain segments of our population (primarily the aged and the poor) to accept cheaper grades of medication that, as we have discussed, may not be equal in quality, safety, or efficacy to the innovator's product. In the event of the passage of proposed legislation to extend Medicare to cover provision of drugs to the elderly on an outpatient basis or to establish one or another of the currently proposed forms of National Health Insurance Programs, the population base for which generic drugs of questionable quality can be mandated will be considerably broadened.

Conclusion

In a general overview of the generic substitution issue, the one theme found to prevail is the uncertainty uncovered each time a major feature of generic substitution is examined. For example, differences in absorption have been identified for many drugs (indeed for most of the drugs studied), but we are still uncertain as to whether the still untested multi-source drugs also might have bioinequivalence problems.

Other than one evaluation indicating that as many as one in ten multi-source drugs have bioinequivalence problems, there are few data defining the frequency with which potentially therapeutically inequivalent generic products can occur. We are, therefore, uncertain as to how often patients would be exposed to generically dispensed drugs that are errratically absorbed and may prove to be therapeutically inequivalent.

Although dramatic examples of both therapeutic failure and toxicity have been described as a result of generic substitution, the severity of the clinical problems that might result from know or unknown absorption differences and the frequency of such clinical effects are difficult to estimate. We are unsure of how often lot-to-lot variability in absorption for any one manufacturer's product could occur. We cannot tell whether differences in absorption among generic products can occur more frequently as a result of prolonged storage of pharmaceutical products. We do not know how valuable our existing standards and safeguards are in assuring the quality, safety, and efficacy of the generic products planned for substitution. We are even uncertain as to whether generic substitution will or will not be cost effective.

In an era when consumer advocacy demands meticulous evaluation of the risk/benefit relationship, it is difficult to understand the tremendous pressures that are being exerted on our society to accept, without substantial evidence, the potentially harmful risks associated with the concept of generic substitution, particulary when its benefits seem so nebulous.

References

Adir, J., and Barr, W.H.: Effect of sleep on bioavailability of tetracycline. J. Pharm. Sci. 66:1000–1004, 1977.

Azarnoff, D.L., and Huffman, D.H.: Therapeutic implications of bioavailability. Ann. Rev. Pharm. Tox. 16:53, 1976.

Chodos, D.J., and DiSanto, A.R.: *Basics of Bioavailability*. Kalamazoo, Michigan, The Upjohn Company, 1973.

Chodos, D.J.: Personal file, 1978.

Gardner, S.: Bioavailability and bioequivalence requirements. Federal Register 42:1624, 1977.

Howie, V.M., and Ploussard, J.H.: Compliance dose-response relationships in streptococcal pharyngitis. Am. J. Dis. Child., 123:18, 1972.

Koch-Weser, J.: Medical intelligence; Drug therapy; Bioavailability of drugs. N. Engl. J. Med., 233:233, 503, 1974.

Manninen, V., Melin, J., and Hartel, G.: Serum-digoxin concentrations during treatment with different preparations. Lancet, 2:934–935, 1971.

Ruedy, J., Davies, R.O., Gagnon, M.A., McLean, W.M., Thompson, W.G., Vitti, T.G., and Wilson, T.W.: Dosage, compliance and bioavailability in perspective. Can. Med. Assoc. J. 117:323–324, 1977.

Wagner, J.G.: Generic equivalence and inequivalence of oral products. In *Biopharmaceutics and Relevant Pharmacokinetics*. Hamilton, Illinois, Drug Intelligence Publications, 1971.

Generic Substitution and Grandma's Secret Recipe

John M. Mazzullo, M.D.
University of Rochester School of Medicine and Dentistry

It has become fashionable to equate "generic prescribing" with the American way, motherhood, and apple pie. Many young physicians inbred with consumerist zeal and antiestablishment prejudice are quick to take up the banner of generic equivalence. The purpose of this article is to examine the validity of this endorsement of generic equivalence.

The crux of the issue is the concept of bioavailability. I define this term as *the ability of a compound to gain access to the blood stream, and subsequently the active receptor site, in an active form.* Given that we know what the active moiety is, and that we can measure it in the blood stream, we are interested in whether this active moiety can survive passage through the acid of the stomach and then disintegrate and dissolve and be absorbed in the proximal small bowel. The absorbed moiety must then traverse the liver. Each of these steps on the way to the active site can be viewed as pitfalls that can dramatically influence bioavailability. For instance, a drug may disintegrate but not dissolve in gastric juice. Or, for example, if the hepatic extraction were unlimited, theoretically bioavailability would be zero.

Many *in vitro* tests have been designed in an effort to assure uniform biologic effects from different pharamaceutical preparations (bioequivalence). The first, and most obvious, is the measurement of the amount of drug in each tablet. Clearly, such "chemical equivalence" is a long way from bioequivalence. The two other tests that attempt to bridge this gap are disintegration and dissolution studies.

Disintegration, a key to bioavailability, depends on many pharmaceutical factors. Most drugs are dispensed in very small quantities—usually in milligrams. To make these drugs into easily handled tablets, the active compound is combined with a supposedly inert binder or filler, called an *excipient.* Three critical variables in the manufacture of any pharmaceutical product are the final crystalline structure of the active moiety, the nature of the excipient, and the pressure exerted by the tablet compressor. The compressor fuses the active drug and the excipient into tablets. If the crystalline structure is improper, the excipient a poor choice, or the pressure too great, the tablet may not disintegrate.

In order to perform a disintegration study, a tablet is placed in a liquid, usually water, and the time it takes for the tablet to fall apart is measured. A tablet may fall apart but the particles thus formed may not go into solution. To compensate for this, dissolution studies are done. In one such study, simulated gastric juice is made and placed in a constant temperature apparatus to keep it at body temperature. The tablet is added, the solution is stirred, and the rate at which the tablet dissolves in the simulated gastric juice is measured.

There is no assurance that two different tablets giving equal results in *in vitro* disintegration and dissolution studies will produce equal biologic effect. There is a much more reliable relationship between equal blood levels and desired biologic effect. Yet the FDA does not require manufacturers to submit lots for blood level testing. They require only *in vitro* testing to meet compendial standards, which are codified by the *United States Pharmacopoeia* (USP) and the *National Formulary* (NF).

There are many logistic problems that need solving before the FDA can require that all marketed drugs must produce a certain blood level. We must have the technologic means to measure the active moiety. Should the drug be given to humans or to experimental animals? To healthy volunteers or to patients with the disease for which the drug is intended? To cite extreme examples, can one give methotrexate to healthy volunteers and a possibly poorly absorbed penicillin to a patient with pneumonia? To compound matters, the attainment of blood levels may not always correlate with clinical efficacy. Even more direct proof of efficacy would be clinical trial data.

For example, in the case of chlorpromazine, we have clinical trial evidence of safety and effectiveness for only one compound—that of Smith Kline and French (Thorazine). In addition, we have many years of post-marketing clinical use to reinforce the original New Drug Application (NDA). Smith Kline and French had a patent on the chemical structure of chlorpromazine for 17 years. What is *not* patented is the manufacturing process. When the patent runs out, the manufacturing process that results in the clinically proven product, Thorazine, does *not* become public knowledge. It's almost as if Grandma tells you what is in her famous chocolate cake but doesn't tell you how to mix the ingredients together or how long to bake the cake. Therefore, each generic drug manufacturer must, in a manner of speaking, recreate Thorazine, and the federal government has no control over how well they succeed. Generic products only meet compendial standards for chemical purity and disintegration and dissolution rates. They are, in effect, attempts to make the chocolate cake without knowing the recipe.

If there is no proof of clinical efficacy for a generic product, why would physicians take a chance and prescribe generically? Generic drugs are supposed to save the patient money. Let us examine this proposition. Richard Horvitz and other colleagues in our department obtained data on this issue. They found, in Rochester, New York, at least, that what primarily determined the final retail price of the drug was not whether the physician prescribed generically but in which kind of pharmacy the drug was purchased (Horvitz et al., 1975). Generic drugs were on the average more expensive at small neighborhood pharmacies. One reason for the higher price may be that the consumer is buying other services at the neighborhood store, such as longer hours, delivery services, and family medication records. Factors of this kind determine price more often than whether or not the physican prescribes a brand name drug. Also, a large chain pharmacy can support its small drug market by the rapid turnover of cosmetic and over-the-counter products. The combination of limited pharmacy services and high-volume turnover produces a lower price for all drugs, generic *and* brand name.

Another potential problem of writing prescriptions for generic products is that every time the patient goes to a pharmacy for a refill, the patient may get a different product from a different manufacturer. Not only is bioavailability likely to vary from company to company but the tablets may look different! Can you imagine the confusion this situtation can produce?

Another difficulty with generic prescriptions is that some generic manufacturers do not have as much quality control in production as one finds in most of the established, well known companies. Perhaps this belief is the result of some high class Madison Avenue brainwashing, but I am convinced that ethical drug firms manufacture medicines "as if people's lives depended on them." Not only do these firms spend a significant percentage of their profits on quality control, but another large percentage is returned to the company for research and development of new drug entities. One reason why the patent laws were developed was to insure that an ethical drug firm was "reimbursed" for its effort in developing the compound. Incentive in our capitalist society for development of new medications is the profit that accrues from the 17-year monopoly of the marketplace. Generic drug manufacturers have no interest in the development of new drugs. If we do not prescribe by brand name, where will the money come from to support development of new drugs?

5

Will Patient Package Inserts Help or Harm?

Patient Package Inserts Will Benefit Consumers

Lawrence Fleckenstein, Pharm. D.

How Appropriate is the Proposed Patient Package Labeling?

William R. Barclay, M.D.

. . . For of this you may be very sure, that if one of those empirical physicians, who practice medicine without science, were to come upon the gentleman physician talking to his gentleman patient, and using the language almost of philosophy—beginning at the beginning of the disease, and discoursing about the whole nature of the body, he would burst into a hearty laugh—he would say what most of those who are called doctors always have at their tongue's end: foolish fellow, he would say, you are not healing the sick man, but you are educating him; and he does not want to be made a doctor, but to get well.

Plato, *Laws*

We do not know the mode of action of almost all remedies. Why therefore fear to confess our ignorance?

Armand Trousseau

I prefer to be called a fool for asking the question, rather than to remain in ignorance.

John Homans

How hard it is for some people in authority to realize the folly of being overbearing and rude to those whom they can control!

Sir W. Arbuthnot Lane

Don't say *things. What you* are *stands over you the while, and thunders so that I cannot hear what you say to the contrary.*

Ralph Waldo Emerson

Introduction

It is alleged by many consumer advocates that patients want to know more about both their diseases and their medicines. Surveys seem in general to support this statement, although there are certain situations in which something less than total disclosure is in the patient's best interest.

Fleckenstein argues for the patient package insert (PPI) as a needed supplement to human communication, which is often lacking or inadequate in health care. He believes that PPIs will lead to better risk-benefit assessments, prevention of adverse drug reactions and interactions, improved patient compliance, and effective warnings about inadvisable drug use.

The arguments against PPIs strike Fleckenstein as unimpressive. Cost should not be excessive, he argues, and demands on the physician's time need not be prohibitive. As for waiting until more research is done on PPIs so as to assess their efficacy and potential for harm before they are widely implemented, Fleckenstein believes that delay can be potentially more harmful than proceeding cautiously but immediately.

Barclay, who reflects the views of many physicians and academicians who have spoken out against PPIs, is more apprehensive. He worries about PPIs that are incomprehensible, and about patients who will be frightened—perhaps to the point where they will fail to take needed medicines. Barclay also is concerned about the reactions of patients who may be "talked into" imagined side effects by reading that they might occur.

An important point is who shall prepare PPIs. If the government does it, the inserts are bound to be out of date, since the FDA moves slowly when revising labeling. Regardless of who prepares them, there will have to be judgments made about the purpose of the insert (warning or balanced presentation?), its length, its level of composition, its language, and its distributor. For many physicians, specially important questions are whether *everyone* will need to get a PPI, or get the *same* one, and whether there can be the sort of flexibility that characterizes good medicine.

One hopes that our society will proceed with appropriate caution and wisdom—with "deliberate speed." It is hard, in any case, to avoid the feeling that PPIs will be with us to an ever increasing extent in the years ahead.

LOUIS LASAGNA, M.D.

Patient Package Inserts Will Benefit Consumers

Lawrence Fleckenstein, Pharm. D.
Alta Bates Hospital, Berkeley, California

The public has a right to be informed about its medicines, and it needs certain instructions in order to use drugs properly. Patients should know the expected benefits of treatment and should be told that in some cases, treatment is only palliative and does not alter the course of the underlying disease. When risks are specifiable, it has long been the hallmark of good medical practice to inform patients of potential problems. In addition, the public should be aware that only some of the risks of drug therapy are known; any treatment involves an element of the unknown.

Patients need to be acquainted with certain basic information in order to utilize medicines to their best effect and to avoid the risk of harm. Generally, this information includes the name of the drug, its nature and uses, its dosage and administration, common side effects (and what to do if they occur), and facts about stability and storage. Access to these facts and the preservation of the right to be informed are fundamental privileges that should be guaranteed for all patients.

Concept of the Patient Package Insert (PPI)

Presumably, physicians, pharmacists, and others are already supplying patients with needed knowledge of drugs. However, indications from a variety of sources reveal that patients are inconsistently instructed about their medicine and in some cases receive little or no guidance. The PPI, a label to be supplied with each prescription, insures that the patient is at least exposed to the basic data concerning the medication. The insert is written in language that is easy for the average person to understand. However, because the insert must be generalized, the need for individual counseling and dialogue between the practitioner and the patient still exists. The PPI is not ideal, but it is a rather good and workable mechanism that provides consumers with more and better information than they now obtain.

Why Have Written Information?

Communication between practitioners and patients is challenging because medical issues are complicated and often must be conveyed in technical and unfamiliar language. Although it is generally agreed that verbal counseling by the physician is the single most effective means of communication with patients, it is also acknowledged that this form of interaction alone is not usually strong enough to maximize patient care. Most physicians are unable or unwilling to allot precious time to giving elaborate instructions or to encouraging patients to ask questions. Many patients receive limited or vague directions, and confusion and misunderstanding result. Furthermore, it is not always easy for a doctor to present the essential information clearly and concisely. Since faulty communication and misapprehension can have serious consequences if unnoticed and uncorrected, the need for clarification and supplementation of information is apparent. The more we rely solely upon a single method of informing patients, without inquiring why it is inadequate or what the alternatives are, the harder it becomes to deal thoughtfully, intelligently, and critically with our pressing problems. It is irrelevant to argue over which method of communication, oral or written, is preferred, since these two methods can and should be used together. The PPI adds another dimension to our approach to improving communication between practitioners and patients.

Benefits of Patient Package Labeling

One of the obvious benefits of patient package labeling is that it will lead to more informed consumers. This will be manifested in many ways, but two important consequences are better risk-benefit assessments and an improved understanding of complex drug issues. Other advantages include better distribution of information, reduction in the number of adverse drug reactions and interactions, improved drug administration techniques, better patient compliance, more open discussion of certain sensitive medical issues, and greater awareness of drug misuse.

Improved risk-benefit assessments. With the use of PPIs, patients will be better informed about medicines and better able to participate in decisions concerning drugs. The decision to use a drug is highly personal, and it should be made by a patient and his doctor together. The risk-benefit assessment is based upon the best available information and the judgment of both the physician and the patient.

Obviously, the outcome of this process is highly dependent on the information available to each. The physician has powerful tools to help him: extensive training, previous experience, learned colleagues, medical textbooks, journals, and the Physicians' Desk Reference (PDR)—a collection of physician-oriented package inserts. For the patient, the situation is quite different. Most have had little medical training or experience and rely heavily on the advice of the physician. There is a lack of readily available and digestible written information for patients on the details of medications. The PPI is a step in the direction of correcting this deficiency and will help patients to make more intelligent choices. Some opponents of PPI argue that giving patients a little information will do more harm than good, because patients will not understand or be able to interpret what they read. Inevitably, given more responsibility, a few patients will make poor decisions, perhaps even some with harmful outcomes. But it is highly unlikely that the harm these errors may cause would approach the harm caused by ignorance or by biased or wrong information.

Better understanding of complex drug issues. More and more drug issues are appearing in the news and are becoming topics of public discussion. Consider how much press coverage has been given to estrogen-associated endometrial carcinoma, the swine flu vaccination program, and the potential of oral contraceptives to induce thromboembolism. The media typically present one side of the story. New accounts of the birth control pill often dwell on the problems associated with these agents rather than on their beneficial aspects. Rarely are the stories tempered by the fact that pregnancy itself carries risks of complications. How can the public be expected to make rational decisions about drug use when the harm that drugs may cause is constantly being thrust before them? In the case of oral contraceptives, emotional and political issues have prevailed; logic and medical perspective have been lost.

In order to discuss such complex subjects, there is a need to raise the level of public understanding by presenting honest and unbiased information. In other words, both sides of the story must be told. The PPI could accurately summarize the essential points involved in risk-benefit assessments, and by so doing could help patients to make sound judgments.

Better distribution of information. Almost everyone would agree that an important advantage of PPIs is that they would make distribution of information more uniform than the present haphazard methods do. Traditional means of informing patients about drugs are unreliable. In some cases, a prescription is issued and dispensed to a third party rather than to the patient for whom it is intended and the patient may never receive verbal counseling. If PPIs are given routinely to patients when medicines are dispensed, the document will be readily and widely available. This would also avoid the current situation in which information is occasionally omitted because of an oversight or a communication gap.

Prevention of adverse drug reactions. Another advantage of PPIs is that they can warn patients about potential adverse drug reactions, some of which are preventable. Some patients suffer drug-related adversities either because they are not aware that such reactions can occur or because they are not instructed in measures of prevention. For example, the rebound hypertension associated with certain antihypertensive medications could be largely avoided if patients were warned not to discontinue treatment abruptly on their own. The phototoxicity of tetracyclines could be prevented or lessened by wearing protective clothing or by using sunscreens during periods of sun exposure. In addition, the severity of some adverse reactions could be lessened by forewarning patients of early signs of toxicity and telling them when to seek medical attention. The patient receiving adriamycin should be warned that his urine will be red for one to two days after administration and that this is not cause for alarm. However, beyond this time red urine may be a sign of hematuria from an excessively low platelet count, in which case the patient should be advised to seek medical attention promptly to lessen the chance of serious problems.

Is it not our duty to undertake every reasonable measure to prevent or to minimize adverse drug reactions? This information is too important to leave to chance, and a written version of it should be dispensed with every prescription.

Prevention of drug interactions. PPIs will warn consumers of potential drug-drug and drug-food interactions. Many important examples can be cited. The combination of warfarin and aspirin can result in serious toxicity. The therapeutic response can be impaired when digoxin is taken together with antacids. Patients on oral anticoagulants or cardiac glycosides should pay strict attention to other medicines, including those that can be purchased without prescriptions.

Alcohol is commonly involved in drug-drug or drug-food interactions. It can exaggerate the effects of other central nervous system depressants and can cause violent reactions in patients taking disulfiram and certain other medicines. The patient on disulfiram treatment should avoid alcohol scrupulously. This is sometimes difficult, because alcohol can be disguised in unexpected forms: elixirs and tinctures of medications; mouthwashes, shaving lotions, and various cosmetics; and many foods, including dessert dishes containing brandy, rum, or liqueur. Patients on disulfiram or undergoing anticoagulant treatment should be familiar with the substantial information that is available, in order to avoid problems.

It takes a great deal of time and effort to develop an appropriate level of awareness of these considerations through oral communication. Whereas oral instructions are necessary and desirable, more often than not it is too time consuming to use this approach exclusively and the end product is a compromise that pleases no one. It is far better to combine oral communication with written information that includes a listing of drugs and foods to avoid, which patients can study at their own convenience.

Since many medicines are prescribed to be taken over a long period, the possibility of forgetting the information is an important consideration. A written document can be maintained as a ready source of reference for periodic review. Increased patient awareness of adverse drug reactions and drug interactions will be one of the most significant benefits of patient package labeling.

Improved drug administration techniques. PPIs will help patients to understand the importance of proper drug administration. The amount, the timing, and the duration of dosage play key roles in the outcome of drug therapy. For example, nitroglycerin must be used judiciously to minimize the development of tolerance and yet obtain maximal relief from anginal pain; antiarrhythmics must be taken on a scheduled basis for sustained beneficial cardiac action; and a full course of antibiotic treatment is necessary to avoid relapse of an infection. Since this information is so vital, its importance should be underscored to the patient, and repetition or reinforcement by the insert is highly desirable.

No matter how effective any drug is, it will not do any good unless it arrives at its site of action. Administration of aerosols, insufflations, nebulizers, eye drops and ointments, various topical preparations, and suppositories is confusing to many patients and to some doctors. Diagrams are readily incorporated into the patient brochure and are especially helpful for demonstrating proper techniques. We spend a lot of money to insure drug quality and potency. Shouldn't we spend a little to develop labeling that will increase the likelihood that drugs are administered correctly?

Improved patient compliance. We hear a great deal today about the issue of patient compliance. The extent of the problem has been documented and some of the contributing causes have been identified. Some investigators feel that if patients know more about their medicines and the reasons for taking them, they would be more likely to follow directions carefully. For that reason, some of the initial strategies for improving patient compliance involved the use of written information about medicines. Unfortunately, the impact that the availability of information has had on patient compliance is not clear-cut. One educational program that included written medical and medication information had no effect upon compliance with antihypertensive drug regimens (Sackett et al., 1975). On the positive side, several studies have shown that written materials can help to improve patient adherence to antibiotic regimens in acute illness (Colcher and Bass, 1972; Sharpe and Mikeal, 1974). Others have found that written information improved compliance when combined with oral reinforcement by the pharmacist (Clinte and Kabat, 1976).

It is becoming increasingly clear that compliance is a complicated problem that is influenced by a number of factors. Supplying written information cannot be expected to eliminate the problem and to render patient compliance a matter of historical interest. However, PPIs should have a favorable influence, and these modest gains should not be overlooked. At the very least, written information will help those patients who are ignorant or misinformed about drug use.

Discussion of sensitive issues. PPIs will help to provide information about sensitive drug issues that are usually not fully discussed with patients. I am aware of an incident in a local institution in which a number of outpatients failed to respond to treatment for lice infestations because of inadequate application of the prescribed pesticide. The pharmacy department neglected to give them the instructions supplied by the manufacturer because the leaflets had been inadvertently discarded by the stock clerk. The patients were too embarrassed to ask questions of their physicians and pharmacists, even though they didn't understand how to use the medicine. The physicians and pharmacists involved in the incident were quite frank in expressing their attitudes about patients with this condition. One physician said he just wanted to "Kwell 'em and get them out of here." Patients were given minimal oral instructions and were not encouraged to ask questions. As a result, therapeutic failure occurred in the face of exposure to a potent chemical. To correct this situation, special written instructions were prepared for Kwell cream, lotion, and shampoo. These are now given routinely to every patient with a prescription for one of these products. Additional failures have not been encountered during the six months that the information sheets have been used.

At Alta Bates Hospital, patient information sheets are used as part of a patient education program for cardiac and cancer drugs. Sheets for cancer drugs have been developed only recently and our experience is quite limited. Up to this point, patients have readily accepted the material and read it, and most have commented that it is a good idea. An unexpected benefit of the information sheets was that patients found it easier to share their experiences with their families by having them read about the medications. Drug descriptions have been reassuring in some cases and have dispelled some of the exaggerated fears patients and family members have had about chemotherapy. Use of the sheets began with a few selected patients in the hospital. Now, most hospitalized cancer patients receive the information, some physicians use it in their private offices, and the head of the cancer program at a nearby institution has asked for permission to reproduce the sheets for the patients there. The point is that when one is faced with a highly sensitive and emotional topic such as cancer, every available resource to improve communication must be utilized.

Warnings of inappropriate use. There are instances in which patients should be warned against the excessive and injudicious use of powerful drugs. To select an obvious example, patients must be made aware that prolonged use of narcotic analgesics or certain hypnotics can produce physical dependence. Here, the primary focus should be on educating patients about rational drug use.

Several factors must be considered before requiring this type of labeling. First, there should be evidence of past misuse of the drug by patients. Second, there should be some element of patient control over the medicine involved. Some aspects of drug abuse are very emotional; warnings chosen for patient package labeling should, therefore, be considered carefully. PPIs should not be used as an indirect legal mechanism to regulate medicine. This is one strong reason for having inserts prepared by experts from academic, medical, and pharmaceutical communities rather than by the FDA. PPIs should have a positive tone that emphasizes patient education. They should not become another tool of the FDA to regulate prescribing or to interfere with intelligent medical practice.

Criticisms of the PPI

What are the arguments against patient package inserts? Are they valid? Some critics cite the lack of patient interest, the increased cost of medication, the need for additional research and for more physician time to counsel patients, and increased reporting of side effects by patients.

Lack of patient interest. Will patients read the insert? Available evidence suggests that patients do read PPIs. Two surveys of oral contraceptive users indicate that over 90 percent of patients who are aware of the insert have read it (Fleckenstein et al., 1976; Morris et al., 1977). If these data can be applied to other drugs, they suggest that PPIs will be widely read and accepted as a source of drug information. A study conducted at the University of Rochester concluded: "People do want to know (about drugs); they want to know a lot and do not want to have to ask for this information" (Joubert and Lasagna, 1975). Thus, the available evidence does not support the notion that patients don't want to know about their medication or won't read the insert. Rather, what emerges is evidence of insufficient available information about drugs. PPIs are favorably received by patients and deserve wider utilization.

Increased cost of medication. Undoubtedly, preparation and distribution of PPIs will result in additional cost, which will probably be passed along to consumers in the form of higher prescription prices. Although this expense is not expected to be staggering, most would agree that there ought to be a favorable cost-benefit ratio in deciding which and how many drugs to label. If, for instance, no benefit can be realized from labeling relatively innocuous digestive enzymes, why label them?

Is cost a real barrier to the development of additional labeling? In the absence of any firm data on this subject, one can only be guided by the development of other forms of labeling. It is hard to detect any rise in the wholesale or retail prices of drugs that have been labeled recently (e.g., estrogens). In addition, cost has not been a notable deterrent to the development of more extensive labeling for physicians or the less extensive labeling prepared for patients with over-the-counter (OTC) drugs. The experience thus far suggests that labeling is an economical and efficient way of supplying drug information. Barring the use of gilded, embossed printing or a dramatic increase in the cost of low quality paper, increases in prescription costs due to PPI's should be minimal.

Need for additional research. It has been suggested that there is a need to prove that PPIs will accomplish what is expected of them and that a favorable relationship exists between risks and benefits (Dorsey, 1977). Further, it is contended that PPIs should be held to the same standard of proof as that required of new drugs. This view seems blindly irrational and unnecessarily extreme. In the first place, PPIs (unlike new drugs) are not inherently efficacious or toxic. Second, patient labeling has a good track record, and there is no evidence that it is doing more harm than good. Third, the controlled clinical trial is a valuable research tool, but it is not the only route to wisdom. Aristotle pointed out long ago that it is a mistake to take the standards of proof appropriate to one particular field and to designate them as universal standards for all other fields.

> It is the mark of an educated mind to expect that amount of exactness in each kind which the nature of the particular field subject admits. It is equally unreasonable to accept merely probable conclusions from a mathematician and demand strict demonstrations from an orator (Nicomachean Ethics, Volume I).

Finally, there are plenty of examples of informational programs for patients that have never been subjected to controlled study: informed consent for experimental drugs or surgery; patient package labeling for OTC drugs; and patient brochures and pamphlets produced by various organizations, including professional groups, government regulatory bodies, and pharmaceutical firms. Why hold PPIs to one standard and these other sources of information to another?

Studying the effects of available medical information for patients is difficult because we are looking for small gains in a number of areas, each of which is influenced by a number of other factors. Compliance, for instance, is affected by some that are known (comprehension, physician-patient relationship, frequency of administration, duration of illness, therapeutic effects, and side effects) and some that are unknown. An additional complication is that many of the beneficial aspects of labeling have hazy endpoints that lend themselves to overstatement or understatement (e.g., increased knowledge, improved decision-making, better risk-benefit assessments, etc.).

Rigorous scientific studies would be a formidable challenge for the most skilled investigator. They would require carefully designed studies using a large number of subjects, and they would be expensive and time consuming. Even the most detailed investigation could be criticised in that the results would not necessarily apply to the general population or to some special population (e.g., the acutely ill, the aged, diabetics, the blind, etc.). Thus if we are to wait for this kind of demonstration, we will wait forever and allow ignorance, misunderstanding, and other evils to go unchallenged for want of full proof that they can be corrected.

A more sensible approach is to develop patient package labeling gradually. A group of interested medical and pharmaceutical experts could prepare an initial draft, with the content agreed upon by the group. Such a method has been used successfully to prepare patient information for OTC drugs (Ad Hoc Working Group, 1977). A surveillance program could be established to determine the impact of the insert and to detect deficiencies. If the initial inserts do not produce the desired results, corrections could be made after experience has been gained. In essence, we would be learning from our own mistakes just as we do in other aspects of patient care. The method I propose is no more risky than blindly assuming that our current methods of informing patients are working satisfactorily. The gradual implementation-surveillance approach is appealing because it is eminently more feasible, more flexible, less expensive, and more rapidly applicable than one requiring rigorously controlled trials.

MORE PHYSICIAN TIME. Some clinicians feel that increased time will be required to discuss insert information with the patient (Fleckenstein, 1977). With oral contraceptives, however, this situation has not been a problem. Physician-patient contact patterns were reported by patients to be generally unaffected by the availability of written information (Morris et al., 1977). Even if this phenomenon does not hold true for other drug categories, increased contact between the patient and physician may be viewed positively, for it is probably this dialogue that will have the greatest influence on patient compliance. The very real possibility exists that increased time spent discussing treatment will later pay off with better patient compliance, resulting in fewer office visits and hospitalizations.

MORE SIDE EFFECTS. To my knowledge, the contribution of PPIs to the incidence of drug reactions has not been investigated. However, there is no doubt that patients will imagine and report more side effects if they are aware that the reactions can occur. Abundant evidence reveals that even patients taking placebos will report adverse effects when the possibility is suggested to them. Subjective reactions, mostly reversible and of relatively minor severity, are the most common side effects encountered with placebos. One would expect the imagined effects attributable to PPIs to involve similar complaints. These should be weighed against the side effects and adverse drug interactions that are prevented or lessened by the availability of the insert. On balance, the increased reporting of subjective side effects (if it does occur), with inherently low morbidity, is a reasonable trade-off for the fewer serious adverse drug reactions that can result from greater patient awareness.

Conclusion

Patient package labeling has far-reaching and desirable benefits. Because current methods of patient education are inconsistent, the need for more and better drug information is apparent. PPI is an appealing concept because it is workable, economical and efficient, and it is a method that is well received by patients. Arguments against the insert are not persuasive; the benefits of labeling far outweigh the potential risks. PPI's will reduce the elements of ignorance and uncertainty about drugs.

The experience with PPI's now available is encouraging, and the gradual development of PPIs and their more widespread use are desirable. The goal is to improve patient understanding about medicines; its importance is the overriding reason to take all reasonable measures to reach this end.

References

Ad Hoc Working Group:'Minimum information for sensible use of self-prescribed medicines. Lancet, 2:1017, 1977.

Clinte, J.C., and Kabat, H.F.: Improving patient compliance. J. Am. Pharm. Ass., NS 16:74, 1976.

Colcher, I.S., and Bass, J.W.: Penicillin treatment of streptococcal pharynigitis. JAMA, 222:657, 1972.

Dorsey, R.: The patient package insert. Is it safe and effective? JAMA, 238:1936, 1977.

Fleckenstein, L., Joubert, P., Lawrence, R., et al.: Oral contraceptive patient information. A questionnaire study of attitudes, knowledge and preferred information sources. JAMA, 235:1331, 1976.

Fleckenstein, L.: Attitudes toward the patient package insert—a survey of physicians and pharmacists. Drug Inform. J., 11:23, 1977.

Joubert, P., and Lasagna, L.: Patient package inserts. I, Nature, notions and needs. Clin. Pharmacol. Ther. 18:507, 1975.

Morris, L.A., Mazis, M., and Gordon, E.: A survey of the effects of oral contraceptive patient information. JAMA, 238:2507, 1977.

Sackett, D.L., Haynes, R.B., Gibson, E.S., et al,: Randomized clinical trial of strategies for improving medication compliance in primary hypertension. Lancet, 1:1207, 1975.

Sharpe, T.R., and Mikeal, R.L.: Patient compliance with antibiotic regimens. Am. J. Hosp. Pharm., 31:479, 1974.

How Appropriate is the Proposed Patient Package Labeling?

William R. Barclay, M.D.
American Medical Association, Chicago, Illinois

Patients generally rely on their physician's knowledge and experience for assurance that the drugs prescribed for them are safe and effective. Most patients do not demand a full written disclosure of their prescription drug's mode of action, indications, and potential hazards. These aspects of therapy have been happily left to the doctor, and patients rightly have assumed that this is part of the professional service for which they are paying.

However, with the introduction of birth control pills came a new type of drug, a pharmaceutical product prescribed for millions of healthy women that caused some serious adverse reactions in a small percentage of those taking it. The fact that its use was widespread and that serious side effects occasionally occurred in young people who were not previously ill resulted in proposals from consumer groups and the Food and Drug Administration (FDA) that appropriate warnings be issued when the birth control pills were dispensed. This was the first major effort to include a patient package insert (PPI) with a prescription drug. What followed was a compromise between the American Medical Association (AMA), which advocates that the physician be the patient's source of medical advice, and the FDA, which desired a new form of drug labeling. The compromise was a pamphlet, "What You Should Know About The Pill," prepared as a cooperative effort by the AMA, the FDA, and the American College of Obstetrics and Gynecology. Initially, the pamphlet was distributed by the physician or, on his direction, by the pharmacist. Evaluation of the response to this type of information disclosed a surprising degree of acceptance, understanding, and appreciation on the part of women who had received the pamphlet. This gave encouragement to those who advocated preparation of consumer information for selected drug products.

The precedent having been established by a PPI for birth control pills, the FDA has now prepared labeling for the general use of estrogens. It also proposed issuing PPIs for most, if not all, prescription drugs. There exist, however, considerable differences in opinion among consumer groups, the general public, pharmaceutical firms, pharmacists, physicians, and the FDA on the value of such labeling, on the form it should take, and on the manner of its distribution.

No adequate data exist concerning the number of patients who would take the trouble to read a PPI, how many of those who read it would comprehend it, and finally how many would heed the warnings and take appropriate action. Unfortunately, those who might benefit the most from reading a PPI will probably make the least use of such documents, either because of poor literacy or personal irresponsibility. Of even more concern to physicians than those who won't read the PPI are those who will take its warnings too seriously and be deterred from taking the medication as prescribed. In addition, there are patients who will develop symptoms through suggestibility and who will blame the physician and the medication for problems that are really caused by the PPI itself.

The form in which PPIs should be published has received much attention. A pamphlet such as "What You Should Know About the Pill" is attractive, easily readable, and reasonably comprehensive. However, it would be expensive to print, cumbersome to store for distribution, and could not possibly be placed inside the package of a medication. Limiting the amount of information given, especially in respect to minor or rare adverse side effects, would contribute to reducing the size of the PPI, but such an approach is opposed by those who advocate complete informational disclosure. Failure to mention some of the alleged toxic effects might also complicate the liability problem for pharmaceutical manufacturers.

Ideally, the PPI should emphasize the effectiveness of the drug and the importance of using it exactly as directed by the physician. Following this statement should be a listing of signs and symptoms that the patient might experience, along with common or major toxic reactions. In any event, the patient should not be expected to act as his own diagnostician and recognize a toxic reaction from its technical description. It would probably be of little help to a patient to learn that the medication prescribed might result in "thromboembolic disease." However, it would be helpful to know that the prescribing physician should be contacted in the event that chest pain, unexplained cough, shortness of breath, or pain and tenderness in the calf muscles developed. The controversy between those who view the PPI as a helpful aid to patients and physicians and those who view it as a legal document for complete disclosure is still unsettled.

Because the nature of the content has not been agreed upon, the group responsible for writing the text also remains unchosen. It is to be hoped that physicians would play a major role in preparation of the text. The United States Pharmacopoeial Convention has proposed that it be officially made responsible for preparation of the text. Whoever is selected to perform this onerous chore, final approval of the text will rest with the FDA, if the PPI is to be regarded as official.

The final issue in the debate over PPIs is who shall distribute them. The FDA would probably favor enclosure of the labeling in every prepackaged unit of drug, with some supplementary system for issuing the label in case drugs are dispensed in forms other than packages prepared by the manufacturer. The pharmacist would presumably favor any system that did not give him total responsibiliy for storing, filing, and dispensing the PPIs for every drug carried in his pharmacy. Physicians would prefer a system over which they could exercise some veto power so that some patients did not receive the PPI. Obviously, no single system can be devised that will please everyone and in fact, the final system may please no one.

One feature that everyone agrees on is the fact that PPIs will cost money to write, update, print, and distribute. Obviously, this cost will be borne by the patients. Since cost is mandated by bureaucratic regulation, quite independently of whether any individual consumer wishes to have the service, it is like the addition of one more tax on an already financially overburdened medical care system.

6

Is Measurement of Drug Blood Levels Helpful in Managing Patients?

Intelligent Use of Drug Blood Level Data is Helpful in Managing Patients

Lewis B. Sheiner, M.D.

Problems in the Use of Drug Blood Levels in Patient Management

R. John Dobbs, M.B., Ch.B., MRCP, and Sylvia M. Dobbs, M.B., Ch.B.

Clinical Response is More Important Than Measurement of Blood Levels in Managing Epileptic Patients

Samuel Livingston, M.D., and Irving Pruce, M.D.

The physician today seems athirst for blood.

Jean Fernel, *Treatise*

In the letting of blood three main circumstances are to be considered, "who, how much, when."

Robert Burton, *The Anatomy of Melancholy*

Let chemistry push her researches into the remotest accessible recesses of the living economy, and let her claim, for her own, every process, every act, every transformation, over which she can establish a legitimate jurisdiction.

Elisha Bartlett, *Philosophy of Medical Science*

Introduction

Until recently, there was little interest in using the measurement of drug levels in biologic fluids as a guide to clinical management. Today, hospital and private commercial laboratories are able to provide such measurements for an increasingly lengthy list of drugs. What is not clear, as these three essays show, is how useful such measurements are in actual practice.

Sheiner proposes a model that is hard to argue with in theory. He also lists some uses for which drug level measurements are of generally accepted value, such as in toxicologic "screens" and attempts to measure compliance or bioavailability. Sheiner then lists some of the irrational uses of drug levels, such as the attempt to make them pathognomonic and unequivocal indicators of "efficacy" or "toxicity."

Those who worship at the shrine of blood level measurements and those who decry their use would be well advised to read with care Sheiner's criteria for the rational use of drug levels for what he calls "intermediate therapeutic endpoints," as well as his list of pitfalls lying in wait for the unwary physician.

The Dobbses have compiled a comprehensive list of their own, with a host of variables that are likely to make the evaluation of blood levels difficult. The enthusiast for measuring anything and everything had better read their contribution carefully and examine and reflect upon the fascinating figures that accompany their essay.

Finally, Livingston and Pruce apply their scalpel to the literature on blood level measurements in epileptic patients. Their essay is valuable for many reasons, not the least of which is the enormous clinical experience of this Baltimore team. Antiepileptic drug levels, like digoxin levels, are very frequently measured by clinicians; Livingston and Pruce suggest that these measurements are often unnecessary or misleading or both. They make a cogent case for the importance of clinical observations, and they propose that when the patient's behavior is at variance with what the blood level would predict, it is generally wise to ignore the blood level.

Even these authors, however, see a need for drug level measurements in some situations, and their list of indications is full of sage advice for the practitioner.

All three essays seem, therefore, to agree that blood levels of drugs can represent an important source of information, but that a blind, unnatural reliance on them reflects poor medical judgment.

LOUIS LASAGNA, M.D.

Intelligent Use of Drug Blood Level Data is Helpful in Managing Patients

Lewis B. Sheiner, M.D.
University of California School of Medicine, San Francisco

Drug levels, like anything else, are good for some things and not for others. I will not discuss at length the unequivocally rational and the unequivocally irrational uses for drug level measurements. In between, however, are uses for drug levels that are genuinely controversial. These will get most of the attention in this essay, as I argue that such uses are, in fact, appropriate and valuable.

By drug level, I mean *one or more measurements of the concentration of drug or drug products in a body fluid.* Because it is not my purpose to discuss the utility of drug levels for scientific inquiry, I further restrict the body fluid in question to one derived from a patient receiving the drug. *Drug level* may thus refer to the concentration of drug or metabolite in blood, sweat, or tears, or in such less poetic fluids as urine, saliva, or blood fractions, notably plasma. The matter for debate is clear. Can such measurements be beneficial?

A convenient conceptual model for drug use states that after choosing a drug whose pharmacologic action is, in principle, likely to benefit a given patient, its benefits can be maximized only if the route of administration, the amount, and the timing of application are properly chosen. Let all these features be termed *dosage.* Dosage will determine ultimate benefit because doses of drug (via any route) give rise to concentrations of drug in blood, which in turn give rise to concentrations of drug in tissues, including those in which the drug is intended to act. Drug at its site of action presumably interacts with "receptors," ultimately to give rise to pharmacologic effects. These, in turn, interact with normal or disease-altered physiologic processes that augment or oppose the drug's effects to give rise finally to net clinical effects. These result in some net benefit (*efficacy*) or harm (*toxicity*) to the patient. In this model—at the crudest level—the greater the dosage, the higher the blood concentration; hence, the higher the tissue and active site concentration, the more receptors "occupied," and the more intense the drug's effects. Thus, because the intensity of drug effect relates directly to efficacy and toxicity, dosage relates directly to patient benefit. It does so, however, through the multi-stage "series" system I have described. Anything that causes variability or uncertainty in any stage of the system can increase variability or uncertainty in the entire system. We may thus be uncertain of the effect of a given dosage of drug on a given patient because we cannot predict (1) the blood concentration (the drug may not be absorbed completely, or it may be eliminated extra-rapidly, or extra-slowly), (2) the tissue concentration (blood supply to the site of action may be altered), (3) receptor occupancy (receptor affinity for drug may be unusual), (4) the pharmacologic effects of a given degree of receptor occupancy (unknown factors may alter the quantitative nature of the linkage), and/or (5) the resultant clinical effects (variable degrees of disease-induced alterations in normal physiologic response may be present).

In this context, it can be proved that anything

that reduces uncorrelated variability or uncertainty in any part of the overall system necessarily reduces uncertainty in the entire system. In particular, knowing the drug concentration in blood reduces uncertainty in the first step of the dosage-clinical effect relationship. This is called *pharmacokinetics*, a term encompassing the quantitative and temporal aspects of drug absorption, distribution, and elimination. Since drug level measurements can reduce pharmacokinetic uncertainty, they can reduce overall uncertainty. Because uncertainty can complicate therapeutic decision making, knowing drug levels can be useful. Stripped of some embellishments and particulars, this is the essence of my argument. It remains for me to show under what circumstances uncertainty about the dosage-effect relationship in fact confuses decisions, and in which such cases those drug level measurements actually available to us can clarify them.

Unequivocally Rational Uses of Drug Levels

Let us consider a few instances in which uncertainty is confusing, and how knowledge of drug levels can definitely clarify the situation.

What Has the Patient Taken? Clearly, when dealing with drug overdose, it is important to know what agent has been ingested. A "toxicologic screen," performed on gastric contents, blood, or urine, can often provide crucial information upon which to base therapeutic choices. Likewise, knowledge of the actual magnitude of the drug concentration in blood may prove prognostically useful if certain other information also is known, such as time of overdose ingestion.

Why is the Regimen Failing? When faced with a therapeutic regimen that appears to be ineffective, the reason may sometimes be pharmacokinetic. For example, a drug may be poorly absorbed or eliminated more rapidly than usual. Drug levels, determined during a carefully supervised and planned "experimental" dosage regimen that is designed to elucidate the relevant pharmacokinetics (Sheiner and Tozer, 1978) can be definitive in resolving the issue. The appropriate therapeutic decision obviously depends on whether inadequate drug has been given, or whether adequate drug is nonetheless ineffective.

Is the Patient Taking the Prescribed Medication? Again, it is obvious that the appropriate therapeutic decision will be quite different depending on whether a therapeutic failure represents inability of the drug to alter the course of the illness or merely refusal on the part of the patient to take prescribed medicine. Drug levels in blood or urine can often provide a definitive answer to this question.

Unequivocally Irrational Uses of Drug Levels

Is the Drug Causing Toxicity? It is important to know whether a drug is causing toxicity or if it is potentially harmful to the patient, and it is tempting to try to use drug levels to resolve this issue. Assuming that some clinical signs suggest, but do not prove, drug toxicity, it seems reasonable to diagnose definite toxicity if the level is in a range usually associated with toxic effects. Conversely, if the drug level is in a range usually unassociated with toxicity, it seems reasonable to conclude that the drug may be safely continued. Finding a toxic or nontoxic drug level may influence the diagnosis of drug toxicity, but it can rarely be definitive. Prudence usually dictates withholding a drug when toxicity is suspected, regardless of drug level, except in the most critical, lifesaving situations (Holford and Sheiner, 1977).

In essence, the variability inherent in the level-effect aspect of the dose-effect relationship means that toxic and therapeutic ranges of drug levels must overlap. Drug levels can, therefore, almost never be pathognomonic of either toxicity or lack of it.* It must be regarded in the same way as any other laboratory test, historical item, or physical sign—it may add to the totality of evidence upon which rational judgment is based, but it cannot substitute for that judgment.

This should be obvious. Still, the general inutility of drug levels for diagnostic purposes need not be accepted on theoretical grounds, as it has been empirically verified for at least one drug (Ingelfinger and Goldman, 1976).

Is the Drug Optimally Effective? This question concerns drug efficacy rather than toxicity. One can no more conclude with certainty that

*In certain extreme circumstances, drug levels can be virtually pathognomonic. If, for example, one can be sure that the blood sample for drug level assay was indeed obtained from the correct patient, and if one can further be certain that the laboratory has not made an error, and if, under these circumstances, the drug level is zero, drug toxicity can virtually be ruled out.

inefficacy is present when the drug level is low than one can assume that toxicity is present when it is high. Again, it is true that the *probability* of inefficacy is greater when the drug level is relatively low, but many other factors influence efficacy, just as they do toxicity. Thus, if the patient's clinical status is satisfactory, it makes little sense to raise dosage solely because of a low drug level. Exceptions to this statement concern certain drugs used for prophylaxis, which will be discussed in the following pages.

Controversial Uses of Drug Levels

When examining both drug efficacy and drug toxicity, if readily observable clinical endpoints are available, drug levels will usually contribute little to useful knowledge. But if clinical endpoints are not available, and this happens more often than might be thought, these measurements can be of value in certain instances.

For example, consider the treatment of pulmonary emboli with anticoagulants. The relevant therapeutic endpoint is the nonoccurrence of another embolus, and the relevant toxic endpoint is abnormal bleeding. The first can only be assessed by the *absence* of an event, and the second is too dangerous to permit to occur. We therefore must substitute an intermediate endpoint, the prothrombin time, and attempt to control that. This is rational because we believe that the prothrombin time correlates, albeit imperfectly, with both efficacy and toxicity. Its advantage relative to the true clinical endpoint is that it is easy to observe and it is continuous rather than all-or-none, and monitoring it carries little risk for the patient. Another instance is the treatment of hypertension, in which the therapeutic endpoint is prevention of stroke, kidney failure, blindness, heart failure, and other disorders. The single toxic endpoint common to most antihypertensive drugs is excessive hypotension (signalled by fainting, for example). Whereas the toxic endpoint can be directly observed, the therapeutic one is again measurable only by the *absence* of an event. It does not provide any ongoing feedback concerning the efficacy of treatment. For hypertension, therefore, an intermediate endpoint—the blood pressure—is chosen and controlled. To do so is rational because the blood pressure correlates with the true endpoint, although again, only imperfectly. If we may use some laboratory test (prothrombin time) or physical sign (blood pressure) in this way, why not the drug level? According to our conceptual scheme the drug level *should* correlate with clinical effect, and in many instances empirical evidence suggests that it does (Sheiner and Tozer, 1978). Like the prothrombin time, the drug level is relatively easy to measure and provides a continous and graded intermediate endpoint. When used as such, drug levels are being employed *prospectively* to increase the probability of benefit and to reduce the probability of harm. This is quite distinct from the *retrospective* use of drug levels for diagnosis. The prospective use is rational when certain criteria are met; the retrospective use seldom is.

All the following must simultaneously hold true if the use of drug levels as intermediate therapeutic endpoints is to be rational (Sheiner and Tozer, 1978).

A Target "Effect" Strategy is not Possible. A target effect strategy is difficult or impossible in a number of circumstances, such as when (1) the true therapeutic endpoint is delayed relative to the time available for accomplishing therapeutic regulation (as in hypertension); (2) lack of efficacy can be confused with drug toxicity, as when a new arrhythmia appears during antiarrhythmic therapy; (3) the true endpoint is not sufficiently quantitative or graded to be useful for subtle but necessary dosage adjustments; or (4) measurement of the true objective is either difficult, risky, or excessively costly.

Another Established Intermediate Endpoint (Such as Prothrombin Time) is not Available.

The Drug has a Small Therapeutic Index. This means that in any given individual, the dosage that will produce toxicity is likely to be only slightly more than that required for efficacy. Moreover, the toxicity that may appear must be of some consequence. Thus, to keep within the narrow range between efficacy and dangerous toxicity, it is important to have fine control over dosage, and a graded endpoint is required. In contrast, for a drug with a wide gap between therapeutic dosage and dosage that can cause toxicity (for example, penicillin, in the absence of allergy to it), we usually simply give somewhat more drug than the least responsive case would require, and we do not carefully monitor toxicity.

Drug Levels Must Directly Relate to Drug Effect at Most Times. The relationship between drug level and drug effect need not be perfect, however, just as that between blood pressure and stroke is not perfect. Some correlations, however, are so imperfect as to be useless, such as the one for "hit and run" drugs. These drugs irreversibly alter cellular function—as, for example, some anticancer agents do. For such drugs, the only level that might relate to drug effect would be the peak level; drug levels at other times would be irrelevant. Additionally, such drugs might have cumulative effects if cell recovery time were slow, so that even if the peak level were known, the drug's effect would be somehow dependent on all previous peak levels, not only on the current one. These complications usually preclude prospective use of drug levels. Thus, the only drugs for which levels have proven useful as an intermediate endpoint are those for which the levels relate to current effects, relatively independently of past effects. Moreover, for such drugs, this relationship holds for most of the time during therapy, so that the exact time of assessing the levels is not crucial.

The Physician Must Know How to Use the Drug Level Properly in Order to Regulate Dosage, and the Laboratory Must Provide Timely, Accurate, and Specific Assay Values to Him. The above criteria are quite restrictive, and only a handful of drugs fulfill them—a number of antibiotics, cardiac glycosides, antiarrhythmics, some psychoactive agents, and some anti-inflammatory drugs. Yet these drugs are quite important, as they are responsible for the majority of dose-related adverse effects of drugs seen in hospitals (Melmon, 1971). It is, however, worth stressing that the target level strategy applies to very few drugs. If the strategy is applied inappropriately to drugs that do not fulfill the above criteria, drug levels will be at best, useless, and at worst, dangerous.

Pitfalls in the Use of Drug Levels for Therapeutic Regulation

I will not engage in an extended discussion of how to use drug levels in the context of a target level strategy; for this the reader is referred elsewhere (Sheiner and Tozer, 1978). However, it is necessary to point out some of the pitfalls in the use of drug levels because inappropriate use, even for "appropriate" drugs, can lead to useless or harmful medical practices. I point out these problems also to show that often, when drug levels appear to mislead us, the mistake may be due to inadequate knowledge on our part rather than to any intrinsic irrationality in the use of drug levels themselves.

The most major and obvious pitfall in the use of drug levels concerns inaccuracy in their measurement or in the associated data necessary for their interpretation. Typical therapeutic plasma concentrations of drugs are usually less than 10 mg per liter, and are often less than 100 μg per liter. Such low concentrations of almost anything are difficult to measure. Therefore, poorly equipped laboratories, or ones with less than meticulous quality control or that rarely perform drug level assays, are especially likely to perform assays inaccurately. Obviously, one can make no sense of a grossly inaccurate assay, and if one proceeds as though the data are exact, great harm can result. Even if the drug assay is factual, past dosage must be known in order to make sense of it. If the dosage history is inaccurate, a wrong interpretation may result and the drug level will appear to be misleading.

In addition to the assay and the dosage history, attention must be paid to the time the assay fluid was drawn in relation to the last previous drug dose. Drug levels drawn shortly after a dose tend to be higher than those drawn midway between doses or just prior to a subsequent dose, not only because drug is eliminated during a dosage interval but because drugs are often rapidly absorbed, reach high concentrations in the blood, and then diffuse (distribute) more slowly out of the blood and into the tissues. Drug levels obtained before distribution is complete are difficult to interpret and usually cannot be used to assess how extensively a patient absorbs or eliminates a drug. This, however, is the most crucial information to be obtained from a drug level; if we know this, we can predict future levels resulting from various choices of future dosage, and we may therefore choose rationally that dosage likely to result in the target level. Drug levels drawn too soon after a dose are therefore almost useless, and if they are interpreted as if they had been drawn later, they will be misleading. This is not to say that drug levels determined soon after a dose may not correlate with drug effect at that time; they may or may not, depending on how rapidly the drug equilibrates between blood and active site. But whichever is the case, measurements taken right after a dose almost never tell us very much about the important aspects of individual pharmacokinetics. Thus, although the exact time of drawing the level is not crucial, it should not be too soon after a dose is administered.

Somewhat less prevalent as a source of confusion in interpreting drug levels are certain pharmacokinetic peculiarities of some drugs. For example, some drugs are extensively bound to serum proteins, often albumin. Drug level assays almost always measure total drug in blood or plasma, not unbound drug. However, it is usually the unbound drug that is free to diffuse to its active site, so that the unbound drug concentration in blood or plasma correlates with effect. Moreover, often only unbound drug is available to its elimination site (usually the liver or kidney) and therefore, drug elimination rate is proportional to unbound drug concentration rather than to total drug concentration. In certain metabolic states, or when albumin is low, the extent of binding of drugs may be decreased. When this happens, and dosage is kept constant, elimination for some drugs will increase until unbound levels fall to their former value. The net effect is that the same unbound drug levels will be present as were present with normal binding, but at a lower total drug level. Since unbound drug levels are the same as usual, so is drug effect. An example of such a drug is phenytoin. Its binding is usually about 90 percent, but it falls to 80 percent or less when uremia is present (Reidenberg et al., 1971). If a physician were to measure a phenytoin plasma level in a uremic patient on a standard dose, find it to be one third to one half the usual therapeutic value (10 to 20 mg per liter), and raise the phenytoin dose for this reason alone, he might cause drug toxicity. The original, apparently subtherapeutic drug level might well have been associated with a therapeutic unbound level.

This is not the only example of pharmacokinetic complexity that must be acknowledged in order to use drug levels intelligently. Some drugs exhibit nonlinear kinetics, which means that changes in drug levels are not proportional to associated changes in dosage. Some drug level assays measure inactive metabolites along with active parent compounds and some assays fail to measure active metabolites. Both situations obscure the relationship between level and effect.

The way to cope with such problems is to be aware of their possibility; ignorance misleads, drug levels do not. If a patient receiving digitalis developed paroxysmal atrial tachycardia with 2:1 block, it could be missed if every alternate P-wave on the ECG were hidden in the T-wave. (The physician could also misinterpret the ECG for another reason). In any event, if the physician then continued to give digitalis and the patient died from digitalis toxicity, would we reject electrocardiograms in general as useless or harmful? The drug level can be rejected as useless for therapeutic regulation in the context of a target level strategy only if empirical evidence concerning intelligent and informed use in such a context reveals no benefit. In fact, available empirical evidence confirms theoretical expectation and indicates the contrary: drug levels can be of considerable benefit in this context.

Empirical Results of Using Drug Levels as a Therapeutic Target

Some evidence is available for phenytoin (Lund, 1974) and certain other drugs, but the best example studied is digoxin. Initial research suggested that the incidence of toxicity with this drug, using then current methods of administration, was close to 20 percent (Beller et al., 1971). When a target level approach was used (although only in the sense that initial dosage was adjusted as far as possible to compensate for expected pharmacokinetic differences between individuals, for example, by lowering dosage in the presence of renal disease), toxicity was decreased by about half (Ogilvie and Ruedy, 1972). When a full target level strategy was used—that is, when initial doses were adjusted for expected individual pharmacokinetic peculiarities and subsequent drug levels were measured (and presumably used to insure achievement of the target) toxicity fell again by half, to about 6 percent (Koch-Weser et al., 1974). These empirical results concerning drug effect confirm others that indicate that if drug levels are measured and dosage is adjusted accordingly, target concentrations can be achieved reasonably accurately (Sheiner et al., 1975). Thus, theory and practice combine to support the use of drug levels as therapeutic targets in appropriate circumstances.

Conclusion

There are unequivocally rational uses of drug levels as well as unequivocally irrational ones. A particular application of drug levels—as intermediate therapeutic endpoints when no other superior one is available—is controversial. I believe that this use is rational and valuable, although it is not a panacea. When intelligently and appropriately used as an intermediate endpoint, drug levels can help us to individualize therapy. By doing so, the benefit-risk ratio for a number of important drugs can be increased.

References

Beller, G.A., Smith, T.W., Abelmann, W.H., Haber, E., and Hood, Jr., W.B.: Digitalis intoxication: a prospective clinical study with serum level correlations. N. Engl. J. Med. 284:989, 1971.

Holford, N., and Sheiner, L.B.: The digoxin concentration: before and after the fact (annotation). Am. Heart J. 94:529, 1977.

Ingelfinger, J.A., and Goldman, P.: The serum digitalis concentration—does it diagnose digitalis toxicity? N. Engl. J. Med. 294:867, 1976.

Koch-Weser, J., Duhme, D.W., and Greenblatt, D.J.: Influence of serum digoxin concentration measurements on frequency of digitoxicity. Clin. Pharmacol. Ther. 16:284, 1974.

Lund, L.: Anticonvulsant effect of diphenylhydantoin relative to plasma levels. Arch. Neurol. 31:289, 1974.

Melmon, K.L.: Preventable drug reactions—causes and cures. N. Engl. J. Med. 284:1361, 1971.

Ogilvie, R.I., and Ruedy, J.: An educational program in digitalis therapy. JAMA 222:50, 1972

Reidenberg, M.M., Odar-Cederlöf, I., Von Bahr, C., Borga, O., and Sjöqvist, F.: Protein binding of diphenylhydantoin and desmethylimipramine in plasma from patients with poor renal function. N. Engl. J. Med. 285:264, 1971.

Sheiner, L.B., Halkin, H., Peck, C., Rosenberg, R., and Melmon, K.L.: Improved computer-assisted digoxin therapy: a method using feedback of measured serum digoxin concentrations. Ann. Int. Med. 82:614, 1975.

Sheiner, L.B., and Tozer, T.N.: Clinical pharmacokinetics—the use of plasma concentrations of drugs. In Melmon, K.L., and Morrelli, H.F., *Clinical Pharmacology*, 2nd editiont Macmillan, Inc., 1978.

Problems With the Use of Drug Blood Levels in Patient Management

R. John Dobbs, M.B., Ch.B., D.C.H., M.R.C.P. (U.K.)
St. George's Hospital Medical School, London, England.

Sylvia M. Dobbs, M.B., Ch.B., M.Sc., M.D.
The Middlesex Hospital Medical School, London, England

When choosing a dosage regimen for a patient, one may base the decision on clinical judgment or on measurement of drug concentrations in body fluids or on a combination of the two. At best, clinical judgment involves the titration of dose against an easily measurable response. At worst, it is a guess made in a situation in which the individual variation in dose requirement is large and titration against response is not possible. In the latter instance, measurement of drug concentrations in the blood for comparison with a recommended range would seem to be indicated. However, such measurements are often a waste of both time and money. Contraindications to measurement of drug concentrations are discussed under the following headings: the drug, the assay, the patient, and the physician.

Even when there is every reason to expect drug concentration measurements to be useful, their value may be negated by practical difficulties. In such circumstances, it would be sensible to turn to prescribing aids that have been formulated from clinical data gathered under more nearly ideal conditions.

The Drug

Contraindications to the use of drug concentrations in the blood involve the response of the body to the drug (pharmacodynamics) and the handling of the drug by the body (pharmacokinetics).

Pharmacodynamics

In some situations, response to a drug is easily measured (making knowledge of its concentration irrelevant), whereas in others, the response is not obviously related to concentration.

Routine administration of a standard dose of a drug to all patients is usually not satisfactory. To obtain the best therapeutic response with minimal adverse effect, the dose of a drug should be adjusted to the needs of each patient. Preferably, individualization of dose should be obtained by the quantitative measurement of both its therapeutic and toxic effects. This may simply involve clinical observation. Drugs for which dose may be titrated against response include antihypertensives, diuretics, anticoagulants, and hypoglycemic agents. For others, such as the psychotropic, narcotic analgesic, and antiinflammatory drugs, measurement of the patient's response is more difficult, but "these problems can only be solved at the bedside and clinical pharmacology will not prosper if its practitioners spend too much time with the gas-chromatograph and too little with the patient" (Dollery, 1973). Much of the literature of clinical pharmacology is concerned with pharmacokinetics, but often no data are given to relate the kinetic measurements to the therapeutic or toxic effects of the drug concerned.

Several factors other than concentration of the drug in the blood may affect response. For example, the observed effect of the drug may be an indirect result of its action, the drug may act irreversibly, or the sensitivity of the tissues to a given concentration may be altered by environmental or pathologic influences.

The clinically desired effect of the oral anticoagulant *warfarin* is an indirect result of its action. Warfarin acts by inhibiting synthesis of vitamin K–dependent clotting factors in the liver but does not affect their catabolism. The concentration of circulating prothrombin complex depends on the rates of both synthesis and destruction of these factors. Prothrombin time, which is the usual index of the therapeutic effect of warfarin, is related to the concentration of prothrombin complex in the blood, but the time course of plasma warfarin concentration and prothrombin complex activity are not directly correlated (Nagashima, O'Reilly, and Levy, 1969). Indeed "serum levels of drugs, whose action is very slow in onset or is not rapidly reversible, are seldom useful guides to the intensity of their pharmacologic activity" (Koch-Weser, 1975).

Drugs may bind irreversibly to receptors or otherwise produce changes that persist long after there are detectable amounts of the agent in the blood. When a drug binds irreversibly to the receptor, there is no relationship between the amount attached and the plasma concentration, making the measurement of blood concentrations futile. Alkylating agents may bind in this way to receptors, and monoamine oxidase inhibitors have a prolonged effect on that enzyme. Drugs that bind irreversibly are dangerous because small repeated doses can have a cumulative effect, even when there is no accumulation of drug in the blood. Their action is persistent, since recovery depends on regeneration of the sites at which they acted.

For cases in which the response to a drug is rapid or the action is reversible, changes in tissue sensitivity may still be more relevant to the response than are blood concentrations. Tolerance to the action of a drug may develop so that increasing concentrations are needed to produce the required effect, or the effect may be no longer obtainable despite the higher concentration. Tolerance may occur because compensatory mechanisms conspire to overcome the effect of the drug. On the other hand, the tissues may be rendered more sensitive to a drug by physiologic or pathologic processes, so that toxicity may occur even when the concentration of the drug in the blood does not appear excessive.

Tissue tolerance is important with such drugs as barbiturates, ethanol, and narcotic analgesics. Although barbiturates and ethanol can induce their own metabolic inactivation by liver enzymes so that a greater dose is required to produce a given concentration in the blood, true tissue tolerance is prominent. Cross-tolerance between related compounds often occurs. Homeostatic mechanisms may overcome the effect of a drug so that the response to a given concentration diminishes or disappears. When diuretics are administered, the renin-angiotensin system is activated. The resulting secondary hyperaldosteronism causes the kidney to retain sodium and water in opposition to the action of the drug. Increased sensitivity of tissues to digitalis may be induced by several factors so that dangerous cardiac arrhythmias can occur even when serum concentrations are within the recommended therapeutic range. These factors include hypokalemia, hypomagnesemia, hypercalcemia, hypoxia, acid-base disturbance, hypothyroidism, and myocardial ischemia. A false sense of security may be derived from a report of the serum digoxin concentration in a seriously ill patient in whom several of these conditions are likely to coexist.

Pharmacokinetics

If the measurement of concentration of a drug in the blood is to be of any value, it should reflect the concentration at the site of action. This relationship may not hold for any of several reasons. If a drug produces an active metabolite, a simple relationship between the concentration of the parent compound and the pharmacologic effect cannot be assumed. Interpretation of drug concentrations in the blood is also difficult if the details of administration are not known.

After a dose has been given, concentration in the plasma may not reflect that at the site of action until distribution of the drug is complete. Even if distribution is complete when the sample is taken, plasma concentration may overestimate (for example, if the drug is highly bound to plasma proteins) or underestimate (when there is active drug uptake) the concentration at the site of action.

A drug may produce active metabolites. In fact, the agent administered may be inactive and all the observed effects caused by its metabolites. The therapeutic effect of at least 40 drugs is known to be mediated, wholly or in part, by metabolites (Drayer, 1976). Also, several drugs, notably the commonly used and easily available analgesic acetaminophen, exert their toxic effects through a metabolite. Metabolites tend to be water-soluble compounds excreted by the kidney, so that toxic metabolites are likely to accumulate if renal function is impaired.

When an active metabolite is formed, measurement of only the parent compound in blood may be of little value and can be dangerously misleading. However, it may be impractical, and certainly would be expensive, to measure several closely related compounds individually. Even if this were practicable, too little may be known about their relative pharmacologic activities to allow interpretation of the results. There may also be important differences in the duration of action of drug and metabolite. For example, the active metabolite of α-methyldopa, α-methylnoradrenalin, accumulates in the adrenergic nerve ending, where it persists long after the parent compound has been eliminated from the body. After a dose of α-methyldopa, hypotension persists for more than 24 hours, although very little methyldopa is present in plasma after eight hours (Sjoerdsma et al., 1963). An active metabolite may be formed in the liver (or intestine) during absorption of an oral dose, but not after intravenous administration, as a result of the "first pass effect." The 6-hydroxymetabolite of propranolol, like the parent drug, has beta-adrenoceptor blocking activity (Paterson et al., 1970). After intravenous administration of propranolol, the effect on exercise-induced tachycardia is proportional to $\log_{10}$ (propranolol plasma concentration), but after an oral dose, a three times greater degree of beta-blockade is seen for a given plasma propranolol concentration (Coltart and Shand, 1970). In studying the effect of propranolol on isoproterenol-induced tachycardia in hypertensives, Zacest and Koch-Weser (1972) found that in a minority of their patients (8 of 28), a given oral dose of propranolol produced a plasma concentration 2.5 times greater than it produced in the rest. However, these eight patients needed 2.6 times the plasma propranolol concentration to produce the same degree of beta blockade as the rest of the group. Presumably, they were not producing the active metabolite.

Formation of active metabolites may, in some instances, explain difficulties in correlating the effect of a drug with its plasma concentration, but such cases may also illustrate the overriding importance of clinical observation. Many physicians had formed the impression that the antiarrhythmic effects of procainamide lasted longer than expected on the basis of its half-life. This may be accounted for by the recently described activity of its major metabolite, N-acetylprocainamide (Elson et al., 1975).

A drug usually reaches its site of action by passive diffusion, but some drugs that act intracellularly may be partitioned between extracellular and intracellular water, according to the difference in pH between these sites. Disturbance in acid-base state may alter the relationship between serum concentration and concentration at the site of action (Hill, 1973).

Some drugs are bound to plasma proteins. The bound fraction is pharmacologically inactive because it cannot diffuse to the site of action. The portion of drug that is free in plasma water can equilibrate with that at the site of action. For drugs that are highly protein-bound, the measured plasma concentrations will largely represent inactive drug. If the relationship between bound and free fractions remains constant, changes in total concentration will reflect those in the active fraction. If the serum albumin concentration is low, if the binding ability of the albumin is impaired, or if there is competition for binding sites, the free fraction will be abnormally large, so that toxic effects may be seen at "therapeutic" total plasma concentrations and therapeutic effects at lower total concentrations. In patients with uremia, the ability of serum albumin to bind drugs is impaired, regardless of whether hypoalbuminemia is also present. In such patients, the unbound fraction of phenytoin is doubled or even tripled (Reidenberg et al., 1971). This may account for the increased sensitivity of uremic patients to phenytoin described by Dundee and Richards (1954). When two drugs with a high affinity for the same binding sites on plasma protein are administered together, they compete for these sites and the free concentration of one or the other may increase. These mechanisms are most important when the drug is highly bound to plasma protein (so that a small decrease in total protein binding causes a relatively large increase in free drug) and the apparent volume of distribution is small. Clinically important examples of drug displacement include that of warfarin by aspirin or phenylbutazone to produce excessive anticoagulant effect, and of tolbutamide by salicylates or phenylbutazone to produce hypoglycemia.

Some drugs reach their site of action by active transport. Since the drug accumulates at the site of action, the concentration there will not be reflected in the plasma. This applies to guanethidine, which accumulates in adrenergic nerve endings (Oates et al., 1971).

INTERACTIONS

If a patient is receiving more than one drug, two drugs may interact and enhance or oppose the action of each other. Often, drug combinations are used deliberately as a therapeutic measure to increase response or to reduce toxicity or both. Drugs may interact at or near the site of action, or more remotely, and still affect the same physiologic system (pharmacodynamic interactions). One drug may also alter plasma concentrations of another by affecting absorption, distribution, biotransformation, or elimination (pharmacokinetic interactions). In the case of pharmacodynamic interactions, measurement of concentrations of the drug involved may be uninformative because it may not be known to what extent the drugs are antagonistic or synergistic.

Pharmacokinetic interactions involving competition for plasma protein binding sites have been mentioned. Biotransformation usually inactivates drugs, so that agents that induce metabolism will reduce plasma concentrations. For example, barbiturates can reduce the effectiveness of oral anticoagulants by inducing their metabolism. Complex interactions may also occur. Phenylbutazone, like the oral anticoagulant warfarin, is highly bound to plasma albumin and is also a potent inducer of warfarin metabolism. When they are given together, phenylbutazone displaces warfarin from its binding sites and the increased amount of free warfarin in the plasma produces a greater anticoagulant effect (O'Reilly and Levy, 1970). Some of this increased amount of unbound drug is metabolized, and the total plasma warfarin concentration becomes reduced in the presence of a still elevated free fraction. Induction of the metabolism of a drug whose activity depends largely on an active metabolite, while reducing the plasma concentration of the compound administered, will increase the pharmacologic effect resulting from its administration. For example, the activity of cyclophosphamide, which itself produces little in the way of cytotoxicity, is mediated by metabolites such as 4-ketocyclophosphamide, which has more than 50 times the cytotoxic potency of cyclophosphamide (Hohorst et al., 1971). In the rat, phenobarbital, which increases the metabolism of cyclophosphamide, more than doubles its toxicity (Cohen and Jao, 1969). Cyclophosphamide toxicity has been observed in patients taking phenobarbital and other anticonvulsants when they were given usual doses of cyclophosphamide (Drummond et al., 1968).

The Assay

When a drug is assayed, an appropriate sample should be provided, the method should be sufficiently selective and sensitive, and the results obtained should be reliable.

If a blood level denotes the concentration of a drug in whole blood, the results must be interpreted with caution. It has already been pointed out that it is only drug free in solution in plasma which can equilibrate with that at the site of action, and that when a drug is substantially bound to plasma protein, the total plasma concentration overestimates the effective concentration. Similarly, drugs may partition unequally between red cells and plasma, so that total blood concentration may give a false estimate of the active concentration. Usually, drugs are taken up by red cells according to their lipid solubility, so that hardly any of a highly polar agent such as quaternary ammonium compound enters red cells (Schanker et al., 1961). The concentration of 6-mercaptopurine in human red cells is less than 1 percent of that in plasma (Loo et al., 1968), whereas that of desmethylimipramine is ten times greater than that in plasma (von Bahr and Borgå, 1971) and that of chlorthalidone is twenty times greater, or more (Sjöqvist et al., 1976).

The method of analysis used to determine the required concentration should be sufficiently sensitive for the purpose, and also sufficiently specific so as not to be interfered with by other compounds, including metabolites of the drug in question and other drugs. The assay may measure inactive metabolites as well as the parent compound and thus give a falsely high concentration, as seen, for example, with certain methods used in the fluorometric estimation of quinidine (Kessler et al., 1974). On the other hand, a specific assay may fail to measure active metabolites. Several other drugs, notably barbiturates, interfere with the spectrophotometric assay of phenytoin. If the history of ingestion of other drugs is not given to the laboratory, falsely high concentrations may be reported. Likewise, if a patient is receiving two antibiotics, and the laboratory is unaware of this, the test organism may be killed or its growth inhibited by the second, when the first is supposedly being assayed.

Laboratories vary in the precision with which they can carry out a measurement and in the accuracy of the results obtained. Internal quality control should help to improve the former and external control the latter. Many laboratories still do not employ internal controls, and workers may be unwilling to cooperate with other groups. The need for quality control has been illustrated by the wide variation in results of phenytoin estimation. In one study (Pippenger et al., 1976), samples containing four antiepileptic drugs were sent to various laboratories in the U.S.A. To insure that they did not receive special attention, the samples were sent as though they were from patients. The reported phenytoin concentration in each specimen ranged from zero to levels that would have resulted from a fatal overdose.

Even if the drug history is known and the laboratory is reliable, there may be considerable delay in the specimen reaching the laboratory. Once it has been received, the assay may take several hours to perform, or the specimen may need to be incubated overnight. In these circumstances, the results may be irrelevant to the management of the patient, especially if he is severely ill from a disease, such as a severe infection, or following an overdose.

The Patient

Before any information derived from the measurement of drug concentrations in the blood can be deemed valid, it must be ascertained whether the patient was or is complying with the dosage regimen. Poor compliance is a major problem in prolonged drug therapy. This is especially true if the therapy has to be maintained indefinitely or if the patient feels that he is not benefiting from it. For example, clinical responses to antidepressants may not occur until after two to three weeks of therapy. In a study of patients for whom antidepressants were prescribed, it was found that 59 percent had stopped taking their tablets within three weeks (Johnson, 1973).

Measurement of drug concentrations are said to be of use in detecting poor patient compliance, but results need to be interpreted with caution, and single estimations are of little value. A low concentration may mean that a patient has been complying with the physician's instructions, but that an inadequate dosage has been prescribed. Conversely, if the doctor is concerned about the adequacy of treatment, a low drug concentration found in a blood sample drawn from a noncompliant patient may lead the physician to prescribe an overdose.

In our experience, patients who have missed a prescribed treatment or dosage may attempt to compensate by taking a "loading dose" before seeing their physician. The resulting high concentration in the blood may lead to an unnecessary reduction in dose prescription, with resulting loss of therapeutic effect. In all cases, patients must be told of the importance of following any drug therapy regimen exactly as prescribed.

In addition to compliance with the dosage schedule, the response of the individual patient to the drug must be considered. Some toxic responses are not dose-dependent, and thus cannot be predicted from measurement of the drug concentration, as in idiosyncratic or allergic reactions. As well as these qualitatively abnormal tissue responses, patients show quantitative differences in tissue sensitivity. Response to some drugs varies widely between individuals and may not be accounted for by differences in drug concentrations.

Variability in response can be exaggerated by disease. Asthmatics may develop attacks at concentrations of nonselective beta-adrenoceptor blocking agents that would not produce bronchoconstriction in normal volunteers or nonasthmatic patients. Figure 6-1 shows the relationship between resting ventricular rate and serum digoxin concentration in patients with atrial fibrillation. Although there was no overall correlation between rate and concentration, when the patients were divided into those without serious atrioventricular conduction impairment and those with such an impairment, a significant correlation was found in each group. The corresponding regression lines are approximately parallel, indicating that those with impaired conduction were not more sensitive than the others to digoxin, in that a given change in digoxin concentration did not produce a larger decrease in rate. However, the absolute heart rate in these patients became unacceptably slow at concentrations recom-

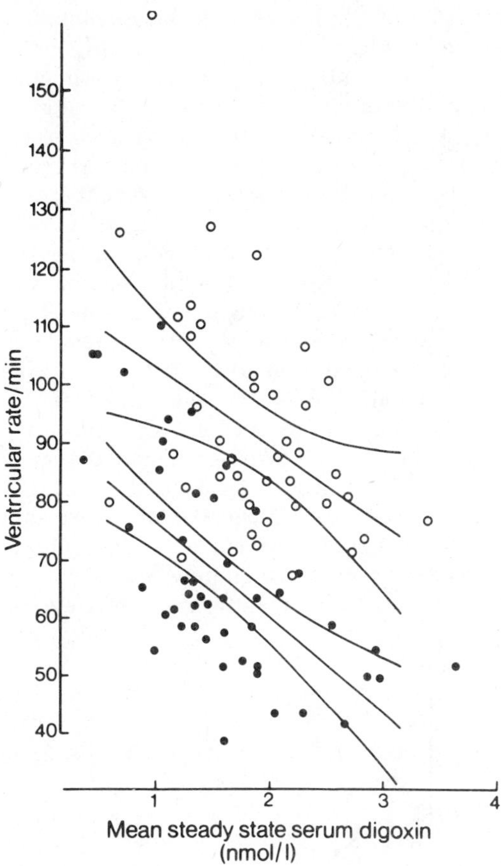

Figure 6-1. Relationship between resting ventricular rate and mean steady state serum digoxin concentration attained in atrial fibrillation. Forty-two measurements of resting ventricular rate and the corresponding serum digoxin concentration are shown in patients without serious impairment of atrioventricular conduction (○) and 49 measurements in those with evidence of impaired conduction (●). (Dobbs et al., 1977).

mended for control of rapid ventricular rates.

What constitutes a therapeutic concentration depends on the patient and on the condition to be treated. Hoeschen and Cuddy (1975) showed a linear improvement in left ventricular function with increasing serum digoxin concentrations toward the upper end of the standard therapeutic range. However, in patients with atrial fibrillation and impairment of atrioventricular conduction treated with digoxin for heart failure, serum concentrations at the lower end of the range are more appropriate because of the aforementioned effect on ventricular rate (Dobbs et al., 1977). The recommended serum concentration of salicylates for prevention of valvular heart disease in patients with rheumatic fever is above 350 mg per liter (Coburn, 1943), but analgesia may be obtained at lower concentrations. Thus, if a therapeutic range defined in one situation is extrapolated too freely to other situations, patients may be exposed needlessly to high concentrations of drug and risks of toxicity. On the other hand, if toxicity was initially observed in a particularly sensitive group, other patients may be deprived of benefits that are only possible at higher concentrations. If tolerance develops to a drug, then not only is there a difference in the therapeutic range amongst individuals but the range will alter with time in the same individual.

The Doctor

As mentioned, it is neither necessary nor useful to measure the concentration in the blood for many drugs. Theoretically, such measurements might be helpful (1) during treatment with drugs that have a small therapeutic ratio, (2) when the response is difficult to judge clinically, and (3) where the therapeutic range of concentrations has been clearly defined. Thus, "the monitoring of plasma levels of hypoglycemic, antihypertensive, and anticoagulant drugs is not justified, while an open mind has to be kept in relation to drugs affecting subjective variables, such as mood and pain, and drugs used prophylactically, such as phenytoin, lithium, and antiarrhythmics. The list of drugs is at present short . . ." (Sjöqvist et al., 1976). However, even when an assay that is both sensitive and selective is available, and the patient is known to be compliant, little can be achieved by measurement of the drug concentration if the doctor is unable to make rational decisions based on the result. He needs to be adequately informed about the drug in general and about the circumstances of the particular case in which measurement of concentration is requested.

If the details of administration of a drug be disregarded or unknown, the interpretation of its concentration in the blood is difficult. If a drug has been taken at regular intervals for a short time and is still accumulating, the concentrations measured will underestimate those obtaining under steady state conditions. It takes about five elimination half-lives for "steady state" to be reached. Samples taken while the drug is accumulating may be misleading as to the effectiveness or the safety of maintenance therapy. The elimination half-life of digoxin in a patient with impaired renal function may be a week. If he is started cautiously on digoxin in the hospital at a maintenance dose, instead of being given an initial loading dose, he may well be discharged before his blood concentrations reach a steady state. The same maintenance dose that resulted in "safe" concentrations in the hospital may cause toxicity after discharge. The concentration in the blood also varies considerably with time following a dose. An overdose of a hypnotic drug generally is a single dose, or several doses taken over a short period. The interval between time of ingestion and time of the blood sample is often uncertain. It is not surprising, then, that the plasma concentrations of barbiturates, glutethimide, and methaqualone found on admission of the patient to the hospital correlate poorly with the depth and duration of coma. A similar poor relationship exists between severity of symptoms of salicylate poisoning and salicylate concentrations. However, if the plasma concentration can be corrected for the time after ingestion, the correlation is greatly improved (Done, 1960).

The relationship between the concentration/time curve of the drug in plasma and the response varies considerably among drugs. It may be different not only for toxic and therapeutic effects of one drug but also for the use of that drug in different situations. In much of the information available about the relationship between response and blood levels, this is not taken into account, or unwarranted assumptions about the relationship are made. In the use of penicillins, it may be advantageous to allow the trough concentration to fall below the *in vitro* minimum inhibitory concentration, since these agents act best against rapidly dividing organisms. However, there are relatively inaccessible situations, such as vegetations on the heart valves in bacterial endocarditis, where the peak and trough concentrations seen in the plasma will not be reflected. Moreover, a very high mean plasma concentration is necessary to achieve adequate bactericidal concentrations at such a site. With aminoglycoside antibiotics, it is commonly recommended that high peak concentrations should be avoided in order to prevent ototoxicity. The inner ear, where the damage occurs, is also a deep or inaccessible compartment. Line, Poole, and Waterworth (1970) using streptomycin, and Dobbs (1973) using gentamicin, have shown independently that the trough concentration bears more relation to the development of ototoxicity than does the peak, presumably because the trough is a better reflector of the total area under the concentration/time curve and therefore of the exposure of the inner ear to blood containing the antibiotic.

It is frequently assumed that by achieving serum digoxin concentrations within the range of 1.3 to 2.6 nmol per liter, the prevalence of all forms of toxicity is greatly reduced. Smith and Haber (1970) found that 87 percent of their patients with electrocardiographic signs of toxicity had concentrations of 2.6 nmol per liter and above, and 90 percent of those without such signs had concentrations below 2.6 nmol per liter. Dobbs and colleagues (1977) titrated dose against concentration in 86 patients, starting from the initial maintenance dose, with the aim of achieving a mean concentration in the lower half of the therapeutic range. Figure 6–2 shows that symptoms occurred frequently at concentrations between 1.3 and 2.6 nmol per liter, but ten patients exceeded this range without developing symptoms. There was no significant difference between the lowest concentration at

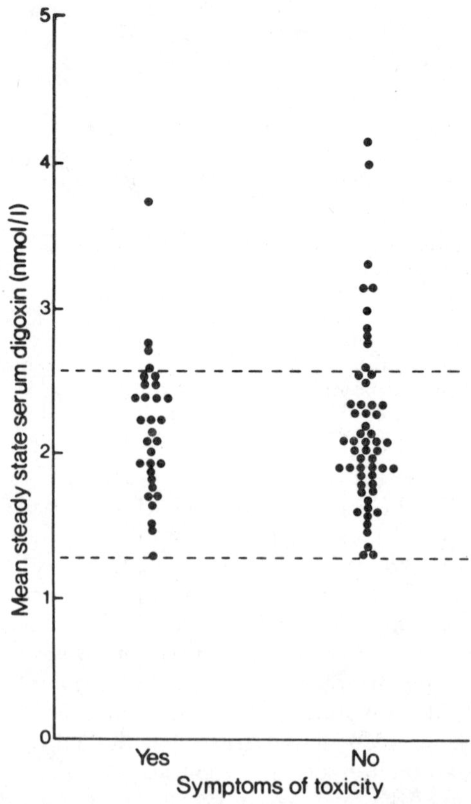

Figure 6–2. Risk of symptoms of toxicity in relation to the mean steady state serum digoxin concentration. The lowest concentration at which 31 patients experienced symptoms of toxicity can be compared with the highest concentrations achieved by the 55 patients who remained symptom-free. The dotted lines enclose the generally accepted therapeutic range. (Dobbs et al., 1977).

which symptoms of toxicity were experienced in 31 patients (2.15 ± 0.09 (1 SE) nmol per liter) and the highest concentrations achieved by the 55 patients who remained symptom-free (2.14 ± 0.08 nmol per liter). Figure 6–3 shows the serum concentration immediately before the daily dose and at one, two, four, and seven hours after the dose in ten of the patients with symptoms other than vomiting. A similar series of samples was taken before and after the largest daily dose given to 10 patients selected randomly from the group without symptoms of toxicity. There was no significant difference between assay results in toxic and nontoxic patients at any of the sampling times. The 31 patients with symptoms of toxicity had a significantly lower serum creatinine concentration and body weight than the 55 patients without symptoms. Since there was no significant difference in creatinine clearance between the groups, it is suggested that toxic patients had lower muscle masses than those who were symptom-free. Thus, in these patients, serum digoxin concentrations would have been of less value in avoiding symptoms than other, more readily available information.

The quoted digoxin concentrations refer either to the mean steady state concentration (i.e., the average serum concentration during the dosage interval) or to an estimate of this. If concentrations are measured in samples taken without regard to their time relationship to the dose, it is hardly surprising that the overlap between cardiotoxic and noncardiotoxic concentrations will be greater than that described by Smith and Haber (1970). Cardiotoxicity is unrelated to peak serum digoxin concentrations. Bertler, Bergdahl, and Karlsson (1974) produced peak concentrations of 35 to 122 nmol/l in 22 patients with suspected or proven myocardial infarction complicated by left ventricular failure. The patients had been given intravenous injections of from 0.75 to 1.0 mg. of digoxin at rates from 0.125 to 0.75 mg per minute. The plasma digoxin concentration remained above 2.6 nmol/l for at least two hours in all patients. No extracardiac symptoms occurred, and the only arrhythmia seen was moderate sinus bradycardia in one patient with sick sinus syndrome. Figure 6–4 shows two of the concentration/time curves.

Whether the response is related to the peak concentration, to the concentration just before the next dose, or to the mean steady state con-

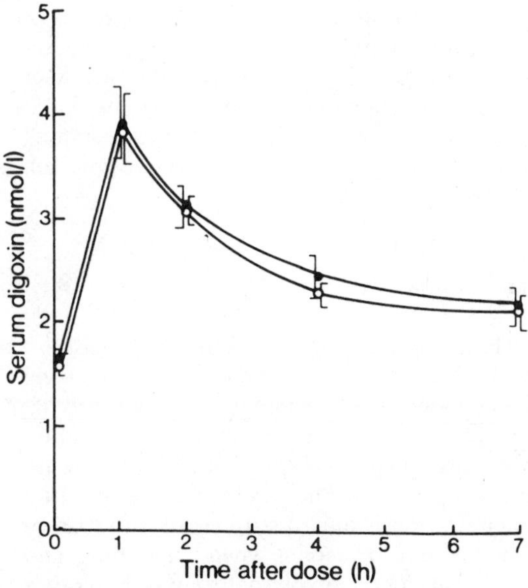

Figure 6-3. Serum digoxin concentration/time curves in 10 of the 31 patients with symptoms of toxicity (•) and 10 of the 55 symptom-free patients (○). The mean concentrations (± 1 s.e. mean) achieved by the two groups are compared at each of five sampling times (Dobbs et al., 1977).

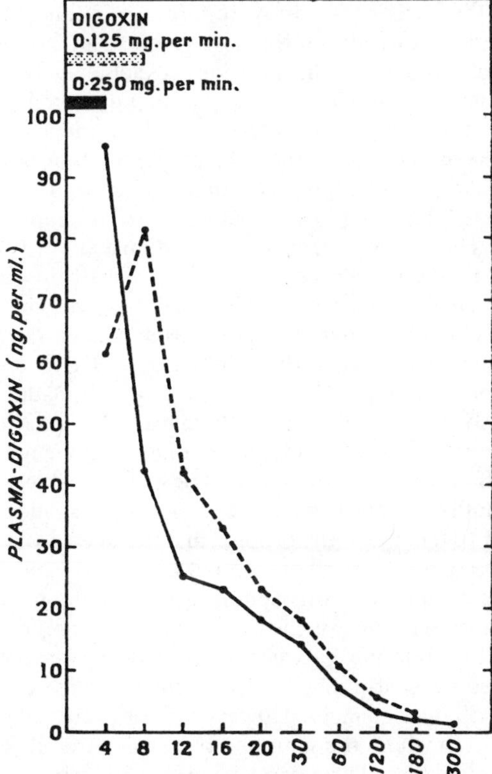

Figure 6-4. Plasma-digoxin concentration after administration of 1 mg of digoxin intravenously at two different injection rates. (Bertler et al., 1974).

centration, if the timing of the sample is ignored, accurate assessment of further dose requirements is impossible and comparison of results between different laboratories becomes meaningless (Smith and Rawlins, 1973). Usually, a single serum sample must suffice as an estimate of the mean steady state concentration. For digoxin, the ability to predict the mean concentration from a single assay result is maximal at about 7 hours after the dose. At this time, the concentration assayed approximately equals the mean concentration (Dobbs et al., 1976). Especially when dealing with outpatients, it is rarely possible to take the sample at a chosen time after the dose, and the most one can hope for is that the time interval between the last dose and the taking of the sample can be established so that an estimate of the mean concentration can be made from the result of the assay. Even when equations relating the concentration at different sampling times to the mean steady state concentration are available, few assay services are sufficiently oriented towards practical patient care to include such estimates routinely in their reports.

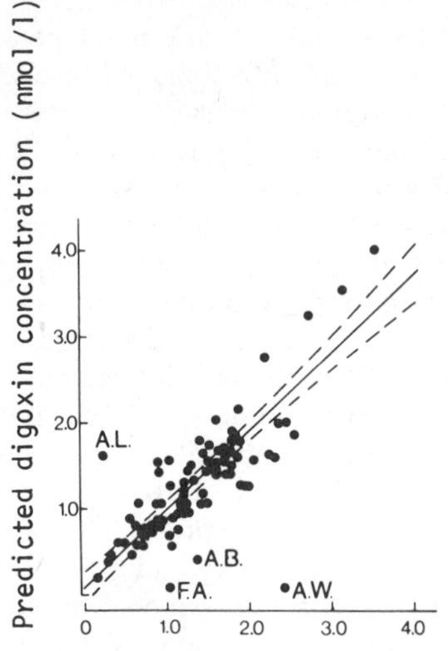

Figure 6-5. Comparison of the serum concentrations predicted following a dosage change with that measured by radioimmunoassay in 87 outpatients. The regression line and its 95 percent confidence limits are shown. (Dobbs et al., 1976.)

When the maintenance dose is to be adjusted on the basis of an assay report, can a linear relationship between the dose given to an individual and the concentration he achieves be assumed? Doubling the dose will not double the steady state concentration if the patient is noncompliant or if the rate of elimination of the drug is constant, i.e., of zero order. If a linear relationship exists between size of maintenance dose and serum concentration achieved, the predicted concentration (P) achieved by a chosen maintenance dose (D_2) will be given by $P = C_1D_2/D_1$, where C_1 is the serum concentration achieved when the original dose (D_1) was given. In Figure 6–5, this prediction (P) is made for 87 patients receiving daily digoxin doses and compared with the measured digoxin concentration achieved by the second dose (D2). Tablet counting revealed that two patients (F.A. and A.B.) did not take the original maintenance dose as prescribed. Another two patients (A.W. and A.L.) admitted retrospectively to noncompliance with one of the two regimes. A significant correlation between predicted and measured concentration was found for the remaining 83 dose changes. However, these were patients in whom the sampling time was carefully standardized. They were receiving digoxin in calendar packs and given every other encouragement to comply. In routine practice, a much larger proportion of patients will not achieve concentrations proportional to the dose given.

Phenytoin is eliminated by first order kinetics at lower plasma concentrations, and by zero order kinetics at higher ones. The limited capacity of the enzymes involved in its metabolism is saturated at higher concentrations. Figure 6–6 illustrates the serum concentrations of phenytoin obtained by a wide range of doses in three patients. In each patient, the effect of a given change in dose varies with the initial serum concentration. The danger of assuming proportionality between dose and concentration achieved is obvious.

Prescribing Aids

There is a substantial difference between what is known about drug therapy and the level of knowledge we commonly apply to solving clinical problems. The primary aim of education in clinical pharmacology should be to ensure that drugs are used as wisely as possible. Drug concentration is only one piece of information to be taken into account when prescribing, and it will only occasionally determine the course of action. Therefore, instruction in how best to use drug assays should be given a relatively low priority.

Theoretically, by monitoring drug concentrations, individual differences in absorption,

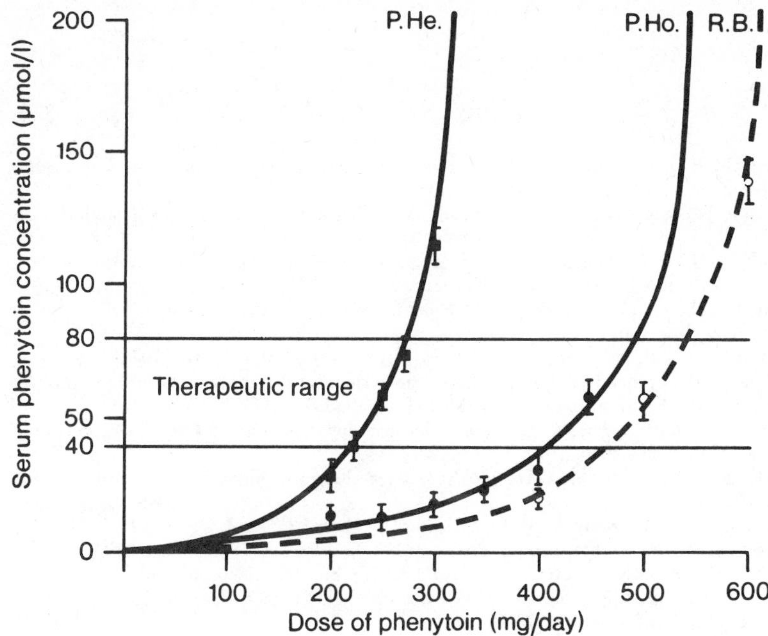

Figure 6-6. The serum levels obtained for three different patients at different doses of phenytoin (Oxley, 1976).

distribution, metabolism, and excretion are bypassed, but as has been pointed out, interpretation of blood concentrations may involve many practical difficulties. Perhaps the greatest of these is the step from the assay result to the choice of dose. In contrast, with the use of prescribing aids, the dose is obtained directly from the patient's characteristics. Ideally, these aids will have been formulated from data on a sufficiently large and varied population for them to include advice as to the different dose requirements of special groups (e.g., patients in atrial fibrillation with impaired atrioventricular conduction). Every effort will have been made to insure maximal compliance, and drug administration and sampling times for assays will have been standardized. The assay will have had adequate quality control. At present, the greatest potential use of prescribing aids is for drugs that are mainly excreted by the kidney, such as aminoglycoside antibiotics and digoxin.

References

Bertler, A., Bergdahl, B., and Karlsson, E.: Plasma digoxin concentrations after an intravenous loading dose. Lancet 2:958, 1974.

Coburn, A.F.: Salicylate therapy in rheumatic fever. A rational therapy. Bull. Johns Hopkins Hosp. 73:435, 1943.

Cohen, J.L., and Jao, J.Y.: Enzymatic basis of cyclophosphamide activation by rat liver. Proc. Am. Assoc. Cancer Res. 10:14, 1969.

Coltart, D.J., and Shand, D.G.: Plasma propranolol levels in the quantitative assessment of β-adrenergic blockade in man. Br. Med. J. 3:731, 1970.

Dobbs, S.M.: Aminoglycoside ototoxicity. M.Sc. thesis. University of Manchester, 1973.

Dobbs, S.M., Kenyon, W.I., and Dobbs, R.J.: Maintenance digoxin after an episode of heart failure: placebo-controlled trial in outpatients. Br. Med. J. 1:749, 1977.

Dobbs, S.M., Parkes, J., and Rodgers, E.M.: Digoxin: linearity between dose and serum concentration. Brit. J. Clin. Pharmacol. 3:940, 1976.

Dobbs, S.M., Rodgers, E.M., Mawer, G.E., and Kenyon, W.I.: Serum digoxin concentrations. Brit. J. Clin. Pharmacol. 3:674, 1976.

Dobbs, S.M., Rodgers, E.M., Kenyon, W.I., Livshin, D., Slater, E., and Godsmark, B.: Digoxin prescribing in perspective. Brit. J. Clin. Pharmacol. 4:327, 1977.

Dollery, C.T.: Pharmacokinetics: master or servant? Eur. J. Clin. Pharmacol. 6:1, 1973.

Done, A.K.: Salicylate intoxication. Significance of measurements of salicylate in blood in cases of acute ingestion. Pediatrics, 26:800, 1960.

Drayer, D.E.: Pharmacologically active drug metabolites: therapeutic and toxic activities, plasma and urine data in man, accumulation in renal failure. Clin. Pharmacokinet. 1:426, 1976.

Drummond, K.N., Hillman, D.A., Marchessault, J.H.V., and Feldman, W.: Cyclophosphamide in nephrotic syndrome of childhood. Can. Med. Assoc. J. 98:524, 1968.

Dundee, J.W., and Richards, R.K.: Effects of azotemia on the action of intravenous barbiturate anesthesia. Anesthesiology 15:333, 1954.

Elson, J., Strong, J.M., Lee, W.K., and Atkinson, A.J.: Antiarrhythmic potency of N-acetyl-procainamide. Clin. Pharmacol. Ther. 17:134, 1975.

Hill, J.B.: Salicylate intoxication. N. Engl. J. Med. 288:1110, 1973.

Hoeschen, R.J., and Cuddy, T.E.: Dose-response relation between therapeutic levels of serum digoxin and systolic time intervals. Am. J. Cardiol. 35:469, 1975.

Hohorst, H.J., Ziemann, A., and Brock, M.: 4-ketocyclophosphamide, a metabolite of cyclophosphamide. Arzneim. Forsch. 21:1254, 1971.

Johnson, D.A.W.: Treatment of depression in general practice. Brit. J. Med. 2:18, 1973.

Kessler, K.M., Loowenthal, D.T., Warner, H., Gibson, T., Brigs, W., and Reidenberg, M.M.: Quinidine elimination in patients with congestive heart failure or poor renal function. N. Engl. J. Med. 290;706, 1974.

Koch-Weser, J.: The serum level approach to individualisation of drug dosage. Eur. J. Clin. Pharmacol. 9:1, 1975.

Line, D.L., Poole, G.W., and Waterworth, P.M.: Serum streptomycin levels and dizziness. Tubercle 51:76, 1970.

Loo, T.L., Luce, J.K., Sullivan, M.P., and Frei, E.: Clinical pharmacologic observations on 6-mercaptopurine and 6-methylthiopurine nucleoside. Clin. Pharmacol. Ther. 9:180, 1968.

Nagashima, R., O'Reilly, R.A., and Levy, G.: Kinetics of pharmacologic effects in man: the anticoagulant action of warfarin. Clin. Pharmacol. Ther. 10:22, 1969.

Oates, J.A., Mitchell, J.R., Feagin, O.T., Kaufmann, J.S., and Shand, D.G.: Distribution of guanidinium antihypertensives: mechanism of their selective action. Ann. NY Acad. Sci. 179:302, 1971.

O'Reilly, R.A., and Levy, G.: Pharmacokinetic analysis of the potentiating effect of phenylbutazone on anticoagulant action of warfarin in man. J. Pharm. Sci. 59:1258, 1970.

Oxley, J.: Drug therapy in epilepsy. Hospital Update 2:327, 1976.

Paterson, J.W., Conolly, M.E., Dollery, C.T., Hayes, A., and Cooper, R.G.: The pharmacodynamics and metabolism of propranolol in man. Pharmacol. Clin. 2:127, 1970.

Pippinger, C.E., Penry, J.K., White, B.G., Daly, D.P., and Buddington, R.: Interlaboratory variability in determination of plasma antiepileptic drug concentrations. Arch. Neurol. 33:351, 1976.

Reidenberg, M. M., Odar-Cederlöf, I., von Bahr, C., Borgå, O., and Sjöqvist, F.: Protein binding of diphenylhydantoin and desmethylimipramine in plasma from patients with poor renal function. N. Engl. J. Med. 285:264, 1971.

Schanker, L.S., Nafpliotis, P.A., and Johnson, J.M.: Passage of organic bases into human red cells. J. Pharmacol. Exp. Ther. 133:325, 1961.

Sjöqvist, F., Borgå, O., and Orme, M.L.: Fundamentals of clinical pharmacology. In Avery, G.S., *Drug Treatment. Principles and Practice of Clinical Pharmacology and Therapeutics.* Littleton, Mass., Publishing Sciences Group, Inc., 1976.

Sjoerdsma, A., Vendsalu, A., and Engelman, K.: Studies on the metabolism and mechanism of action of methyldopa. Circulation 28:492, 1963.

Smith, T.W., and Haber, E.: Digoxin intoxication: the relationship of clinical presentation to serum digoxin concentration. J. Clin. Invest. 49:2377, 1970.

Smith, S.E., and Rawlins, M.D.: *Variability in Human Drug Response,* 1st edition. London, Butterworth and Co., Publishers, 1973.

von Bahr, C., and Borgå, O.: Uptake, metabolism and excretion of desmethylimipramine and its metabolites in the isolated perfused rat liver. Acta Pharmacol. Toxicol. 29:359, 1971.

Zacest, R., and Koch-Weser, J.: Relation of propranolol plasma level to β-blockade during oral therapy. Pharmacology 7:178, 1972.

Clinical Response is More Important than Measurement of Blood Levels in Managing Epileptic Patients

Samuel Livingston, M.D.
Johns Hopkins Hospital Epilepsy Clinic

Irving Pruce, M.D.
Samuel Livingston Epilepsy Diagnostic and Treatment Center

Since almost any and all medical data may be of some potential diagnostic, therapeutic, or prognostic value, no one would dispute the claim that anticonvulsant blood levels may be helpful in the treatment of the patient with epilepsy. However, the concern of physicians today is whether successful management of the epileptic patient mandates that serum concentration examinations be performed at regular intervals throughout the course of anticonvulsant drug therapy.

Our experience over the past 15 years with thousands of phenobarbital and phenytoin (Dilantin) serum levels, and that with hundreds of carbamazepine (Tegretol), ethosuximide (Zarontin), and primidone (Mysoline) blood levels during relatively recent times, has demonstrated that it is unnecessary to perform these examinations in the overwhelming majority of patients and, with the exception of an occasional instance, that effective therapeutic regimens can be established and maintained solely on clinical bases. Serum levels have little to offer when the patient responds to drug therapy and when the physician is cognizant of the side effects and some of the basic pharmacokinetics of antiepileptic medications.

Others are in agreement with our findings (Fincham and Schottelius, 1973; Herberg, 1975). We also call attention to recent monographs by various authorities in which treatment procedures are based almost entirely on clinical grounds (Farmer, 1975; Gold and Carter, 1972; Menkes, 1975; Nelhaus, 1976). In addition, we would be remiss if we did not acknowledge the monumental results achieved in the treatment of epileptic seizures prior to the advent of quantitative drug concentration techniques by such eminent American epileptologists as Aird, Bridge, Keith, Lennox, Merritt, Peterman, and Putnam (to name but a few), whose successes were attributable to the utilization of sound and frequently brilliant clinical methodology.

Although procedures for the measurement of phenobarbital and phenytoin in the blood had been available since 1948 and 1956 respectively, anticonvulsant serum levels were not extensively used until the introduction of gas-liquid chromatographic techniques for the simultaneous determination of multiple drug blood levels. This process led some physicians to believe that the treatment of epilepsy would not only be revolutionized but rendered relatively simple, so that in this new "era of pushbutton epileptology," the administration of anticonvulsants could be so "scientifically individualized" that almost all patients would have their seizures satisfactorily controlled with little or no toxicity. Enthusiasm approached fanaticism in some instances, and many authors dogmatically proclaimed that blood level determinations were indispensable in the management of patients with seizure disorders. Practitioners were frequently confronted with such admonitions as "Monitoring of plasma DPH concentrations, as with other anticonvulsants, is essential in the therapy of the epilepsies" (Sherwin et al., 1974). It has even been claimed that gas-liquid chromatography "has changed the outlook for epileptic patients" (Kutt and Penry, 1974). The following ignominious affront to the clinician merits repetition because of its sheer absurdity: "Unless the physician knows the serum level he cannot now make rational adjustments in therapy" (Freeman and Lietman, 1973). Suffice it to state at this point that time and experience have not confirmed these theories—at least not in the general epileptic outpatient population.

It is frequently asserted, without documentation, that blood levels enable the physician to (1) individualize and tailor the dosage of medication for each patient (2) adjust the dosage much more accurately and scientifically, and (3) minimize or prevent untoward reactions. Some illustrative statements follow.

> The availability of gas chromatographic means of measuring blood levels of the most common anticonvulsant drugs has been a powerful weapon for the clinician, who can now adjust dosage much more scientifically and accurately (Scheinberg, 1977).

> . . . With the general availability of laboratory methodology to determine the concentrations of anticonvulsants in serum, dosages of these drugs can be individually tailored to the requirements of the patient rather than having the same dose administered to each patient. In this way the differences in metabolic rates between patients will be taken into consideration and side effects will be minimized (Committee on Drugs, American Academy of Pediatrics, 1973).

> . . . In a significant number of cases, tolerance to clinical manifestations of toxic drug concentrations may exist, making clinical assessment alone not an efficient indicator of drug concentrations capable of exerting untoward reactions in nervous system, bone marrow, liver, etc. These reactions can now be avoided by monitoring the serum concentration of each drug at appropriate intervals (Glaser, 1973).

We reject claims that monitoring of antiepileptic drugs now allows the individualization of dosage because of the implication that prior to the development of techniques for measuring serum concentrations, dosage schedules were not adapted to each patient's particular requirements. Twenty-five years ago, we stressed that the dosage of anticonvulsant medication varies from patient to patient and that "the proper dosage is that amount which controls a patient's seizures and does not produce untoward reactions to the extent that they interfere with his general well-being" (Livingston, 1954). At that time, we also emphasized that "the administration of Dilantin requires careful supervision because the dose producing a therapeutic effect frequently approaches that at which unpleasant side effects appear." The individualization of dosage has always been a basic principle of antiepileptic therapy in our practice, and we have signified its importance repeatedly throughout the years. "Each patient requires exact and painstaking individual titration of the dosage of antiepileptic medication appropriate for the specific type of epilepsy . . ." (Livingston, 1966). We have found it necessary to monitor blood levels only occasionally in order to provide a "custom tailored" treatment program.

We also repudiate the allegation that adjustments in dosage based upon the results of serum drug levels are "much more scientific" than those made on clinical grounds, and we offer the following resume of a case history, which was cited as an example of the value of blood levels (Fincham and Schottelius, 1973), in support of our position:

> A patient with uncontrolled seizures was receiving phenytoin (300 mg) daily, and had a blood level of 2.5 mcg per ml. The dosage was increased to 400 mg daily, and the serum level rose to 8.2 mcg per ml, but the seizures persisted. The daily dosage was increased to 500 mg and the corresponding blood level of 15.5 mcg per ml was associated with improved seizure control.

We propose that the same increases in dosage with resultant seizure benefit could have been accomplished without having performed even one blood level determination—although we would have raised the dosage in smaller increments—and at a considerable saving to the patient in time, convenience, and expense. We fail to understand how adjustments in dosage predicated on clinical assessment can be labeled "less scientific" than identical dosage changes made on the basis of blood levels, unless one regards the brain as a "less scientific" instrument than a laboratory procedure.

Neither do we accept the assertion that monitoring blood levels enables the physician to regulate the dosage "much more accurately," with the *possible* exception of infants receiving phenytoin and some infants receiving phenobarbital, and alterations of the dosage of phenytoin when the serum concentration is within the "therapeutic range." It has been our general experience that dosage adjustments based on good clinical analysis are as accurate and effective as those predicated on serum concentration values.

Based on the use of phenytoin in approximately 4000 patients, most of whom were children, we concluded in 1956 that it "is not a very valuable drug for the treatment of convulsive disorders of infants and young children since it is frequently impossible to determine the maximal tolerated dosage" (Livingston, 1956). Our experience during the ensuing 23 years, which included serum level measurements in hundreds of infants and young children, has confirmed and even reinforced our earlier evaluation, and we have recommended for many years that phenytoin not be prescribed as the initial anticonvulsant to patients of these ages (Livingston, 1968). We have found that phenytoin blood levels in infants may establish whether the concentration is within the nebulous "therapeutic range," but they are of little value in proving intoxication, unless, of course, clinical signs of overdosage such as extreme drowsiness or unconsciousness are apparent. One cannot be positive that a blood level within the "therapeutic range" in infants is unassociated with side effects such as ataxia or diplopia, or conversely, that a value in the "toxic range" is actually accompanied by symptoms of toxicity. Moreover, it has not even been definitely established that the "therapeutic ranges" are the same for both children and adults; this, of course, is also true for the "toxic ranges." Most physicians have merely extrapolated the adult "therapeutic" and "toxic" values to children, but supportive data are generally lacking or inadequate.

Very few practicing physicians are cognizant of the tenuous quality and the instability of blood levels in the phenytoin "therapeutic range," i.e., that small alterations in the dose when the serum concentration is in this area may cause dramatic changes in the blood level and result in either an increase in seizure frequency or in symptoms of intoxication. It should be clearly understood that even an increase of 25 mg of phenytoin daily may thrust a blood level from the therapeutic zone well into the toxic range. Therefore, it is obvious that even if one routinely performs phenytoin serum levels, accuracy of dosage regulation is not assured unless the physician is intimately familiar with the drug's pharmacokinetics, and even then accuracy is certainly not guaranteed. For example, it has been reported recently that a patient receiving 225 mg of phenytoin daily, with a serum concentration of 14 mcg per ml, experienced clinical signs of intoxication and presented a blood level of 48 mcg per ml following an increase in dosage of 25 mg per day (Johannessen, 1975).

Although our work with phenytoin blood levels was limited in 1966, we had achieved sufficient clinical practice to appreciate that the relationship between the phenytoin dose and the serum concentration was not linear and that the blood level rose with increasing steepness as the dose was elevated. We recommended, therefore, that increases in phenytoin dosage above the conventional amount be made in small increments such as 30 or 50 mg daily (Livingston, 1966). If this procedure is employed, it is generally unnecessary to monitor the phenytoin blood level, even if the serum concentration should be in the "therapeutic range."

Statements implying that untoward reactions can be prevented or minimized by adjusting the drug dosage according to the blood level are appealing, but they grossly oversimplify complex pharmacodynamic and pharmacokinetic phenomena. As stated previously, phenytoin blood levels in the "therapeutic range" are highly unstable, and many factors not under the control of the prescriber, such as increased bioavailability, can cause an elevation into the toxic range with concomitant side effects. Since there is great interindividual variation in the limits of the so-called "toxic range," some patients may become intoxicated at very low serum concentrations, whereas others remain free of clinical signs of toxicity despite blood levels well in excess of the upper boundaries of the "therapeutic range." It should also be noted that the "toxic range" for children may be quite different from that of adults, as previously stated, so that blood levels that are nontoxic in children may be associated with a significant incidence of intoxication in adults (Livingston, 1966; Melchior et al., 1971). In addition, "even if one maintains optimal drug therapy and avoids intoxication by adequate monitoring of serum levels, unwanted side effects may accumulate over the years" (Meinardi et al., 1977).

We disagree with the assertion that untoward reactions in bone marrow and liver, for example, "can now be avoided by performing blood level determinations at appropriate intervals" (Glaser, 1973). There is no correlation between the height of the serum concentration and the occurrence of side reactions in systems other than the central nervous system. In the case of phenytoin, but not with other anticonvulsants, there appears to be a fair to good relationship between the blood level and untoward reactions in the central nervous system in most patients. On the other hand, with phenobarbital for example, the blood level that is associated with drowsiness varies so much from patient to patient that it is generally unreliable as an indicator of intoxication, and we employ clinical assessment almost exclusively in determining toxicity in patients receiving this drug.

The primary objective in the treatment of epilepsy is to attain complete control of seizures or at least to reduce their frequency to the extent that the patient may lead an essentially normal life. It is not surprising, therefore, that the "promise"' of a significant increase in the proportion of controlled patients by virtue of routine blood level determinations had enormous impact and led many physicians to adopt serum concentrations as the major weapon in their antiepileptic arsenals. The following "promising" expressions are representative. "Data from several prospective studies indicate that therapy guided by monitoring of blood levels has decreased by as much as 50% the number of patients whose seizures are poorly controlled, as compared with empirical treatment periods" (Kutt and Penry, 1974); "The ability to monitor the serum level enables the clinician to tailor the patient's dose to produce a concentration within the therapeutic range, and there is now evidence that, for phenytoin at least, the improvement can be substantial" (Editors, Lancet, 1975).

The investigations cited in support of these and similar statements invariably include those of Dawson and Jamieson, Sherwin et al., and Lund, and it is worthwhile to review these reports. In the first study, only 25 percent of the patients presented blood levels within the therapeutic range at the start of the investigation, whereas 80 percent of the subjects had therapeutic phenytoin concentrations at the end of the survey. The authors concluded that the increase in seizure control was due to improvement in *compliance* and correction of *inadequate* dosage regimens (Dawson and Jamieson, 1971). Of 37 ambulatory patients with uncontrolled petit mal attacks in the second study, 14 (38 percent) had drug plasma levels below the 95 percent tolerance limit in contrast to 5 (9 percent) of the controlled group. This difference, due to *noncompliance,* was eliminated by regular monitoring of the blood concentration (Sherwin et al., 1973). In the third study, phenytoin plasma levels were determined monthly to bimonthly for three years in a group of 32 ambulatory patients (Lund, 1974). The mean drug blood levels increased from 6.1 mcg per ml the first year to 11.7 mcg per ml the second year and to 15.0 mcg per ml during the third year, and the annual mean number of grand mal seizures per patient decreased from 5.8 to 4.1 to 1.6, respectively. The author attributed the improvement in seizure control to three factors: elevation of *inadequate* doses, increased *bioavailability* following the change from the acid to the sodium dosage form, and cautioning the patient to avoid *irregular drug intake.*

The article published by Sherwin et al. in 1973, "Improved control of epilepsy by monitoring plasma ethosuximide," was widely distributed to physicians in the U.S., and its title suggested to many, if not most, that blood level determinations represented an innovative procedure in the treatment of epilepsy. The titles or summaries of the other two reports conveyed essentially the same message, and only a minority of physicians realized that, in actuality, improvement in seizure control described in each of these articles was due primarily to the identification of *noncompliant patients* or those who were receiving *insufficient drug dosages.* Needless to say, noncompliance can be minimized or prevented and effective dosage schedules can be established on clinical grounds alone if the physician allots the proper time and approach to consideration of these factors.

The initial enthusiasm for serum level measurements was not limited to the medical profession but also affected many epileptic patients who learned of the new "miracle" through newspapers and magazines. Overzealous articles in publications sponsored by epilepsy organizations engendered undue optimism in a large number of individuals with refractory disorders, and many of them were convinced that control of seizures was "just a blood test away."

During the past several years, the initial eagerness and optimism concerning the essentiality and even the value of blood levels have diminished considerably. Now, most authorities concur that clinical assessment is more important than serum analysis in adjusting antiepileptic drug dosages, a precept that we first offered in 1970 (Livingston, 1970a) and repeatedly thereafter (Livingston et al., 1975). Others, too, realized the limitations of blood levels in the early 1970's, and one study cautioned that "therapeutic decisions should never be based solely on the drug concentration in serum . . . drug level determinations cannot substitute for careful medical observation and judgment and must always be interpreted in the context of all clinical data" (Koch-Weser, 1972). Ardent protagonists of blood level examinations have recently published acknowledgments of the prime importance of clinical evaluation in the treatment of epilepsy: "Clearly, the best therapeutic results will be obtained when clinical judgment is combined with laboratory information" (Kutt and Penry, 1974); "Drug level monitoring is valuable when used to supplement clinical observation, but it is no substitute for it" (Richens, 1977).

That practicing physicians have become increasingly disenchanted with routine monitoring of blood levels and that these examinations have not confirmed early appraisals of their value has been aptly noted: "When a new investigation or drug is introduced there often ensues a honeymoon period in which their advantages are emphasized to the neglect of their limitations . . . the honeymoon phase [of blood levels] is passing" (Brett, 1977). Although everyone knows that "water seeks its own level" and that the same holds true for new medical procedures and the efficacy of newly discovered medications, it is profitable to explore the reasons why, in our opinion, the initial "promise" of blood level determinations remains largely unfulfilled.

First, blood level examinations have not remedied on a scientific laboratory basis most of the causes for treatment failure in epileptic patients, the majority of which can be precluded or rectified on clinical, albeit empirical, grounds. The following significant reasons for treatment failure were enumerated by the AMA Department of Drugs in 1973: noncompliance, insufficient doses of appropriate drugs, not using two or three drugs concomitantly when indicated, improper classification of the seizure type, use of the wrong drug, failure to recognize progressive neurologic disease, too frequent changes in drug therapy, premature withdrawal of drugs, poor indoctrination of patients, and failure to recognize the social and economic needs of patients.

Although noncompliance and insufficient drug dosage problems can be identified by blood monitoring, these situations can be obviated and managed successfully by utilization of clinical methods. It should be reiterated that if, for example, a daily dose of 300 mg of phenytoin does not control a patient's seizures, the clinician would increase the dose accordingly. The "academician" would perform a blood level determination that, in all probability, would reveal a "subtherapeutic" concentration, and he would then also elevate the dosage. Of what value was the serum concentration result over and above that of the information derived from clinical assessment? The answer, of course, is none.

Differentiation of a progressive neurologic disorder from a case of drug intoxication is a well documented indication for measuring blood levels, although it should be borne in mind that drug toxicity suggestive of neuropsychiatric disease is not always associated with high drug serum concentrations (Ambrosetto et al., 1977). Too frequent changes in drug therapy can usually be precluded by blood level analyses, but they can also be avoided more surely and more easily by employing clinical precepts—i.e., no medication should be regarded as ineffective until it has received an adequate trial at the maximally tolerated dosage (Livingston, 1963).

It is often recommended that a drug prescribed in dosage sufficient to yield a blood level within or at the upper segment of the "therapeutic range" but that failed to control seizures satisfactorily be considered ineffective and be either withdrawn or supplemented by a second medication (Borofsky et al., 1972; Editors, Lancet, 1975; Reynolds, 1975; Scott, 1975; Shorvon and Reynolds, 1977). We believe that this policy of withdrawal denies the patient a potentially valuable drug, because many cases require the administration of medication in dosage sufficient to produce a blood level that exceeds the average "therapeutic range." Many of our patients were uncontrolled with serum concentrations considered therapeutic, but they were subsequently controlled or markedly improved without clinical signs of intoxication when the serum concentration was raised above the average range. That many patients require and can tolerate serum levels well above the therapeutic range has also been documented by others (Booker, 1972; Troupin, 1976). In some cases, one may have to compromise and accept control of seizures at the expense of minor toxicity such as drowsiness.

Blood level determinations have played no role in the remedy or the prevention of the remainder of the factors cited by the AMA Committee as contributing to the failure of treatment. Though often neglected, proper indoctrination of patients (Livingston, 1970b) and consideration of the socioeconomic aspects of epilepsy (Livingston, 1963, 1972; Gordon, 1976) are exceedingly important principles in the management of the epileptic patient.

Second, there is considerable concern regarding the unreliability factor in the determination of antiepileptic blood levels. Richens (1975) directed attention to the fact that there was no agreement as to the true concentration of drugs in specimens submitted to five laboratories that offered a routine service for these examinations. Subsequently, Pippenger and associates (1976) mailed three pooled sera containing ethosuximide, phenobarbital, phenytoin, and primidone to various laboratories in the U.S. They reported that for each specimen, the results ranged from 0 to levels so high as to be consistent only with massive overdosage. The coefficients of variation ranged from 38 percent to 505 percent. Such unacceptable results could have easily led the physician to adjust drug dosages in the wrong direction. Apparently, analyses performed in hospitals are equally deficient, since "in some hospitals, drug intoxication would be diagnosed on the same specimen that produced a subtherapeutic level in another hospital" (Richens, 1975).

Third, the general lack of concordance regarding the specific therapeutic ranges for antiepileptic medications has constituted a serious problem for many physicians, because "measurements of blood levels of a drug become useful guidelines for dosage adjustments only when the therapeutic range has been defined by controlled, careful clinical studies in a large number of patients" (Koch-Weser, 1972). The anticonvulsants that have been investigated the longest and the most intensively by means of blood levels are phenobarbital and phenytoin, and yet precise definition of therapeutic ranges for these medications has not been elucidated, so that the upper and lower values vary from clinic to clinic and from one commercial laboratory to another. For example, Borofsky et al. (1972) have adopted a rigid upper boundary of 20 mcg per ml for the phenytoin therapeutic range; Buchthal and Lennox-Buchthal (1972) state that the therapeutic range is "over 10 mcg per ml, probably over 15 mcg per ml in adults, and occasionally over 20 mcg per ml" and probably "on the order of 15 to 25 mcg per ml" when phenytoin is given regularly; Richens (1976) recommends a therapeutic zone of 10 to 25 mcg per ml whereas Jeavons (1976) prefers a therapeutic range of 7 to 17 mcg per ml in his clinic; and Troupin (1976) does not hesitate to extend the upper value of his range to 35 mcg per ml. It is, therefore, not difficult to understand why physicians who have not had extensive experience with phenytoin serum concentrations may have some trouble in deciding whether a modest blood level value is in the subtherapeutic zone or at the lower end of the therapeutic range, or whether a more substantial level, 23 mcg per ml, for example, is within the toxic range or at the upper end of the therapeutic index. Such situations illustrate the desirability of employing clinical methods rather than laboratory tests in the treatment of epileptic patients.

We, like most others, have found the usual therapeutic range for phenobarbital to be 10 to 30 mcg per ml (Livingston et al., 1975), but it differs considerably from patient to patient. It is difficult to predict the upper therapeutic limit with any degree of accuracy in most cases because of the large interindividual variation in tolerance to the side effects (especially drowsiness) of the drug. We do not believe that there has been sufficient experience to permit the designation of reliable "therapeutic" or "toxic" blood level ranges for other standard antiepileptic drugs such as carbamazepine, diazepam, ethosuximide, or primidone, although preliminary values have been published (Kutt and Penry, 1974; Richens, 1976). Substantive data regarding the serum concentrations of secondary anticonvulsive agents such as ethotoin (Peganone), metharbital (Gemonil), and methsuximide (Celontin) are virtually nonexistent.

The situation concerning primidone blood levels is unique because the drug undergoes biotransformation to two active metabolites, phenobarbital and phenylethylmalonamide (PEMA), and it is frequently difficult to relate anticonvulsant activity (or the lack thereof) or toxicity to the level of primidone, phenobarbital, or PEMA, or various combinations thereof. In addition, there seem to be considerable interpatient differences in the amount of phenobarbital that appears in the blood subsequent to a specific mg per kg dose of primidone; moreover, we have observed that higher serum concentrations of primidone-derived phenobarbital seem to be less intoxicating than similar levels resulting from the administration of phenobarbital itself. Therefore, except in unusual cases, we generally do not utilize primidone blood level determinations in the management of our patients.

Therapeutic range is generally determined by the intensity of the epileptic disorder—usually, it is lower in patients with mild epilepsy and higher in those with severe cases. It is interesting to note, however, that Jeavons (1976) has stated that most adult patients in his clinic do not attain phenytoin blood levels within the generally accepted therapeutic range of 10 to 20 mcg per ml (28 of 43 patients had levels below 7 mcg per ml) although serum concentrations of other anticonvulsants have been within normal limits. Conversely, Troupin (1976) found it necessary to maintain serum levels of at least 25 mcg per ml in a large number of patients receiving only phenytoin.

As previously described, another factor that compromises the validity of therapeutic range values is the disturbing observation that the therapeutic zone in children may not be the same as that for adults with any of the anticonvulsive agents.

More importantly, since it is not known to what extent the administration of additional antiepileptic medication alters the therapeutic range of an initially prescribed drug, Richens (1976) raised the possibility that "monitoring serum levels is an aimless exercise if several drugs are being given together." Schmidt (1977) studied a group of patients to determine if comedication influences the therapeutic level, and he concluded that "it is not useful to extrapolate therapeutic concentrations from patients treated with one drug to those on co-medication. This limits the use of this concept for practical clinical purposes as the majority of patients still receive more than one antiepileptic drug."

Fourth, many factors, most of which are uncontrollable by the prescriber, may affect the serum concentration of a drug. They have been enumerated by Koch-Weser (1972) as (1) host factors that affect the extent of gastrointestinal absorption, (2) distribution through fluid compartments, (3) body size and composition, (4) binding at inactive sites, (5) rates of metabolism and excretion, and (6) bioavailability of the dosage form prescribed. He stated that "all these determinants are subject to much individual and temporal variation due to genetic and environmental factors, to consequences of disease, and to concomitant administration of other drugs." To these variables may be added age, since it is well known, for example, that infants eliminate antiepileptic drugs such as phenobarbital and phenytoin more rapidly than do adults, and sex, because it has been demonstrated that females on the average achieve lower phenytoin blood levels than do males from the same mg per kg dose (Sherwin et al., 1974).

Because the circumstances that affect blood levels are so numerous and variable, especially the rates of metabolism and elimination, one must question the reliability and the actual significance of a single random serum concentration determination. Van der Kleijn et al. (1975) studied clinical pharmacokinetics in monitoring chronic treatment with antiepileptic drugs, and they identified the factors that specifically influence the relevance of blood level determinations as (1) time of sampling, (2) food intake, (3) comedication, (4) environmental stability, (5) patient compliance, (6) intercurrent disease, (7) pharmaceutical quality, (8) assay quality, (9) chemical stability, and (10) possibility of, and accuracy in, measuring therapeutic effect. Unfortunately, most of these factors are also not under the control of the physician.

Some of the disruptive effects of the factors that modify blood level analysis validity can be minimized, at least theoretically, by meticulous regulation of each variable or by monitoring the serum concentration repeatedly during a 24-hour interval, but in ordinary private outpatient practice, these procedures are not feasible. Actually, one blood specimen per office visit is usually the maximum that can be obtained, and although a single sample may adequately reflect the serum concentration of drugs with long plasma half-lives such as phenobarbital, in adults who metabolize anticonvulsants at rates consistent with established "average" values, it may be meaningless in patients whose positions are at the upper or lower portions of drug half-life scales. As an illustration, since the mean plasma half-life of phenytoin in adults is approximately 23 hours, but the range varies from seven to 56 hours, one may have difficulty in interpreting a phenytoin blood level in a patient who metabolizes the drug so rapidly that the half-life is only 12 hours. In addition, it has been found that the difference between peak and trough phenytoin serum concentrations in adults may vary as much as 50 percent (Wilder et al., 1972) within a 24-hour period, so that one should appreciate that a single phenytoin blood level may not be representative of the mean daily blood level. Because some anticonvulsants—e.g., carbamazepine and primidone—have relatively short plasma half-lives, the hourly variation in the blood concentration may be considerable and therefore, the results of a single serum level examination may be of dubious value, if not plainly misleading.

The reliability and value of a single blood level are even more suspect and tenuous in children, and especially so in infants, because the rates of elimination and metabolism are more rapid and erratic. Consequently, the hourly variation in the serum concentration is greater than that in adults. The study of phenytoin kinetics by Curless et al. (1976) poignantly demonstrates the hazards that may be associated with the obtaining of one blood level in children. Since 10 of their 11 patients exhibited very brief phenytoin half-lives, ranging from 1.2 to 6.7 hours, the authors cautioned that although children with short plasma half-lives may present adequate average blood levels, they "also may have toxic peak levels and subtherapeutic trough levels." How then can the private practitioner be sure that a single blood level determination result does reflect the average serum concentration between dosage intervals and not a transient high or low level? Obviously, he can't. Attainment of meaningful and representative serum concentrations in infants and young children requires that blood level examinations be performed serially throughout the period of investigation. Needless to say, the undesirability of such procedures because of their adverse physical and psychologic effects upon the child is clear, not to mention, of course, the anxiety, money, and time involved for both patients and parents. Brett (1977) aptly emphasizes that "there are strong arguments against frequent blood-letting in young children, if only because it can turn what should be a pleasurable visit to the clinic or hospital into a dreaded ordeal. This may lead to an increase in defaulters, since parents need to be convinced that a painful procedure is essential if they are to tolerate it for their children."

When contemplating the relevance of serum concentration determinations in a private outpatient practice, the time of sampling may be a very influential factor, but only a few physicians and a minority of commercial laboratories are fully aware of its significance. For example, Meijer (1975) reported that blood levels of carbamazepine analyzed before and after the morning dose differed by as much as 100 percent. Most practitioners send the patient directly from the office to the laboratory for a serum concentration examination, or an appointment is scheduled at the convenience of the laboratory, without, in either instance, any consideration of the optimal sampling time. Except for phenobarbital, which presents a relatively stable blood level pattern in adults, serum concentrations may vary considerably during a 24-hour interval, and it therefore becomes important to obtain the blood level at the proper time. Since each anticonvulsant may have its own appropriate sampling time (van der Kleijn et al., 1975), the situation can become rather complex in patients receiving multiple drug therapy.

In our opinion, the greatest value of blood levels is to be found in the research laboratory, where serum concentration investigations have yielded a wealth of knowledge, especially in the field of pharmacokinetics, so that we now have a much better understanding of drug metabolism. In addition, the ability to measure drug blood levels has confirmed, and sometimes disproved, prior clinical impressions. For example, it has corroborated (Svensmark and Buchthal, 1964) the clinical observation that infants and young children require relatively large doses of antiepileptic medication to produce an anticonvulsant effect (Livingston, 1954), but rejected (Buchthal and Lennox-Buchthal, 1972) the theory of synergistic multiple drug activity. Anticonvulsant blood level research has supplied answers to some questions of significance to the clinician (Buchthal and Svensmark, 1971), the most important of which are (1) the length of time required for the serum concentration to become constant, (2) the plasma half-life, (3) the time of peak concentration following various routes of administration, (4) rates of metabolism and elimination in children and adults, (5) dosage schedules for acute situations that mandate unconventional regimens, and (6) the presence and intensity of drug interactions.

Indications for Determination of Drug Blood Levels

Clinical response is unequivocally the most important criterion in regulating the dosage of antiepileptic medication. However, we have found serum concentrations to be helpful in the management of some patients, most commonly in those who do not respond to maximal doses or who manifest symptoms of intoxication while receiving small or conventional dosages of anticonvulsant agents.

On the basis of 15 years' experience in the investigation of antiepileptic blood levels in thousands of patients, we have found the following indications to be both significant and practical.

Whether or not a Patient is Taking His Medication as Prescribed is the Most Important Indication for Monitoring Serum Levels. In a large number of patients who were not responding to maximal doses of antiepileptic drugs and were referred to our center for evaluation and possible change of their ineffective regimens, a blood level determination disclosed either the complete absence of anticonvulsant material or so low a concentration with respect to the prescribed dosage that we were convinced that they were either taking their medication on an irregular basis or not at all. Initially, many of these patients, who were primarily teenagers, emphatically insisted that they had taken their medications exactly as instructed, but after intensive interrogation and confrontation with the results of their blood level examinations, they admitted to noncompliance with their dosage schedules. Following supervised administration of their drugs, either by hospital staff or by parents, each of these patients achieved satisfactory serum concentrations.

We have, however, observed reliable patients who displayed very low phenytoin blood levels while receiving relatively large doses of the drug. Kutt and McDowell (1968) offer, in addition to noncompliance, two reasons for this phenomenon: malabsorption of phenytoin from the gastrointestinal tract and increased metabolism of phenytoin. It has also been reported that uremic patients present exceptionally low phenytoin blood levels, despite average or maximal dosage (Odar-Cederlöf et al., 1970). Medication error, such as the ingestion of 30 mg phenytoin capsules instead of the 100 mg capsules that had been prescribed, was responsible for low serum levels in several of our patients. We are also cognizant of similar situations that resulted from the pharmacist's dispensing the weaker (30 mg per 5 ml) instead of the regular (125 mg per 5 ml) potency of phenytoin suspension. Such medication mistakes are not, of course, limited to phenytoin, but have occurred with all the antiepileptic drugs that are available in more than one potency per dosage form, especially phenobarbital and primidone.

More frequently encountered, however, are findings of high blood levels in association with conventional drug doses due to medication error or intentional manipulation of doses by the patient or the parent. Intoxication due to medication mistake has been reported to occur most often with the ingestion of 100 mg phenytoin capsules instead of the weaker strength that had been ordered (Clow et al., 1973) and occasionally, in our experience, with the dispensing of 250 mg primidone tablets rather than the 50 mg potency that had been specified. Intentional intoxication of children by parents has been reported, and Solow and Green (1972) cite the case of a six-year-old boy on a daily regimen of 80 mg phenobarbital and 100 mg phenytoin whose mother maintained a dosage schedule sufficient to produce a phenytoin serum concentration of 88 mcg per ml "because the 'sedation' made him easier to care for." We are also aware of intoxication resulting from the use of a tablespoon instead of a teaspoon during chronic administration of anticonvulsants in liquid dosage forms. Because of the inherent dosage hazards and inaccuracies (Livingston, 1963), and the large number of cases of accidental intoxication associated with improper administration (generally insufficient agitation) of anticonvulsant liquid preparations, particularly phenytoin suspension (Lagos, 1972), we do not employ liquid dosage forms in our practice.

Manipulation of drug dosages by the patient without medical consultation is not uncommon, particularly during the initial stages of therapy, because of the popular misconception that "if 2 is good, 3 is better, and 4 is still better." Since many individuals become impatient for success early in the treatment program and may attempt to accelerate the therapeutic process by increasing the drug dosage, we endeavor to preclude such situations by informing them that the establishment of an optimal antiepileptic regimen is not generally achieved overnight. We stress that anticonvulsant medication must be prescribed in a systematic manner. If so approached, the appropriate therapy may be ascertained in some patients after a short trial on one drug, whereas in others it may take a longer interval, since several medications may have to be administered in maximal dosage individually or in combination before a satisfactory treatment program is constructed. In addition, we explain to each patient that a significant period may be required for an antiepileptic drug to exert its anticonvulsant activity—for example, two weeks in the case of phenytoin and three to four weeks for phenobarbital. We also caution patients, particularly those receiving multiple drug therapy, not to diminish any drug dosage because of symptoms of toxicity until we specifically instruct them to do so, because patients frequently reduce the dose of the wrong medication, with possible adverse consequences.

Although noncompliance, particulary involving irregular or reduced drug intake, appears to be a prevalent practice and a primary reason for treatment failure, it has not been a significant problem in our patients because we direct ourselves energetically and comprehensively to this subject at the initial consultation and at every subsequent office visit. We fully explain the absolute necessity of adherence to the therapeutic regimen exactly as prescribed and caution against even the slightest manipulation of dosage without authorization. We impress upon each patient (or the parents) the hazards associated with erratic drug ingestion and stress that the occurrence of a seizure may result from the omission of even a single dose of medication. The relationship between the abrupt discontinuance of antiepileptic drug therapy and the precipitation of seizures or grand mal status epilepticus is specifically emphasized.

At times, teenagers may present a formidable challenge to a policy of strict compliance, and we have been successful in the attainment of satisfactory cooperation in these patients by additionally informing them that the performance of a blood level examination will rapidly resolve the question of whether they are taking their medication as instructed. We also mention, mostly for the benefit of the parents, that serum concentration analyses are not inexpensive, and may have to be repeated on a regular basis if we seriously suspect noncompliance. We also stress that motor vehicle operators' licenses are issued only to patients whose seizures are completely controlled, and that freedom from attacks is seldom, if ever, achieved in individuals who do not comply precisely with their dosage schedules. These factors, in combination with the previously cited admonitions, are, in our experience, major incentives to teenagers and generally stimulate sufficient motivation to assure compliance.

In Patients Who Manifest Symptoms of Intoxication While Receiving Small or Conventional Drug Doses, It is Essential (1) to Determine the Cause, e.g., Progressive Neurological Disease That May not Have Been Apparent or was Overlooked at the Initial or Subsequent Visits; (2) to Determine Whether the Medication is Indeed the Etiologic factor; and (3) to Make Remedial Adjustments in the Dosage Schedule if Necessary. In such instances, we also investigate the possibility of medication error due to a dispensing mistake or to patient manipulation of drug dosage.

Signs of phenytoin overdose in association with small or average dosages have been reported in the case of congenital deficiency of the hepatic parahydroxylation enzyme system, liver disease, coexisting disease of the central nervous system, impairment of elimination mechanisms, and interaction of drugs (cited in Livingston, 1972).

Attention is directed to the fact that patients who have taken phenytoin for prolonged periods without any symptoms of toxicity may suddenly and inexplicably become ataxic or diplopic, and we caution against the immediate reduction of phenytoin dosage, whether predicated on clinical assessment or on blood level results, unless the intoxication persists longer than three or four days. We have observed this phenomenon, which is probably due to temporary increased bioavailability, in many cases, and almost without exception, the symptoms resolved spontaneously without any reduction in dosage or neurologic sequelae (Livingston, 1956).

The Specific Offending Agent Must be Determined in a Patient Receiving Multiple Drug Therapy who Manifests Evidence of Drug Intoxication, (e.g., ataxia in someone taking both phenytoin and primidone).

It Must be Ascertained Whether the Failure of a Multiple Drug Regimen is Due to Interaction, Whereby One Medication Accelerates the Metabolism of Another or Conversely, if Intoxication is due to Impairment of Metabolism of One Drug by Another (Table 6–1).

Hepatic enzyme induction, with consequent anticonvulsant drug interaction or altered drug metabolism, is a subject of intense interest, as evidenced by the large number of articles appearing within recent years. In our opinion, the enthusiasm of some authors for the topic of antiepileptic drug interaction tends to overemphasize the significance of this pharmacologic phenomenon in clinical practice. With relatively few exceptions, the reader is led to believe that hepatic enzyme induction or inhibition by anticonvulsant drug therapy occurs universally, with predictable results on drug interaction and metabolism. Based on our experience, we can state that this is definitely not so, and that we have encountered altered hepa-

Table 6-1. *Drugs Reported to Alter Phenytoin Metabolism*

Impairment	Acceleration
Bishydroxycoumarin (Dicumarol)	Carbamazepine*† (Tegretol)
Chloramphenicol (Chloromycetin)	Phenobarbital*
Chlordiazepoxide*† (Librium)	
Chlorpromazine*† (Thorazine)	
Diazepam*† (Valium)	
Diazoxide†	
Disulfiram (Antabuse)	
Ethosuximide*† (Zarontin)	
Halothane† (Fluothane)	
Isoniazid	
Methylphenidate*† (Ritalin)	
Phenobarbital*†	
Phenylbutazone† (Butazolidin)	
Phenyramidol (Analexin)	
Prochlorperazine*† (Compazine)	
Propoxyphene† (Darvon)	
Sulfaphenazole† (Sulfabid)	
Sulthiame* (Conadil; Ospolot)	

* We have prescribed this drug to hundreds of patients receiving phenytoin, and we have not observed clinical proof of altered phenytoin metabolism or an adverse effect on seizure control in any case.

† Evidence for drug interaction resulting in an adverse clinical effect is generally lacking or so meager as not to allow definite conclusions.

tic enzyme activity with resultant adverse clinical effects only in very rare instances. Although we have observed changes in some laboratory test values that were attributable to the interaction of drugs, the respective patients exhibited little or no alteration in their clinical status, particularly of seizure control or drug intoxication. In many instances, reports of anticonvulsant drug interactions are contradictory and confusing and generally are of little but academic importance, except to emphasize the fact that these reactions are extremely inconsistent and variable from one patient to another.

The Possibility of Drug Toxicity Must be Investigated in a Patient who Exhibits Symptoms that may Also be Manifestations of Another Disorder, Such as a Neurodegenerative Disease in a Patient Receiving Phenytoin. A syndrome known as "phenytoin encephalopathy," characterized by ataxia, change in character or increase in frequency of seizures, choreoathetoid movements of the limbs and trunk, dystonic posturing, facial grimacing, mental changes, and mouthing movements, has been described in recent years (McLellan and Swash, 1974; Ahmad et al., 1975), generally in association with blood levels of approximately 40 mcg per ml or above and usually in patients with a previous neurologic deficit.

The Possibility of Drug Intoxication in Infants and Mental Retardates Receiving Phenytoin Should be Investigated. Since the clinical recognition of phenytoin overdosage in infants (Livingston 1956) and mentally retarded patients (Iivanainen et al., 1977) is frequently difficult, it is recommended that the blood concentration of drug be determined at regular intervals to insure that toxic levels have not been achieved.

Conclusion

In summary, we emphasize that clinical response is the most important criterion in regulating the dosage of anticonvulsant drugs, and that although serum concentration determinations may be occasionally helpful in patient management, it is generally unnecessary to perform such examinations on a routine basis. Buchthal and Svensmark (1971) remind us that "the wise physician was able to get along without knowing his patient's blood level by increasing the dose slowly until convulsions either are controlled or until toxic symptoms appear." We believe that this is still practicable today.

References

Ahmad, S., Laidlaw, J., Houghton, G.W., and Richens, A.: Involuntary movements caused by phenytoin intoxication in epileptic patients. J. Neurol. Neurosurg. Psychiatry 38:225, 1975.

AMA Department of Drugs: *AMA Drug Evaluations.* Acton, Mass., Publishing Sciences Group, Inc., 1973.

Ambrosetto, G., Tassinari, C.A., Baruzzi, A., and Lugaresi, E.: Phenytoin encephalopathy as probable idiosyncratic reaction: case report. Epilepsia 18:405, 1977.

Booker, H.E.: Phenobarbital, mephobarbital, and metharbital: relation of plasma levels to clinical control. In Woodbury, D.M., Penry, J.K., and Schmidt, R.P., eds., *Antiepileptic Drugs,* New York, Raven Press, 1972.

Borofsky, L.G., Louis, S., Kutt, H., and Roginsky, M.: Diphenylhydantoin: efficacy, toxicity and dose-serum relationships in children. J. Pediatr. 81:995, 1972.

Brett, E.: Implications for measuring anticonvulsant blood levels in epilepsy. Dev. Med. Child. Neurol. 19:245, 1977.

Buchthal, F., and Lennox-Buchthal, M.: Diphenylhydantoin; relation of anticonvulsant effect to concentration in serum. In Woodbury, D.M., Penry, J.K., and Schmidt, R.P., eds., *Antiepileptic Drugs,* New York, Raven Press, 1972.

Buchthal, F., and Svensmark, O.: Serum concentrations of diphenylhydantoin (phenytoin) and phenobarbital and their relation to therapeutic and toxic effects. Psychiat. Neurolog. Neurochirurg. 74:117, 1971.

Clow, D., Stephenson, J.B.P., Logan, R.W., and Jamieson, E.C.: Errors in phenytoin dosage. Lancet 2:256, 1973.

Committee on Drugs, American Academy of Pediatrics: Comment on: amphetamines in epilepsy. Pediatrics 52:754, 1973.

Curless, R.G., Walson, P.D., and Carter, D.E.: Phenytoin kinetics in children. Neurology 26:715, 1976.

Dawson, K.P., and Jamieson, A.: Value of blood phenytoin estimation in management of childhood epilepsy. Arch. Dis. Child. 46:386, 1971.

Editorial: Drug levels in epilepsy. Lancet 2:264, 1975.

Farmer, T.W.: Convulsive disorders, syncope, and headache. In Farmer, T.W., ed., *Pediatric Neurology.* Hagerstown, Md., Harper and Row, Publishers, 1975.

Fincham, R.W., and Schottelius, D.D.: The role of antiepileptic blood levels in the treatment of patients with epilepsy. J. Iowa Med. Soc. 63:433, 1973.

Freeman, J.M., and Lietman, P.S.: A basic approach to the understanding of seizures and the mechanism of action and metabolism of anticonvulsants. In Schulman, I., ed., *Advances in Pediatrics,* Chicago, Year Book Medical Publishers, Inc., 1973.

Glaser, G.H.: Paroxysmal disorders: convulsive disorders. In Merritt, H.H., ed., *A Textbook of Neurology,* Philadelphia, Lea and Febiger, 1973.

Gold, A.P., and Carter, S.: Pediatric neurology. In Shirkey, H.C., ed., *Pediatric Therapy,* St. Louis, The C.V. Mosby Co., 1972.

Gordon, N.: The control of anti-epileptic drug treatment. Dev. Med. Child. Neurol. 18:535, 1976.

Herberg, K.P.: Delayed and insidious onset of diphenylhydantoin toxicity. South. Med. J. 68:70, 1975.

Iivanainen, M., Viukari, M., and Helle, E.P.: Cerebellar atrophy in phenytoin-treated mentally retarded epileptics. Epilepsia 18:375, 1977.

Jeavons, P.M.: Serum-phenytoin. Lancet 1:491, 1976.

Johannessen, S.I.: General discussion. In Schneider, H., Janz, D., Gardner-Thorpe, C., Meinardi, H., and Sherwin, A.L., eds., *Clinical Pharmacology of Anti-Epileptic Drugs.* Berlin-Heidelberg, Springer-Verlag, 1975.

Koch-Weser, J.: Serum drug concentrations as therapeutic guides. N. Eng. J. Med. 287:227, 1972.

Kutt, H., and McDowell, F.: Management of epilepsy with diphenylhydantoin sodium: dosage regulation for problem patients. JAMA 203:969, 1968.

Kutt, H., and Penry, J.K.: Usefulness of blood levels of antiepileptic drugs. Arch. Neurol. 31:283, 1974.

Lagos, J.C.: Diphenylhydantoin risks in children. JAMA 220:726, 1972.

Livingston, S.: *The Diagnosis and Treatment of Convulsive Disorders in Children.* Springfield, Ill., Charles C Thomas, Publisher, 1954.

Livingston, S.: Treatment of epilepsy with diphenylhydantoin sodium (Dilantin sodium). Postgrad. Med. 20:584, 1956.

Livingston, S.: *Living With Epileptic Seizures.* Springfield, Ill., Charles C Thomas, Publisher, 1963.

Livingston, S.: *Drug Therapy for Epilepsy.* Springfield, Ill., Charles C Thomas, Publisher, 1966.

Livingston, S.: Treatment of grand mal epilepsy: phenobarbital versus diphenylhydantoin sodium. Clin. Pediatr. 7:444, 1968.

Livingston, S.: Seizure disorders. In Gellis, S.S., and Kagan, B.M., eds., *Current Pediatric Therapy,* Philadelphia, W.B. Saunders Co., 1970a.

Livingston, S.: The physician's role in guiding the epileptic child and his parents. Am. J. Dis. Child. 119:102, 1970b.

Livingston, S.: *Comprehensive Management of Epilepsy in Infancy, Childhood and Adolescence.* Springfield, Ill., Charles C Thomas, Publisher, 1972.

Livingston, S., Berman, W., and Pauli, L.L.: Anticonvulsant drug blood levels: practical applications based on 12 years' experience. JAMA 232:60, 1975.

Lund, L.: Anticonvulsant effect of diphenylhydantoin relative to plasma levels. Arch. Neurol. 31:289, 1974.

McLellan, D.L., and Swash, M.: Choreo-athetosis and encephalopathy induced by phenytoin. Br. Med. J. 2:204, 1974.

Meijer, J.W.A.: Report on worksheet collected after WODADIBOF I. In Schneider, H., Janz, D., Gardner-Thorpe, C., Meinardi, H., and Sherwin, A.L., eds., *Clinical Pharmacology of Anti-Epileptic Drugs,* Berlin-Heidelberg, Springer-Verlag, 1975.

Meinardi, H., van Heycop ten Ham, M.W., Meijer, J.W.A., and Bongers, E.: Long-term control of seizures. In Penry, J.K., ed., *Epilepsy: The Eighth International Symposium.* New York, Raven Press, 1977.

Melchior, J.C., Buchthal, F., and Lennox-Buchthal, M.: The ineffectiveness of diphenylhydantoin in preventing febrile convulsions in the age of greatest risk, under three years. Epilepsia 12:55, 1971.

Menkes, J.H.: *Textbook of Child Neurology.* Philadelphia, Lea and Febiger, 1975.

Nelhaus, G.: Neurologic and muscular disorders. In Kempe, C.H., Silver, H.K., and O'Brien, D., eds., *Current Pediatric Diagnosis and Treatment,* Los Altos, Calif., Lange Medical Publications, 1976.

Odar-Cederlöf, I., Lunde, P., and Sjöqvist, F.: Abnormal pharmacokinetics of phenytoin in a patient with uraemia. Lancet 2:831, 1970.

Pippenger, C.E., Penry, J.K., White, B.G., Daly, D.D., and Buddington, R.: Interlaboratory variability in determination of plasma antiepileptic drug concentrations. Arch. Neurol. 33:351, 1976.

Reynolds, E.H.: The value of serum diphenylhydantoin (phenytoin) in the management of epilepsy. Proc. R. Soc. Med. 68:102, 1975.

Richens, A.: Results of a phenytoin quality control scheme. In Schneider, H., Janz, D., Gardner-Thorpe, C., Meinardi, H., and Sherwin, A.L., eds., *Clinical Pharmacology of Anti-epileptic Drugs,* Berlin-Heidelberg, Springer-Verlag, 1975.

Richens, A.: clinical pharmacology and medical treatment. In Laidlaw, J., and Richens, A., eds., *A Textbook of Epilepsy,* Edinburgh, Churchill Livingstone, 1976.

Richens, A.: Precise adjustment of phenytoin dosage. In Penry, J.K., ed., *Epilepsy: The Eighth International Symposium,* New York, Raven Press, 1977.

Scheinberg, P.: *Modern Practical Neurology.* New York, Raven Press, 1977.

Schmidt, D.: Variation of therapeutic plasma concentrations of phenytoin and phenobarbital with the type of seizure and co-medication. In Penry, J.K., ed., *Epilepsy: The Eighth International Symposium,* New York, Raven Press, 1977.

Scott, D.F.: Drug levels in epilepsy. Lancet 2:514, 1975.

Sherwin, A.L., Robb, J.P., and Lechter, M.: Improved control of epilepsy by monitoring plasma ethosuximide. Arch. Neurol. 28:178, 1973.

Sherwin, A.L., Loynd, J.S., Bock, G.W., and Sokolowski, C.D.: Effects of age, sex, obesity and pregnancy on plasma diphenylhydantoin levels. Epilepsia 15:507, 1974.

Shorvon, S.D., and Reynolds, E.H.: Unnecessary polypharmacy for epilepsy. Br. Med. J. 1:1635, 1977.

Solow, E.B., and Green, J.B.: The simultaneous determination of multiple anticonvulsant drug levels by gas-liquid chromatography: method and clinical application. Neurology 22:540, 1972.

Svensmark, O., and Buchthal, F.: Diphenylhydantoin and phenobarbital: serum levels in children. Am. J. Dis. Child. 108:82, 1964.

Troupin, A.S.: The choice of anticonvulsants—a logical approach to sequential changes—a comment from an American neurologist. In Laidlaw, J., and Richens, A., eds., *A Textbook of Epilepsy.* Edinburgh, Churchill Livingstone, 1976.

van der Kleijn, E., Guelen, P.J.M., van Wijk, C., and Baars, I.: Clinical pharmacokinetics in monitoring chronic medication with anti-epileptic drugs. In Schneider, H., Janz, D., Gardner-Thorpe, C., Meinardi, H, and Sherwin, A.L., eds., *Clinical Pharmacology of Anti-Epileptic Drugs,* Berlin-Heidelberg, Springer-Verlag, 1975.

Wilder, B.J., Streiff, R.R., and Hammer, R.H.: Diphenylhydantoin: absorption, distribution, and excretion. In Woodbury, D.M., Penry, J.K., and Schmidt, R.P., eds., *Antiepileptic Drugs,* New York, Raven Press, 1972.

7

Are Carcinogenicity and Teratogenicity Tests Useful?

THE PREDICTION OF HUMAN DISEASES FROM LABORATORY AND ANIMAL TESTS FOR TERATOGENICITY, CARCINOGENICITY, AND MUTAGENICITY

Robert L. Brent, M.D., Ph.D.

ARE CARCINOGENICITY TESTS USEFUL?

David Salsburg, Ph.D.

I owe my reputation to the fact that I use digitalis in doses the text books say are dangerous and in cases that the text books say are unsuitable.

K.F. Wenckebach

While there are several chronic diseases more destructive to life than cancer none is more feared.

Charles H. Mayo

Ah, the paradise that awaits us in 1984! . . . For every ill a pill. Tranquilizers to overcome angst, pep pills to wake us up, life pills to ensure blissful sterility. I will lift up mine eyes unto the pills whence cometh my help.

Malcolm Muggeridge

Some drugs have been appropriately called "wonder drugs" inasmuch as one wonders what they will do next.

Samuel E. Stumpf

There are no really "safe" biologically active drugs. There are only "safe" physicians.

Harold A. Kaminetzky

Introduction

There is a school of thought that argues on behalf of more and more testing in animals as the best way to avoid the unpleasant surprises of drug toxicity. The truth of the matter is that animals are not people, and predictions from animal studies will never cover all the things (good or bad) that drugs can do in humans.

Brent has supplied a thoughtful and detailed exposition of the current state of the art in predicting genetic, teratologic, and carcinogenic damage. He examines critically the available data and dogmas and finds them lacking, at least in part.

However, Brent is well aware that the problems currently being attacked suboptimally in the laboratory deserve society's attention. He believes that the public will be best protected if scientists seek new knowledge about cancer, mutations, and congenital anomalies; if new and better experimental protocols are evolved; if we engage in better epidemiologic surveillance; and if we try to *prevent* cancer, mutations, and malformations. His paper is reasonable, provocative, and instructive.

Salsburg addresses the issue of carcinogenicity testing, and he believes that the current protocols, whose application grows daily, are not only doomed to generate a high rate of falsely indicted "carcinogens" but may cause us to overlook real chemical hazards.

Cancer is an emotionally loaded word, and it is not surprising that both scientists and laymen find themselves behaving irrationally and inconsistently in trying to deal with its terrors. My own reading of the literature on "threshold" doses of carcinogens has led me to the opinion that such discussions represent the modern version of the ancient scholastic game of "how many angels can balance on the head of a pin?"

If Salsburg's indictment is correct, we had best bestir ourselves and search for methods that are less costly—or at least less misleading!

Louis Lasagna, M.D.

The Prediction of Human Diseases from Laboratory and Animal Tests for Teratogenicity, Carcinogenicity, and Mutagenicity*

Robert L. Brent, M.D., Ph.D.
Jefferson Medical College,
Thomas Jefferson University, Philadelphia

Defining the Issues

There is no doubt that exposure of human populations to some drugs and chemicals is associated with an increase in congenital malformations and the development of tumors. Likewise, many scientists believe that extrinsically produced mutagenesis is occurring in the human population, although no one has demonstrated that mutations in humans have been produced by chemicals or drugs. Nevertheless, one cannot deny the possibility that some human mutations are the result of drug or chemical exposure.

The controversy with regard to teratogenicity, carcinogenicity, and mutagenicity is not concerned with whether environmental drugs and chemicals can contribute to these problems. Debate does exist in two areas:

1. What is the magnitude of the contribution of environmental chemicals and drugs to human teratogenesis, carcinogenesis, and mutagenesis?
2. What is the value of animal or laboratory tests in predicting the presence and magnitude of the hazard to the human?

Before attempting to answer these questions, one must recognize that these are complex issues because they involve interactions among the scientific community, industry, government, and the media. Thus, it is often difficult to keep the discussions objective and calm. Also, cancer and congenital malformations are emotional subjects. If one suggests that industrial chemicals, drugs, or food additives may be contributing to these diseases in the human, one is aggravating an already troublesome situation.

The most fundamental problems about teratogenicity, mutagenicity, and carcinogenicity are the following:

1. What are the biochemical, physiologic, and structural alterations that are responsible for teratogenesis and carcinogenesis?
2. Are there threshold exposures for carcinogens, teratogens, and mutagens, below which an increased incidence above background would not be expected?
3. How important are repair mechanisms in reversing and protecting against the effects of carcinogens, teratogens, and mutagens?
4. At very low exposures to carcinogens and mutagens, is there a linear or exponential reduction in effect?

* Supported by NIH HD 630, 11038, ERDA.

5. Can we develop animal models that predict with a reasonable degree of certainty the teratogenic, mutagenic, and carcinogenic effects of chemicals and drugs in humans?

The disturbing aspect of this subject is that decisions regarding regulation and protection of patients, consumers, and employees have to be made, regardless of whether sufficient understanding or pertinent data as to the hazards are available. In most instances, society favors the conservative approach. But now, and in the future, the attempt to reduce risks to the population may become a financial burden that our economy cannot support. Thus, the risk versus benefit concept is difficult to apply in the real world. The balance can vary considerably, depending on one's point of view. In a democratic society, groups or individuals who decide that a known or unknown risk is hazardous can attempt to eliminate the risk. In the recent past, a cranberry crop was destroyed and cyclamates were removed from food products because of potential, but unproven, human risks. It appears that most errors will be in the direction of protecting the public from chemical harm. Certainly, if errors are to be made, this is the direction they should take. On the other hand, pressure groups can behave erratically, as is evidenced by their support for Laetrile and their outcry against the FDA's attempt to ban saccharin, since the saccharin and cyclamate situations were quite comparable.

Table 7-1. *Estimated Contribution of Various Factors to Developmental Defects in Humans*

Condition	Percentage of Abnormalities at Birth
Cytogenetic Abnormalities	5
Recessive and Dominant Genes	20
Polygenic Inheritance Multifactorial Relationships Spontaneous Errors in Embryogenesis	65
Exposure from Day 12 Until Term	
Radiation	< 1
Maternal Disease States	4
Chronic Alcoholism Diabetes Phenylketonuria Endocrinopathies Trauma Others	
Intrauterine Infection	4
Syphilis Toxoplasmosis Cytomegalic Inclusion Disease Rubella Herpes Simplex Amnionitis Other	
Drugs and Chemicals	1

Teratogenicity Testing

We know more about the combined incidence and etiology of human congenital malformations than we do about mutations and tumors in humans. Table 7-1 lists the relative contribution of known and suspected factors to the occurrence of malformations. The largest category is a conglomerate of three important factors: polygenic inheritance, multifactorial relationships, and spontaneous (intrinsic) errors of embryogenesis. Multifactorial relationships include the interaction of environmental factors and unique genetic susceptibility. This susceptibility might pertain to a species, strain, or individual. The induction by cortisone of cleft palate in mice reflects both species and strain susceptibility, since some strains of mice are much more susceptible to cortisone-induced cleft palate than are others. Differences among similar species have been observed with acetazolamide-induced teratogenesis (Green et al., 1973). Multifactorial relationships are much more difficult to analyze in the human population, since it is extremely difficult to recognize individuals with unique susceptibilities to potential environmental teratogens because the population is so genetically heterogeneous.

The relationship of drug exposure to teratogenesis involves confounding factors. Table 7-1 lists maternal disease states and intrauterine infection as significant contributors to teratogenesis, whereas drugs and chemicals are listed as less important. One would expect an increase in drug usage during pregnancy, if the mothers had infection, signs of infection, or some other medical illness. Therefore, when drugs are associated with teratogenesis, it may not be a causal relationship, especially if the disease state being treated is also associated with an increased incidence of congenital malformations (Koskimies et al., 1978).

Although it appears that drugs and chemicals are minor contributors to the malformation problem, we cannot be certain, because so many malformations have no known etiology. Furthermore, new drugs and chemicals that may have teratogenic potential will be introduced. It is for this reason that there are continued attempts to improve the predictive ability of animal testing.

The establishment of drug testing protocols for teratogenic screening resulted primarily from the thalidomide episode. Although many laboratories throughout the world had developed their own methods for studying potential teratogenic agents, the quality of these investigations ranged from very good to very bad. In the 1960s, numerous publications by committees and individuals reported or suggested various protocols for screening drugs for teratogenicity. One must remember that a protocol for such screening is *empirically* derived, primarily because many of the basic mechanisms of teratogenesis in mammals are unknown.

Before concentrating on the problems of drug testing, it is worthwhile to consider some of the opinions expressed in the July 1963 edition of the Commission on Drug Safety Bulletin concerning the entire problem of the prenatal effects of drugs (Warkany et al., 1963). In 1963, experts in the field knew that drug testing in animals would not guarantee drug safety to the unborn child. Their report emphasized the lack of knowledge in teratology and the need for more basic research support. More sophisticated studies dealing with drug metabolism in the fetus and mother and the use of isotopically labeled drugs were suggested. These suggestions have been only partially implemented. The report included two points that, in retrospect, might be faulted. First of all, it did not stress the importance of epidemiology programs in preventing further thalidomide-type episodes, and it suggested the utilization of empirical *in vitro* studies for screening procedures, which only further confuse the potential effects of a drug in the human embryo.

A World Health Organization (WHO) document published in 1967 reiterated many of the points made in 1963, and it made a plea for more epidemiologic studies (Baker et al., 1967). The conclusions of this group are recorded as follows:

(1) At present no method of preliminary screening in animals can provide absolute assurance against the occurrence of a teratological reaction in human pregnancy. Nevertheless, it is believed that it should be possible to greatly reduce the risk by improved preclinical screening for teratogenic effects, especially with the exercise of sufficient care in the choice of appropriate species, time of testing and effective dosage levels.

(2) The predictive value of teratological screening can be enhanced by observing the procedures recommended in this report and by avoiding the sources of error described. Further improvement of the predictive reliability of tests can be expected when research provides the necessary information on basic mechanisms of teratogenesis. Because of the lack of key information in several areas related to teratology, extensive programmes of research must be undertaken if teratogenic risk to man is to be reduced to the lowest possible level.

(3) The limited knowledge of the fundamental developmental processes and the mechanisms of teratogenic drug action on the one hand and the need for internationally acceptable criteria and methods for testing on the other necessitate internationally organized, multidisciplinary research efforts of long-range character.

(4) Teratological studies in primates should occupy a prominent place in research efforts.

(5) Since animal tests cannot with certainty predict teratogenic drug effects in man, it is essential that drugs be kept under close surveillance for several years after their introduction.

(6) Epidemiological studies of congenital malformations are an indispensable supplement to drug-monitoring activities.

(7) Further efforts must be made to inform the medical profession of the teratogenic risks presented by drugs in spite of their clearance through approved screening methods.

(8) In women, the balance between the therapeutic benefit and the teratogenic risk of a drug should be carefully assessed at all times during the reproductive span, especially when the possibility of pregnancy cannot be excluded.

Teratogenicity Test Protocols

One must realize that drug testing protocols have been empirically designed (Lorke, 1963; Brent, 1964, 1969, 1972; Cahen, 1964; Loosli et al., 1964; Zbinden, 1964; Gottschewski, 1965; Wilson, 1965; Frohberg and Oettel, 1966; Baker et al, 1967; Bertrand et al., 1972; Tuchmann-Duplessis, 1972, 1973; Grice et al., 1975; Berry and Barlow, 1976; Fraser, 1977). The reliability of a particular testing protocol is demonstrated only after years of correlating the animal and human data. For mutagenicity, carcinogenicity, and teratogenicity, it has been very difficult to establish testing procedures in animals whose results would be acceptable to regulatory agencies as guaranteeing safety in humans.

Table 7–2 lists the factors that one should consider in evaluating the effects of a drug in a teratologic animal experiment. The three litter tests of the U.S. Food and Drug Administration (FDA) include many of the parameters mentioned in Table 7–2, but do not request information dealing with fetal metabolism, placental transfer, or the mechanism of teratogenesis. Points 10, 11, and 12 of the table are important criteria for evaluating drugs that might be given to pregnant women. In most instances, if we were aware of the metabolic fate of a drug and its mechanism of action, many empirical drug testing procedures could be eliminated.

Current protocol for teratogenicity testing apparently makes the FDA more comfortable, although it probably provides the pharmaceutical companies with few useful procedures. In fact, if the information derived from testing procedures were the only criterion utilized in evaluating a drug, thalidomide could be shown to be nonteratogenic in two species, and therefore, it could be marketed today! But test results in animals are not the only criteria, and in the United States, most new drugs carry a warning about their potential harm to the fetus, even when no effects have been demonstrated in animal teratology studies. Today, it is less likely than ever that the thalidomide situation would be repeated—not because of the introduction of drug testing in pregnant animals, but because almost all new drugs carry a warning about their use in pregnant women and because patients and physicians are less likely to use drugs of any kind during pregnancy.

What is the purpose of teratogenic testing in experimental animals? These tests do not determine whether drugs are safe in human beings. You might ask why the FDA would establish a test to determine whether a drug is teratogenic and then ignore the results when determining whether the drug should or could be used in pregnant women. The answers are very complicated. Zbinden summarized the general consensus about teratologic testing in an issue of the Newsletter of the Environmental Mutagen Society:

> Those of us who have experienced the FDA-enforced rush of teratogenicity testing of drugs, new and old, as an aftermath of the thalidomide tragedy, know only too well that premature and arbitrary fixation of difficult experimental methodology is bound to produce a lot of useless results. Millions of dollars were spent on chronic reproduction studies before somewhat more appropriate methods were suggested. Consequently, all drugs had to be retested at great cost but still with unsatisfactory results. If part of this enormous effort had been spent on method development, experimental teratology might be better off than it is now.

Why is it that empirically established animal teratogenic testing is not a reliable predictor of the human response? Why are these tests not valid? Other empirically contrived animal test procedures have been acceptable to the FDA, the drug industry, and the scientific community. Teratogenesis, however, is not a single response. It does not result from one series of pathologic processes; a multitude of variable factors determine whether these events will occur in a particular species. Most important, we do not know the basic mechanisms involved in the induction of many malformations. What we have learned has only made us realize even more that the transfer of animal teratologic data to the human situtation is unreliable. This is so because:

1. Pure strains of animals may have a narrower response to drugs than the human population because they are more genetically homogeneous than the human population

Table 7–2. *Factors to be Considered in Establishing a Teratogenic Drug Testing Procedure*

1. Species of Animals
2. Number of Litters (Litter Effect)
3. Stages of Administration
4. Route of Administration
5. Dosage Schedule
6. Dosage Range
7. Controls
8. Examination of Fetuses after Cesarean Section at Term:
   - Malformation Rate
   - Term Fetal Weight (Presence of Growth Retardation)
   - Resorption Rate
9. Examination of Fetuses Allowed to Deliver Spontaneously:
   - Growth
   - Behavior
   - Biochemical and Physiologic Development
10. Fetal and Maternal Drug Metabolism
11. Placental Transport
12. Determination of Mechanism of Action

2. Variations in diet and metabolism between animals and humans may mean that environmental agents will be metabolized entirely differently in these species

3. Presence of obesity in the human population could affect the metabolism and storage of toxic compounds

4. Variation in placental function may be important in determining which drugs get to the fetus and whether some environmental factors are teratogenic.

Also, important variabilities within the human species might make certain individuals more susceptible than others to the toxicologic effects of some drugs. These include genetic heterogeneity that affects body metabolism, differences in diet and size (malnutrition and obesity), antecedent or concurrent disease, concurrent drug ingestion, and variability in placental transfer. It is literally impossible to account for all the factors when applying teratogenic testing data to the human species.

Zbinden feels that we could improve the value of animal test data if we evaluated the biochemical and pharmacologic aspects of the chemical in question more extensively:

> If we could always know how the drug acts, how it is absorbed, how it interacts with essential enzyme processes, and how it is detoxified and excreted, we would hardly need a toxicity test. It follows that if we want to improve our toxicological evaluations, and nobody will dispute that improvement is needful, we have to do more work on the mechanism of action (Zbinden, 1964).

The problem with this concept is that the human species has immense genetic heterogeneity. Unless we can predict the pharmacodynamics of a drug or a chemical in all variants of the human species, we will still have difficulty in applying animal data to humans. We are aware of many genetic traits that magnify the risk of environmental hazards (xeroderma pigmentosa, maternal phenylketonuria, Bloom's syndrome, Fanconi's anemia). How many unknown genetic variants also contribute to susceptibility to environmental hazards? Unless we understand the genetic correlation between the test animal and the human population, with regard to the response of a pregnant animal to a drug or a chemical, we cannot even begin to transfer the data. There are also instances in which animal data have no applicability at all to humans. This could be due to genetic differences in drug metabolism or to differences in placentation or placental transport (Brent et al., 1961, 1971; Brent, 1969, 1971). Available data support these concepts. There are approximately 20 known teratogens in humans and almost 1000 in mice and rats. Many rodent teratogens do not interfere with human development; some human teratogens do not interfere with rodent development. Obviously, reproductive tests in animals should be only one aspect of protecting the public from teratogenic hazards.

Carcinogenicity and Mutagenicity Testing

Recent studies have indicated that the basic processes and mechanisms involved in carcinogenesis and mutagenesis overlap significantly. In fact, several authors have attempted to determine whether there are common mechanisms involved in carcinogenesis, mutagenesis, and teratogenesis, but the consensus is that teratogenesis, although it may have some similar mechanisms, is quite different from the other processes (Kalter, 1975; Magee, 1977). No one has claimed that all mutagens are carcinogenic, but there are investigators who have reported that 90 percent of chemicals proven to be animal carcinogens are also mutagens (McCann et al., 1975). These same investigators claim that agents that have proven not to be carcinogenic are rarely mutagenic in the Salmonella/microsome test.

It would simplify matters if all carcinogens could be discovered by mutagenicity testing. But some known mechanisms for carcinogenesis exist, such as (1) drugs and chemicals acting as carcinogens, (2) oncogenic viruses, (3) immunosuppression from disease, drugs, or genetic constitution, (4) hereditary tumors, (5) somatic mutations, and (6) combined factors (i.e., genetic susceptibility plus carcinogen). Chemical agents, such as asbestos or certain metals, are thought to function differently from the usual mutagens. Similarly, suppression of the immune system by various means (exogenous drugs and hormones, intrinsic genetic immunologic disease) can result in tumor formation in animals and man. It is very likely that multiple events are involved in oncogenesis, but we are ignorant of how these factors interact and whether other mechanisms are involved.

Although there has been an interest in experimental oncogenesis for many years and in mutagenesis since Muller's work of 1928, this interest heightened in the 1960s. A series of anxiety- and thought-provoking statements appeared in the press and the medical literature, strongly warning the public of the dangers of caffeine, the threat of genetic damage, the impossibility of predicting "safe" levels of drugs or chemicals in humans, the hazards of environmental carcinogens, and the difficulty (and possibility) of acting against chemical mutagens. It is obvious that there was disagreement among scientists about the contribution of chemicals and drugs to the occurrence of cancer and mutation in the human population. During the past two decades, protocols were developed for testing drugs and chemicals for oncogenicity and mutagenicity.

Mutagenicity Test Protocols

Standards for oncogenicity testing in animals have been described in great detail (Grice et al., 1975). These chronic studies can determine whether a particular exposure to an agent can produce tumors, and they reveal that there is a marked difference in species and strain susceptibility to carcinogens. For example, some strains of rats did not respond to 7, 12-dimethylbenzanthracene, whereas another strain showed a 100 percent incidence of mammary tumors (Boyland and Sydnor, 1962). Sex differences have also been noted. Therefore, if a chemical is proved carcinogenic in an animal species, there are problems in applying the information to humans, including the determination of threshold and oncogenic doses.

The development of protocols for testing mutagenicity has been very controversial. Interested scientists had little difficulty in developing complex protocols, although there was some disagreement about how to interpret the results. Researchers concerned with mutagenicity also argued about the value of different testing procedures. Through discussion and development of new information, mutagenicity protocols have evolved and their assets and liabilities have become clearer. Some of the tests now utilized to evaluate drugs and chemicals are described.

Specific locus test. This test was used by Russell (1951) to determine mutation rates in a group of recessive loci following radiation exposure. The method consists of mating treated and untreated mice that are homozygous wild type at multiple loci to mice that are homozygous recessive for those multiple loci. The recessive traits are easily detectable in the homozygous state. Thus, spontaneous mutation rates and induced mutation rates can be determined *in vivo.* Although this test has been extremely important in determining the quantitative aspects of radiation mutagenesis, it is a tedious and expensive test that prohibits its use in mass screening. Specific locus tests clearly demonstrate that a reduction in dose rate decreases the mutagenic effect of x-ray, although the total dose is the same. Some critics claim that this test is insensitive when compared to some of the *in vitro* tests, but it also may be more appropriate for evaluating a chemical's mutagenic potential in the human.

In vivo somatic mutation production. This method is reported by Russell (1977) and involves the exposure of C 57B1 females mated to T males on day 10.25 after copulation. The occurrence of some skin spotting is believed to be due to somatic mutations. The authors believe that this test may be a useful screen for germinal specific locus mutations. Although the somatic reproduction test is not a direct measure of germinal cell mutations, it is less tedious than the specific locus test. It does have several disadvantages for chemical mutagenic testing. First, the chemical or drug has to cross the placenta. Second, the metabolism or handling of the agent at the cellular level may be different in embryonic cells. This technique requires more evaluation before its appropriate place in mutagenicity testing can be determined.

Cytogenetic analysis. Tests to evaluate chromosomal damage can be performed on cells treated *in vitro* or *in vivo.* Furthermore, analysis of the chromosomes can consist of (1) scoring metaphase plates for chromosomal aberrations with and without banding techniques (Cattanach et al., 1968; Rohrborn and Basler, 1977; Frank et al., 1978), (2) determining the incidence of sister chromatid exchanges (Taylor et al., 1957; Kato, 1974), or (3) determining the incidence of micronuclei (Schmid, 1976). The scoring systems and the interpretation of results have created much disagreement. There may be less significance to gaps, breaks, and reunions in the *in vitro* test systems because the normal process of repair may be compromised. Similarly, *in vivo* cytogenetic studies present problems in interpretation because we are not certain of the relevance of these test results to the occurrence of human disease. Significant cytogenetic alterations include transmittable translocations produced in germ cells. There is little difficulty in viewing this finding as significant in man. Nichols (1973) believes that "there has been a high correlation between the induction of chromosomal abnormalities and the induction of gene mutation produced by irradiation and chemicals," but Auerbach (1976), when discussing the relationship between chromosome breakage and gene mutation, says "Results with chemical mutagens discourage the assumption of a close correlation." Data exist that support Auerbach's view. Malic hydrazide and 8-ethoxy caffeine induce chromosome breaks but no mutations (Sobels, 1977). Natarajan et al. (1976) reported that absence of chromosomal aberrations does not necessarily prove absence of genetic damage.

Host-mediated assay (Gabridge and Legator, 1969). In this test, a microbial indicator organism is injected into the peritoneal cavity of a mammalian organism, which is then treated with the test drug or chemical. After several hours, the organisms are harvested from the peritoneal cavity and the number of mutants is scored. By comparing the mutation rate in control organisms—subjects exposed to the chemical in an isolated culture—with those exposed in the host-mediated assay system, one can determine whether (1) the chemical is mutagenic, (2) the metabolic products are mutagenic, and (3) whether the mammalian organisms have the capacity to detoxify or amplify the mutagenic properties of the chemical. In addition to special strains of Salmonella, other microorganisms and mammalian cells have been used. Scoring has included backward and forward mutation, and the frequency of chromosome aberrations (Fahrig, 1974; Hill, 1976; Mohn, 1977).

The host-mediated assay was an important innovation. Although the chemical or drug is metabolized by a mammalian organism, the mutagenic potency is measured in cells artificially placed in the peritoneal cavity. If one is interested in carcinogenic potential or mutagenic effects in somatic cells, one must realize that the target organs are not included in the test. Similarly, if one is interested in germ cell mutations, interpretation of the mutagenic potential of drugs or chemicals may not be appropriate unless the drug has been metabolized by the germ cells. It is possible that the cells in the target organs might behave substantially different from the test cells or organisms selected for the host-mediated assay.

Salmonella/mammalian microsome mutagenicity test (Ames et al., 1973; Ames, 1974). A set of tester strains of *Salmonella typhimurium,* which is described by Ames as "supersensitive," are mutants caused by a known type of DNA damage (base pair substitutions and various kinds of frameshift mutations) incurred for detecting mutagens by a back mutation test. A deletion of one of the genes of the excision repair system has made the test organisms hundreds of times more sensitive to most mutagens. Other organisms have been developed for testing forward mutations. Test organisms are coupled with a microsomal hydroxylase system from rat or human liver. It is believed that the microsomal fraction can activate many classes of carcinogens and mutagens. This test has been modified in order to evaluate the presence of mutagens in human urine (Durston and Ames, 1974; Yamasaki and Ames, 1977). A urine concentrate from smokers has been demonstrated to contain mutagens, whereas no mutagens were present in nonsmokers.

The Salmonella microsome test has been heralded by many scientists as an important advance in mutagenicity and carcinogenicity testing. One of its advantages is the ability to screen large numbers of compounds very rapidly for mutagenicity. It has also demonstrated that a high percentage of proven animal carcinogens are also mutagenic. The test "amplifies" the mutagenicity of many polycyclic hydrocarbons and aromatic amines. Although this amplification of sensitivity may seem beneficial to some scientists, it might indict many compounds that are not mutagenic in humans. Since some compounds may produce cytogenetic abnormalities but not point mutations, this test could miss some agents that have mutagenic potential. Finally, it is possible to overlook the mutagenic activity of a compound if it happened to have high affinity for A or T bases, and if the mutant site of the tester strain contained only GC base sequences.

Since the determination of carcinogenesis in this assay is primarily based on rodent experiments, the association between mutagenesis and carcinogenesis relates to animal tumors. Therefore, the predictive value of this mutagen assay is related to animal and not human carcinogenesis. It is also important to recognize that there appears to be a variable correlation between carcinogenic and mutagenic potency in rodents (Brusick, 1977; Ashby and Styles, 1978).

Dominant lethal test. This test measures the induced incidence of embryonic death in the preimplantation and early organogenetic stages following exposure of developing ova or sperm to toxic agents prior to conception

(Bateman, 1960).

Either male or female animals can be exposed to potential environmental teratogens. Historically investigators have preferred males, since the toxic effects of a chemical may indirectly affect embryonic survival in a treated mother, thus complicating the analysis of embryonic loss. The dominant lethal test is not a good screening procedure for testing chemical agents for mutagenesis because it is relatively insensitive (Generoso et al., 1974). Several known chemical mutagens, such as nitrogen mustard and dimethylnitrosamine, have not been positive in the dominant lethal test (Epstein et al., 1972). Furthermore, there appear to be differences in species susceptibility to chemicals used in this procedure.

Goldstein and Spindle (1976) have modified the dominant lethal test by examining the embryos on the second day of gestation rather than after the period of organogenesis. They also superovulated the female mice so that the number of ova in each experiment was larger. Thus, their index is the ratio of cleaved to noncleaved embryos, and it involves direct observation of the embryos. Regardless of the method used to test for dominant mutations, it is believed that chromatid deletions are the cause of the dominant lethality (Generoso et al., 1975). It should be emphasized that the spectrum of chromosomal damage responsible for embryonic death is not completely understood. It has been stated that an agent that was evaluated by a group of genetic tests and was positive only in the dominant lethal assay would not contribute to human disease in the F_1 generation, since the affected embryos would die. This concept is a reflection of some investigators' willingness to transfer animal data to man and the fact that few studies have investigated the F_2 and F_3 generations following the dominant lethal test.

Somatic mutations in cultured mammalian cells. This line of investigation for developing testing protocols using isolated mammalian cells is relatively new and may eventually offer the possibility of studying numerous human cell lines in culture. Although the results may be difficult to interpret in the early years, testing protocols using human cell lines offer many advantages over bacterial systems. Furthermore, there is a great opportunity for expanding our knowledge about the process of mutation in human cells.

Other mutagenicity screening tests. It is certain that other genetic screening tests will be developed, based on applications of new genetic information or attempts to mimic more accurately the response of the human organism. The possibility of accomplishing these goals will be discussed. Two newer tests, which should contribute important basic information, involve DNA repair and the reactions of DNA with chemicals and drugs. DNA repair can be measured by inducing unscheduled DNA synthesis and measuring the incorporation of labeled thymidine or deoxycytidine into the DNA in control and into chemically exposed DNA. The nature of the incorporation following mutagen exposure may indicate the type of lesion produced by the mutagen. Although *in vitro* or *in vivo* DNA repair studies do not measure genetically transmissible damage, the damage can be demonstrated in somatic or germinal cells. Thus, the tests should contribute to our understanding of the process of mutagenesis.

An understanding of the chemical reactions between potential mutagens and DNA would be extremely valuable but would not provide quantitative information on the mutagenic potential of compounds reacting with DNA.

Applicability of Mutagenicity Tests to Humans

Each researcher who has developed a mutagenicity testing protocol has emphasized the positive aspects of the protocol with regard to its potential for predicting mutagenicity and/or carcinogenicity in humans. Auerbach (1976) reviewed some important questions concerning mutagenesis and their bearing on testing. If she is correct,we are far from being able to predict quantitative mutagenic effects in humans. Auerbach concludes that:

1. Results with chemical mutagens discourage the assumption that there is a close correlation between chromosome breakage and gene mutation.
2. Tests for deletions have to be carried out in eukaryotes in order to be applicable to man.
3. The dominant lethal test has limited value for the assessment of genetic hazards.
4. The relationship between deletions and point mutations is variable from mutagen to mutagen and not predictable for a particular mutagen.
5. Chromosome breakage, which is a genetic risk, and recombination, which is not a genetic risk, should be studied in order to determine

whether correlation for their occurrence exists.

6. The concepts of premutational lesions and repair are not emphasized in mutation testing protocols because the dosages used are frequently very high and the test substance may be interfering with repair only at high exposures, thus exaggerating its mutagenic effect.

Investigators who are firmly convinced of the importance of mutagenicity testing admit that "the use of cytogenetics, host-mediated assay and dominant lethal test for the detection of mutagenic substances was based on the belief that a single mutagenic test system could not detect all genetic events of relevance to man" (Green et al., 1976).

Sobels (1976) suggested that "regulatory measures ought to be postponed until verification has been obtained from a battery of different test systems." He thus admits that he is not prepared to select the test systems. The dilemma facing scientists involved in the regulation of drugs and chemicals found to be mutagenic in one or another test is reflected in this ambiguous and confusing statement: "As scientists, we are obliged to carry our scientific integrity with us as far as is humanly possible and then make it quite clear when we are leaving the scientific realm and entering the realm of finding workable and useful formulations in the service of society which is in need of protection from adverse effects of environmental chemicals" (Sobels, 1976). The concept of "don't just stand there, do something" is being applied to the field of teratogenic, carcinogenic, and mutagenicity testing.

The inability to predict the impact of a chemical suggested to be mutagenic or carcinogenic by some testing procedure is further amplified by the fact that the dose-response relationship of mutagens is not linear and, therefore, extrapolation of results at high doses to low exposures is not valid (Sobels, 1975).

The Controversy

Let us now return to the questions asked at the beginning of this essay. *What is the magnitude of the contribution of environmental chemicals and drugs to human teratogenesis, carcinogenesis, and mutagenesis?*

It appears that environmental chemicals and drugs are the least important primary teratogens, although it is difficult to determine whether they act as multifactorial agents. Furthermore, there is minimal, if any, controversy regarding the contributions of drugs and chemicals to human teratogenesis (Table 7–1).

On the other hand, there is marked disagreement about the role of chemicals, drugs, and other environmental agents in the production of mutagenicity and carcinogenicity in humans. Epstein (1977) has stated that there is "a growing scientific consensus that most human cancers are environmental in origin." It is more important to have facts than a consensus. In reality, we are aware of approximately 20 human carcinogens. Some are industrial chemical products and some are drugs and medical therapies with a known carcinogenic and/or mutagenic risk (Tomatis et al., 1978). It is imperative that we know much more about the process of mutagenicity and carcinogenicity before we can assess the importance of such etiologic factors as environmental carcinogens, immunologic defects, intrinsic genetic factors, viruses, and other yet-to-be discovered mechanisms. If one accepts the "consensus" that most human cancers are environmental in origin, one is accepting a hypothesis as fact. In the meantime, the scientific and industrial community must consider methods of reducing exposure to toxic agents, but not under the delusion that this will solve the cancer problem, for this is just not so.

Studies of the Japanese in Hiroshima and Nagasaki emphasize the difficulties in examining mutagenic and carcinogenic agents in humans. Although radiation is believed to be a potent carcinogen and mutagen, the results in the Japanese population were surprising. Exposures absorbed by the Japanese population were many times greater than those of a worldwide fallout, diagnostic radiation, or contamination from nuclear power plants. It is significant that whereas there was no significant genetic effect, there was a definite carcinogenic effect. These human studies raise a plausible hypothesis that should be tested. In the human, is carcinogenesis a more sensitive measure of the presence of an environmental hazard than is mutagenesis? Environmentally induced carcinogenesis is a "real" situation in the human; chemical mutagenesis has never been documented in man. Since carcinogenesis is an irreversible endpoint in a sequence of pathologic processes, it is easy to measure the impact of the result. Mutations have the possibility of repair, negative selection, and self-destruction. The quantitative aspects of radiation-induced mutations are well known (Russell, 1951, 1977), and it is therefore reassuring that the human population in Hiroshima and Nagasaki did not exhibit significant genetic effects. This may speak well for the human organism's ability to diminish the final effect of environmental mutagens.

What is the value of animal or laboratory tests in predicting the presence and magnitude of mutagenic, carcinogenic, and teratogenic hazards in the human?

It is known that these nonhuman testing procedures can result in false positive and false negative results. Some animal teratogens are less active in the human; some human teratogens are less active in the laboratory. Since we have little information on evironmental human mutagens, it is difficult to evaluate the accuracy of laboratory mutagenicity testing in humans. However, there are data on human carcinogenesis and, therefore, it is possible to correlate animal carcinogenesis studies with human epidemiologic studies. Investigators have made great strides in this area. It is unfair to criticize the developers of testing protocols because the results of the tests may not be directly applicable to the human or may be, in some instances, erroneous. Remember that some testing protocols have been developed because they were mandated by legislation. Others have been developed as by-products of sound basic research in these fields. Thus, even the scientists who have developed them recognized their deficiencies.

Animal or laboratory testing cannot predict with reasonable accuracy qualitative or quantitative carcinogenic, mutagenic, or teratogenic effects in humans. Although most researchers support this concept, some disagree. Epstein (1977) states that "there is an overwhelming consensus in the qualified scientific community that data derived from valid and well-conducted animal experiments yield carcinogenicity data with a high degree of presumptive human relevance." Apparently, Epstein has not followed the controversy about saccharin carcinogenicity. Saccharin studies were performed by highly competent scientists, and the controversy in the scientific community was concerned with applying the data to humans. In defense of Epstein's stand, it is true that carcinogenicity testing may be further developed than teratogenicity or mutagenicity testing.

The emotionality of this topic is reflected in the statement, "There can be no possible justification, scientific or otherwise, for leading industrial representatives or regulatory officials to insist that animal data must be validated by human experience before regulatory action can be taken" (Epstein, 1977). This is both inflammatory and inaccurate. Many leading members of industry and regulatory agencies are more than willing to base decisions on animal testing in an effort to protect the public, even though they are not convinced that a human hazard exists.

The most important reason for the lack of predictability of animal testing is the genetic heterogeneity of the human population. Unless one can determine the contribution of various genetic loci to animal testing results and the nature of these genetic loci in the human population, one cannot guarantee the applicability of the results to humans. Furthermore, no laboratory testing procedure accounts for additional variations in the population. For example, a majority of the world population is lactose intolerant, and a very few individuals may develop a fatal bloody diarrhea in infancy following ingestion of milk. No one suggests that milk should be eliminated from everyone's diet. We have a similar situation in the field of carcinogenesis. Miller (1976) pointed out that certain individuals are more susceptible than others to the carcinogenic effect of x-rays. Patients with ataxia telangiectasia have an exaggerated response to radiation (Galloway, 1977). We know that patients with xeroderma pigmentosa are unusually susceptible to the carcinogenic effect of solar radiation. We are ignorant of how many variations in human genetic loci may contribute to altered susceptibility to mutagens, carcinogens, and teratogens. Therefore, every testing protocol utilizing cells or animals will only be relevant to a portion of the human population. In some instances, it will not be relevant to *any* of the human population, as in the case of thalidomide testing in pregnant rats. In only a few instances will a testing protocol be relevant to the entire human population.

It should be apparent that regardless of how we refine our tests for teratogenesis (Brent, 1964, 1972; Grice et al., 1975), carcinogenesis (Grice et al., 1975), or mutagenesis (Bridges, 1974), the results cannot be applied quantitatively to the human population. Khera (1976) concluded: "Comparative studies on the metabolism and teratogenicity of food chemicals in a range of species are not available to the extent that firm conclusions can be drawn." Bridges (1974) suggested that the three-tier approach to mutagenesis testing will provide information giving a "quantitative indication of the potential risk to man followed by a risk-benefit assessment." Russell (1977) is critical of anyone's ability to accomplish this feat and is hypercritical of the concept of a radiation equivalent dose. Until we know much more about mammalian genetics, it would be naive to think that a radiation equivalent dose for chemical mutagens has any significance.

Solutions

The solutions to the problems of human mutagenesis, carcinogenesis, and teratogenesis will come from four areas: new knowledge, better testing protocols, population monitoring, and prevention.

New Knowledge

New knowledge will come from extensive programs in basic research dealing with the mechanisms involved in teratogenesis, mutagenesis, and carcinogenesis. Although the use of established protocols for testing rarely develops new knowledge, new concepts derived from basic research will measurably improve the predictive value of laboratory testing procedures. It is evident that a great investment in time and resources will be necessary to understand these problems more clearly. The more we learn about a particular process, the more we recognize the pitfalls of testing protocols.

For example, we have long known that many agents that are teratogenic in mice or rats are not teratogenic in humans. Recent studies dealing with the yolk sac in the rodent have revealed that yolk sac dysfunction may be a factor in rodent teratogenesis (Brent et al., 1961; Brent, 1969, 1971; Brent et al., 1971). Thus, drugs or chemicals that affect the rodent by interfering with the yolk sac may have no effect in the human. A second example involves cleft palate in the mouse. Our laboratory has demonstrated that high doses of many drugs interfere with rodent embryonic development simply by reducing the appetite of the pregnant mouse during gestation (Szabo and Brent, 1974, 1975). The cleft palate induced by these drugs had little to do with the human situation because the dosage used in the human is hundreds of times lower.

Basic research will be one way to answer questions dealing with threshold, linear response, and repair following low exposures. It is likely that a threshold exists for many teratogenic effects. Thus, most well known teratogens will affect the embryo at doses covering three $\log_{10}$ ranges. Death or severe malformations will occur at the highest exposure, and nothing will be seen at the lowest exposure. For many drugs and chemicals, the range from threshold to maximal effect covers only two $\log_{10}$ scales. Since it is impossible to prove a negative finding, we are left with the concept that although it appears that teratogenic effects have a threshold, we cannot prove it for all such effects. It is even more difficult to prove the existence of a threshold for carcinogenic or mutagenic effects. In fact, when establishing permissible or safe levels, one usually assumes a linear dose-response relationship. In all probability, because repair can occur more readily at low exposures, it is likely that low exposures have less of an effect than one would predict from extrapolating data from carcinogenic or mutagenic experiments utilizing high exposures.

In the meantime, we must extrapolate animal data to humans utilizing the most conservative approach, even though the extrapolations may be gross exaggerations of the hazards.

New Protocols

Better testing protocols will be by-products of new information. Besides attempting to predict human effects, animal testing can provide a means of understanding mechanisms or of supporting an association reported in humans. Thalidomide was demonstrated to be teratogenic in humans, but it was difficult to develop an animal model to support the human finding (Brent, 1969). Spray adhesives were reported to be mutagenic and actually were removed from the marketplace, but later studies indicated that the original reports were erroneous and that no cytogenetic defects were produced by exposure to spray adhesives (Osterberg et al., 1975; Lubs et al., 1976). When bacterial and single-cell systems were used to evaluate the mutagenicity of hycanthone, the drug was reported to be mutagenic (Ong and de Serres, 1975). Because of the importance of hycanthone, Russell (1975) was asked by the WHO to evaluate hycanthone by utilizing mammalian systems. He used the dominant lethal test, x-chromosome loss, and gene mutations, and he reported that hycanthone had no genetic effects, even at dosages well above those used clinically.

Despite enthusiasm for bacterial and other single-cell systems because of their rapidity and low cost, one should be concerned about the many pitfalls in nonmammalian systems.

Protocols of the future may have little resemblance to the ones we are utilizing today. It is to be hoped that they will be based on concepts yet to be conceived. Regardless of the quality and innovativeness of the newer protocols, however, they will never be able to predict risks for the entire human population.

Population Monitoring

Although the Center for Disease Control (CDC) has initiated a congenital malformation surveillance program, we could monitor the occurrence of malformations, cancer, and mutation in a much more sophisticated manner if the resources were provided. The expertise and equipment are available but the effort would have to be greatly expanded.

Congenital malformation and cancer surveillance at a national level would provide baseline data on the incidence and trends of these diseases. Legislation would have to be passed in order to make available to the epidemiologists medical history, genetic history, and history of environmental exposure. This information should be computerized so that a surveillance program could call attention to new statistical correlations and significant changes in incidence of disease. Such a program would have almost immediate benefits, but they would also improve with time as the epidemiologic data become more accurate. A simple manual punch card system would have uncovered the association between thalidomide and limb malformations after less than 15 cases, rather than after the 5000 that occurred.

Establishment of clinical surveillance programs is not a new idea. In 1964, I suggested, "At the present time, the most reliable method of protecting the public from all harmful effects of drugs is through strict clinical surveillance programs." In 1965, Ingalls and Klingberg published the same message. Clinical surveillance is expensive and tedious, and it will take years to educate physicians, the public, and administrative agencies to comply with the regulations. But if we had started the program in 1964, it would be operational today.

Population surveillance programs for genetic disease are more difficult to conceive and to implement than are programs to monitor the incidence of cancer and congenital malformations. One could survey for changes in the sex ratio or the incidence of clinical genetic disease, but these are very insensitive. Neel et al. (1969; Neel, 1970) suggested that we monitor the structure of serum proteins from human umbilical cord blood and evaluate the amino acid structure of a score of serum proteins. This is the most promising method for monitoring human populations.

Potential benefits of genetic monitoring are many. We would begin to gather vast amounts of genetic information about humans, and we would be able to document the existence of genetic hazards (Sutton, 1976). Drug testing procedures alone will never do this. There is now not enough information to know whether environmental mutagenesis is an important problem. In a later paper, Neel (1974) suggested that population monitoring will provide information about mutation rates in civilized versus uncivilized populations. This may be important in determining the variability of the human population's sensitivity to environmental mutagens.

The plea is not for expanded surveillance programs but for expanded high quality programs. There are many poor epidemiologic studies. For example, a report by Milkovich and van den Berg (1974) indicated that meprobamate and chlordiazepoxide were human teratogens. On the basis of this report, the FDA advised that these drugs not be administered during pregnancy. The study had a half dozen serious errors that actually refuted the conclusions. If we had sound national epidemiologic programs, reports could be immediately checked, thus preventing erroneous decisions from being made.

I cannot emphasize sufficiently the importance of expanding and improving population monitoring for malformations, mutations, and cancer. Although all environmental causes of human congenital malformations have to date been reported by alert physicians or scientists, accurate surveillance programs may in the future contribute to our understanding of etiology (Miller, 1975).

Prevention

Prevention of cancer, mutations, and malformations involves the (1) elimination of offending agents, (2) elimination of affected embryos, (3) treatment of affected embryos, and (4) use of eugenics. Each method offers proven and hypothetical solutions to the problems under discussion but also raises controversial ethical, social, economic, and political issues.

Elimination of offending agents. This may seem easy to accomplish until a particular agent is selected. Consider that approximately 100,000 people die each year from lung cancer, and that a substantial number of these victims have cigarette smoking as a primary factor. Yet a substantial number of smokers and the tobacco industry have resisted most attempts to eliminate this hazard. Chemical and industrial pollutants are by-products of an industrial society. Elimination of certain industries or attempts to reduce the population exposure level may cause economic hardships that some may consider worse than potential health hazards. The concept of cost versus benefit will not be analyzed further here because it involves expertise beyond the realm of biomedical science.

A reduction in the use of drugs during pregnancy seems simple to accomplish because physicians are aware of the sensitivity of the embryos and mothers are concerned about congenital malformations. Limiting the drug exposure of pregnant women is usually a decision that is based on "clinical judgment." With the increase in negligence litigation, physicians are less likely to use drugs during pregnancy because malformations may be traced to the drug (Brent, 1967, 1977). Some industries are faced with a dilemma when hiring women of reproductive age because the employer is not in a position to guarantee the safety of the working environment. Thus, the safest policy would be to prevent these women from working in potentially hazardous environments. On the other hand, affirmative action proponents might pursue the philosophy that industrial firms should not eliminate women from the working place, but they should make every effort to protect employees from hazards. These problems can have an enormous impact on the health and welfare of our citizens.

Elimination of affected embryos. This is another method of reducing genetic disease and malformations. It is likely that almost all heterozygous and homozygous recessive states will be diagnosable *in utero*. Furthermore, all cytogenetic and morphologic abnormalities will be readily diagnosed in the first trimester, and thus the vast majority of malformed or genetically affected embryos can be eliminated early in pregnancy. It would even be possible to destroy embryos carrying single recessive genes in an effort to eradicate common recessive diseases such as cystic fibrosis or sickle cell disease in just a few generations. Since abortion is currently a controversial matter, only the future will determine whether the elimination of abnormal fetuses will become an important factor in decreasing the incidence of genetic disease and malformations in liveborn offspring.

Treatment of affected embryos. This procedure may become possible in the future. In the meantime, diseases such as erythroblastosis and intrauterine infections can be treated *in utero*. It is within the realm of possibility that genetic disease may be treatable *in utero*.

Eugenics. As genetics becomes more sophisticated, it will be possible to describe each individual's genetic makeup and, in many instances, to provide couples with information on the risk of genetic disease, malformations, and even malignancy in their offspring. Whether this information will be used in planning families is at present a matter for conjecture.

Conclusion

The role of chemicals and drugs in producing genetic disease, cancer, and malformations is far from clear. Although evidence indicates that a very small percentage of human cancers are primarily related to drugs or chemicals, there is no evidence that drugs and chemicals have changed the mutation rate in man. Furthermore, the percentage of malformed children resulting from drug and chemical exposure is extremely small. The problem is that since most cancers and malformations do not have a known etiology, environmental factors may be playing some role in their development. Because environmental factors can be controlled (more or less), it would be prudent to determine which ones have the greatest potential for harm and should be removed from, or reduced in, our environment.

The development of protocols for animal and laboratory testing of drugs and chemicals for teratogenicity, mutagenicity, and carcinogenicity has been reviewed. It is obvious that these tests cannot predict with certainty the qualitative and quantitative effects of drugs and chemicals in humans. There are instances in which even the laboratory tests disagree. This is especially true with regard to teratogenicity and mutagenicity. Since these tests frequently cannot predict whether a drug or chemical is safe or harmful, the regulatory agencies have a difficult time utilizing the information obtained. For example, the FDA warns that all new drugs have not been proven safe in pregnant women, even when animal teratogenicity tests are negative. At the same time, drugs that have been utilized for decades with no reported malformations in humans remain on the market, even though they are potent animal teratogens (e.g., acetylsalicylic acid). Despite these shortcomings, animal and laboratory screening of drugs and chemicals for teratogenesis, mutagenesis, and carcinogenesis should continue because valuable information and experience has resulted. It is distressing that many harmless compounds will be suspected of adverse effects as a result of false positive tests, but this is the price we must pay, since we do not have a better understanding of these processes.

Although we are trapped into utilizing testing protocols despite their lack of predictiveness of human disease, I am optimistic about our ability to understand and to prevent the harmful effects of environmental agents. We can prevent and treat intrauterine disease; the options are now available to us as citizens. The future use of eugenic principles may also decrease the incidence of malformations, cancer, and genetic disease. Important contributions in this area will come from the results of basic biomedical research and sophisticated large scale epidemiologic surveillance.

Data indicate that the induction of carcinogenesis may be a more sensitive barometer to the presence of environmental hazards than is the induction of mutagenesis. If it can be substantiated, this concept could be an important aspect of population monitoring. Both basic research and epidemiologic monitoring should provide information about the mechanisms of disease development, the incidence of these diseases, and the etiologies of cancer, malformation, and mutation.

Finally, despite the fact that many have warned that pollution, environmental chemicals, and drugs are or will be major causes of cancer and mutation, I think this is very unlikely. The phenomena of selection, repair, and cell death will in all likelihood prevent the occurrence of marked increases in the mutation rate or the production of viable cells markedly different from the parent cells. Furthermore, genetic epidemiologic studies patterned after the suggestions of Neel should provide us with the knowledge that drastic changes in human DNA are not occurring. Although many people have spoken pessimistically about the harmful effects of environmental agents, I believe we have the tools and resources to understand and to manage the problem of environmental carcinogenesis, mutagenesis, and teratogenesis. I wish I could be as optimistic about some of the other social and economic problems that confront our culture.

References

Ames, B.N., Lee, F.D., and Durston, W.E.: An improved test system for the detection and classification of mutagens and classification of mutagens and carcinogens. Proc. Natl. Acad. Sci. USA 70:782–786, 1973.

Ames, B.N.: A combined bacterial and liver test system for detection and classification of carcinogens as mutagens. Genetics 78:91–95,1974.

Ashby, J., and Styles, J.A.: Does carcinogenic potency correlate with mutagenic potency in the Ames assay? Nature 271:452–455, 1978.

Auerbach, C.: Some old problems in mutagenesis and their bearing on mutagen testing. Mutat. Res. 41:3–6, 1976.

Baker, J.B.E., et al.: Principles for testing of drugs for teratogenicity. Die Pharmazeutische Industrie 29:759–763, 1967.

Bateman, A.J.: The induction of dominant lethal mutations in rats and mice with triethylmelamine (TEM). Genet. Res. 1:381–392, 1960.

Berry, C.L., and Barlow, S.: Some remaining problems in the reproductive toxicity testing of drugs. Br. Med. Bull. 32:34–38, 1976.

Betrand, M., Levet, E., Girod, J., and Leperco, M.F.: L'Embryotoxicite des medicaments. Les Cahiers de Medecine Veterinaire 2:1–26, 1972.

Boyland, E., and Sydnor, K.L.: The induction of mammary cancers in rats. Br. J. Cancer 18:731–739, 1962.

Brent, R.L., Averich, E., and Drapiewski, V.A.: Production of congenital malformations using tissue antibodies. I, Kidney antisera. Proc. Soc. Exp. Biol. Med. 106:523–526, 1961.

Brent, R.L.: Drug testing in animals for teratogenic effects: thalidomide in the pregnant rat. J. Pediatr. 64:762–770, 1964.

Brent, R.L.: Medicolegal aspects of teratology. J. Pediatr. 71:288–298, 1967.

Brent, R.L.: Implications of experimental teratology. Excerpta Medica International Congress Series No. 204:187–195, 1969.

Brent, R.L.: The effect of immune reactions on fetal development. Advances in Bioscience 6:421–455, 1971.

Brent, R.L.: Johnson, A.J., and Jensen, M.: The production of congenital malformations using tissue antisera. VII, Yolk sac antiserum. Teratology 4:255–276, 1971.

Brent, R.L.: Protecting the public from teratogenic and mutagenic hazards. J. Clin. Pharmacol. 12:61–70, 1972.

Brent, R.L.: Litigation-produced pain, disease and suffering: an experience with congenital malformation lawsuits. Teratology 16:1–14, 1977.

Bridges, B.A.: The three-tier approach to mutagenicity screening and the concept of radiation-equivalent dose. Mutat. Res. 26:335–340, 1974.

Brusick, D.J.: In vitro mutagenesis assays as predictors of chemical carcinogenesis in mammals. Clin. Toxicol. 10:79–109, 1977.

Cahen, R.L.: Evaluation of the teratogenicity of drugs. Clin. Pharmacol. Ther. 5:480–514, 1964.

Cattanach, B.M., Pollard, C.E., and Issacson, J.J.: Ethyl methanesulfonate induced chromosome breakage in the mouse. Mutat. Res. 6:297–307, 1968.

Durston, W.E., and Ames, B.N.: A simple method for the detection of mutagens in urine: studies with the carcinogen 2-acetylaminofluorene. Proc. Nat. Acad. Sci. 71:737–741, 1974.

Epstein, S.S., Arnold, E., Andrea, J., Bass, W., and Bishop, Y.: Detection of chemical mutagens by the dominant lethal assay in the mouse. Toxicol. Appl. Pharmacol. 23:288–325, 1972.

Epstein, S.: Cancer and the environment. Bull. Atom. Sci. 33:22–30, 1977.

Fahrig, R.: Development of host-mediated mutagenicity tests. I, Differential response of yeast cells injected into testes of rats and peritoneum of mice and rats to mutagens. Mutat. Res. 26:29–36, 1974.

Frank, D.W., Trzos, R.J., and Good, P.I.: A comparison of two methods for evaluating drug-induced chromosome alterations. Mutat. Res. 56:311–317, 1978.

Fraser, F.C.: Relation of animal studies to the problem in man. In Wilson, J.C., and Fraser, F.C., *Handbook of Teratology,* Vol. 1, New York, Plenum Press, 1977.

Frohberg, H., and Oettel, H.: Method of testing for teratogenicity in mice. Indus. Med. Surg. 35:113–120, 1966.

Gabridge, M.G., and Legator, M.S.: A host-mediated microbial assay for the detection of mutagenic compounds. Proc. Soc. Exp. Biol. Med. 130:831–834, 1969.

Galloway, S.M.: Ataxia telangiectasia: the effects of chemical mutagens and X-rays on sister chromatid in blood lymphocytes. Mutat. Res. 45:343–349, 1977.

Generoso, W.M., Russell, W.L., Huff, S.W., Stout, S.K., and Gosslee, D.B.: Effects of dose on the induction of dominant-lethal mutations and heritable translocations with ethyl methanesulfonate in male mice. Genetics 77:741–752, 1974.

Generoso, W.M., Preston, R.J., and Brewen, J.G.: 6-Mercaptopurine, an inducer of cytogenetic and dominant-lethal effects in premeiotic and early meiotic germ cells of male mice. Mutat. Res. 28:437–447, 1975.

Goldstein, L.S., and Spindle, A.I.: Detection of x-ray induced dominant lethal mutations in mice: an in vitro approach. Mutat. Res. 41:289–296, 1976.

Gottschewski, G.H.M.: Konnen Tierversuche zur losung der frage nach der teratogenen wirkung von medikamenten auf den menschlichen embryo beitragen? Arzneim. Forsch. 15:97–104, 1965.

Green, M.C., Azar, C.A., and Maren, T.H.: Strain differences in susceptibility to the teratogenic effect of acetazolamide in mice. Teratology 8:143–146, 1973.

Green, S., Zeiger, E., Palmer, K.A., Springer, J.A., and Legator, M.S.: Protocols for the dominant lethal test, host-mediated assay, and in vivo cytogenetic test used in the Food and Drug Administration's review of substances in the GRAS (generally recognized as safe) list. J. Toxicol. Environ. Health 1:921–928, 1976.

Grice, H.C., et al.: *The Testing of Chemicals for Carcinogenicity, Mutagenicity, Teratogenicity.* Canada: Marc Lalonde, Minister of Health and Welfare Canada, 1975.

Hill, B.F.: Testing chemical mutagens: the host-mediated assay. Charles River Digest 25:No. 3, 1976.

Ingalls, T.H., and Klingberg, M.A.: Implications of epidemic embryopathy for public health. Am. J. Public Health 55:200–208, 1965.

Kalter, H.: Some relations between teratogenesis and mutagenesis. Mutat. Res. 33:29–36, 1975.

Kato, H.: Induction of sister chromatid exchanges by chemical mutagens and its possible relevance to DNA repair. Exp. Cell Res. 85:239–247, 1974.

Khera, K.S.: Significance of metabolic patterns in teratogenic testing for food safety. Clin. Toxicol. 9:773–790, 1976.

Koskimies, O., Lapinleimu K., and Saxen, L.: Infections and other maternal factors as risk indicators for congenital malformations: a case-control study with paired serum samples. Pediatrics 61:832–838, 1978.

Loosli, Von R., and Theiss, E.: Methodik und problematik der medikamentos-experimentellen teratogenese. Bull. Schweiz. Akad. Med. Wiss. 20:398–416, 1964.

Lorke, D.: Method for the investigation of embryotoxic and teratogenic effects on rat. Naunyn-Schmiedeberg's Arch. Pharmacol. 246:147–151, 1963.

Lubs, H.A., Verma, R.S., Summitt, R.L., and Hecht, F.: Re-evaluation of the effect of spray adhesives on human chromosomes. Clin. Genet. 9:302–306, 1976.

Magee, P.N.: The relationship between mutagenesis, carcinogenesis and teratogenesis. In Scott, D., Bridges, B.A., and Sobels, F.H., *Progress in Genetic Toxicology,* Elsevier/North-Holland Biomedical Press, 1977.

McCann, J., Choi, E., Yamasaki, E., and Ames, B.N.: Detection of carcinogens as mutagens in the Salmonella/microsome test: assay of 300 chemicals. Proc. Nat. Acad. Sci. 72:5135–5139, 1975.

Miller, J.R.: Some epidemiological aspects of teratogen detection. Mutat. Res. 33:45–54, 1975.

Miller, R.W.: The feature in common among persons at high risk of leukemia. In Yuhas, J.M., Tennant, R.W., and Regan, J.D., *Biology of Radiation Carcinogenesis,* New York, Raven Press, 1976.

Milkovich, L., and van den Berg, B.J.: Effects of prenatal meprobamate and chlordiazepoxide hydrochloride on human embryonic and fetal development. N. Engl. J. Med. 291:1268–1271, 1974.

Mohn, G.R.: Actual status of mutagenicity testing with the host-mediated assay. Arch. Toxicol. 38:109–133, 1977.

Natarajan, A.T., Tates, A.D., van Buul, P., Meijers, M., and De Vogel, N.: Cytogenetic effect of mutagens/carcinogens after activation in a microsomal system in vitro. I, Induction of chromosome aberrations and sister chromatid exchanges by diethylnitrosamine (DEN) and dimethylnitrosamine in CHO cells in the presence of rat-liver microsomes. Mutat. Res. 37:83, 1976.

Neel, J.V., and Bloom, A.D.: The detection of environmental mutagens. Med. Clin. North Am. 53:1243–1256, 1969.

Neel, J.V.: Evaluation of the effects of chemical mutagens on man: the long road ahead. Proc. Nat. Acad. Sci. 67:908–915, 1970.

Neel, J.V.: Developments in monitoring human populations for mutation rates. Mutat. Res. 26:319–328, 1974.

Nichols, W.W.: Cytogenetic techniques in mutagenicity testing. Agents Actions 32:86–92, 1973.

Ong, Tong-man, and DeSerres, F.J.: Mutagenic evaluation of antischistosomal drugs and their derivatives in neurospora crassa. J. Toxicol. Environ. Health 1:271–279, 1975.

Osterberg, R.E., Murphy, J.E., Bierbower, G.W., and Sauro, F.M.: An evaluation of the mutagenic potential of an aerosol spray adhesive in the rat. Mutat. Res. 31:169–173, 1975.

Rohrborn, G., and Basler, A.: Cytogenetic investigations of mammals: comparison of the genetic activity of cytostatics in mammals. Arch. Toxicol. 38:35–43, 1977.

Russell, W.L.: X-ray-induced mutations in mice. Cold Spring Harbor Symp. Quant. Biol. 16:327–336, 1951.

Russell, W.L.: Results of tests for possible transmitted genetic effects of hycanthone in mammals. J. Toxicol. Environ. Health 1:301–305, 1975.

Russell, L.B.: Validation of the in vivo somatic mutation method in the mouse as a prescreen for germinal point mutations. Arch. Toxicol. 38:75–85, 1977.

Russell, W.L.: The role of mammals in the future of chemical mutagenesis research. Arch. Toxicol. 38:141–147, 1977.

Schmid, W.: The micronucleus test for cytogenetic analysis. Chem. Mutagens. 4:31, 1976.

Sobels, F.H.: Some problems associated with the testing for environmental mutagens and a perspective for studies in "Comparative Mutagenesis." Mutat. Res. 46:245–260, 1977.

Sobels, F.H.: Charlotte Auerbach and chemical mutagenesis. Mutat. Res. 29:171–180, 1975.

Sobels, F.H.: Some thoughts on the evaluation of environmental mutagens. Mutat. Res. 38:361–366, 1976.

Sutton, H.E.: The impact of induced mutations of human populations. Mutat. Res. 33:17–24, 1976.

Szabo, K.T., and Brent, R.L.: Species differences in experimental teratogenesis by tranquillising agents. Lancet: i:565, 1974.

Szabo, K.T., and Brent, R.L.: Reduction of drug-induced cleft palate in mice. Lancet 1:1296–1297, 1975.

Taylor, J.H., Woods, P.S., and Hughes, W.L.: The organization and duplication of chromosomes as revealed by autoradiographic studies using tritium-labeled thymidine. Proc. Nat. Acad. Sci. 43:122, 1957.

Tomatis, L, Agthe, C., Bartsch, H., Huff, J., Montesano, R., Saracci, R., Walker, E., and Wilbourn, J.: Evaluation of the carcinogenicity of chemicals: a review of the monograph program of the International Agency for Research on Cancer (1971 to 1977). Cancer Res. 38:877–885, 1978.

Tuchmann-Duplessis, H.: Teratogenic drug screening. Present procedures and requirements. Teratology 5:271–286, 1972.

Tuchmann-Duplessis, H.: Teratogenic screening methods and their application to contraceptive products. Meeting on pharmacological models to assess toxicity and side effects of fertility regulating agents. Geneva, September 17–20, 1973.

Warkany, J., et al.: Conference on prenatal effects of drugs. Commission on Drug Safety Bull., June 1963.

Wilson, J.G.: Embryological considerations in teratology. IV, Drugs and the mammalian embryo. Ann. NY Acad. Sci. 123:219–227, 1965.

Yamasaki, E., and Ames, B.N.: Concentration of mutagens from urine by adsorption with the non-polar resin XAD-2: cigarette smokers have mutagenic urine. Proc. Natl. Acad. Sci. 74:3555–3559, 1977.

Zbinden, G.: The problems of the toxicologic examination of drugs in animals and their safety in man. Clin. Pharmacol. Ther. 5:537–545, 1964.

Are Carcinogenicity Tests Useful?

David Salsburg, Ph.D.
Senior Statistician, Pfizer Inc.

The major points that will be made in this essay revolve around the term *useful*, and they can be simply stated. It is impossible to use lifetime feeding studies in rodents to determine if a new drug will "cause cancer in man," because those studies are too badly designed to answer any clear-cut questions about the way in which a drug might be involved in the carcinogenic process. If the data from those studies are treated by the blind applications of statistical methods, there is a 20 to 50 per cent probability that a new drug will be "shown" to cause cancer when, in fact, the pattern of tumors is the result of pure chance. Furthermore, one can discover whether a drug is a "weak carcinogen" only if the study uses 10^{12} animals per dose. If, on the other hand, the data are examined with biologic "common sense," the concept of carcinogenicity is so ill defined that a large number of biologically active substances appear to be "carcinogenic" at high doses. Thus, my thesis is that the tests as now designed are *not* useful, because the rate of false positives (both statistical and biologic) is so great that they cannot be used to discover if a drug will cause cancer in man.

My attention is restricted to a specific kind of carcinogenicity test—the lifetime feeding study in rodents. There are a number of short-term tests whose value and interpretation are still open to considerable disagreement. Some of these examine for drug-induced changes in the nucleic acid of living cells (such as the Ames test in Salmonella and the unscheduled DNA repair tests that use *in vitro* preparations of mammalian cells). Other tests that have been proposed build on the initiator-promoter concept and examine the test compound's effect when used with varying combinations of known carcinogenic substances. Most of these short-term tests have a major advantage over the lifetime studies in that they have well defined endpoints and are well designed. However, they deal with biologic events that may be only incidental to the process of cancer. Until we can work with a more precise definition of carcinogenicity, such tests are open to the suspicion that they cover only a small spectrum of the biologic events that worry society. The lifetime study, on the other hand, has been proposed and is widely recognized as the only test that includes most of the aspects of what we now call *carcinogenicity*.

Background

During the past four or five years, both new and old drugs have been subjected to a toxicology "screen" involving a procedure that (1) has never been fully evaluated to determine its relevance to man, (2) has a high probability of producing false positive results, and (3) adds about a quarter of a million dollars and up to three extra years to a drug's development. The procedure also violates fundamental principles of good biologic experimentation, and it can easily produce results that cannot be analyzed without serious statistical bias and a resulting confusion between direct carcinogenesis and extraneous biologic events.

This procedure has cast suspicion on a list

of marketed drugs that includes a widely used sedative (phenobarbital), the major defensive agent in the treatment of tuberculosis (isoniazid), a standard treatment for trichomoniasis (metronidazole), a potent diuretic (spironolactone), and a whole class of psychotherapeutic agents (the phenothiazines). A poll taken at the Biopharmaceutical Subsection of the American Statistical Association meetings in 1976 indicated that, up to that time, at least 10 new drugs had been withdrawn from investigation in the U.S. owing to findings from such studies, when less than 30 such studies were completed.

Why would a scientifically advanced nation introduce such a major and unevaluated stumbling block to the development of new drug therapy? The answer lies in one word—cancer.

Prior Research

Early in the 1930s, it was discovered that if certain coal tar derivatives were painted on the shaven skin of mice with repeated applications, skin tumors would be induced in about 12 to 14 weeks (see Shubik and Hartwell, 1969, for a description of these early experiments). In an attempt to discover the nature of carcinogenesis, experiments were run during the following 30 years to establish what kinds of chemical compounds would cause cancer in this fashion. The more the researchers looked, the more complicated the matter became. Tumor yields could be increased, for instance, by combining the carcinogenic substance with a "promoter" such as croton oil. It appeared early in these studies that slight molecular modifications of some of these compounds reduced or even eliminated their carcinogenic potential. For instance, one of the most widely studied classes of compounds was the benzpyrenes, and it seemed for a time as if slight shifts in the arrangements of the rings or the use of specific side chains produced noncarcinogens.

As a statistician looking at most of these experiments in retrospect, I can see that I could account for the failure to find carcinogenesis by pointing to the small numbers of animals used (often less than 25 mice in a single experiment). Furthermore, since one purpose of those early experiments was to discover a cancer model in rodents that could be used for the evaluation of antineoplastic therapy, most of the effort on chemical carcinogenesis before 1965 dealt with known carcinogens rather than with the search for new agents. For instance, Supplement II of the Shubik and Hartwell paper lists over 700 experiments done from 1945 to 1960 dealing with 9,10-dimethyl-1, 2-benzanthracene, and only two experiments with phenobarbital! It is interesting to note that the two experiments on phenobarbital were run by the same investigator; he used only 20 mice per experiment, had no controls, and concluded that the compound was not carcinogenic.

Eventually, the most effective animal screens for antineoplastic agents became those using transplanted tumors. Some of the more massive experiments aimed at establishing chemical screens for carcinogenicity (Shimkin et al., 1967) became part of the history of scientific digressions. However, the shibboleth remained that only a small percentage of chemical compounds cause cancer and that slight molecular modifications are often sufficient to turn a carcinogen into a noncarcinogen. This underlying assumption led the International Union Against Cancer to recommend, at its 1956 meeting in Rome, that carcinogens be banned from the food supply. From this came the Delaney Amendment to the U.S. Food and Drug Law.

It should be noted that this conclusion was based almost entirely on skin painting experiments, plus a scattering of experiments in which the animals were injected with the suspect compound and a smaller number in which they were fed the suspect compound. (A description of some of the earliest feeding studies can be found in Oser, 1973.) No attempt was made in these earlier studies to consider the effects of long-term feeding with toxic doses.

Throughout the 1960s, evidence began to accumulate from long-term feeding studies that both drugs and widely used agricultural chemicals could increase the rate of tumors or cause rare tumors in animals. The suggested effects of agricultural chemicals led the National Cancer Institute to contract for a lifetime feeding study of 120 herbicides, pesticides, and acaricides in mice. A preliminary note describing this study was published by Innes et al. (1969). By 1972, concern over the carcinogenic potential of beta-adrenergic blocking agents led the Food and Drug Administration (FDA) to ask each drug company with such a compound in clinical testing to subject the drug to lifetime feeding studies in mice and rats.

Protocol Development

As far as I can determine, the Innes study of agricultural chemicals and the studies resulting from the FDA request of 1972 represent the first examples of lifetime feeding studies with many similar chemicals that used controls and whose results were subjected to careful scrutiny. This is not to say that there were no previous lifetime studies, but with these two efforts, an attempt was made to standardize the protocols so that similar compounds could be compared. Both positive and negative controls were introduced, and the data that resulted were carefully analyzed by both the experimenting facility and the governmental agencies that had ordered the studies. In contrast, most of the previous work had been done by independent investigators who could choose whether or not to publish the results of their studies and who were the only ones to examine the raw data.

Even with these standardized protocols, variations existed among the studies. The Innes study of agricultural chemicals used only 19 animals per group, treated the animals via both oral and parenteral routes (although only the oral results were published), and used two strains but only one species. The FDA request (1) did not specify the number of animals to be used (although most drug companies settled on a minimum of 50 per dose as a result of conversations with FDA officials), (2) required that the animals be fed for 18 months and then followed (an additional six months for rats, three months for mice), and (3) required that two species of randomly bred strains of rodents be used.

The lifetime feeding study that has become standard for testing new drugs has gradually taken shape from those initial protocols. Current drug testing protocols use four dosage levels: an untreated control group, a low dose of test compound that is a small multiple of the maximum human dose, a high dose that is sufficient to produce subnormal weight gain in about 10 percent of the animals, and a middle dose between those two. Animals are fed on a dose per kilogram basis from weaning until death or until 18 months for mice and 24 months for rats. Most companies use at least 50 animals per sex per dose. Some companies use two control groups; some use 100 animals at each dose group. Sometimes, additional groups that receive intermittent dosing are added.

Although there is a standard drug testing protocol, many serious questions still remain. In particular, there is doubt about the meaning of tumors induced by high and toxic doses of the test compound. However, somehow the idea has evolved that lifetime feeding studies represent a "definitive assay" of carcinogenicity. In 1974, for instance, the Health Research Group of Washington, D.C., an organization funded by Ralph Nader's Public Citizen, Inc., petitioned the FDA to require such studies of all new drugs before they could be used in humans. The Commissioner of Food and Drugs rejected their petition, but the petition presents the usual arguments for such a requirement and can be looked upon as one of the most complete cases made so far for the position that carcinogenicity testing be required for new drugs. A fundamental flaw in that petition is the assumption that the lifetime feeding study is a well defined bioassay of carcinogenesis. It would be useful, therefore, to determine if it is possible to use the lifetime study, as it is now designed, for a bioassay. To answer this question, let us first look at what a bioassay should be.

The Lifetime Study as a Bioassay

In general, one can think of a bioassay as a rigid, stereotyped procedure in which one provokes a measurable biologic response with varying amounts of compound in order to characterize the activity of that compound. A typical bioassay measures biologic response at several different doses of the investigational compound. These values are then compared with a similar sequence of responses produced by a compound of known activity or with a standard curve evolved from earlier experiments. Comparisons are made within the framework of a mathematical model whose structure has been established by prior experimentation. The result is a statement about the relative potency of the unknown compound or a statement that the unknown mixture contains a certain amount of standard compound (or has activity equivalent to a certain amount of standard compound). In addition, all bioassays have thresholds—that is, there is a level of biologic measurement below which the assay cannot distinguish the presence of the material or activity sought. The operating characteristics of a good bioassay are usually known, so it is possible to include that threshold of response as one of the parameters of the mathematical model.

Sometimes, a bioassay is used primarily to detect the presence of activity above the level of that threshold. If the lifetime feeding study is a bioassay, this would seem to be its major purpose. We seek to detect the presence of a biologic activity called *carcinogenesis*. If so, what is the well defined mathematical model whose structure has been established by prior experimentation?

A MODEL FOR CARCINOGENESIS

A model is implicit in many researchers' statements (see, for instance Nelson et al., 1971; Shubik et al., 1977; and the U.S. Federal Register, October 4, 1977, in which the Department of Labor proposed standards for identifying carcinogens in the workplace). The model has been made more explicit by Mantel and Schneiderman (1975), among others. It assumes that there is a well defined endpoint in a given animal—i.e., the observance of a tumor. The probability that an animal will be observed with a tumor is thought of as a function of (1) an inherent characteristic of the compound at test, (2) the dose of the compound, if it has that characteristic, and (3) the amount of time the animal is exposed to the compound, if it has that characteristic. Those who propose *in utero* exposure will add a fourth dimension to the domain of that function: the reduction of an animal's defenses against cancer.

Since we are looking for an increase in the probability of an event, and since each animal can supply us with only a "yes" or "no" response, the model implies that there is a threshold of observation in the sense that with a given number of animals, we can be reasonably sure of picking up an increase in probability only if it exceeds a certain amount. Figure 7–1 displays the curve of the number of animals we need to be 90 percent sure of finding at least one with a tumor, plotted against the probability of tumor for a given dose of the carcinogen. For very low probabilities,we need an unrealistically larger number of animals. If the model is correct, we can increase the proportion of animals with tumors by increasing the dose and/or the time of exposure, and, hence, be able to detect the inherent characteristic of carcinogenesis with a smaller number of animals.

Unfortunately, the model does not fit reality. First of all, there is a considerable amount of background random noise. That is, animals that

Figure 7–1. Number of animals needed to be 90 percent sure of having at least one animal with tumor, assuming no background incidence.

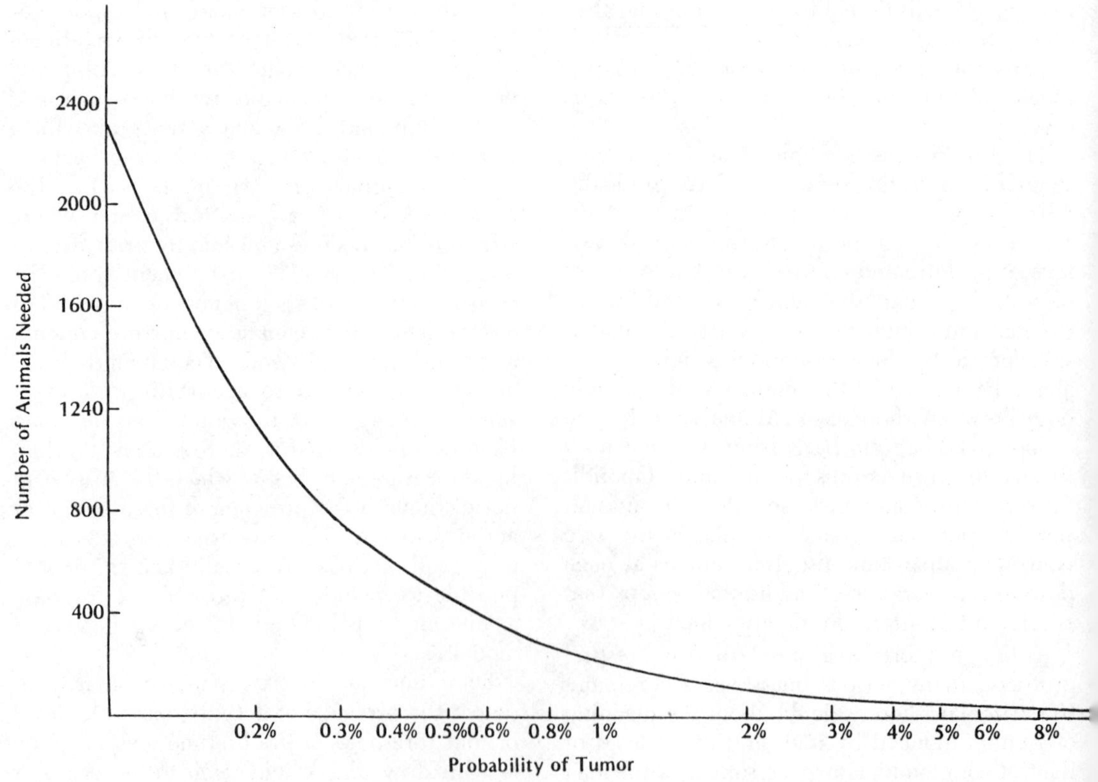

are not treated with the compound in question but are kept as controls tend to have tumors too. The pattern and frequency of such tumors change with species, strain, location of trial, and even time of year (Mackenzie et al., 1972; Sher, 1972). The bioassay must therefore detect an increase in probability of tumor above that shown in the controls. The tradeoff between the number of animals and the ability to detect a difference becomes more difficult. Figure 7–2 displays the curve for the number of animals versus difference in probability needed to be 90 percent sure of seeing such an effect, when 10 percent of the control animals tend to have tumors.

As before, we can increase the sensitivity for a given number of animals if we can increase the difference in probability of tumor between the control and the treated animals. However, we can do this by extending the period of exposure only if extending exposure does not also increase the background rate to the same or greater extent. If extending exposure increases the background rate, it could easily make detection even more difficult.

Proposals have also been made to modify the definition of what will be called a *tumor-bearing animal* (Shubik et al., 1977). This has led to arguments over whether one should consider only malignant tumors, all tumors, all hyperplastic lesions, only gross tumors, or both gross and microscopic ones. Many of these arguments seem to flow from a failure to think in terms of this mathematical model. From the stand-

Figure 7–2. Number of animals needed per group to be 90 percent sure of detecting added probability of tumor when 10 percent of controls have tumors (α = 5 percent).

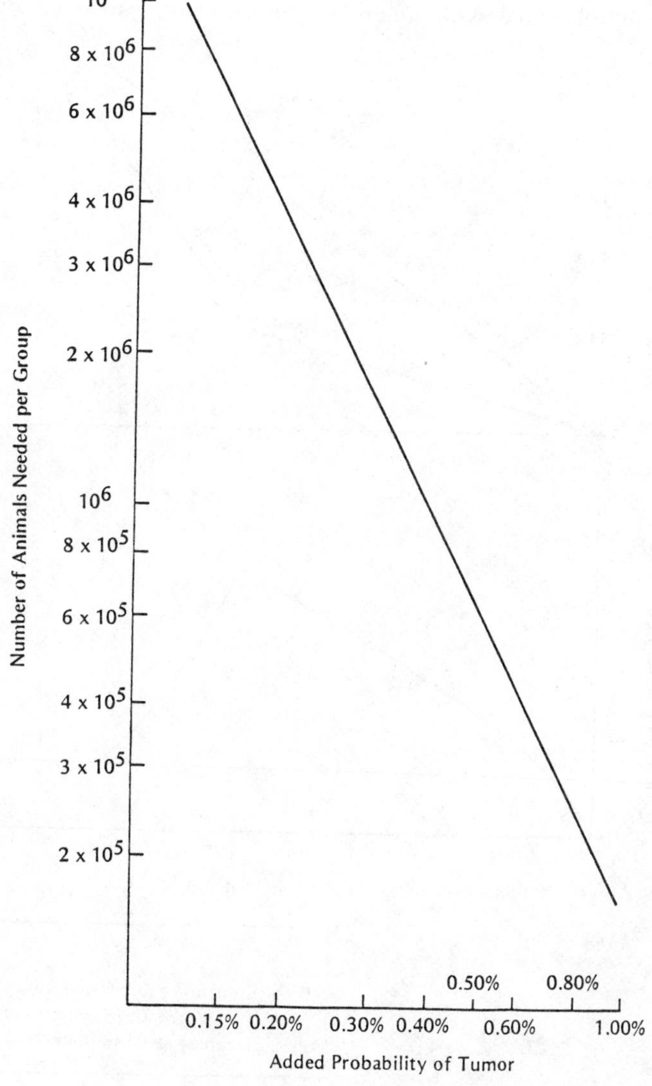

point of the model, it is clear that these techniques will increase the sensitivity only if they increase the difference in probability between controls and treated subjects that an animal will be counted as tumor bearing.

In order to know if extending exposure or modifying the definition of a tumor-bearing animal will increase the difference in probability, we will have to examine data from experiments already run and construct a series of careful experiments that will further refine the mathematical model by allowing us to sketch in the algebraic form of this dose-time-definition-dependent probability function. My own analysis of data from lifetime studies suggests:

1. For both rats and mice, there is some point (about 18 months for the Sprague-Dawley rat) up to which there is a very low level of background noise and beyond which the number of control animals with tumors in certain organs increases very rapidly. If this is true, the curves of tumor probability versus time of exposure may look like Figure 7–3. This has also been noticed by Mantel (1977).

2. As we allow the definition of a tumor-bearing animal to include lesions that are not life threatening or can be seen only under the microscope, we begin to have a large number of competing events and can conceivably find that a true carcinogen shows a lower probability of "tumor" than the controls. I will return to this idea later.

The mathematical model has other errors in it, which I will also come back to. For the moment, however, let us consider a bioassay based on that model in which we compare the proportion of tumor-bearing animals on various doses of compound with the proportion of tumor-bearing animals in the controls. One way to avoid some of the complications is to restrict

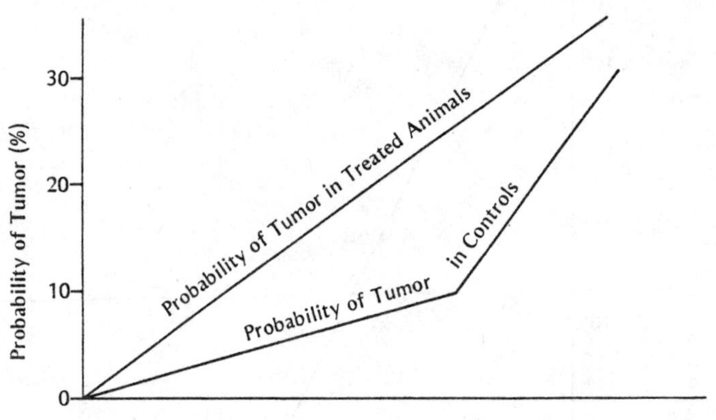

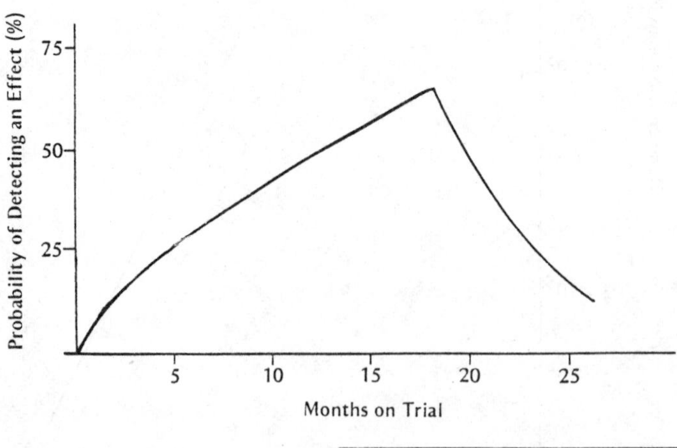

Model:

Prob {Controls} = .0056 (months) + .0215 (months -18)$^{+}$

Prob {Treated} = .0142 (months)

Figure 7–3. Probability of detecting a tumorigenic effect when controls change in rats at 18 months.

our attention to rare tumor types. We would then have an assay designed to discover compounds with a biologic activity that induces an animal to have a tumor in an organ not normally prone to tumor. In our mathematical model, the probability of such a tumor increases with increasing dose and with increasing time of exposure, but the probability of such a tumor in the controls remains relatively constant as we allow for increasing exposure time. We can now calculate the threshold of such an assay.

The Rare Tumor

Figure 7–4 shows the tradeoff between the number of animals per dose and the increase in tumorigenesis, assuming that the control incidence is less than or equal to 0.1 percent. I have plotted this on log-log paper and have shown the extreme end of the curve. Note that a direct consequence of the model is that no matter how many animals are put on test, an undetectable additional probability of tumor remains. If this model is correct, society is forced to make decisions—we must be willing to find a tradeoff point. How much in the way of scientific resources will we expend for a given compound, and how fine-tuned a difference do we wish to detect? In a very simplistic view of that tradeoff, to be 90 percent sure that a compound at test will *not* cause one cancer in a population of N people, we will have to test the compound in $0.02N^2$ animals per group. If

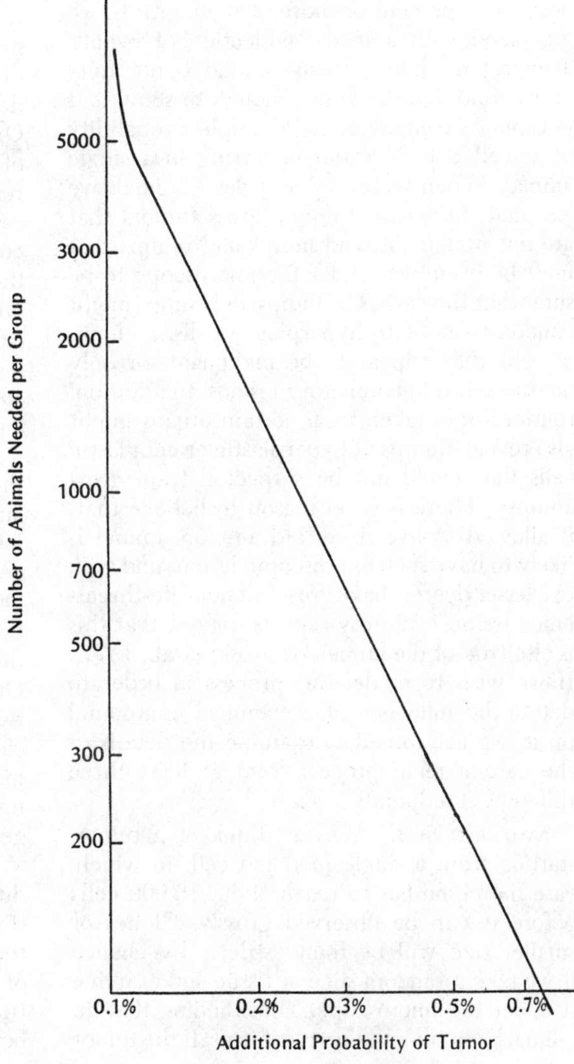

Figure 7-4. Number of animals needed per group to be 90 percent sure of detecting added probability of tumor when 0.1 percent of controls have tumors ($\alpha = .05$).

N is 20 million people (the number of potential patients that might require chronic use of an antiinflammatory drug, for instance), the number of animals needed is more than 10^{12}.

If the mathematical model is correct, those involved in making regulatory decisions should have a clear understanding of this tradeoff. Before we spend $200,000 or more on a carcinogenic study of a given compound, it is worth considering how much safety we are in fact buying.

Other Tumor Types

Once we get beyond the compound that induces a rare tumor type, the mathematical model breaks down completely as a descriptor of reality. When we start looking at tumors that occur in 5 percent or more of the controls, we are faced with a mixed collection of events. Tumorigenesis in a living animal is not fully understood, but we know enough to show that it cannot be modeled as a simple probability of a well defined event occurring in a single animal. When we examine a dead animal, we can find malignant tumors, gross tumors that are not malignant, and lumps and bumps that must be examined under the microscope to be sure what they are. The lumps and bumps might contain tissue with hyperplastic cells, a clump of cells that appear to be malignant, or only nontumorous inflammatory lesions. In addition, routine slices taken from certain organs might also reveal clumps of hyperplastic or neoplastic cells that could not be suspected from gross autopsy. There is good reason to believe that, if allowed to live to an old age, an animal is likely to have such microscopic lesions and will, to a lesser degree, have gross but non-life-threatening lesions. Autopsy reports suggest that this is also true of the human (Huyoshi et al., 1977). If we wish to model this process in order to detect the influence of a chemical compound on it, we are forced to examine the details of the carcinogenic process from at least three different standpoints.

Sampling bias. We can think of a tumor starting from a single modified cell, in which case the clone has to reach about 10,000 cells before it can be observed grossly. Clones of smaller size will be found strictly by chance if we take a random slice of tissue and examine it under the microscope. Thus, finding that an animal has a tumor takes two forms. If the tumor is gross, we can be fairly certain of finding it, but if the tumor is microscopic, the probability that we will find it is a function of the way in which we sample the tissues of the animal. Suppose our sampling rule is to take a standard slice of each of several organs plus a slice of all grossly observable lumps and bumps. Suppose further that in both the control and treated animals, microscopic tumors can be found scattered with equal probability in a given tissue but that one of the effects of the compound is to cause nodules of normal tissue to grow in that organ or to induce cysts within the tissue. These nodules and cysts will be found and sampled, along with small bits of surrounding tissue, thus increasing the probability that a microscopic tumor will be found—even if the compound has had no effect on those tumors.

Indirect action. The compound might not have any effect on carcinogenesis *per se,* but it might cause these microscopic tumors to grow more rapidly (as occurs with continual dosing of ultraviolet light) so that there are a larger number of gross tumors in the treated animals. Or, the compound might enhance the growth of one type of tumor, leading to a higher occurrence of metastatic tumors. Both these events can be considered serious enough to indict the compound, but they are distinctly different from the concept of a carcinogen that causes a heritable change in a single cell and starts an irrevocable process of cancer. The other effects could conceivably be solely due to the high doses used, and it might be possible to estimate a "no-effect" dose.

Time-to-tumor. For some tumor types, there is strong evidence that almost all control animals would develop a tumor if they lived long enough. Test compounds could cause a decrease in the median time for such a tumor. Or, by killing off enough "weak" animals at the higher and toxic doses, they could increase the median time at which tumors are observed. Or, they might produce a combination of these two effects. The way in which such a compound causes a change in median time may involve initial heritable modifications of the cells or may involve nothing more than a change in the general rate of metabolism for the entire animal. We may never be able to distinguish among different causes, but if we attempt to model this type of observation in terms of time-to-tumor, we shall have to include measurements of the size and severity of the lesion, since tumors continue to grow in living animals beyond the time of their initial appearance.

Alternative Approaches

We can, of course, continue to use the simplistic mathematical model of tumorigenesis as a probability that is a function of dose and time, and we can apply this to the large variety of possible observations we get when we deal with tumor types that occur in the controls. If we do so, however, the assay is no longer specific. Instead, we will find ourselves on a hunting expedition in which we are comparing all possible combinations of tumor types and sites.

Table 7-3 (Salsburg, 1977) shows what can happen with such a hunting expedition. If we examine the usual number of tissues in each animal and have three doses of compound compared with controls, using 50 animals per sex per dose, we end up making more than 70 comparisons of controls and treated subjects. If we blindly apply 5 percent tests of statistical significance to these comparisons, the table shows how often we can be wrong and indict an innocent compound strictly by chance alone. These estimates are based on a Monte Carlo study I ran using the incidence of commonly occurring tumors from long-term studies conducted at Pfizer.

It has been proposed that we can adjust the statistical tests to declare significance at the 1 percent level and reduce this false positive rate. However, we still label many compounds as carcinogens when the activity observed may be simply tumor enhancement rather than true tumorigenesis. It may turn out that such tumor enhancement is relatively common when we apply high doses of biologically active substances to rodents for their entire lifetimes. If so, we will soon find ourselves with a large catalog of carcinogenic compounds without being able to distinguish between those that are dangerous at any dose and those that are tumor enhancing only at exaggerated doses.

Table 7-3. *Monte Carlo Estimates of False Positive Probability (Nominal Alpha Level 5 Percent)*

Species	Length of Study (Months)	No. Organs/ Tumor Types	% False Positives
Male rats	24	5	51.2
Female rats	24	4	19.6
Male mice	18	5	21.5
Female mice	18	5	13.6
Male hamsters	19	3	12.1
Female hamsters	19	4	12.5
Male mice	20	5	57.3
Female mice	20	5	50.2

At the same time, we might miss some very carcinogenic compounds whose effect occurs early in the animal's life but is then swamped by similar events that occur in the controls just prior to sacrifice. If the effect is life-threatening, of course, we will see it in the early tumor-related deaths of the dosed animals. But one can conceive of a situation in which the early tumors induce a higher level of clinical morbidity but one not severe enough to bring about early sacrifices that might uncover the event.

If we are going to consider tumor types that occur in the controls, and if we still wish to avoid either indicting 20 to 50 percent of all biologically active compounds (as appears to be happening now) or failing to catch the disease-producing but not fatal compounds, we will have to model the process with more complicated mathematics. From the more complex model, we will have to derive modified experimental designs. I have suggested a few such designs (Salsburg, 1977), but they are based on my own speculation about what might be useful mathematical models.

In particular, we need to construct a series of experiments whose design evolves as we develop the models that best describe the process. Past experimentation in carcinogenesis was aimed primarily at causing the process with a few well studied compounds in order to understand how to cure it. We now need experiments that examine the relationship between the process of cancer and much broader classes of compounds in order to understand how ingestion of toxic or near toxic doses of chemicals influences that process. Some of these experiments can be relatively short term. For instance, we will need to sketch in the effects on lesions seen with aging, and we can probably start with older animals, or we may want to look at the induction of microscopic tumors in animals in the prime of health. Some of these studies may have already been done but are buried in the vast flood of uncoordinated experimentation that plagues the field of cancer research. But in the end, we will need to conduct a series of well designed lifetime experiments, with the two- to three-year delay involved in each one of them. If these experiments could be organized from a central planning body or bodies, the time needed to derive usable mathematical models might be shortened, but we are still talking in terms of years.

Conclusion

We are very far from having a definitive assay for carcinogenesis. Instead, by requiring that new drugs be subjected to a still unevaluated toxicologic experiment, we stand a very real chance of producing answers to questions no one knows how to ask properly. If the 12 of 30 positive results found up to 1976 are indicative of the future, we can expect that from 20 to 50 percent of all new drugs will appear to be carcinogenic in such studies.

Medical science has entered a new extension of drug therapy. Using modern biochemistry, it is possible to construct compounds with very narrow spectra of activity that can be used to ameliorate the disabilities of chronic illnesses like angina, diabetes, asthma, and emphysema. They will have to be taken for the remainder of the patient's lifetime, and they pose all the unknown risks of long-term chronic therapy. Among those risks is that they may induce or speed up the process of cancer. It should be possible to use the tools of toxicology to get some estimate of those risks, but the tools will have to be more finely tuned than the lifetime study as it is now designed. If we continue using current models, not only will we be unable to estimate those risks but we will go a long way toward discouraging further drug development in those areas in which there is a high probability that the lifetime study will show something or in which the additional cost and uncertainty outweigh the expected return.

Are carcinogenicity tests useful? If we had a good one, the answer would be yes. Unfortunately, so long as we must depend upon the lifetime feeding studies now in use, the answer is no. In fact, the lifetime study not only is of questionable use in current drug development but has the potential to destroy the very nature of that development.

References

Huyoshi, Y., et al.: Malignant neoplasms found by autopsy in Hisayama, Japan during the first ten years of a community study. J. Natl. Cancer Inst. 59:13–19, 1977.

Innes, E.B., Ulland, B.M., et al.: Bioassay of pesticides and industrial chemicals for tumorigenicity in mice: a preliminary note. J. Natl. Cancer Inst. 42:1101–1114, 1969.

MacKenzie, W., et al.: Comparisons of neoplasms in six sources of rats. J. Natl. Cancer Inst. 50:1243–57, 1972.

Mantel, N., and Schneiderman, M.: Estimating "safe" levels, a hazardous undertaking. Cancer Res. 35:1379–1386, 1975.

Mantel, N.: Affidavit presented to the hearing clerk of the Food and Drug Administration, U.S. DHEW, in the matter of actions and procedures for evaluating assays of carcinogenic residues in edible products in animals, March 21, 1977.

Nelson, N., et al.: FDA advisory committee on protocols for safety evaluation: panel on carcinogenesis report on cancer testing. Toxicol. Appl. Pharmacol. 20:419–438, 1971.

Oser, B.L.: An assessment of the Delaney Claims after 15 years. Food Cosmet. Toxicol. 11:1–6, 1973.

Salsburg, D.: The use of statistics when examining life-time studies in rodents to detect carcinogenicity. J. Toxicol. Environ. Health 2:613, 1977.

Sher, S.: Mammary tumors in control rats; Literature tabulation. Toxicol. Appl. Pharmacol. 22:562–588, 1972.

Shimkin, M.B., Weder, R., Marzi, D., Gubaroff, N., and Sientzeff, V.: Lung tumors in mice receiving different schedules of urethane. In Le Cam, L.M., and Neyman, J., eds., Proceedings of the 5th Berkeley Symposium, University of California Press, 1967.

Shubik, P., and Hartwell, J.: *Survey of Compounds Which Have Been Tested for Carcinogenic Activity.* PHS Publication No. 149, U.S. Gov't Printing Office, 1969. (Subsequent volumes were prepared on contract with the NCI and bring the survey up to 1975.)

Shubik, P., et al.: General criteria for assessing evidence for carcinogenicity of chemical substances; Report of the subcommittee on environmental carcinogenesis, National Cancer Advisory Board. J. Natl. Cancer Inst. 58:461–3, 1977.

8

Are Fixed Ratio Combination Drugs Good or Bad?

The true polypharmacy . . . is the skillful combination of remedies.

Sir William Osler

Better a tried remedy than a new-fangled one.

Ambroise Paré

Introduction

Few therapeutic issues engender more heat than the controversy over fixed ratio combinations (FRCs). Weintraub argues strongly in favor of their use, pointing out that FRCs are more convenient and cheaper than single agent drugs, and that they increase the accuracy of drug-taking, decrease the risk of adverse effects and incompatibility of ingredients, diminish the dangers of imprecise diagnosis, and increase the efficacy of treatment. Weintraub asserts that reliance on tested combinations is preferable to idiosyncratic combinations devised by individual physicians.

MacCannell and Giraud are clearly not doctrinaire opponents of FRCs. They remind the reader of the traditional arguments against FRCs but acknowledge that theory and fact do not always coincide. They also, however, do not buy the commonly cited arguments in favor of FRCs, and they conclude by arguing that most FRCs "could disappear without injury to therapeutics."

LOUIS LASAGNA, M.D.

Fixed Ratio Combinations—Pro Position

Michael Weintraub, M.D.
University of Rochester School of Medicine and Dentistry

We must accept the premises that (1) more than one medication may be necessary to achieve a particular therapeutic goal and (2) these medications may need to be given simultaneously.

Why are these premises tenable? No single medication may possess all the properties necessary to treat a condition; a variety of drugs acting on different symptoms may be needed. Drugs acting by different mechanisms or on different aspects of the same condition may both increase effectiveness and decrease adverse effects. Medications acting on the same process at the same point may provide additive effects not necessarily achieved by simply raising the dose of one drug. Decreasing the number of drug administration maneuvers, such as intramuscular injections or eye drops, may either decrease potential morbidity or improve the outcome. In many cases, the etiology of a clinical presentation is not clear and several possible disorders must be treated simultaneously. Drug resistance is less likely to occur with some specialized combinations—namely, those for malaria prophylaxis and tuberculosis. Sometimes, use of a combination drug can reduce toxicity with no loss of efficacy, as when pyridoxine is combined with isoniazid, or with an increase in efficacy, as in combinations of narcotic analgesics and central nervous system stimulants (Forrest et al., 1977).

I hope to show that, given the practice of simultaneous use of several medications, fixed ratio combinations (FRCs) are more logical than concomitant innovations concocted by conservative consultants, conscientious and competent though they may be.

In Favor of FRCs

The advantages of FRCs can be thought of as "the nine Cs": Convenience, Cost savings, Compliance, Controverting of adverse drug effects, Compatibility, Communality, Comprehensiveness, Components, and Confidence. After discussing each of these topics, I then discuss several criticisms that have been raised against the use of FRCs and show that the benefits of FRCs outweigh their deficiencies.

Convenience

The importance of convenience in determining the outcome of pharmacotherapy cannot be denigrated. FRCs provide convenience for physician, pharmacist, and patient. Any innovation that decreases paperwork and leaves more time for physician-patient interaction not only improves physician productivity but, by promoting discussion of the regimen, establishes rapport and understanding. FRCs diminish errors and work on the part of the prescribers, who need not memorize the most efficacious doses and ratios of ingredients in designing a multiple drug regimen.

Patients will need to take less time away from their work because fewer appointments will be necessary to check for dose changes or to correct misdiagnosis. Patients appreciate not having to carry a variety of bottles with them on forays out of the home. Medication errors resulting from hunting through a pill box containing several types of small white or yellow pills decrease if the disparate medications are combined (Mazzullo and Lasagna, 1972). It is also more likely that an undesirable drug-drug interaction will arise from patient-scheduled simultaneous drug ingestion than from pharmaceutically combined medications.

FRCs provide convenience for the pharmacist by decreasing the potential for compounding and filling errors. Instead of counting and typing, the pharmacist can discuss the medication with the patient (such discussion is mandated in several states) and take time to examine the patient profile for possible interacting medications or allergies.

The time saved by the use of FRCs can increase the productivity of both physician and pharmacist, enabling them to see more patients and to provide services at the highest level of their training. Better medical care will thus be provided at lower cost.

Cost

Filling prescriptions for the individual drugs of an FRC increases the total cost under the pharmacist's fee-for-service billing system. A charge of $2.80 would be assessed at a typical medical center (such as Strong Memorial Hospital) outpatient pharmacy for *each* of the ingredients in a vasodilator-diuretic-sympatholytic antihypertensive regimen. Providing the same drugs in comparable doses but as a single FRC instantly saves the patient at least $5.60. And this is only the final charge in the producer-to-consumer chain. There will be savings at each level; the drug wholesaler will save labor expenses because he needs to handle only one preparation from one supplier and deliver that one medication to the retailer. The manufacturer may charge less for the combination because he increases his market share, often without concomitant decrease in sales of single entity products. The latter point has been discussed in detail by Kemp (1975). Although drug costs are a small percentage of total health care expenditures, the amount of money involved is large and can represent a significant outlay for an individual patient (Weintraub, 1976). If a comparable standard of care can be obtained at a lower cost, it makes sense to use a drug product providing that advantage.

Compliance

Many factors determine the extent to which patients will actually take prescribed medication. Leaving aside arguments on whether strict adherence to the therapeutic plan always benefits the patient, let us examine how FRCs can affect compliance. We would naturally assume that patients will take convenient medications more faithfully than inconvenient ones. It has, in fact, been demonstrated that the more complex the regimen, the less likely patients are to follow it (Gately, 1968; Weintraub et al., 1973). FRCs immediately simplify the therapeutic plan by decreasing the number of medications that have to be ingested. (Just think of the effect it would have on compliance if multivitamin preparations, oral contraceptives, or combination antihypertensives were prescribed as the individual ingredients!) FRCs also diminish the confusion involved in taking several different capsules or tablets, especially when some of them resemble one another. Mazzullo, Lasagna, and Griner (1974) have documented the effect that confusing prescription directions have on compliance. FRCs decrease such confusion. Faced with many medications and a complex administration schedule—and perhaps not remembering what had been taken when—a patient has several choices: (1) he may not take any more of any medication, perhaps losing the therapeutic effect; (2) he may take one or more of the remaining medications, perhaps ingesting an excessive dose; or (3) he may call the physician for advice, wasting both his own and the doctor's time. None of these possibly detrimental courses of action would be necessary with the FRC.

In my own study of digoxin compliance, some patients mentioned financial considerations as factors in taking medications as prescribed (Weintraub et al., 1973). Since FRCs cost less than the individual ingredients, they can help to improve compliance.

Still another way in which FRCs may promote patient adherence to the therapeutic plan is by decreasing undesirable effects attributed to the medication. Frequently, patients are justified in discontinuing the use of a drug because of symptoms of drug-related toxicity. It is the physician's job to find out whether the patient has stopped or decreased the medication and why. Strict adherence to a regimen that causes major or minor toxicity is not good therapeutics. Altering doses or stopping therapy for irrational reasons is also not good therapeutics. Instead of these undesirable options, the patient and the physician should discuss the regimen, including its unpleasant aspects. Improved compliance, a more desirable therapeutic outcome, and less drug toxicity should result from this sort of communication (Weintraub, 1978).

Controverting Adverse Effects

By combining small doses of medications that have different undesirable effects, well constructed FRCs could have less dose-related toxicity than a single drug given in the amount necessary to achieve the same therapeutic effect. Combining a vasodilator with a diuretic and a sympatholytic agent for the treatment of hypertension exemplifies how smaller amounts of any one drug will be needed to lower blood pressure. Dose-related effects such as headache, dehydration, postural hypotension, or even a lupus-like syndrome can be prevented when the three drugs are combined in an FRC. Because toxicity profiles differ among the components of the FRC, maximal doses can be used in hard-to-treat patients without overwhelming adverse effects.

FRCs may contain medications that directly counteract an undesirable effect of the primary therapeutic agent. Examples of such advantageous combinations are isoniazid-pyridoxine, potassium-sparing and potassium-wasting diuretic combinations, and combinations of narcotics and central nervous system stimulants. In addition to decreasing adverse drug reactions, FRCs improve the safety of treatments in other ways.

Compatibility

The ingredients, excipients, coatings, and compounding of an FRC have been proven, in both laboratory and clinical tests, not to cause an undesirable interaction. Such proof cannot be produced for the extemporaneous combinations created by physicians or pharmacists. Furthermore, each time a series of prescriptions is filled for individual preparations, as opposed to one for an FRC, a new possibility of a drug-drug interaction arises. The pharmacist may fill the prescriptions with different manufacturers' products. Changing suppliers can create or alter the type of drug interaction. For example, imagine that in a multiple-drug regimen, the excipient of medication *A* binds drug *B*, decreasing its absorption. The physician and patient had titrated the individual agents for maximum benefit, but the next time the prescriptions are filled, either a different formulation (A') or another manufacturer's product (A'') is used, neither of which binds drug *B*. By allowing greater absorption, this will immediately increase the active amount of medication *B*. In the reverse situation, what amounts to a decrease in dose will occur. Use of an FRC prevents the problem of a pharmaceutical incompatibility interaction altering the "dose" of individual drugs.

There is no guarantee that the ratios of individual medications created by physicians will be the most effective combinations pharmacologically, either in general or for a particular patient. Additionally, given the difficult problem of fitting medication schedules into one's life, a new ad hoc ratio frequently will be established by the patient. For example, although a ratio of 10 mg of carbidopa to 100 mg of L-dopa may be optimal if they are taken together in an FRC, taking the drugs at different times may mean that the peak effect of carbidopa in blocking dopa decarboxylation will occur at a time least likely to be of benefit—i.e., when serum L-dopa levels are low, creating an inefficient ratio. Thus, the work and expense of adjusting the inhibitor to the patient's level of decarboxylase activity may be undermined by a simple change in administration schedule. The flexible regimen then becomes valueless for the patient for whom it was created. Furthermore, the physician will not be able to apply the experience he has gained from the work of this dose adjustment to the care of other patients.

Communality

The doses and ratios contained in FRCs are intended to apply to a broad range of patients with a particular disorder. The amounts and proportions chosen are constrained on the high side by the need to avoid toxicity and on the low side by the need to insure effectiveness, but they are based on both experimental and clinical trial results. Some patients have special conditions that affect their response to medications, necessitating careful dose adjustment. Most often, however, one of a series of FRCs should apply to the majority of patients with a particular disease or symptom complex. Additionally, since clinical presentations may have one of several causes, a mixture of medications will be appropriate to treat the most likely etiologies without omitting other major causes.

Comprehensiveness

FRCs enable physicians to "cover their bets." Organs have a limited way of responding to insults. It is difficult for an ophthalmologist, for example—even with direct inspection of the diseased tissue—to distinguish between an allergic and an infectious process. In order to include both possibilities in the treatment plan, the ophthalmologist can select an FRC containing both antiinflammatory and antibiotic agents. Certainly, with laboratory tests or other studies, a precise etiology may be ascertained. Although costly and time-consuming, making a specific diagnosis would obviate the need for multiple medications.

As occurs so often, unfortunately, one process (infection) may provoke another (allergic reaction), or one (allergy) may increase the likelihood of another (infection) by decreasing host defenses or altering the tissue environment. A precise diagnosis made at the first visit thus becomes less precise (or incorrect) a short time later. Use of an FRC right away not only covers both possibilities initially with less cost and begins treatment of the second problem, but may avert return visits as well. This is just one example of how an FRC, with its multiple approaches, can improve therapeutic outcome.

COMPONENTS

Several therapeutic rationales underlie the combination of two or more individual agents into an FRC. Many signs and symptoms are physical covariates, occurring together as part of the disease picture, and several different medications may be needed to treat each part of a disease. There may not be a unitary cause for all aspects of the clinical picture nor any way that a single drug will influence every disease feature. In an FRC, effective components that can treat simultaneously several different aspects of a disease are administered together.

Medications such as trimethoprim and sulfamethoxazole act on different steps along the same biochemical pathway. Combining them in fixed, appropriate proportions results in synergistic rather than just additive effects. Although only some FRCs can work in this way, most provide additive effects that at least allow lower doses of drug to be effective and decrease the risk of unwanted effects.

Dollery (1977) discussed the value of using FRCs in the treatment of hypertension. He sees each component acting to inhibit partially one of several hypertensive mechanisms, and he foresees most mildly or moderately hypertensive patients being treated with FRCs, including as yet unmarketed formulations.

The use of FRCs may also block the development of bacterial or tissue resistance. Although the time course and reasons for the development of opioid tolerance are not simple, the addition of a central nervous system stimulant to a narcotic in an FRC seems to delay the development of such tolerance. Delayed tolerance may be a consequence of improved efficacy of the FRC, resulting in lower doses needed for pain relief, or there may be a specific explanation for this observation that has not been found.

FRCs are convenient, have proven bioavailability, have no undesirable interactions, allow for simultaneous multiple approaches to a complex disease process, allow for several possible diseases to be treated at one time, cost less, have fewer adverse effects, and are effective. It is no wonder that they have been in honored use for many years and have imparted a feeling of confidence in the therapeutic outcome.

CONFIDENCE

Practitioners have developed confidence in the most popular FRCs through their favorable experiences with them. Improved compliance, decreased cost, and lowered toxicity with the use of FRCs have undoubtedly contributed to this. In addition, the patient perceives the physician's confident attitude and responds to it. In this way, the health professional's confidence becomes part of the therapeutic process, promoting the placebo effect of the treatment and facilitating therapeutic success.

Criticisms of FRCs

What about the criticisms of FRCs? Just how compromised, for example, is the ability of the practitioner to adjust medication doses to the patient's need? There are many conditions for which precise tailoring of the regimen is not necessary or is intrinsically difficult. In these situations, FRCs perform very well. Also, the wide range of dose sizes may even make dosing flexibility easier. The ratios of ingredients are based on commonly used regimens, again decreasing the need for careful dose adjustment. Compounding special mixtures or cutting tablets is often made unnecessary by the use of FRCs.

Do FRCs Encourage Sloppy Diagnosis? Often, a specific diagnosis cannot be made when the patient first presents because organs respond in similar fashion to different insults. Nonetheless, treatment seems appropriate at this time. What is the practitioner to do but choose medications that begin treatment for any of several potential diseases or that make the patient more comfortable, regardless of diagnosis? FRCs provide the necessary broad approach. One physician's sloppy therapeutics is another physician's way of "covering all bets."

Recently, experts in hypertension have been discouraging the use of the "million-dollar workup" of patients with hypertension. Tailoring therapy to renin status is going out of vogue. Adherents of this new philosophy take an empirical approach to diagnosis and therapy, using various FRCs as the basis for antihypertensive treatment.

Academic physicians may disparage the use of FRCs because their view of the patient is different from that of the primary care physician. Academicians do not usually see the FRC successes; they usually see the patient at a time when the diagnostic signs of the disease have developed more completely–i.e., after several days or weeks of symptoms. They search for a specific diagnosis more often than primary care physicians do because referral to a tertiary level of care demands such precision. Precise diagnosis allows for and requires specific therapy. Depending on which part of therapy each feels is important, the primary and tertiary care physicians perceive different values in FRCs. Primary care personnel see how FRCs can increase their efficiency, decrease the cost of medical care, and treat patients for several possible disease causes, perhaps diminishing the number of visits needed. At the tertiary care level, physicians often subordinate such efficiency to diagnostic and therapeutic rigor.

Do FRCs Increase Toxicity Because of Unnecessary Ingredients? We are learning that drug toxicity is not a raging epidemic. Except for the predictable adverse effects due to a drug's basic effects or to inappropriate patient self-administration, medications really cause little harm. How FRCs affect the balance between toxicity and therapeutic effect must be measured before any firm statement on their deficiencies can be made. Unfortunately, data necessary to judge the risks and benefits of FRCs versus single agents do not always exist. When the data have been obtained, analysis reveals, at the very least, equivalent risk with improved therapeutic outcome. Studies of single agents pushed to maximal benefit versus FRCs have, to my knowledge, not been made. We do know that the lower amount of drug needed in FRCs reduces the risk of dose-related toxicity, rendering FRCs safer rather than more toxic than single agents.

What is the Risk That Physicians, not Knowing the Ingredients of FRCs, May Prescribe a Drug That the Patient Should not Take? Although theoretically this may occur, we do not know how often it actually does. The major problem of lack of knowledge on the part of the physician or the pharmacist (or even the patient) cannot be attributed to the preparations, especially because many of the brand names clearly indicate the ingredients. The answer to this objection to FRCs is not to deprive patients of needed medications but to educate health professionals about therapeutics–including how to learn the components of FRCs.

What About Pharmacokinetic Differences Between the Agents in an FRC? Discouraging the use of FRCs because the components have different half-lives or peak absorption times ignores two important problems with prescribing individual agents. If physicians who use FRCs are assumed not to know the ingredients in them, can they be assumed to know the optimal doses, ratios, and times for dosing of single agents in relation to the patient's pharmacokinetics? Even if the individual drugs are prescribed correctly, the likelihood is strong that patients will take them together anyway. Or, patients may take the single drugs at variable intervals, with resultant fluctuation between increased and diminished levels of the desired effect. Whatever pharmacokinetic inequalities FRCs encompass, they provide the constancy of simultaneously administered components. This should mean a more predictable result. We cannot, however, base the FRC dose interval on the FRC component with the shortest half-life, as some have recommended. Using such a system may result in undesirable accumulation of the agents with the longer half-life.

Conclusion

The conclusion of this analysis is that FRCs are preferable to unproven, intuitive, potentially interacting, and irrational improvisations. FRCs have many positive attributes, and the objections raised to their use should not deter physicians from prescribing them when indicated.

References

Dollery, C.T.: Pharmacologic basis for combination therapy of hypertension. Ann. Rev. Pharmacol. Toxicol. 17:311, 1977.

Forrest, W.H., Brown, B.W., Jr., Brown, C.R., Defalque, R., Gold, M., Gordon, H.E., James, K.E., Katz, J., Mahler, D.L., Schroff, P., and Teutsch, G.: Dextroamphetamine with morphine for the treatment of postoperative pain. N. Engl. J. Med. 296:712, 1977.

Gately, M.S.: To be taken as directed. J. R. Coll. Gen. Prac. 16:39, 1968.

Kemp, B.A.: Some economic considerations of combination products—and their withdrawal. In Lasagna, L., ed., *Combination Drugs: Their Use and Regulation,* New York, Stratton Intercontinental Medical Book Corporation, 1975.

Mazzullo, J.M., and Lasagna, L.: Take thou . . . but is your patient really taking what you prescribed? Drug Ther. 8:11, 1972.

Mazzullo, J.M., Lasagna, L., and Griner, P.F.: Variation in interpretation of prescription directions. JAMA 227:929–932, 1974.

Weintraub, M.: Drug costs. Drug Ther. Sept. 1976, pp. 178–180.

Weintraub, M.: Toward creative compliance. In Beber, C.R., and Lamy, P.P., eds., *Medication Management in the Elderly,* Amsterdam, Excerpta Medica, 1978.

Weintraub, M., Au, W.Y.W, and Lasagna, L.: Compliance as a determinant of the serum digoxin concentration. JAMA 224:481–485, 1973.

Fixed Ratio Drug Combinations—Sense and Nonsense

Keith L. MacCannell, M.D., Ph.D., F.R.C.P.(C), F.A.C.P.

George Giraud, B.Sc. (Pharm.)

University of Calgary, Alberta, Canada

... The existence of thousands of fixed combinations makes the drug market indiscernible and useless. They obscure the relatively few essential drugs and make it difficult for the doctor to find his way amongst the mass of offered medicaments. Few drug combinations are justifiable. These are well known and should be permitted as before. All others should be banned until it has been shown that their advantages are greater than their disadvantages
(Herxheimer, 1975).

... The trouble with combined preparations on the market today is that they rarely combine the right things. Why, for example, can we not have a preparation containing digoxin, furosemide and potassium in one tablet? Or an orciprenaline-and-tetracycline combination? ... If the pharmaceutical industry put as much effort into devising useful combination products as it puts into the production of tetracyclines for children and barbiturates for the suicidal, we might have more success in the art of therapeutics
(Zermansky, 1972).

Two physicians, two arguments—one for generic purity, the other for expanded therapeutic miscegenation. Which, if either, is correct?

The Use of Fixed Ratio Combination Products

It is estimated that in 1972, retail sales of prescription drugs in the United States totaled $10 billion—representing approximately 2.5 billion prescriptions (Silverman and Lee, 1974). Of the 200 most widely used prescription drugs in the United States, 37 percent are fixed dose combination products (Dengler and Lasagna, 1975). In any given year, therefore, American physicians write hundreds of millions, if not billions, of prescriptions for combination drugs. Although comparative data are not available, a high degree of utilization of combination drugs probably exists in most developed countries. It is claimed, for example, that 21 percent of prescriptions written under the United Kingdom's National Health Service are for combination drugs (Cromie, 1974).

Self-medication must also be considered in assessing the usage of fixed dose combination drugs. Most nonprescription (over-the-counter or OTC) products are combination drugs. This is verified in Table 8–1, which has been developed from data presented in the Handbook of Non-Prescription Drugs (American Pharmaceutical Association). Again, the magnitude of usage of such OTC products is immense. In 1972, for example, retail sales of OTC laxatives, antacids, internal analgesics, and antidiarrheal preparations in the United States were said to be worth $212.7 million, $116.7 million, $136.0 million and $75.6 million respectively (Silverman and Lee, 1974).

Much of this self-medication with OTC combination drugs is generated by advertising directed to consumers. However, pharmacists stock these products and counsel customers on

Table 8-1. *Popularity of Combination Drugs*

Classification	Number of Products Listed	Number Containing >1 Ingredient*	Percent Containing >1 Ingredient	Mean Number of Ingredients per Product
Antiemetic	7	0	0.0	1.0
Laxative	102	63	61.8	1.9
Antacid†	75	61	81.3	2.2
Analgesic	86	52	60.5	2.4
Antitussive	114	98	86.0	2.8
Cold/allergy product	77	72	93.5	3.1
Antidiarrheal	24	24	100.0	4.2

* Not included as ingredients: flavoring, coloring, sweeteners, preservatives, solubilizers

† Included as ingredients: "buffering agents"

Data have been collated from the *Handbook of Non-Prescription Drugs*, 5th edition, Washington, D.C., American Pharmaceutical Association, 1977.

selection. Clearly, the pharmacist, like the physician, accepts combination products.

The Professional's Knowledge of Combination Drugs

One does not expect the consumer of OTC preparations to survey the contents of all the remedies before choosing a specific product. However, our level of expectation is considerably higher for physicians and pharmacists; one does not expect a physician to prescribe a combination product unless he knows its constituents, nor does one expect a pharmacist to dispense a product without similar information. But do physicians and pharmacists actually know enough about the fixed ratio combinations (FRCs) they promote?

We are aware of no detailed study that has examined this question, but Biron and his colleagues, in small surveys done in Quebec, Canada, explored the knowledge of physicians and hospital pharmacists regarding common combination drugs (Biron, 1973; Gagne et al., 1975). These pilot studies provided disturbing information, some of which is presented in Table 8–2. If these observations can be extended to the general population of North American physicians and pharmacists (and there is no reason to suspect that they cannot be), they indicate that physicians are prescribing—and pharmacists dispensing—combination drugs with a remarkable degree of ignorance about them. Arguments that FRCs are prescribed as an exercise in rational therapeutics are significantly weakened when the prescriber does not know what he is actually prescribing.

The "Margin of Safety" that Protects the Physician from Therapeutic Ignorance

The experienced physician is well aware of several important elements of therapeutics:

1. Most diseases are of limited duration and the patient will recover with or without medications (although medications may alter the course of the disease).

2. Most drugs have a very favorable therapeutic ratio—i.e., there is considerable difference between the dose producing desired pharmacologic response and the dose producing toxic effects.

3. The "placebo response" is frequently an important determinant of therapeutic response.

All these factors help to explain the wide popularity of OTC drugs. Most of these preparations have limited therapeutic efficacy, but when used as treatment for acute illness, they have an unquantified but probably limited potential for doing harm.

Many, probably most, prescribed combination drugs are also used for acute illnesses. Moreover, such products rarely contain a drug with a narrow therapeutic margin. (We are aware, for example, of no combination product containing cardiac glycosides, antiarrhythmics, or anticonvulsants.) Like the average person, the physician usually can obtain satisfactory results with combination drugs in the treatment of acute illnesses without knowing the composi-

Table 8-2. *Professionals' Understanding of Combination Drugs*

Combination Drug	Constituents	Percent of Hospital Pharmacists Correctly Identifying Constituents*	Percent of Physicians Correctly Identifying Constituents*
Aldactazide®	Hydrochlorothiazide Spironolactone	86	60
Azo Gantrisin®	Phenazopyridine Sulfisoxazole	61	45
Dyazide®	Hydrochlorothiazide Triamterene	86	65
Etrafon®	Amitriptyline Perphenazine	87	50
Ornade®	Chlorpheniramine Phenylpropanolamine	3	0
Supres®	Chlorothiazide Methyldopa	15	33

Data were abstracted from Biron (Can. Med. Assoc. J. 109:35–39, 1973) and from Gagne et al. (Ann. Int. Med. 82:680-2, 1975.)

* 60 physicians (residents, general practitioners, and specialists) were asked to name at least 3 fixed dose drug combinations they had prescribed in the last year and to indicate the number and identity (generic or trade name) of the ingredients in each. Data were presented on 24 combination drugs. 71 hospital pharmacists were asked to provide the same information on drugs they had "recently dispensed." Data were presented on the same 24 combination products.

tion of the product he is using. The patient gets well with or without the medication; sometimes, perhaps, despite the medication.

However, the "margin of safety" is not as great for the physician as for the lay person. Prescription combination drugs are frequently used by physicians in the treatment of chronic illnesses. They are also not inherently as "safe" as OTC combination drugs—if they were, they would not be available only as prescription drugs. Moreover, they are frequently given to patients who may have an intercurrent disease that requires modification of therapy.

The physician who uses single entity drugs—and indeed the physician who uses combination drugs but knows their composition—maintains a margin of safety by being able to match patient with drug product and by being alert to drug toxicity. The physician who is not knowledgeable about the combination products he is using—and who therefore is functioning at the level of any person who walks into a pharmacy and selects an OTC product from the shelf—is prescribing blindly. This is as remote from good therapeutics as "fast foods" are from good nutrition.

If the physician is unaware that a combination product contains a specific drug, he cannot possibly assess whether the product is contraindicated for his patient. For example, one must be concerned about the unwitting use of combination drugs containing a pressor sympathomimetic amine in a hypertensive patient. (However, we are aware of no data that indicate that such therapeutic adventures contribute to morbidity or mortality.)

Proponents of combination drugs argue that the wide acceptance and use of FRCs indicate their safety, even when prescribed without full knowledge of their contents and when they are administered for chronic ailments. However, one sees what one looks for. The surprisingly high incidence of adverse effects from single entity drugs has been appreciated only in the last decade. Most studies on the epidemiology of adverse drug reactions have been done in teaching hospitals, where good drug histories are common and the use of combination drugs is minimal. Knowledge of the pharmacology of constituent drugs leads one to expect that the incidence of adverse effects with combination drugs would be found to be high if patients receiving these preparations were systematically examined. There are few internists who have not seen complications of combination drug therapy, such as aspirin-induced asthma attributable to the salicylate in a FRC cold remedy. However, we simply do not know the incidence of adverse reactions to combination drugs. So far as we are aware, there is only one study that touches peripherally on this point (Clark and Troop, 1972). In this study, the use of a hydralazine-reserpine-hydrochlorothiazide combination in hypertensive patients was said to be associated with no greater incidence of side effects than when the constituents were given singly.

Traditional Arguments Against Fixed Ratio Combination Drugs

Let us ignore for the moment the evidence to the contrary and assume that physicians do know the composition of FRCs and therefore select and use them with some degree of logic. Are there still arguments against their use? How valid are these arguments?

Inflexibility of dosage. The major argument against fixed dose combination drugs has been that these agents do not permit the physician to adjust the dose of one constituent without simultaneously modifying the dose(s) of the other constituent(s). This contention does not have much strength. As noted previously, most combination products contain drugs that have a wide therapeutic margin, the doses of which do not have to be titrated individually. Even when precise titration is necessary, one can frequently titrate each component drug individually and then find, from amongst the large number of combination products available, one or more that contains the individual drugs in concentrations closely approximating the individually computed doses. This latter point assumes, of course, that the bioavailability of a drug is similar when combined with other drugs and when given singly. Considering the many problems of formulation, there is no *a priori* reason why this should be so, but data on this point are lacking.

Administration of unnecessary drugs. It is certainly true that many patients who are given combination drugs will receive drugs they do not require. It makes little sense to give a mild hypertensive patient a combination drug containing hydralazine, reserpine, and a thiazide diuretic when perfectly adequate control can be obtained with a thiazide alone. In such circumstances, one would be unnecessarily exposing the patient to the significant toxicities of hydralazine and reserpine. A contrary argument is that the use of a combination drug might enable one to impose a lesser total daily dose of two or more active ingredients, thereby minimizing toxicity from each constituent. There is no evidence for this potentially favorable aspect of combination therapy; even if it were true, it would minimize only dose-related toxicity, and not toxicity related to hypersensitivity or to idiosyncrasy.

Another valid argument against most combination drugs is that the consumer might be exposed unnecessarily to drugs with unknown teratogenic or carcinogenic effects. Many drugs are inadequately evaluated with respect to these (witness the current saccharin controversy). Unquestionably, with the thousands of chemical entities available to us, we must already have drugs on the market that do have such adverse effects. (One wonders, for example, whether thalidomide would not still be marketed as a sedative had congenital heart lesions been the major teratogenic effect rather than the highly visible phocomelia.) Such risks, however small, are magnified when a combination drug containing multiple ingredients is prescribed in a situation for which a single chemical entity would be appropriate. There is no justification for exposing any patient needlessly to drug-related risk. This is particularly true for women of childbearing age, who seek medical attention more frequently and receive more prescriptions (presumably including prescriptions for combination drugs) than do men.

The argument is also made that combination drugs expose the patient to potential drug interactions. It is unquestionably true that the incidence of adverse drug reactions increases markedly in a nonlinear fashion with the number of drugs taken. At the same time, originators of FRCs are careful not to combine two ingredients with known interactions. One would expect that the incidence of drug interactions would be greater when multiple drugs are given independently than when drugs are given in combination for the simple reason that the physician is less cognizant of drug interactions than are pharmaceutical manufacturers.

Proponents of combination therapy argue, presumably on the basis of this reasoning, that the use of combination drugs actually *reduces* the possibility of drug interactions. However, one important point is overlooked: the patient may be taking not *one* combination drug but two or more—in terms of constituents, perhaps five or six different drugs. Clearly, under such circumstances, the potential for drug interactions is greatly increased rather than decreased.

Illogical combinations. In 1966, panels set up under the auspices of the American National Academy of Sciences and the National Research Council evaluated 1200 combination drugs marketed prior to 1962. Of these, only 45 were rated as "effective" (Crout, 1974). The rest were questioned on the basis of safety, efficacy, or inclusion of unnecessary ingredients. American guidelines for acceptance of combination drugs—which have been accepted to greater or lesser degree elswhere—specify that (1) each component must make a contribution to the claimed therapeutic action, either by increasing the additive or synergistic effect, enhancing the safety of a major active ingredient, or minimizing the potential for abuse and (2) the dose must be such that the drug is safe and efficacious for a "significant population" requiring concurrent therapy. Obviously, such guidelines are imprecise, yet they resulted in the virtual disappearance in North America of most of the illogical combinations (for example, adrenocortical steroids plus aspirin and/or antihistamines and "cold remedies" containing antibiotics). In most cases, combination drugs have a greater claim to legitimacy than they did a decade ago, but unfortunately, that claim is still marginal for many preparations.

A parallel argument is advanced that many combination drugs are illogical not because of the choice of constituents but rather because they contain drugs with different half-lives and different bioavailabilities. There is some merit to this argument, but it can be applied equally well to individually administered drugs. The skillful therapist is knowledgeable about half-lives and uses appropriate dosage schedules for individual agents, but his less skilled colleague generally uses drugs without respect to half-lives. In such situations, it matters little whether he uses them in combination or as single entities. Moreover, bioavailability is rarely of great significance with drugs possessing reasonable therapeutic margins, unless the bioavailability is very aberrant.

Arguments for Fixed Ratio Combination Drugs

Significant arguments for fixed dose drug combinations are frequently overstated but nonetheless should be evaluated carefully.

Adherence to therapeutic regimens. Factors that influence a patient's drug compliance are only now being examined, and data are still incomplete. (For a review of drug compliance, see Sackett and Haynes, 1976.) It seems reasonably certain that good compliance is correlated with the duration of therapy—the shorter the duration, the greater the compliance (Haynes, 1976). Since many combination drugs, particularly OTCs, are taken for acute illnesses, it would follow that compliance should be reasonably good. However, in this circumstance of short-term therapy, there is no reason to suspect that compliance with a combination drug should be any better than that with a single entity drug. Similarly, there appears to be a negative correlation between the number of daily doses and compliance, with the best compliance occurring with once-daily dosing (Porter, 1969). If this is so, one would expect that compliance would be improved if a combination drug could be taken once a day as an alternative to taking an individual drug more frequently. However, most combination drugs do not lend themselves to less frequent dosing. Compliance with respect to combination drugs, should, therefore, be similar to compliance for single entity drugs if both are given on the same dosage schedule.

Finally, it appears that compliance correlates inversely with the number of different medications taken (Malahy, 1966; Clinite and Kabat, 1969). It has also been claimed that the incidence of medication errors increases with the number of different medications taken daily, these observations being made both in hospitalized patients (Vere, 1965) and in outpatients (Malahy, 1966). Such observations support the use of combination drugs.

On the basis of these incomplete studies, one would expect the use of combination drugs to offer advantages in terms of patient compliance only if it resulted in less frequent dosing and a simplified dosage schedule. Substitution of a combination drug given three times a day should offer no major advantage over two or more single entity drugs, all of which are also given three times a day. Well designed studies to ascertain whether combination therapy actually does improve compliance are very much needed.

Convenience to physician and patient. Convenience to the patient is consistently advanced as an argument for FRC drug therapy, yet this argument fails if combination therapy does not reduce the number of needed doses. It is a convenience to the patient and probably an aid to drug compliance if an FRC can be taken three times a day as an alternative to taking several single entity drugs, each of which is taken according to a different schedule. However, with single entity prescribing, it is surprisingly easy, with appropriate selection of drugs, to bring the dosage schedule of the various drugs into harmony. Common dosage schedules of many single entity drugs cannot be justified by their pharmacokinetics, and many drugs that are traditionally given *t.i.d.* can just as readily be given on a *q.i.d.* schedule and vice versa.

Convenience to the physician is a more solid argument for use of combination drugs. The physician who uses combination drugs can write one rather than two or more prescriptions. Moreover, it is surely easier for the practitioner to instruct the patient on the use of one tablet or capsule than to provide instructions on the use of separate medications. However, this latter consideration does not apply if the physician selects his single entity drugs so they can be given on the same dosage schedule.

Improved efficacy. It is apparent that some combination drugs are more effective than their individual constituents given singly. Obvious examples of this are the combination oral contraceptive agents. Here, there is an excellent rationale for administering estrogen and progestin together; titration of the constituents is unnecessary and undesirable since the titration endpoint is pregnancy. At the same time, a variety of preparations containing different ratios of active drug is available to suit the needs of individual patients. Moreover, the combination can be given once a day. It would be difficult to argue against the validity of such drugs. Another example is provided by the combination of sulfamethoxazole and trimethoprim. Here, two drugs with similar half-lives influence the bacterial synthesis of tetrahydrofolic acid at different points. The apparent rationale of this approach has been lessened recently by suggestions that the major therapeutic benefit of this combination is due to trimethoprim. If this is so, the administration of trimethoprim alone would be more reasonable, since sulfa drugs have a high incidence of toxicity. Another apparently valid FRC is the combination of L-dopa and a dopa decarboxylase inhibitor that minimizes the peripheral effects of L-dopa treatment. However, even here, one cannot be entirely enthusiastic about the combination product, since many patients have no need for the dopa decarboxylase inhibitor.

Except for a few such examples, one can find little support for the claim that therapeutic results can be obtained more readily with combination drugs than with single entity preparations. We are aware of only one study that examined the efficacy of combination therapy compared with that of single agent therapy. Clark and Troop (1972) compared the combination drug Ser-Ap-Es (reserpine 0.1 mg, hydralazine 25 mg, hydrochlorothiazide 25 mg) with its constituents when administered singly and in various combinations. It was claimed that more satisfactory lowering of diastolic blood pressure occurred in hypertensive patients treated with the combination drug. This study appears to have been based on retrospective chart review; moreover, it is not clear whether patients were followed by the same physicians or whether standardized protocols for blood pressure recording were observed. Nevertheless, it is a most interesting study and should be extended to other FRC products.

Cost of therapy. It has been suggested that fixed dose drug combinations generally cost about 20 percent less than single components separately purchased (McMahon, 1971). There is no reason to doubt this statement; certainly, if savings in production and distribution costs were passed on to the consumer, it should be true. However, this assumes that the patient requires all the components of the combination. A financial saving will not ensue if a patient needs a single drug and is receiving three or more in a combination. Because of this, and because of bulk purchasing and the variable cost of similar drugs produced by different companies, there appears to be no valid way of determining whether combination drugs are truly less expensive. Something that one does not need and that has a potential for toxicity is not a bargain at any price.

Improving the performance of inadequate physicians. There is one argument in favor of combination drugs that is not advanced, even by their supporters, but is nevertheless valid: a physician who is less than competent in diagnostic or therapeutic skills may have a greater chance of "hitting the mark" with combination drugs than with single entity drugs. When a patient is being treated by a physician whose skills are inadequate, he may be better served by a combination antibiotic than by a single entity antibiotic that is completely off target. Such "wide-spectrum" combination drugs are becoming less and less common. Antibiotic combinations and antibiotic/sulfa drug combinations are rapidly disappearing. The same is true of combination psychoactive agents. Even so, the unskilled physician would still probably be safer with most of the combination antihypertensive agents than with some of the very potent single entity drugs that are available.

Conclusion

Several conclusions can be drawn from the arguments for and against combination drugs:

1. The argument that combination drugs have no place in therapeutics is not valid.
2. Sales of specific combination drugs that cannot be justified on the basis of composition or dosage schedules indicate excessive prescribing of combination drugs.
3. Factors that determine the popularity of combination drugs have been poorly defined. Certainly, the use of combination drugs does not appear to be based on knowledge of their composition.
4. The use of combination drugs imposes a burden of unnecessary chemical exposure on patients.
5. Arguments that rational drug combinations may improve therapeutic response through improved drug compliance and additive effects of subtoxic doses of constituents cannot be documented.
6. Theoretical arguments for the use of combination drugs disappear when, as is frequently the case, two or more combination drugs are prescribed, frequently on different dosage schedules.
7. The incidence of adverse drug reactions to combination drugs is unknown, and more work has to be done in relating short- and long-term toxicity to possible advantages in terms of improved compliance.
8. The contention that FRCs restrict the physician's ability to titrate the composition of individual agents is not a strong one because of the generous therapeutic margin of most constituents.
9. Most combination drugs could disappear without weakening practical therapeutics. Combination drugs which *are* composed of active components that *do* contribute to the therapeutic effect could be improved through greater attention to the choice of constituents and the matching of constituents in terms of half-lives.

References

Biron, P.: A hopefully biased pilot survey of physicians' knowledge of the content of drug combinations. Can. Med. Assoc. J. 109:35–39, 1973.

Clark, G.M., and Troop, R.C.: One tablet combination drug therapy in the treatment of hypertension. J. Chronic Dis. 25:57–64, 1972.

Clinite, J.C., and Kabat, H.E.: Prescribed drugs . . . errors during self administration. J. Am. Pharm. Assoc. 9:450–452, 1969.

Cromie, B.W.: Drug combinations. Curr. Med. Res. Opin. 1:78–86, 1972.

Cromie, B.W.: Combination products. Postgrad. Med. J. 50:103–106, 1974.

Crout, J.R.: Fixed combination prescription drugs: F.D.A. policy. J. Clin. Pharmacol. 14:249–254, 1974.

Dengler, H.J., and Lasagna, L.: Report of a workshop on fixed ratio drug combinations. Eur. J. Clin. Pharmacol. 8:149–154, 1975.

Gagne, J., Biron, P., and Morson, R.: A survey of hospital pharmacists' knowledge of the content of drug combinations. Ann. Int. Med. 82:680–2, 1975.

Haynes, R.B.: A critical review of the "determinants" of patient compliance with therapeutic regimens. In Sackett, D. L., and Haynes, R. B., *Compliance with therapeutic Regimens,* Johns Hopkins University Press, 1976.

Herxheimer, H.: The danger of fixed drug combinations. Int. J. Clin. Pharmacol. Biopharm. 12:70–73, 1975.

Malahy, B.: The effect of instruction and labelling on the number of medication errors made by patients at home. Am. J. Hosp. Pharm. 23:283–292, 1966.

McMahon, F.G.: Drug combinations: a critique of new federal regulations. JAMA 216:1008–1013, 1971.

Porter, A.M.W.: Drug defaulting in a general practice. Br. Med. J. 1:218–222, 1969.

Silverman, M., and Lee, P.R.: *Pills, Profits and Politics.* Berkeley, University of California Press, 1974.

Vere, D.W.: Errors in complex prescribing. Lancet 1:370–373, 1965.

Zermansky, A.G.: Letter to the editor. Lancet 2:919, 1972.

SECTION II

Specific Problems

9

Are Drugs Useful in Treating Obesity?

The Myth of the Usefulness of Amphetamines in the Long-term Management of Obesity

Thaddeus E. Prout, M.D.

Drugs Are Useful in Treating Obesity

W. L. Asher, M.D.

Persons who are naturally very fat are apt to die earlier than those who are slender.

Hippocrates, *Aphorisms*

Patient (dissatisfied with dietary restriction): "Say, Doc, I'm blamed if I'm going to starve to death, just for the sake of living a little longer."

A.S. Daggy, *Harper's Weekly*, 1887

I see no objection to stoutness, in moderation.

William S. Gilbert, *Iolanthe*

Imprisoned in every fat man a thin one is wildly signalling to be let out.

Cyril Connolly, *The Unquiet Grave*

Introduction

Obesity, for some, is a socially catastrophic condition. To others, it is simply a result of poor moral fiber and requires only a little will power for its correction. Still others focus on the negative impact of obesity on health (diabetes, hypertension, heart disease, etc.). We are, as a society, currently "thin-oriented" as opposed to being admirous of "robust, portly" types, as were previous generations and other cultures.

Each physician has to judge for himself how vigorously to reduce patients' weights and, indeed, what is an acceptable definition of *overweight.* Each has to come to grips not only with the grotesquely mammoth patient but also with the "Twiggy-type" who wants to be even more cadaveric than she already is.

Prout is obviously not a fan of amphetamines (or of any anorectic drugs). He considers them of trivial import as aids to weight control, and dangerous to boot. At best, he believes that they deserve only short-term usage. Delighted with the decrease in amphetamine usage as a result of federal production quotas and the negative publicity these drugs have gotten, he is not, one suspects, totally pleased with the switch to other anorexiants. (One wishes he had said more about the efficacy of nondrug approaches to weight reduction. Dietary advice often works poorly, and I anticipate that the dramatic early successes of behavioral modification in reducing weight will be replaced by more sober assessments with the passage of time.)

In contrast, Asher obviously sees a very real role for drugs as *part* of an obesity control program. He quite properly stresses both the pharmacologic and the psychologic effects of drug treatment. He, too, steers away from amphetamines now, but only because of the bad press they have received. (Other doctors stress the nuisance of prescriptions for Schedule II drugs, which are dispensed under strict federal controls.)

As a pharmacologist, I can second Asher's unwillingness to stick with a fixed and arbitrary dosage, and I share his concern for individual rather than "average" performance of a drug. A drug rarely can be used optimally if its application is made identical for all patients. Asher also stresses the need for proper timing of dose, and he sees no need to discontinue the use of an anorexiant if it is well tolerated and continues to have a beneficial effect. He is apparently not overwhelmed by side effect complaints or the specter of drug abuse.

For agents other than anorexiants, he sees little use except for thyroid preparations. Asher also emphasizes the toxic potential of anorexiants if misused. (Digitalis, one might add, is neither effective *nor* safe for weight reduction.)

Prout represents one extreme of the profession in his degree of negativism about appetite suppressants. Asher is by no means at the other extreme, which is represented by those who believe that such drugs are the *answer* to obesity. Most doctors, like Asher, fall in between, using drugs in a battle against a problem that some do not even consider to be medical in nature and one that is often lost by both physician and patient.

Louis Lasagna, M.D.

The Myth of the Usefulness of Amphetamines in the Long-Term Management of Obesity

Thaddeus E. Prout, M.D.
Johns Hopkins University School of Medicine

Although some reviews on the use of amphetamines in the treatment of obesity speak out strongly against them and point out inherent dangers (Edison, 1971), and others are neutral (Silverstone, 1967), many reports and advertising campaigns deliver positive therapeutic messages in favor of amphetamine use, even in the absence of substantiating evidence (Bray and Greenway, 1976). Such reviews bedazzle the reader with truisms on tyrosine metabolism and, having established an air of authority, go on to recommend some of the available pharmaceutical agents while neutralizing adverse conclusions from other sources. One of the important critiques of modern drug usage in the treatment of obesity comes from a committee of the Food and Drug Administration (FDA) that was convened to study the safety and efficacy of anorectic agents (Prout, 1972). Laudatory reviews of amphetamines do not do justice to these recommendations and are likely to misrepresent them. Thus, it will be the purposes of this article to (1) note the conditions under which it became necessary to convene the FDA panel, (2) state the conclusions and recommendations of the committee, and (3) bring the reader up to date on some of the recent steps that have been taken to control the inappropriate use of amphetamines in view of their continued promotion.

Background of Amphetamine Usage

The history of the inappropriate use of amphetamines dates nearly to the time of their discovery. A decade after the synthesis of amphetamines by Alles (Alles, 1927), they were found to be useful agents in the treatment of patients with narcolepsy, and some of these patients were noted to lose weight (Prinzmetal and Bloomberg, 1935). The drugs were then tested specifically as aids in the treatment of obesity (Lesses and Myerson, 1938) and, in less than three years, over 300 references appeared on the uses of amphetamines (Ivy and Krasno, 1941). It was recognized that the drugs were powerful psychic stimulants that increased the patient's sense of well being and energy (Weiss and Laties, 1962). For this reason, it was not surprising to find the diversion of amphetamines from medical to nonmedical use less than 15 years after the first description of their medical applicability.

Early in 1950, Congress became aware of the problems of amphetamine abuse; in 1954, Congressional hearings on this subject were begun. As a result of these hearings, the FDA was urged to begin action to prevent further abuse, but it was not furnished with the power to carry this out. In 1960, explosive street traffic in amphetamines spurred renewed interest in curtailing nonmedical use while continuing to make these agents available by prescription. By 1965, it was clear that the FDA lacked enforcement capability under existing statutes, so the Drug Abuse Control Amendment was enacted, giving the agency greater authority with which to tackle the problem. Enforcement was still not possible, however, and the responsibility was finally transferred to an agency of the Justice Department which, since 1973, has been named the Drug Enforcement Administration (DEA) (Federal Register, 1977).

Amphetamine Studies and Experiments

Since the safety and efficacy of amphetamines and the related congeners remain unproven in the treatment of obesity (Edison, 1971), the FDA ruled that all such drugs would have to be reviewed under a new drug application procedure. Pharmaceutical companies responded, anxious to protect their financial stakes in this lucrative field, and eventually 100 new applications with supporting data were received by the FDA. The evidence presented by pharmaceutical firms included over 1000 volumes of data concerned with 12 so-called anorectic drugs. Computer programs were written to digest this mass of material, and the useful portion of this evidence on safety and efficacy consisted of approximately 200 double-blind controlled studies carried out on almost 10,000 subjects. These were submitted to the consultants on anorectic drugs of the FDA for their review and recommendations.

By August 1972, this group of consultants had completed the review of the material offered. It was found that few studies were available for periods longer than eight weeks and that most of the studies were further marred by the fact that frequently, more than 50 percent of the patients dropped out of the study and were not included in the analysis. Obviously, exclusion of the dropouts led these studies to conclude greater success, since the dropout numbers largely represent treatment failures. In brief, although pharmaceutical agencies were asked to put forward their best effort, it was far from satisfactory. Representative studies have been summarized in Table 9–1.

Although other analyses have been made showing the continuous and increasing efficacy of the active agents over the placebo with time (Bray and Greenway, 1976), such data must have included studies that were not accepted by the committee. There was very little evidence of increasing weight loss over time in any of the studies accepted for review, and as in all studies involving obesity, the greatest weight loss was found during the early part of the study in both the control and the active drug treatment groups. The difference in weight loss for the two groups rapidly decreased as the study progressed. Few studies over eight weeks in duration were acceptable because of design deficiencies.

In a few of these studies, it was also possible to determine the percentage of patients who experienced specific side effects. Approximately 20 percent of patients on the active drug experienced restlessness, insomnia, fatigue, or euphoria. This may be compared to a finding of similar complaints in less than 2 percent of the control group. Other evidence confirmed the fact that congeners of amphetamines, like the parent compound, caused increased motor activity, elevation of blood pressure, tachyphylaxis, drug tolerance, and central nervous system

Table 9–1. *Data on Amphetamine Studies Submitted to the FDA for Review*

Duration in Weeks	Number of Studies	Starting Participants*	Pounds Lost Per Week		Total Difference
			Test Drug	Control	
4	20	1200	1.73	1.05	0.68
8	18	1000	1.44	1.09	0.35
52	1	95	0.1	0.1	0.0

* The appropriate numbers of patients in the study were divided between control patients and patients on the test drug. Note should be taken of the fact that in these studies, the dropout rates were as high as 50 percent. The information listed here, nevertheless, is a summary of the best of the material offered.

stimulation. It is the last effect that apparently leads to abuse of these drugs as stimulants; drugs that lack this effect are unlikely to find their way into street sale and illegal use. Although there are different patterns of illicit usage in various countries, there is reason to believe that this phenomenon is more closely related to supply routes than it is to intrinsic differences among these drugs.

Thus, on the basis of a comparative analysis of double-blind experiments between test drugs and their control groups that had been made available by pharmaceutical firms for the express purpose of showing both efficacy and safety of these drugs, the FDA advisory committee submitted its final conclusions to the Commissioner of the FDA in August 1972 (Prout, 1972).

Conclusions of the Advisory Committee of the FDA on Anorectic Agents

1. Adult obese subjects who are instructed in dietary management and treated with anorectic drugs on the average tend to lose more weight than those treated with placebos and restricted diets in relatively short-term trials.

2. The amount of weight loss associated with the use of an anorectic drug varies from trial to trial. Possible origins of increased weight loss due to the various drug effects are not established, because weight loss appears to be related to variables other than the drug prescribed, such as the physician investigator, the population treated, and the diet prescribed. Studies do not permit conclusions as to the relative importance of the drug and nondrug factors on weight loss.

3. The magnitude of increased weight loss of drug-treated patients over placebo-treated patients was only a fraction of a pound per week. Rate of weight loss was greatest in the first weeks of therapy for both groups of subjects and tended to decrease in succeeding weeks.

4. The natural history of obesity is measured in years, whereas the studies cited are restricted to a few weeks' duration. Thus, the total impact of drug-induced weight loss over that of diet alone must be considered clinically trivial.

5. The limited usefulness of these agents must be measured against any possible risk factors inherent in their use, such as nervousness, insomnia, and drug habituation.

6. Amphetamines, including methamphetamine, have been widely abused in numerous populations. It is thus in the best interests of the public health to limit usage as far as is compatible with adequate therapy. This is both to minimize the risk of dependence in susceptible patients and to decrease the amount of drugs being distributed, since widespread prescription of a dependence-producing drug inevitably increases the possibility for diversion to nonmedical use and abuse.

7. Evidence presented for newer anorectic congeners of the amphetamine family and for nonamphetamine drugs do not set them apart as having higher benefits or lower risks than older drugs. The risk potential of fenfluramine may be an exception to this general statement.

8. There was no evidence in the data reviewed that showed that combination of an anorectic agent with other drugs increases the benefits or reduces the risk of the anorectic agent.

9. There are no clinical data to support the parenteral use of these drugs in the treatment of obesity, nor is obesity an indication for use of these agents.

Recommendations

On the basis of the data reviewed and all the evidence at hand, the FDA formulated several recommendations.

1. All anorectics reviewed (dl-amphetamine, d-amphetamine, methamphetamine, benzphetamine, phentermine, chlorphentermine, clortermine, phenmetrazine, phendimetrazine, fenfluramine, mazindol, and diethylpropion), with the exception of fenfluramine, should be placed on Schedule II on the basis of abuse potential. (Schedule II drugs are kept under close surveillance by the FDA, and their production is strictly controlled.)

2. In the case of anorectics in combination with other drugs, the preparation should be evaluated in accordance with FDA policy on combination drugs, and each constituent of the combination drug must contribute to the total effect claimed for the preparation. Both combination drugs that are currently available and those that are proposed for the future should be subjected to these criteria, in view of the lack of demonstrated efficacy of those constituents already reviewed.

3. Amphetamines prepared for or in a form suitable for parenteral use should not be approved for use in the treatment of obesity.

4. Single-entity oral anorectic preparations including amphetamines should be permitted to be labeled for restricted use in obesity, provided that they are used in association with a specific weight reduction program and that the clinically trivial contribution of these drugs to the overall weight reduction is properly emphasized. To carry out the latter recommendation, statements such as those made in points 3, 4, and 5 of the conclusions of the FDA investigation should be included in all labeling and in all promotional products. Moreover, these agents can only be recommended for use in the treatment of obesity in a carefully monitored and specified weight reduction program under the care of a physician.

5. Approval of all anorectic drugs prepared for future use should be based on demonstration of efficacy as measured by statistical superiority of the drug over a placebo in trials using FDA recommended protocols. These include provisions for, among others, tests on a specific target population, specification of a minimum duration trial to assure clinical relevance of the study, and consideration of the patient dropout factor.

6. Appropriate summary data derived from efficacy studies should be presented in labeling and in all promotional material in order to indicate the degree of weight loss that was shown. For this purpose, the aforementioned labeling guidelines should be supplemented by the addition of the relevant facts found for the drug under consideration.

Other studies. Research interest in these drugs has, of course, continued, but more recent information in addition to that made available to the FDA does not show that administration of these drugs under different conditions is likely to lead to a higher level of efficacy (Chlouverakis, 1975).

Mann (1971) and Seltzer (1966) have pointed out that an increased mortality rate related to obesity is found only in patients whose weight is 30 percent over the ideal. Obesity played a negligible role in mortalities in females in the Framingham Study, unless it was accompanied by elevated blood pressure and increased serum cholestrol (Kannel et al., 1967). In effect, this means that any treatment that is proposed for the cosmetic improvement of body weight, so often deemed desirable by the patient, must be measured against the risk of that therapy. Thus, procedures for relief of obesity and the attendant risks should be considered only in individuals whose body weight is 30 percent or more in excess of the desirable amount. In addition, other health hazards must be given a much higher priority than obesity if one is attempting to decrease mortality or morbidity in the patient population. Hypertension is clearly a more significant risk factor than is obesity, and drugs that increase the risk of hypertension in a futile attempt to reduce body weight are clearly contraindicated.

Effects of the FDA Study on Amphetamine Usage in Obesity

The practical impact of the recommendations of the advisory committee on the use of amphetamines has been of interest in relation to (1) the patterns of drug abuse, (2) the conscience of the involved pharmaceutical companies, and (3) the effects on patient care.

Effects on patterns of drug abuse were predictable. It was recognized that elimination of the popular drugs would only turn attention to other drugs with similar pharmacologic effects on the central nervous system. This became particularly likely when the FDA made a subtle distinction in the recommendations by the advisory committee and thereby altered their practical applications. The FDA took the position that *potential* abuse was not sufficient cause for placing a drug in Schedule II, under which prescription use and production are tightly restricted. Drugs for which *actual* abuse had not been shown were placed in Schedule III or Schedule IV; therefore, significant prescription limitations or production quotas were deemed unnecessary. As predicted, there was a shift of focus from the drugs in Schedule II to the other drugs, which required little change in the prescribing habits of the physicians. More importantly, extraordinary efforts were made by certain companies to document the need for high production quotas. Drugs not previously abused became prominent in isolated areas. In 1973, for example, the use of phenmetrazine increased at least threefold in Washington, D.C. This began at approximately the same time that pharmaceutical promotional campaigns were started, and it was also coincidental with a sharp decline in methamphetamine use, which was not encouraged as phenmetrazine was. At the same time, there was a tripling of phenmetrazine production by the manufacturers of this drug, which was continued through March 1975. In fact, use of phenmetrazine exceeded use of heroin among drug-positive hospital admissions during the first part of 1974. In contrast to the trend for phenmetrazine, use of both amphetamine and methamphetamine declined in 1973 and continued to do so through March 1975 (Kozel and DuPont, 1976).

The effect of the FDA recommendations on the pharmaceutical industry as a whole is less easy to see. In some instances, increased sales of amphetamines led to reinvestigation of this problem by the Subcommittee on Monopoly of the Senate Small Business Committee (Federal Register, 1977). The Pennwalt Corporation, which produces a resinated preparation of phentermine, was cited as having unusual sales because production of the drug appeared to be far in excess of any potential medical need. According to the testimony of F.A. Rody, Jr., of the Drug Enforcement Administration (DEA), the Pennwalt Corporation exported large quantities of their amphetamine materials to Mexico. So much of this was smuggled back into the country and sold on the black market that the DEA had to set up "Operation Blackjack" to bring pressure on Pennwalt and force them out of the export business (Holden, 1976). This is another striking example of the fact that what industry considers good for itself is not necessarily good for the population.

The more important effect on industry has been the continued search for agents that possess anorectic action without causing the side effect of central nervous system stimulation. Fenfluramine is such an agent but unfortunately can cause the opposite side effect, owing to its capacity to precipitate depressive symptoms. Because of the tendency of depression to follow cessation of treatment with this drug, it has been recommended that fenfluramine be used continuously rather than intermittently in order to avoid repeated risks of this side effect. Fenfluramine is contraindicated in patients with a history of severe depression, but it is notably useful in the management of obesity in psychiatric patients who have been maintained on long-term treatment with phenothiazine compounds. This latter fact has excited a great deal of interest from the point of view of treatment for obesity, since this suggests that the central nervous system control of obesity can be altered pharmacologically. In addition, there is some evidence that fenfluramine has a lipolytic effect in that it is able to mobilize fat from fat depots, but this important observation needs to be explored further (Dannenburg and Kardian, 1967). It is not certain whether other molecular manipulations could lead to the development of anorectic agents without significant side effects of any kind, but clearly there should be a greater effort on the part of the pharmaceutical industry to develop a safe and effective agent for long-term use.

The effect of the advisory committee recommendations on patient care is not demonstrable in either a positive or negative sense (Ashwell, 1973). In 1972, Canadian physicians led their government to prohibit the use of amphetamines for the treatment of obesity. Many individual American states, including Maryland, have also denounced the acceptability of amphetamines and related compounds for the treatment of obesity. There is no information that suggests that these actions have caused any hardships on obese patients in the areas cited.

One important effect on patients has been the redirection of concern toward more fundamental aspects of health care for the obese. There is renewed interest in dietary instructions, and it has been pointed out that intense training for up to 25 hours over a period of one year is needed for patients with obesity complicated by diabetes (Davidson, 1975; Davidson, 1977). This is but a practical application of a behavioral approach to obesity that has proved to be of great importance to our understanding of this complex problem (Penick et al., 1971; Foreyt, 1977). Among the more successful studies of behavioral modification is that reported by McReynolds et al. (1976), in which 19 patients who were treated with behavioral management lost an average of 18.6 pounds at the end of a 15-week program, and 22 pounds by the end of three months. At six months, these patients were still holding a loss of 20.4 pounds. Reviews of other studies in this field may be found in the report of Stunkard and Mahoney (1976).

Conclusion

In our concern about the treatment of patients, we must now be ready to take the same step that Canadian physicians took in 1972. Use of products with trivial therapeutic benefits but serious potential harm to society must be carefully controlled. Anecdotal reports and testimonials of individual successes are easily found for obese patients and can be equally easily "documented" for the OTCs that can be bought without prescription but clearly have no scientific merit. Such reports cannot be considered valid excuses for some members of the medical profession to propagandize their peers into support of relatively worthless drugs that continue to jeopardize society as a whole. This is equally true for the reports from well established investigators working in the field whose results, although enthusiastically reported, cannot be replicated by the practicing physician. Better education of physicians is clearly needed (Lasagna, 1973), but anecdotal and unsubstantiated reports are not the proper vehicle.

The Pennwalt Corporation has a way of saying what we all want to hear, and this was recently demonstrated in their full page advertisement in Newsweek (February 6, 1978) that stated, in part:

> . . . whenever we find that our story is not getting across, we tend to blame the other guy. We point the finger . . . to everyone, in fact, except ourselves. Unfortunately people see through these inconsistencies . . . they don't really believe us anymore. We think it is time . . . to try a totally new approach: Candor. We hope it catches on.

Frankly, so do we, especially in the reporting of the results of so-called anorectic drugs used for weight reduction. It might even lead us back to those ancient dicta *Veritas* and *Primum non nocere*.

References

Alles, G.A.: Comparative physiological action of phenylethanolamine. J. Pharmacol. 32:121, 1927.

Ashwell, M.A.: A survey of patient views on doctors' treatment of obesity. Practitioner 211:653, 1973.

Bray, G.A., and Greenway, P.L.: Pharmacological approaches to treating the obese patient. Clin. Endocrinol. Metab. 5:455, 1976.

Chlouverakis, C.: Dietary and medical treatment of obesity: an evaluative review. Addict. Behav. 1:3–21, 1975.

Dannenburg, W.N., and Kardian, B.C.: Fed. Proc. 26:399, 1967.

Davidson, J.K.: The FDA and hypoglycemic drugs. JAMA 232:853, 1975.

Davidson, J.K.: Plasma glucose lowering effect of caloric restriction in obesity+individual insulin treated diabetes mellitus. Diabetes 26:355, 1977.

Edison, G.W.: Amphetamines: a dangerous illusion. Ann. Int. Med. 74:605–610, 1971.

Federal Register, DHEW, FDA, Amphetamine Public Hearing, Part 3. Friday, Oct. 14, 1977.

Foreyt, J.P.: Obesity. In Williams, R.B., Jr., and Gentry, W.D., eds., *Behavioral Approaches to Medical Treatment,* Cambridge, Mass., Ballinger Publishing Co., 1977.

Holden, C.: Amphetamines, tighter controls on the horizons. Science 194:1027–28, 1976.

Ivy, A.C., and Krasno, L.R.: Amphetamine sulphate: a review of the pharmacology. War Med. 1:15, 1941.

Kannel, W.B., LeBauer, E.J., Dawber, T.R., and McNamara, P.M.:Relations of body weight to development of coronary heart disease. The Framingham Study. Circulation 35:734, 1967.

Kozel, N.J., and DuPont, R.L.: Criminal charges and drug use patterns of arrestees in the District of Columbia. Technical Paper, 1976.

Lasagna, L.: Attitudes toward appetite suppressants: a survey of U.S. physicians. JAMA 225:44, 1973.

Lesses, M.F., and Myerson, A.: Benzedrine sulphate as an aid to the treatment of obesity. N. Engl. J. Med. 218:119, 1938.

Mann, G. V.: Obesity: the nutritional spook. Am. J. Public Health 61:1491, 1971.

McReynolds, W.T., Lutz, R.N., Paulsen, B.K., and Kohrs, M.B.: Weight loss from two behavior modification procedures with nutritionists as therapists. Behav. Ther. 7, 1976.

Penick, S.B., Filion, R., Fox, S., and Stunkard, A.J.: Psychosom. Med. 33:49–55, 1971.

Prinzmetal M., and Bloomberg W.: The use of benzedrine for the treatment of narcolepsy. JAMA 105:2051–2054, 1935.

Prout, Thaddeus E., Chairman of FDA Consultants on Anorectic Drugs (1972): Hearings before the SubCommittee on Monopoly of the Select Committee on Small Business Competitive Problems in the Drug Industry. Safety and efficacy of anti-obesity drugs. Part 31, Nov. 9, 10, 11, 18, and 19, 1976, pp 15064–15065.

Seltzer, C.C.: Some re-evaluations of the build and blood pressure study, 1959, as related to ponderal index, somatotype and mortality. N. Engl. J. Med. 274:254, 1966.

Silverstone, J.T.: The treatment of obesity. Hosp. Med. 1:594, 1967.

Stunkard, A.J., and Mahoney, M.J.: Behavioral treatment of eating disorders. In Leitenberg, H., ed., *Handbooks of Behavior Medification and Behavior Therapy,* Englewood Cliffs, N.J., Prentice-Hall, 1976.

Weiss, B., and Laties, V.C.: Enhancement of human performance by caffeine and amphetamines. Pharmac. Rev. 14:1–36, 1962.

Drugs Are Useful in Treating Obesity

W. L. Asher, M.D.
American Society of Bariatric Physicians

When I was approached by the editor to take the "pro" position for the question "Are drugs useful in treating obesity?" I agreed on the condition that I might modify the question to "Are drugs useful in the treatment of obesity?" He agreed.

Drugs, I believe, are of minimal value in treating obesity per se, but if used as one of the modalities in the overall treatment program of obesity, they frequently add a significant dimension thereto.

In 1963, I became acquainted with the frustrations of bariatric medicine when I treated a 345-pound male patient who, with intensive therapy, succeeded in losing 60 pounds, only soon to regain it. Since that time, I have seen several thousand obese patients in private practice, a fair portion of whom have been considerably more successful than was my initial patient, but many of whom have been equally unsuccessful. Since 1969, I have also been involved with the American Society of Bariatric Physicians, for several years as Executive Director and, more recently, as Director of Professional Affairs. Thus, my background is principally practice-oriented. I have also engaged in a few clinical and rat studies pertaining to obesity.

It should be pointed out that although I am involved with a society of physicians who have a special interest in the treatment of obesity, the views that I express are my own and do not necessarily reflect those of the society or other physician members. Approaches to treating obesity vary greatly among the society members and range from strongly drug-oriented to totally non drug-oriented. Most favor a multimodal approach and, with perhaps a few exceptions, rely heavily upon modification of eating behavior.

This presentation will draw in a minor way upon the literature in the field, in some instances upon generally acknowledged precepts, and, more frequently, upon results of my own clinical experience. It is particularly in the last category that I would expect the reader often to be skeptical. If this skepticism generates some additional clinical trials in this area, which frequently lacks data, it will have served a useful purpose.

Inadequacies of Current Treatments

All the modalities we currently use in the treatment of obesity are inadequate, but unless we choose to abandon our patients, we must do the best we can until something better comes along. Generally speaking, the least effective treatment modalities are also the least expensive and the least risky; the most effective are the most expensive and the most risky. At one end of the spectrum are "Do it yourself" programs to take off 5 or 10 pounds in a few days, which appear in magazines. At the other extreme are gastrointestinal bypasses, which are generally quite effective, rather expensive, and relatively risky. Somewhere between the two—and usually used in conjunction with diets—are drugs, behavior modification, and exercise. With the exception of the gastrointestinal bypass, successful weight reduction programs require conscious efforts at modification of eating habits and general changes in lifestyle. Complete or modified fasts, and in some cases, behavior modification programs for the treatment of obesity, have generally not been very successful. A survey of the literature (Stunkard and McLaren-Hume, 1959) on the treatment of obesity showed that in the studies of those "experts" reporting in the literature in such a way that their results could be analyzed, only about 25 percent of all patients lost 20 pounds or more and about 5 percent lost 40 pounds or more. When we analyzed the practices of six bariatric physicians treating overweight patients, we found somewhat better results (Asher and Dietz, 1973). Of the 1409 patients who were treated for obesity by this group, 38 percent lost 20 pounds or more and 10 percent lost 40 pounds or more. It should be noted that some patients who enroll in treatment do not need to lose 20 pounds and many do not need to lose 40 pounds. Be that as it may, overall treatment results are frequently "underwhelming."

Generally, the group of therapists studied by Stunkard and McLaren-Hume were not drug prescribers, whereas the bariatric physicians whom we analyzed were drug prescribers. Presumably, other factors may have accounted for the additional success of the bariatric physicians, but it also seems conceivable that the drugs used were helpful in the short-term success of these patients.

In any program, a good many patients who are "successful" on a short-term basis regain their lost weight, given a little time. Lest the therapist be too prone to self-flagellation in this matter, it must be remembered that many of those who seek the help of a physician are "hard core" patients who have failed in their efforts at self-treatment. Beside the common cold, obesity is probably one of the most common self-treated conditions, and I rather suspect that in a good percentage of people, self-treatment is successful. Thus, it is frequently the self-help failures who seek the aid of physicians.

Effects of Drugs in Treatment of Obesity

In January 1977, the American Society of Bariatric Physicians asked its members who used appetite suppressants in the treatment of obesity to complete a questionnaire. Of 475 members, 176 (37 percent) responded. (Supposedly, some of the nonrespondents also use appetite suppressants in treatment programs.) Responses to one question are shown in Table 9–2. Insofar as appetite suppressants are concerned, a fair portion of our membership find them not only of use but of value, sometimes for considerable periods. A survey of physicians' views in general about anorectic drug usage (Lasagna, 1973) revealed that 78 percent of general practitioners, 57 percent of obstetrician-gynecologists, and 50 percent of internists prescribe appetite suppressants. Of these physicians, 25 percent will prescribe anorexiants for longer than three months.

Direct and Indirect Effects

Drugs have two types of effects—direct, which can be illustrated by the appetite-suppressing action of the anorectic drugs, and indirect, which is less apparent (for example, inducing the patient to return regularly for treatment). Often, the medication becomes the factor that lures the patient back in, and without getting him back, the probability of therapeutic success is considerably reduced. If the physician is somewhat softhearted, patients frequently are lost to treatment after they make a successful telephone plea to have prescriptions refilled at the pharmacy because they can't possibly get into the doctor's office.

Bariatric physicians who concentrate principally on the treatment of obesity frequently dispense drugs from their offices. The advantages of this are saving patients some money,

Table 9–2. *How Long Do Patients Receive Appetite Suppressants?*

	Number of Physicians	Percent of Physicians
3 months or less	48	29.6
3 to 6 months	50	30.9
6 to 12 months	18	11.1
1 to 2 years	6	3.7
As long as needed	30	18.5
Other answers*	10	6.2
TOTAL	162	100.0

* Some of the "Other answers" indicated alternate days, or 15 days of intermittent therapy, or 50 percent of time on program.

helping the doctor to pay some of his overhead, and, more importantly, getting the patient to return for treatment. The patient has no choice but to see the physician before more medications are dispensed, and this contact with the physician and his assistants can set the stage for ongoing reeducation programs.

Drugs will be discussed in the following categories: (1) anorectic agents, (2) bulking agents, (3) diuretics, (4) thyroid drugs, (5) digitalis, (6) placebos, and (7) human chorionic gonadotropin.

Anorectic Agents

Literature and Clinical Experience

The era of the appetite suppressants began in the late 1930s. Smith Kline & French has been marketing amphetamines for appetite suppression since 1938. During World War II, amphetamines were used frequently during military maneuvers by both Allied and Axis troops endeavoring to stay awake and alert for more than the usual periods. They were the only appetite suppressants on the market until the late 1950s and early 1960s, when several other drug companies, as a result of their search for a less stimulating appetite suppressant, received approval from the Food and Drug Administration (FDA) to market their products. Those coming on the market at that time included phentermine (Ionamin, Wilpo), phendimetrazine (Plegine), phenmetrazine (Preludin), and diethylpropion (Tenuate). Except for chlorphentermine (Pre-Sate), which was approved in the late 1960s, no other new anorectic drugs were approved after the early 1960s by the then resistant FDA, until 1973, when three new ones finally ran the gauntlet of FDA bureaucracy and were approved. They were fenfluramine (Pondimin), the first appetite suppressant with a sedative rather than a stimulating effect; mazindol (Sanorex), the first appetite suppressant that is chemically unrelated to the amphetamines; and clortermine (Voranil), which is closely related chemically to chlorphentermine. No new anorectic drugs have been approved since 1973. However, Beecham-Massengill has obtained approval for Fastin, which is phentermine in a 30 mg timed-release form.

In the mid-1960s, increased drug abuse in the streets led to the classification of amphetamines as *controlled* drugs. In 1971, both amphetamines and Preludin were named Schedule II, controlled drugs, permitting the FDA to set quotas on the amounts of these drugs that can be produced. Because of increased regulation and diminished supply, usage of these two classes of drugs has declined. In 1972, the balance of the appetite suppressants were classified as Schedule III or Schedule IV drugs. Although there are some restrictions with these drugs, quotas are not required. Usage of these "non-amphetamine" drugs has increased as amphetamine usage has decreased.

Frankly, based on my experience with the various appetite suppressants and the modest number of studies that I have done, I doubt that there is a significant difference in the effect of the various anorectics, provided the dosage is properly set. However, certain of the appetite suppressants do seem to have significantly more side effects than others, and therefore, suggested dosage levels may well have been set a little lower in comparison to those for other anorectics. Beside stimulation, amphetamines seem to be relatively free of side effects. Even though amphetamines are good drugs, I have discontinued their use owing to the continued "bad-mouthing" they get because of their illicit street use. I have switched to other appetite suppressants for patients who need them.

I fear that there has been a tendency on the part of both the FDA and the pharmaceutical companies to set relatively low dosage levels for appetite suppressants (and perhaps other drugs) to avoid side effects. In so doing they have set the suggested dosage levels so low that sometimes, the anorectic effects are modest at best. However, by proper titration of the drug dosages, significant benefit can be obtained in a considerable portion of the patient population for long periods.

I personally am not very enamored of the long-acting appetite suppressants, but many of my colleagues, both in and out of the bariatric profession, find this drug form quite useful. Generally, I have not found that the appetite-suppressing effects of the long-acting forms have coincided well with the periods in which they were most needed. Ordinarily, a strong appetite-suppressing effect is most needed at mealtime. Therefore, I use the short-acting drugs and give them approximately one hour before meals (a half hour before is not enough lead time for some patients). A few patients may even need to take them 1.5 hours before meals. Generally, the peak of action of the shorter-acting drugs is somewhere around two hours after administration, with the majority of the activity being complete after four hours. I now use predominantly phentermine and phendimetrazine.

Recommended Treatments

I rarely recommend an appetite suppressant before 11:00 A.M. Generally, if patients are hungry, I prefer to have them eat in the morning, particularly if they eat protein foods. Ordinarily, the obese patient eats a very modest breakfast and doesn't need much appetite suppression in the morning. If necessary, I give the usual morning dose in the middle of the afternoon or add it to the dose before the evening meal. In rare cases, this may cause a problem with insomnia, which is usually remedied with a sedative such as phenobarbital.

For patients who need some appetite suppression earlier, I generally prescribe 8 mg of phentermine one hour before the noon meal and 8 mg one hour before the evening meal. This dosage then can be increased after a few weeks to 16 mg before the evening meal. One can double this dosage and still be within the suggested range, so that in some patients, I may end up using 16 mg before the noon meal, 16 mg in mid-afternoon, and 16 mg before the evening meal. (Generally, I have found phentermine to be one of the less stimulating anorectics.) My next step for those who seem to need a little more appetite suppression and are having no problems with jitters or nerves is to change to 35 mg phendimetrazine tablets in lieu of the 8 mg phentermine tablets. In some cases, this transition is made earlier in the treatment regimen, instead of increasing the phentermine dosage. Thus, patients who need appetite suppression may end up taking 35 to 70 mg of phendimetrazine before the noon meal and from 70 to 140 mg either before the evening meal or spread out during mid-afternoon (before the evening meal). I believe that 35 mg of phendimetrazine has a little more anorectic effect than 8 mg of phentermine.

Dosages are titrated, depending upon the patient's need. Many patients won't need maximum doses. For those who do, I usually don't prescribe a maximum dose until 12 to 16 weeks or more of treatment. With dosages increased to maximal levels, many patients will be helped for quite long periods.

It should be pointed out that not all patients need appetite suppression, particularly if the eating program they are following is fairly low in carbohydrates—i.e., in the range of 40 to 60 grams per day. Frequently, with low levels of carbohydrate, patients have little hunger. If appetite suppressants are used in conjunction with a low-carbohydrate diet, both physician and patient tend to believe that the drugs cause lack of hunger. In the double-blind study of mazindol (Sanorex) that I did a number of years ago, the patient who lost the most weight (some 46 pounds in 16 weeks) was quite delighted with the new drug that we were testing. I don't recall whether the patient or I was more surprised when, after breaking the double-blind code, we found that the patient had been on a placebo. It turned out that he had put himself on a 600-calorie diet that was fairly restricted in carbohydrates.

As indicated earlier, I feel that appetite suppressants should be used as long as the patient needs them and furthermore, that short-term use is totally irrational. It makes no more sense to take the patient who is benefiting from an appetite suppressant off of it after a few weeks than it does to take the patient who is responding to antihypertensive therapy off the antihypertensive agent after a few weeks. If the patient needs the help, is responding, and is not having problems with side effects, then I see absolutely no reason for the therapy to be discontinued. (Interestingly enough, narcoleptics have taken doses of amphetamine up to 50 to 100 mg per day for years on end without any particular problem.) It has been my own observation that as the "target" effect decreases, side effects also do so. Increasing the dosage does not necessarily increase the level of the side effects relative to the therapeutic effect of a drug. If one increases the dosage significantly, he is back at the starting point insofar as the relationship of target effect to side effect is concerned. This relationship is really of more clinical importance than the milligram dosage per se.

OTHER STUDIES

Although some tolerance to anorectics ordinarily develops, many patients will continue responding for a long time. Scoville (1973), in a Herculean undertaking, computerized data from 10,000 patients who had been involved in 200 double-blind studies submitted to the FDA. He found that the patients taking an active drug lost approximately 0.5 pound per week more than those taking a placebo. This formal presentation does not include additional data presented by Scoville at the 1973 John E. Fogarty International Center Conference of the National Institute of Health (Scoville, 1973), which indicated that of those studies in which the patients had been followed in a double-blind manner for as long as 20 weeks, the patients taking anorectics lost or kept off significantly more weight than patients taking placebos for periods of up to 20 weeks.

In the study by Munro et al. (1968), patients who continued to take phentermine for a 36-week period lost significantly more weight than the patients on placebos (average 27 pounds vs. 10.5 pounds). McKay (1973) found that patients taking diethylpropion lost significantly more weight over a 25-week period than patients on placebos (average 25.8 pounds vs. 5.4 pounds). (There have been few other long-term studies of the appetite suppressants and certainly more are needed.) Interestingly enough, in the study by Munro et al., a group of subjects alternating one month on placebo and one month on phentermine lost an average of 28.7 pounds, or about the same as the group who were on phentermine consistently. A more recent study (Steel et al., 1973) found that the alternating phentermine-placebo group did as well as the consistent fenfluramine group and as well as a group alternating phentermine and fenfluramine. The group alternating fenfluramine and placebo did not do as well. In this last group, there was a problem of depression about four days after the patients stopped taking fenfluramine (Steel and Briggs, 1972). In a 16-week double-blind study, I found that the alternating mazindol (Sanorex)-placebo group did as well as the continuous mazindol group. Thus, it appears that intermittent therapy with anorectics (excluding fenfluramine) warrants further consideration.

Certain patients seem to respond well to the appetite suppressants, whereas others do not. Silverstone and Stunkard (1968) found a considerable variation in obese patients' sensitivity to dextroamphetamine. Presumably, this also applies to other anorectic drugs. Recently, Munro and colleagues found that when fenfluramine doses were increased to as much as 160 mg or to maximum tolerance levels, some patients responded with appetite suppression and others did not (Innes et al., 1977). Plasma samples indicated that the responders were those who had the higher levels of plasma fenfluramine. Thus, it appears that the nonresponders may absorb fenfluramine poorly or may metabolize it more rapidly than the responders. This raises the interesting possibility that one might be able to determine why some patients respond to appetite suppressants and others do not.

The majority of over-the-counter appetite suppressants contain phenylpropanolamine, which is chemically related to the amphetamines. In contrast to the amphetamines, however, it has a significant nasal drying effect. Hence, it has been used in quite a number of over-the-counter cold remedies. A recent study seemed to indicate some modest degree of appetite suppression from phenylpropanolamine (Hoebel et al., 1975). It seems doubtful that a significant degree of appetite suppression could be attained and sustained over a reasonable period without running into problems with the drying side effect.

Bulking Agents

At times, agents that provide bulk to the gastrointestinal tract have been tested in the treatment of obesity. Probably the most notable of these is methylcellulose. Generally, these agents have not seemed to be of any particular value. Share et al. (1952) found that giving calorically inert bulk (gum arabic, celluflour) to dogs intragastrically did not inhibit food intake unless large amounts were given just before oral feeding. More recently, however, a study of Pretts (a combination of alginic acid and sodium carboxymethylcellulose), an over-the-counter product, seems to indicate that this bulking agent reduces intensity of feelings of hunger and helps patients adjust to reduced food intake (Marquette, 1976). However, it is difficult to carry out such a study in double-blind fashion.

Diuretics

Although diuretics have gained some acceptance in the treatment of obesity, they have no known impact upon appetite or fat stores, and their usage would seem to be contraindicated, except in cases of water retention. Usually, water retention is not a significant problem if carbohydrate intake is kept relatively low, since there is usually some subsequent salt and water loss. If diuretics are needed, they should, in general, be used intermittently. Diuretics should be used with considerable caution in patients on less than 800- to 1000-calorie diets, since the electrolyte loss secondary to low calorie diets can be further aggravated by diuretics. With fasting regimens, the problem becomes even more acute.

If diuretics are used, the potassium-sparing ones such as Aldactone, Aldactazide, Dyrenium, or Diazide should be considered.

Thyroid Hormone

Through the years, the use of thyroid in the treatment of the euthyroid obese patient has remained controversial. Putnam (1893) was the first to report feeding of thyroid glands to control previously uncontrollable symptoms of myxedema. During the 1890s various conditions, some associated with myxedema, were treated by feeding the thyroid gland, and obesity was no exception. Up to 15 grains of desiccated thyroid per day in the treatment of obesity (Anders, 1907) was advocated in the early 1900s in Osler's *Modern Medicine.*

A decreased metabolic rate was commonly thought to be associated with obesity in the early 1900s. However, calculations of the basal metabolic rate at the time were based on body weight. When these calculations were later based on surface area, few obese patients appeared to have reduced metabolic rates. As the 1930s ended, the era ascribing obesity to a glandular problem drew to a close. Since then, there have been a number of studies concerned with the use of pharmacologic doses of thyroid in the treatment of obesity, but for the most part, they have been poorly controlled. Generally, it appears that the usage of one or two grains of thyroid or the equivalent in other thyroid analogs has little effect on the euthyroid obese individual. However, at three grains of desiccated thyroid per day or the equivalent, there seems to be some enhancement of weight loss in patients receiving thyroid hormones in addition to amphetamines compared with taking amphetamines alone (Gelvin et al., 1959; Kaplan and Jose, 1970). Recent studies, in which thyroid hormone was used without appetite suppressants, have indicated that dosages in the range of 6 to 14 grains of thyroid per day or the equivalent do indeed enhance weight loss in euthyroid obese individuals (Cornman and Alexander, 1965; Bray, 1969; Drenick and Fisler, 1970; Hollingsworth et al., 1970; Lamki et al., 1973). These large doses were given initially to patients not taking any thyroid hormone; subsequently, three patients of Drenick and Fisler developed angina and one of Hollingsworth et al. developed atrial fibrillation. My own clinical experience indicates that patients seldom have problems if thyroid doses are started at one to two grains per day and are gradually increased.

Certainly, administration of initial large doses should be reserved for the carefully controlled study situation. Thyroid hormone should be used with extreme caution in obese patients with any significant cardiac problems. Deaths have occurred in patients receiving "diet pills" (Henry, 1967; Jelliffe et al., 1969). It was felt that these deaths followed hypokalemia-induced myocardial irritability aggravated by thyroid hormone and digitalis, and that the hypokalemia resulted from decreased food intake (secondary to the amphetamines) and from diuretics and laxatives. These deaths occurred in a geographic area in which physicians had prescribed up to six grains of digitalis leaf per day and 20 grains of thyroid per day (Henry, 1968). I studied 7286 overweight patients who received "diet pills" for varying periods and found no increase in the death rate while patients were receiving diet pills, including thyroid pills, compared with when they were not receiving them (Asher, 1972). The patients in this trial were well supervised, which did not generally seem to be the case for the studies in which the deaths occurred.

In clinical practice, thyroid hormone, if started at one to two grains per day, is ordinarily well tolerated by obese euthyroid individuals. There seems to be little indication for increasing the dosage level above this (which for most patients is probably a pharmacologically inert level) if patients are doing well. Some patients experience an extremely slow weight loss after a certain period. At least a portion of this may be due to metabolic slowing secondary to the calorically low food intake. Ancel Keys (1950), in his classic work after World War II, demonstrated a slowing of metabolic rate of up to 30 percent in normal-weight volunteers receiving about 1600 calories per day instead of their usual 3000+ calories. One explanation is that the body has a remarkable ability to maintain homeostasis. Recent work (Portnay et al., 1974; Croxson et al., 1977) suggests a possible mode of action for this phenomenon. The final active form of thyroid hormone in the body causing the end organ metabolic responses is triiodothyronine. The body is capable of converting thyroxine either to active triiodothyronine or to the inactive reverse triiodothyronine. During starvation a relatively larger than normal amount of thyroxine is converted to reverse triiodothyronine. This appears to contribute to the metabolic slowing seen when calorie intake is low. It would seem from this study that triiodothyronine (Cytomel) might be the drug of choice.

In general, I have found that starting the typical healthy euthyroid obese individual on one to two grains of desiccated thyroid per day with a gradual increase causes no problems. Patients should be carefully monitored. Over the years, we have done repeated ECG's on patients, but probably the best initial indications of potential problems are the physician's (1) eliciting from the patients a history of palpitations or (2) finding tachycardia in a patient who did not previously have it. Also, a resting, sitting pulse rate of over 100 may indicate some effect of thyroid on cardiac status.

For those patients who suffer metabolic slowing and a subsequent decrease in the rate of weight loss, increasing the thyroid at monthly intervals by perhaps one grain per day (up to as much as five grains per day) may be helpful. I have rarely seen problems in patients receiving this dosage. Proof of long-term safety and effectiveness of this adjunctive therapy will have to await well controlled, long-term studies. Certainly there is a need for a 12-month or longer double-blind study of comparable groups receiving (1) placebo, (2) no placebo and no drugs, (3) appetite suppressants, (4) thyroid, and (5) thyroid and appetite suppressants. Some authorities have been concerned about enhanced protein loss when obese euthyroid patients receive thyroid. Recent work (Lamki et al., 1973) seems to indicate that this is not a problem if the patients maintain adequate protein intake.

Digitalis

Anders, writing in successive editions of Osler's *Modern Medicine* (1907, 1914, and 1926), advocated digitalis as an agent to guard the heart when pharmacologic doses of thyroid were employed in the treatment of obesity. From that time until the late 1960s, digitalis was used in some "diet pill" mixtures, presumably in an attempt to control the pulse rate when thyroid was given. We have done a double-blind study (Asher and Dietz, 1973) on digitalis leaf added to other diet pills and found that in doses up to the customary 1.5 grains per day of digitalis leaf, there was no effect over that of a placebo on weight loss, blood pressure, or pulse. Therefore, digitalis does not seem to be indicated in the treatment of the obese patient unless clear-cut cardiac indications for its use are present.

Placebo

Double-blind studies have made us aware that patients frequently respond favorably to what they think a medication is supposed to do. The obese patient is no exception, and no comments on the use of drugs in the treatment of obesity would be complete without a discussion of placebos. Medications, either active or inactive, perform two valuable ancillary services in addition to any true pharmacologic activity they may have. Medications help to get the patient in to see the physician so that further counseling is possible, and they also constantly remind patients that they are under treatment and that they should be following the dietary admonitions of the counselor. Patients are reminded of this each time they take a pill or capsule. In a sense, medication is the "doctor away from the office." At times, physicians have used totally inactive pills or capsules—true placebos—while suggesting to the patient that the pills reduce the desire to eat. Although some patients respond favorably to these placebos, the doctor-patient relationship is jeopardized if the patient finds out that he is taking "sugar pills." Pharmacologically active placebos probably are more acceptable from this standpoint (e.g., methylcellulose and vitamins). Although the grain or two of thyroid hormone frequently prescribed by physicians may be of questionable pharmacologic value, it may well perform a useful placebo function in the treatment of the obese patient.

Human Chorionic Gonadotropin

Simeons introduced the use of human chorionic gonadotropin (HCG) in the treatment of obesity (Simeons, 1954, 1956). Controversy over whether the 125 IU daily dose that he advocated had any effect on the treatment of obesity continued for a number of years. We did a double-blind study that suggested that HCG might have more value than a placebo

(Asher and Harper, 1973). More recent studies by Greenway and Bray (1977), partially funded by the American Society of Bariatric Physicians, and those of Stein et al. (1976) and Young et al. (1976) seem to indicate that HCG has no activity in the treatment of obesity. Presumably, HCG could be considered a placebo and, although no significant side effects seem likely at the 125 IU per day dosage level, it is suggested that dosage be reduced to a few IU per day if it is to be used. Simeons' program did have some merit in that the patients came in six times per week for their injections, which served as a valuable opportunity for the physician or his assistant to give additional counseling.

Conclusion

Drugs, if properly used, can be helpful in the treatment of obesity. Although obesity is primarily physiologic, its treatment is primarily psychologic. In my clinical practice we rely heavily on behavior modification and nutrition reeducation. However, in the treatment of such a chronic, persistent condition as obesity, no modality should be overlooked. This includes the drugs we now have. Perhaps in the future the mysteries of obesity can be further unraveled. With better understanding, new pharmacologic agents might be developed so that the treatment of obesity would become primarily pharmacologic rather than psychologic.

References

Anders, J.M.: Constitutional disease. In Osler, W., *Modern Medicine,* Philadelphia, Lea Brothers, 1907.

Asher, W.L.: Mortality rate in patients receiving "diet pills." Curr. Ther. Res. 14:525, 1972.

Asher, W.L., and Dietz, R.E.: Effectiveness of weight reduction involving "diet pills," Curr. Ther. Res. 14:510, 1973.

Asher, W.L., and Harper, H.W.: Effect of human chorionic gonadotropin on weight loss, hunger, and feeling of well-being. Am. J. Clin. Nutr. 26:211, 1973.

Bray, G.A.: Effect of diet and triiodothyronine on the activity of sn-glycerol-3-phosphate dehydrogenase and on the metabolism of glucose and pyruvate by adipose tissue of obese patients. J. Clin. Invest. 48:1413, 1969.

Cornman, H.D., and Alexander, F.: Effects of L-triiodothyronine alone in the treatment of obesity. Fed. Proc. 24:189, 1965.

Croxson, M.S., Hall, T.D., Kletzky, O.A., Jaramill, J.E., and Nicoloff, J.T.: Decreased thyrotropin secretion induced by fasting. J. Clin. Endocrinol. Metab. 45:560, 1977.

Drenick, E.J., and Fisler, J.L.: Prevention of recurrent weight gain with large doses of synthetic thyroid hormones. Curr. Ther. Res. 12:570, 1970.

Gelvin, E.P., Kenigsberg, S.M., and Boyd, L.J.: Results of addition of T3 to a weight-reducing program. JAMA 170:1507, 1959.

Greenway, F.L., and Bray, G.A.: Human chorionic gonadotropin (HCG) in the treatment of obesity. A critical assessment of the Simeons method. West. J. Med. 127:461, 1977.

Henry, R.C.: Weight reduction pills (Letters). JAMA 201:217, 1967.

Henry, R.C.: Statement at Hearings before the Subcommittee on Antitrust and Monopoly of the Committee on the Judiciary, United States Senate (Diet pill industry). Washington: U.S. Government Printing Office, 1968.

Hoebel, B.G., Cooper, J., Kamin, M.C., and Willard, D.: Appetite suppression by phenylpropanolamine in humans. Obes. Bariat. Med. 4:192, 1975.

Hollingsworth, D.R., Amatruda, T.T., Jr., and Scheig, R.: Quantitative and qualitative effects of T3 in massive obesity. Metabolism 19:934, 1970.

Innes, J.A., Watson, M.L., Ford, M.J., Munro, J.F., Stoddart, M.E., and Campbell, D.B.: Plasma fenfluramine levels, weight loss, and side effects. Br. Med. J. 2:1322, 1977.

Jelliffe, R.W., Hill, D., Tatter, D., et al: Death from weight-control pills. A case report with objective postmortem confirmation. JAMA 208:1843, 1969.

Kaplan, N.M., and Jose, A.: Thyroid as an adjuvant to amphetamine therapy of obesity. A controlled double-blind study. Am. J. Med. Sci. 260:105, 1970.

Keys, A., Brozek, J., Henschel, A., et al.: *Biology of Human Starvation.* Minneapolis, University of Minnesota Press, 1950.

Lamki, L., Ezrin, C., Koven, I., and Steiner, G.: L-thyroxine in the treatment of obesity without increase in loss of lean body mass. Metabolism 22:617, 1973.

Lasagna, L.: Attitudes toward appetite suppressants. A survey of U.S. physicians. JAMA 225:44, 1973.

Marquette, C.J.: Effects of bulk-producing tablets on hunger intensity in dieting patients. Obes. Bariat. Med. 5:3, 1976.

McKay, R.H.G.: Long-term use of diethylpropion in obesity. Curr. Med. Res. Opin. 1:489, 1973.

Munro, J.F., MacCuish, A.C., Wilson, E.M., Duncan, L.J.P.: Comparison of continuous and intermittent anorectic therapy in obesity. Br. Med. J. 1:352, 1968.

Portnay, G.I., O'Brian, J.T., Bush, J., Vagenakis, A.G., Azizi, F., Arky, S.H., Ingbar, S.H., and Braverman, L.E.: The effect of starvation on the concentration and binding of thyroxin and triiodothyronine and serum on the response to TRH. J. Clin. Endocrinol. Metab. 39:191, 1974.

Putnam, J.J.: Cases of myxoedema and acromegalia treated with benefit by sheep's thyroids. Am. J. Med. Sci. 106:125, 1893.

Scoville, B.A.: Review of amphetamine-like drugs by the Food and Drug Administration: clinical data and value judgements. In Bray, G.A., ed., *Obesity in Perspective,* John E. Fogarty International Center for Advanced Study in the Health Sciences Conference, National Institutes of Health, 1973 (DHEW Publication No. NIH 75–708).

Share, I., Martynuik, E., and Grossman, M.I.: Effect of prolonged intragastric feeding on oral food intake in dogs. Am. J. Physiol. 169:229, 1952.

Silverstone, J.T., and Stunkard, A.J.: The anorectic effect of dexamphetamine sulphate. Br. J. Pharmacol. 33:513, 1968.

Simeons, A.T.W.: The action of chorionic gonadotropin in the obese. Lancet 2:946, 1954.

Simeons, A.T.W.: Chorionic gonadotropin in geriatrics. J. Am. Geriatr. Soc. 4:36, 1956.

Steel, J.M., Munro, J.F., and Duncan, L.J.P.: A comparative trial of different regimens of fenfluramine and phentermine in obesity. Practitioner 211:232, 1973.

Steel, J.M., and Briggs, M.: Withdrawal depression in obese patients after fenfluramine treatment. Br. Med. J. 3:26, 1972.

Stein, M.R., Julis, R.E., Peck, C.C., Hinshaw, W., Sawicki, J.E., and Deller, J.J., Jr.: Ineffectiveness of human chorionic gonadotropin in weight reduction: a double-blind study. Am. J. Clin. Nutr. 29:940, 1976.

Stunkard, A., and McLaren-Hume, M.: The results of treatment for obesity. Arch. Intern. Med. 103:79, 1959.

Young, R.L., Fuchs, R.J., and Woltjen, M.J.: Chorionic gonadotropin in weight control. A double-blind crossover study. JAMA 236:2495, 1976.

10

What Is the Best Antacid?

Birgir Gudjonsson, M.D., and Howard M. Spiro, M.D.

Unfortunately, only a small number of patients with peptic ulcer are financially able to make a pet of an ulcer.

William J. Mayo

The view that a peptic ulcer may be the hole in a man's stomach through which he crawls to escape from his wife has fairly wide acceptance.

J.A.D. Anderson, *A New Look at Social Medicine*

The healthy stomach is nothing if not conservative. Few radicals have good digestion.

Sydney Smith, *Notebooks*

it is a cheering thought to think that god is on the side of the best digestion

Don Marquis, *archy does his part*

Introduction

Antacids are among the most widely used medicines. Often, to be sure, they are taken as a result of self-diagnosis and self-treatment, and the trigger for buying and taking an antacid is not based on structural abnormalities but on symptoms. Patients take antacids to feel better rather than to heal an ulcer. And, indeed, as Gudjonsson and Spiro point out, the correlation between symptoms and evidence of actual ulceration is not a tight one.

The authors' review of published studies on the effects of therapeutic agents in patients with peptic ulcer disease is informative in many ways. It shows, for example, the remarkable tendency for healing to occur with placebo therapy (even with saline injections). Second, the review shows an enormous variation in the response of patients to placebos. So variable is this reaction that it illustrates dramatically the foolishness of trying to use "historical" controls as a substitute for contemporaneous comparison of treated patients with a properly constituted control group.

"Placebo effects" have their origin in two components. One is what most people mean by "placebo effect"—psychologically determined benefit that results from anticipation, faith in medicine or doctors, and the like. The second derives from spontaneous change as a result simply of the passage of time. Many symptoms improve spontaneously, with or without the taking of a remedy.

Benefits that accrue from spontaneous remission, therefore, will be experienced without taking anything. However, benefits attributed to the first component require that the patient ingest (or at least be given) a "remedy," preferably something in which the patient (and doctor?) has faith. Thus, even if antacids were *pharmacologically* inert, the need to supply a vehicle for the placebo effect still exists.

Recent work on "heartburn" (which is what a lot of patients take antacids for) suggests some added subtleties. Heartburn is now thought to be related at least in part to esophageal reflux of gastric contents. To the extent that this is the case, it places an extra premium on taking something that is swallowed and raises the question of whether an oral placebo is really a physiologic cipher.

A simple classification of the studies reviewed by Gudjonsson and Spiro into those in which placebo outperformed active treatment and those in which the opposite is true (regardless of the magnitude of the difference) shows an interesting fact: the great majority of studies favor active treatment. Even for antacids, the breakdown is 10 to 5 in favor of active treatment. Not all completed studies are published, however, and it is too bad that we cannot know whether this pro-drug ratio is for real or just a fluke. Either way, the statistics are provocative.

LOUIS LASAGNA, M.D.

What Is the Best Antacid?

Birgir Gudjonsson, M.D.

Howard M. Spiro, M.D.

Yale University School of Medicine

The answer to this question is still as unclear as the causes of ulcer and what the therapeutic aims of ulcer treatment should be. Since Abercrombie proposed the acid peptic theory of "peptic" ulcer in 1845, duodenal exposure to excessive amounts of acid has been generally accepted as the cause of duodenal ulcer. This has been held to be the result of (1) excessive gastric secretion of acid and (2) rapid emptying of the acid into the duodenum, together with (3) defective buffering of acid within the duodenum and even (4) a defective mucosal protective mechanism (Wormsley, 1974). Despite such an apparently solid pathophysiologic base, an ulcer comes and goes unpredictably, judged by symptoms at least. The reasons for this unpredictability have never been clear. Kothari and Kothari (1977) have suggested that "peptic" ulcer has too specific an etiologic implication and should be replaced by "dyspeptic" ulcer, which is not a bad idea! In any case, support for the importance of acid and pepsin in the genesis of duodenal ulcer lies in the observation that duodenal ulcer is not often seen in patients with achlorhydria. As acid has seemed to be the main culprit in the pathogenesis of duodenal ulcer, antacids have been the mainstay of therapy. In the discussion that follows, we look at the role of antacids both in relieving symptoms and in promoting healing of gastric and duodenal ulcers.

Common Preparations

Theoretically, antacids should be useful not only because they reduce acidity but also because the increased pH that they bring about lowers peptic activity (Harvey, 1975). Most common gastric antacids (1) contain a weakly basic portion, (2) work by neutralizing or absorbing gastric acid, and (3) can be divided into systemic and nonsystemic types. The basic portion of a systemic antacid is absorbed in appreciable amounts and therefore may lead to metabolic alkalosis, whereas the cationic portion of a nonsystemic antacid forms insoluble basic compounds that remain in the intestinal lumen and are excreted. Sodium bicarbonate, calcium carbonate, magnesium hydroxide, and aluminum hydroxide are among the most frequently used preparations.

SODIUM BICARBONATE. This compound was the "saleratus" of another generation. It is highly soluble and exerts a rapid antacid action in the stomach. The reaction of sodium bicarbonate with hydrochloric acid produces carbon dioxide and water. Much of the carbon dioxide is emitted with a satisfying belch, which may contribute to the therapeutic effect. Any excess carbon dioxide empties rapidly into the small intestine, where it is absorbed and may lead to alkalosis if sodium bicarbonate is taken in large amounts. As it also has a very short-lived action, sodium bicarbonate is rarely advised therapeutically today, although it still has a justifiable place in the home medicine cabinet.

CALCIUM CARBONATE. This preparation has a rapid onset of antacid effect and a duration more prolonged than that of sodium bicarbonate. As it is generally considered to be constipating and to cause significant "acid rebound" (Fordtran, 1968) through gastrin release (Barreras, 1973; Levant et al., 1973), calcium carbonate lately has fallen into disrepute as a prescribed drug for duodenal ulcer. Its merit as a symptom reliever in small and not overly frequent amounts should be kept in mind. The constipating effects of calcium carbonate have been questioned in a commodious review (Clemens and Feinstein, 1977), which suggests that double blind studies are necessary to prove this long-accepted belief.

Magnesium hydroxide. Although this antacid has a prompt and more prolonged neutralizing action than does sodium bicarbonate, its osmotic effects lead to diarrhea in most people. Magnesium hydroxide has thus been relegated to a cooperative role with other antacids, usually aluminum hydroxide.

Aluminum hydroxide. These compounds have the lowest neutralizing capacity on a weight basis, and they vary greatly in their ability to neutralize acid because of differing solubilities (Littman, 1967). Aluminum hydroxide delays gastric emptying (Hurwitz et al., 1976), which may have some theoretical value in prolonging acid neutralization. It causes constipation in most patients and has been associated with relatively dramatic, although fortunately infrequent, side effects such as phosphorus depletion and osteomalacia (Lotz et al., 1968). For a long time, aluminum in antacids was considered nonabsorbable, but it is now known that small amounts are absorbed (Kaehny et al., 1977) and may play a role in the "dialysis encephalopathy syndrome" (Alfrey et al., 1976) as well as in other brain diseases (Crapper et al., 1976).

In 1950, aluminum hydroxide was found to cause reduced absorption of tetracycline (Waisbren and Hueckel). Since that time, it has been learned that various antacids interfere with absorption of many other drugs, including anticholinergic agents (Blaug and Gross, 1965), digoxin (Khalil, 1974; Brown and Juhl, 1976), and naproxen (Segre et al., 1974). Curiously enough, on the other hand, magnesium hydroxide can increase the absorption of bishydroxycoumarin (Ambre and Fischer, 1973) through an unknown mechanism.

Acid Neutralization

Antacids have been used to relieve pain, to promote healing, and occasionally (and with the least justification) to prevent recurrence of ulcer. How much acid has to be neutralized and for how long are still not known. Yet the chemistry of acid neutralization and the ways to bring it about are becoming quite clear (Myhill and Piper, 1964; Fordtran et al., 1966, 1973; Littman, 1967), even if the importance of such acid neutralization remains, in our opinion at least, relatively undefined.

Morrissey and Barreras (1974) emphasized that the goals of neutralization have rarely been defined. If neutralization means bringing the pH to 7.0 and maintaining it there, neutralization is beyond the capacity of most antacids *in vivo*. *Neutralization* is a useful clinical term only when it is taken to mean a decrease in gastric acidity. To neutralize half the acid in a given amount of gastric juice at pH 1.3, the pH only has to be raised to 1.6. Raising the pH further to 2.3 will eliminate 90 percent of the acid, and at 3, all but 1 percent of the acid will be removed. Endpoints of pH 4.4 or pH 7 mean that 99.9 or 99.999 of the hydrogen ion in 0.1 normal hydrochloric acid would have been neutralized; partial neutralization obviously is of major importance.

Piper and Fenton (1964) noted that the amount of antacid required for effective neutralization is determined at least by the variables of gastric secretion, gastric emptying, and the neutralizing capacity of the antacid. For complete neutralization, they concluded that an antacid given every hour had to have neutralizing capability eight times the basal secretion. When the secretion rate was unknown, they suggested that doses of 50 mEq/hr for men with duodenal ulcer and 26 mEq/hr for women were effective in 90 percent of patients. Piper and Fenton found that the amount of aluminum hydroxide in commercial antacids needed to neutralize 50 mEq of hydrochloric acid was 750 ml!

Fordtran and his colleagues (1966, 1973) studied gastric acidity with different stimulants. After a regular meal, gastric acidity remained at relatively low levels for 90 minutes, even though acid was presumed to be secreted at a near maximal rate during this period. Thereafter, acidity rose rapidly to an average maximum of 65 mEq/L. Taking 156 mEq of antacids one hour after a meal led to a striking lowering of gastric acidity to near zero for two hours after ingestion of the antacid, rising to about 3 mEq/L by the end of three hours. The pH of the gastric contents 30 minutes after taking the antacid was about 5.8, as compared with 2.2 half an hour after drinking water.

Fordtran et al. compared the effect of varying amounts of antacids on hypersecreters, whose peak response to histamine was greater than 25 mEq/hr, with that of hyposecreters. The absolute reduction of acidity after 15 ml (39 mEq) of antacid was about the same for both groups (13 mEq/L), but the fractional reduction was obviously much greater in patients whose acid levels were lower to begin with. Fordtran's group recommended giving antacids one and five hours after meals for maximal acid reduction. Studying the neutralizing capability of various antacids, however, they found that the neutralizing capability of 1 ml of the most potent compound (Ducon) was 70.4 mEq, whereas that of the weakest (Phosphaljel) was only 4.2 mEq. To reduce the acidity fivefold for two hours in a patient with a duodenal ulcer, 156 mEq of antacid was necessary in most patients. To give this amount of antacid would require 22 to 371 ml of the commercially available antacids!

Morrissey and Barreras (1974) appropriately feared that such large doses of antacids might be dangerous because of their magnesium content and the inevitable diarrhea (with fluid and electrolyte loss) that may occur. They recommended smaller doses of antacids on an hourly basis during the acute phase of the disease. The question that must be examined, however, is whether there is any benefit from such precise determination of gastric acid and from its subsequent neutralization. In this lie most of the problems to be discussed.

Antacids and Pain Relief in Peptic Ulcer

It has been generally accepted that antacids are effective in the relief of pain associated with duodenal ulcer, but the effect of placebo therein has not been thoroughly evaluated or appreciated.

In looking at studies of pain relief, it is well to keep in mind that "pain relief" is used to mean many different things, including (1) how quickly individual doses of antacids relieve a single spontaneous or induced attack of pain, (2) how many days of therapy it takes for a patient to have complete relief of pain, (3) how many pain-free days the patient may have in a week, (4) how often the patient is free of nocturnal pain, and, most often, (5) how many patients are pain free at specified intervals after the start of therapy. Patients have been asked to grade their pain and relief thereof on various scales such as from 1–6+ or even as a line on a 10 cm scale. It should be clear that these results represent separate effects.

The studies of Lawrence (1952) and Doll and associates (1956), which have been quoted as showing antacids to relieve pain more effectively than placebos, have serious limitations. For example, Lawrence compared three antacids—aluminum hydroxide, magnesium carbonate, and magnesium trisilicate—using barium sulfate as a placebo, in patients with peptic ulcers. Although one can question whether barium sulfate, which may be recognized by the patient with peptic ulcer, is a valid placebo, only magnesium carbonate and magnesium trisilicate were significantly superior to it in these tests. Thirteen percent of the patients had complete abolition of pain with barium sulfate, 42 percent had partial relief, but 45 percent had no pain relief at all. Fifty-three percent of patients had complete relief with magnesium trisilicate, 34 percent had partial relief, and 13 percent experienced no effect at all. Aluminum hydroxide relieved the pain completely in 30 percent of patients, partially in 20 percent, and was ineffective in 15 percent.

Doll's study, which has been interpreted by Piper (1967) as showing an effect of antacids on pain relief, does not actually lead to that conclusion. Doll's report was entitled "Continuous intragastric milk drip in treatment of uncomplicated gastric ulcer." Patients in one group were kept in bed and given a standard medical regimen; patients in the other group received the same treatment along with a milk drip. The patients receiving milk were subdivided into two groups, one being given an additional 40 mEq of soda bicarbonate in milk. Of the patients on the milk treatment, 50 percent were completely free of pain, as compared with 35 percent in the control group. Within the milk treatment group, however, 49 percent of those who received antacids and 53 percent of those that received no additonal antacids were pain free. Nowhere in this paper do Doll and his associates claim that antacids are more effective than milk alone in relieving pain, as had been suggested.

Several other investigators have taken a look at the effect of antacids in pain relief, and the results rarely have been impressive. Hollander and Harlan (1973) gave 16 outpatients with gastric ulcers and 50 patients with duodenal ulcers either placebo or 420 mg of calcium carbonate tablets every hour. At the end of four weeks, all eight patients with gastric ulcers taking antacids were pain free, but only half the patients receiving placebo were pain free. However, 24 of 31 (83 percent) duodenal ulcer patients treated with antacids obtained relief, a difference not statistically different from the 17 of 26 (65 percent) who were pain free on placebo. Butler and Gersh (1975) evaluated the efficacy of antacids on healing and later on pain relief in hospitalized patients with gastric ulcers, and they found that within 72 hours, all patients, whether receiving placebo or antacids, were free of pain.

In a group of 10 patients with duodenal ulcers in a hospital, Sturdevant et al. (1977) compared the pain relief from 15 ml of antacid capable of buffering 30 mEq of HCl with the relief from a similar-appearing placebo. The patients received medication every 30 minutes until they were free of pain. There was no difference in pain relief in the two groups. Even comparing the effect of a larger dose of highly potent antacid with a placebo on a single pain episode, Sturdevant and his colleagues could not find any difference in pain relief in 20 patients, much to their surprise. They had to conclude that factors other than gastric acid neutralization are important in relief of ulcer pain.

Littman et al. (1977) also studied the effect of antacids and placebo on spontaneous and induced pain in patients with duodenal ulcers. The antacid was aluminum hydroxide, 5 ml of which would neutralize 140 mEq of 0.1 normal HCl; the placebo was aluminum hydroxide gel without neutralizing capacity. An important dividend from this study was the demonstration that patients at different hospitals showed great differences in results. At one institution, 8 patients studied 44 times for relief of spontaneous pain obtained relief 79 percent of the time with antacid but only 45 percent of the time with placebo. Elsewhere, however, patients obtained relief in only 17 percent of cases with antacid gel and in 25 percent of cases with placebo. In separate trials in the same study, which were intended to evaluate the efficacy of antacids upon pain induced by instillation of acid, there was no difference between antacid and placebo—63 percent of patients obtained relief with antacids and 62 percent with placebos. Overall, when all tests were evaluated, 53 percent of patients had relief with either compound, and the authors had to conclude that their extensive efforts could not prove that antacids relieved duodenal ulcer symptoms better than placebos did.

Similar results were evident in the sophisticated diagnostic studies of Peterson et al. (1977), who gave 74 patients with endoscopically proven duodenal ulcers either 30 ml of antacid (with neutralizing capacity of 144 mEq HCl) or an identical inactive placebo seven times a day. At the end of four weeks, 69 percent of patients in the antacid group and 63 percent in the placebo group were pain free.

Physicians have known for a long time that the correlation between the presence of an ulcer crater and ulcer pain is poor. Although it has been well documented by barium studies, this poor relationship between ulcer and pain has been proved once again by several endoscopic studies of which the one by Peterson et al. is the most recent. In that study, an ulcer was still present in 16 of 49 (33 percent) patients who were free of pain at four weeks, whereas the ulcer had healed in 12 of 25 (48 percent) patients who were still complaining of pain.

However much they may wish, clinicians and investigators have so far not been able to prove convincingly the superiority of antacids over placebos for pain relief. The notion of Baume and Hunt (1969) that "it is likely that any white medicine sold as an antacid will give relief from ulcer pain" is still valid.

Placebo and Pain Relief

Obviously, attempts at observation may affect results, but studies of other modes of therapy support the notion of a strong placebo effect on pain relief in peptic ulcer. It is interesting in this regard to look at studies of other therapeutic agents to see how often striking results have been obtained by placebo therapy. For example, in 1936, Flood and Mullins treated with saline injections 12 outpatients with duodenal ulcers, 10 of whom had a "stubborn recurrence." During a 30-day period in which they followed a regular diet, 67 percent of the patients obtained complete relief of pain, in most cases after three or four injections of saline. The investigators felt that the relief of peptic ulcer pain in such circumstances emphasized the importance of the placebo effect. In 1947, Gill studied the lack of relationship between the presence of a gastric ulcer and the pain associated with it, and even more important, he raised questions about the factors that cause an ulcer to heal. All but one of 20 patients (95 percent) with symptomatic gastric ulcers whom he treated with daily hypodermic injections of 1 ml of distilled water, an unrestricted diet, and no other therapy became "pain-free within a few days and the ulcers healed in the usual time." He felt, therefore, that the "essential factor is the patient's belief that his treatment is going to be successful," and that "he must find himself in a sympathetic environment and be protected from protracted anxieties."

The response rate in placebo-treated groups has been no less impressive when agents other than antacids have been studied in peptic ulcer patients (Table 10–1). For example, anticholinergic agents have shown a range of 48 to 80 percent for pain relief; patients treated with placebo in the same studies have obtained pain relief in 30 to 80 percent of cases. In carbenoxolone studies, the range of pain relief in placebo-treated patients has been 0 to 54 percent, and in a study of patients treated with colloidal bismuth, it was 60 percent. In these studies,

Table 10–1. *Pain Relief Effect of Placebo and Therapeutic Agent*

Author	Country	Year	Percentage of Patients Free of Pain from Placebo	Therapeutic Agent	Percentage of Patients Free of Pain from Therapeutic Agent
DUODENAL ULCER					
Lawrence	UK	1952	13	Antacid	30–53
Hollander and Harlan	USA	1973	65	Antacid	83
Peterson et al.	USA	1977	63	Antacid	69
Littman et al.	USA	1977	42	Antacid	79
Littman et al.	USA	1977	25	Antacid	17
Littman et al.	USA	1977	63	Antacid	62
Sturdevant et al.	USA	1977	°	Antacid	°
Montgomery et al.	UK	1968	36	Carbenoxolone	26
Amure	Nigeria	1970	0	Carbenoxolone	57
Brown et al.	UK	1972	54	Carbenoxolone	81
Feldman and Gilat	Israel	1971	46	Deglycyrrhizinated Liquorice	52
Melrose and Pinkerton	UK	1961	30	Anticholinergics	48
Trevino et al.	USA	1967	55	Anticholinergics	53
Kaye et al.	UK	1970	80	Anticholinergics	80
Salmon et al.	UK	1974	60	Colloidal Bismuth	90
Pounder et al.	UK	1975	52	Metiamide	76
Binder et al.	USA	1978	3 days 39 4 weeks 59	Cimetidine	63 71
Flood and Mullins	USA	1936	67	Saline injection	
GASTRIC ULCER					
Doll et al.	UK	1956	53	Antacid	49
Hollander and Harlan	USA	1973	50	Antacid	100
Butler and Gersh	USA	1975	100	Antacid	100
Gill	UK	1947	95	Water injection	
Bader et al.	France	1977	2 weeks 39 4 weeks 57	Cimetidine	67 75
Dyck et al.	USA	1978	°	Cimetidine	°
Englert et al.	USA	1978	°	Cimetidine	°

° No difference found but percentages not calculated.

the results for the therapeutic agent, although by themselves often impressive, often have been statistically insignificant because of the favorable response rate in the placebo-treated groups.

Similar difficulties are evident in studies with the newer H_2 antagonists metiamide and cimetidine. In the first study published on pain relief in duodenal ulcers with these agents, Pounder et al. (1975) found 76 percent response rate with the drug and 52 percent with the placebo. On the other hand, Binder et al. (1978), in the cooperative study on duodenal ulcer patients, found significant differences between cimetidine- and placebo-treated groups only at three days, when 63 percent of patients receiving cimetidine and 39 percent of patients receiving placebo experienced relief. At any other point in the study, the differences were not statistically significant. For instance, at four weeks, 71 percent of patients on cimetidine and 59 percent on placebo were pain free. Bader et al. in France (1977) found that 67 percent of patients with gastric ulcers obtained pain relief on cimetidine by day 14, but only 37 percent of the placebo treated group had relief. On day 28, however, 75 percent had obtained relief from cimetidine along with 57 percent of patients treated with placebo. Neither Dyck et al. (1978) nor Englert et al. (1978) could find any statistical differences in pain relief among patients with gastric ulcers receiving either cimetidine or placebo in a double blind fashion.

Healing Rate of Gastric Ulcer

Doll et al. (1952) studied the effects of inpatient and outpatient therapy. They compared results of patients treated with diet, antacids, and bedrest in the hospital with results of a similar group treated with the same antacids and diet but who remained outpatients. After one month, 5 of 32 (16 percent) patients in the hospital group had complete radiographic healing of the ulcer, contrasted with 3 of 32 (9 percent) in the ambulatory group. The apparent benefit of bedrest was even greater when patients in whom two thirds of the ulcer had healed were included in the healed group. Then, 18 of 32 (56 percent) of the patients treated in hospital were improved, but only 7 of 32 (22 percent) of the outpatients benefited. Three months after the start of therapy, 12 (38 percent) of the hospital group had healed their ulcers, in contrast to only 5 (16 percent) of the ambulatory group; when those with two-thirds healing were included, the figures rose to 22 of 32 patients (69 percent) for the hospital group and 13 of 32 (41 percent) for the outpatient group. These studies generally have been accepted as showing that a most important factor in the healing of gastric ulcer is bedrest in hospital but they are remarkable for the low healing rate in the ambulatory group. In 1956, Doll and his colleagues found no differences in ulcer healing in patients being treated with milk with or without antacids or diet alone when they evaluated hospital patients with gastric ulcers and the effect of continuous milk drip; 70 percent of ulcers healed in either group.

Generally, most studies fail to show any statistically significant benefit of antacids over placebos in the healing of gastric ulcers, with the exception of one by Hollander and Harlan (1973) (Table 10–2). In 1969, Baume and Hunt compared the effect of calcium carbonate tablets with that of inactive aluminum hydroxide in outpatients 21 days after therapy, using x-ray as the criterion. The antacid potency of calcium carbonate taken every hour during the day was 50 mEq. The control group received inactive aluminum hydroxide tablets five times a day. Of the 13 patients treated with calcium carbonate, 4 (31 percent) had complete healing at the end of three weeks; 6 of the 15 patients (40 percent) receiving placebos had complete healing at that time. The mean reduction in ulcer size for the patients receiving calcium carbonate was 29 percent; that for the placebo group was 56 percent. Baume and Hunt suggested that elevation of gastric juice pH, even by potent antacids, was unlikely to lead to improvement in ulcer healing rates of outpatients. In 1975, Butler and Gersh had similar results in hospitalized patients with gastric ulcers; 73 percent of patients receiving a commercial liquid antacid and 77 percent of patients receiving a similar placebo every two hours while awake showed healing of gastric ulcer at the end of three weeks. Littman et al. (1977), studying 18 patients with gastric ulcers presumably as outpatients, could not show any significant benefit of antacid over placebo; at the end of four weeks, five of nine patients (56 percent) in the antacid-treated group and four of nine (44 percent) patients in the placebo-treated group had healed their ulcers.

As already noted, only the outpatient study of Hollander and Harlan has suggested any benefit of antacids. They gave 16 outpatients

Table 10–2. *Healing Rate of Gastric Ulcer: Effect of Placebo and Therapeutic Agents*

Author	Country	Year	Percentage of Healed Ulcers from Placebo	Therapeutic Agent	Percentage of Healed Ulcers from Therapeutic Agent
Doll	UK	1956	70°	Antacid	70°
Baume and Hunt	Australia	1969	40 (56°)	Antacid	31 (29°)
Hollander and Harlan	USA	1973	50	Antacid	100
Butler and Gersh	USA	1975	77	Antacid	73
Littman et al.	USA	1977	44	Antacid	56
Doll et al.	UK	1965	39°	Carbenoxolone	78°
Turpie and Thomson	UK	1965	17	Carbenoxolone	33
Horwich and Galloway	UK	1965	24	Carbenoxolone	81
Bank et al.	S. Africa	1967	54	Carbenoxolone	64
Turpie and Thomson	UK	1965	34°	Carbenoxolone	78°
Cocking and MacCaig	UK	1969	64	Carbenoxolone	93
Hampel et al.	W. Germany	1973	29	Carbenoxolone	83
Doll et al.	UK	1962	5	Liquorice Compound	37
Turpie et al.	UK	1969	6 (34°)	Deglycyrrhizinated Liquorice	44 (78°)
Bader et al.	France	1977	37	Cimetidine	69
Ciclitera et al.	UK	1977	50	Cimetidine	80
Dyck et al.	USA	1978	41	Cimetidine	61
Scheurer et al.	Switzerland	1977	83	None	—

° Percentage of ulcer size healed.

with gastric ulcers either two tablets of 420 mg of calcium carbonate each hour or an identical-appearing placebo. All eight patients receiving calcium carbonate, but only four of the eight patients receiving placebo, showed complete x-ray healing of the ulcer at the end of 30 days.

The variation in the rate of gastric healing with placebo therapy is an important factor in evaluating all these studies and thus will be considered separately.

Healing Rate of Duodenal Ulcer

For duodenal ulcer there is discrepancy between the endoscopic and radiologic evaluation of healing. In one series (Salmon et al., 1972), 17 percent of patients who were x-ray negative still showed duodenal ulceration at endoscopy. The literature on antacids and duodenal ulcers to date (Table 10–3 and 10–4) contains only three double blind studies evaluating the effect of antacids, and only one of these was an endoscopic study. Peterson's group (1977) gave 36 patients 30 ml of antacid 7 times a day for a total neutralizing capability of 1008 mEq. A control group of 38 patients received an identical-looking placebo without neutralizing capacity. Evaluation at the end of four weeks by endoscopy showed that 28 (78 percent) of the antacid-treated group had healed ulcers, in contast to 17 (45 percent) of the placebo-treated group. Despite intensive antacid therapy, 22 percent of patients had ulcers still unhealed after four weeks. The authors concluded that their large dose antacid regimen hastened the healing of duodenal ulcer, and they suggested that Hollander and Harlan's earlier study (1973) had shown no benefit from antacids because they had used insufficient amounts (only 2 tablets per hour with a neutralizing capability of 8.2 mEq, to a total of 131 mEq daily, as contrasted with their 1008 mEq daily).

Peterson et al. further suggested that the acid rebound of calcium carbonate might have led to therapeutic failure. To assess ulcer healing, the study used endoscopy, which presumably is more accurate than the radiographic methods of the Hollander and Harlan study. Yet, in the latter study, 50 ambulatory patients received

Table 10-3. *Healing Rate of Duodenal Ulcer: Radiographic Studies*

Author	Country	Year	Percentage of Healed Ulcers from Placebo	Therapeutic Agent	Percentage of Healed Ulcers from Therapeutic Agent
Villalobos et al.	Mexico	1970	63	Antacid	80
Hollander and Harlan	USA	1973	74	Antacid	89
Craig et al.	UK	1967	21	Carbenoxolone	87
Montgomery et al.	UK	1968	5	Carbenoxolone	26
Cliff and Milton-Thompson	UK	1970	29	Carbenoxolone	31
Amure	Nigeria	1970	0	Carbenoxolone	57
Hampel et al.	W. Germany	1972	50	Carbenoxolone	57
Hunt et al.	UK	1973	50	Carbenoxolone	91
Doll et al.	UK	1962	21	Liquorice Compound	81
Friedlander	UK	1954	21	Anticholinergics	20
Lennard-Jones	UK	1961	31	Anticholinergics	18
Amure	Nigeria	1965	0	Anticholinergics	71
Nitter et al.	Norway	1976	27	Trimipramine	100

Table 10-4. *Healing Rate of Duodenal Ulcer: Endoscopic Studies*

Author	Country	Year	Percentage of Healed Ulcers from Placebo	Agent	Percentage of Healed Ulcers from Therapeutic Agent
Peterson et al.	USA	1977	45	Antacid	78
Eshelman et al.	USA	1978	62	Antacid	Not given
Brown et al.	UK	1972	31	Carbenoxolone	81
Davies and Reed	UK	1977	22	Carbenoxolone	69
Sahel et al.	France	1977	20	Carbenoxolone	65
Nagy	Australia	1978	30	Carbenoxolone	87
Blackwood et al.	UK	1976	25	Cimetidine	66
Bodemar and Walan	Sweden	1976	36	Cimetidine	90
Gray et al.	Scotland	1977	25	Cimetidine	85
Celestin et al.	UK	1975	25	Metiamide	67
Bank et al.	S. Africa	1976	42	Cimetidine and Metiamide	82
Semb et al.	Norway	1977	60	Cimetidine	85
Gillespie et al.	UK	1977	28	Cimetidine	85
Bardhan et al.	UK	1977	29	Cimetidine	72
Northfield and Blackwood	UK	1977	19	Cimetidine	62
Hetzel et al.	Australia	1978	38	Cimetidine	84
Binder et al.	USA	1978	2 weeks 26	Cimetidine	46
Binder et al.	USA	1978	4 weeks 48	Cimetidine	57
Binder et al.	USA	1978	6 weeks 63	Cimetidine	80
Landecker et al.	Australia	1976	59	Depepsen	72
Wetterhus et al.	Norway	1976	46	Trimipramine	75
Scheurer et al.	Switzerland	1977	73	None	–

either calcium carbonate as already noted or an identical placebo every two hours, and 24 of the 27 patients (89 percent) receiving antacids healed the ulcer in 30 days. But the study did not reach statistical significance as 17 of 23 (74 percent) patients on placebo therapy also healed the ulcer, at least according to x-ray. The problem of the Hollander and Harlan study, then, was not lack of response to the active ingredient but *too good a response to the placebo.* Comparison of these two studies is important because of the obvious conclusions, but it raises the question as to whether a lower dose antacid therapy might not have led to the same benefit. To our knowledge, only one other study of the effect of antacids on the healing of duodenal ulcers has been carried out in a double blind fashion. Villalobos et al. (1970) gave two groups of 30 patients either skim milk with antacids or regular milk. The healing rate in the antacid group was 80 percent, but in the group treated with milk it was 63 percent, a difference not of statistical significance.

The point we wish to make is that Peterson's study is the most thorough one on antacids in duodenal ulcers thus far, but it reaches statistical significance to show that antacids are superior to placebos simply because the placebo healing rate was much lower than in other antacid studies, again emphasizing the large variation of the response of duodenal ulcers to therapy and the importance of considering placebo healing rates.

Healing Rate of Peptic Ulcer With a Placebo

We have earlier commented that criteria for pain relief vary tremendously. The observed endpoints for healing of peptic ulcers vary no less in all the published literature. No uniform time exists for assessment of healing; authors report on healing at two, three, four, five, six, and twelve weeks and even longer. When radiologic evidence only was used for assessment of healing, authors evaluated the number of ulcers healed at any one time or the percentage of ulcer size healed in the total number of patients. More recently, most authors rely on endoscopy for assessment of healing, especially in duodenal ulcers. One might have expected that endoscopy would lead to an unequivocal and uniform method of assessment, but that does not seem to be so. Ippoliti et al. (1978) give two figures, depending on degree of healing. In general, placebo healing rate in peptic ulcers seems be to lower in the United Kingdom than in other countries (for example, the U.S.) but very few clinical studies are available from most other countries.

Variations in placebo healing rates are pertinent in evaluating the effect of antacids or any other therapeutic agent on gastric and duodenal ulcer healing. Placebo healing rates in various studies on gastric ulcers (Table 10–2) range from Doll et al.'s 5 percent (1962) to Scheurer et al.'s 83 percent (1977), with other authors having noted a percentage healing rate in their placebo-treated patients as high as 50 (Hollander and Harlan, 1973; Ciclitera et al., 1977), 54 (Bank et al., 1967), 64 (Cocking and MacCaig, 1969), and 77 (Butler and Gersh, 1975), all of which compare favorably with the results of some therapeutic agents.

It is of interest also to note the therapeutic effects of several specific agents such as carbenoxolone, which in general seems to be considered effective for gastric ulcers. The range has been from 33 percent (Turpie and Thomson, 1965) to 93 percent (Cocking and MacCaig, 1969), with an average of approximately 61 percent. The range of placebo effect in that specific group has been from 5 percent (Doll et al., 1962) up to 64 percent (Cocking and MacCaig, 1969), with the average approximately 30 percent. Studies with cimetidine have shown therapeutic effects from 61 percent (Dyck et al., 1978) to 80 percent (Ciclitera et al., 1977), with an average of 70 percent; the range in the placebo-treated group was from 37 percent (Bader et al., 1977) to 50 percent (Ciclitera et al., 1977), with an average of 42 percent. In two of these (Dyck et al., 1978; Ciclitera et al., 1977), the differences were not statistically significant.

In looking at duodenal ulcer studies, one must remember that endoscopists have found duodenal bulb ulcers in 15 to 20 percent of patients in whom radiographic studies were normal (Salmon et al., 1972). One might therefore expect that placebo-treated groups studied by endoscopists would have lower proven healing rates than those studied by radiography alone. It could be speculated, for example, that the use of endoscopy would lead to an apparently lower healing rate in Peterson's group than in Hollander's, assuming that all other factors were equal, but this should affect both groups equally. On the other hand, in 13 controlled studies using radiography, the average healing rate was 30 percent, but in 21 more recent studies using endoscopy, the average healing rate was 37 percent by placebo (higher than might have been expected). Does the endoscope affect the results? That is, does the act of submitting to endoscopy favorably (or unfavorably) affect healing? The range of healing in the placebo-treated group radiographically studied has been from 0 to 74 percent (Table 10–3), compared with 22 to 73 percent in the endoscopically studied group (Table 10–4). Surprisingly, the healing rate in the study by Scheurer et al. is 73 percent with placebo only.

Of interest also is the range of effect of a specific therapeutic agent, such as carbenoxolone, with which healing rates in patients with duodenal ulcers have been reported from 18 to 91 percent. In some of the studies on carbenoxolone and related compounds, the results in both groups have been very similar (Cliff and Milton-Thompson, 1970; Hampel et al., 1972; Doll et al., 1962), but in others, the difference has been striking, leaving many to conclude that carbenoxolone is a very effective agent for treatment of duodenal ulcers.

The range with cimetidine has been smaller than that with carbenoxolone—57 to 90 percent (Table 10–4). The range in the placebo group in the cimetidine studies has been from 19 to 63 percent. Most studies with cimetidine show statistical significance, but not all. The study by Semb et al. (1977) showed an 85 percent response rate in the cimetidine-treated group and a 60 percent rate in the placebo-treated group, which is not a significant difference. In a large American multicenter study (Binder et al., 1978), the only significant difference was after two weeks in both inpatient and outpatient studies, but the difference at four and six weeks in the study was not statistically significant: at four weeks, 48 percent of the placebo-treated patients and 57 percent of the cimetidine-treated group had healed, and at six weeks, 63 percent of the placebo group and 81 percent of the cimetidine group had healed. On the other hand, Northfield and Blackwood (1977) found the differences to be significant at all times *except* at two weeks!

Comparing the overall results from these three main agents—antacids, cimetidine, and carbenoxolone—in duodenal ulcer treatment, one notes that the average result in the carbenoxolone group is 61 percent, with an average placebo response in that group of 25 percent. Results with cimetidine are better, with an average of 74 percent, but overall, the placebo effect is 40 percent. Compare this with the results from antacids, where active therapy leads to an average 82 percent healing rate and an overall placebo healing rate of 61 percent. Is antacid a more effective placebo? Should antiulcer drugs be judged by combined pharmacologic and placebo results? Such comparison may not be scientifically valid, but perhaps no less so than when authors emphasize with optimism the numerical differences in their studies, when statistical significance has not been achieved.

Of further interest (but perhaps confusing) is a look at studies in which specific agents are compared with each other. Englert et al. (1978) reported 59 percent healing at six weeks in cimetidine-treated patients, but 61 percent in antacid-treated patients with gastric ulcers. No difference was found between hospitalized patients and outpatients, but unfortunately, no placebo group was included. Ippoliti et al. (1978) compared cimetidine and antacids in duodenal ulcer patients but did not obtain a statistically significant difference; 62 percent healing in the cimetidine group and 52 percent in the antacid group. Hunt et al. (1977) compared cimetidine and carbenoxolone in gastric ulcer treatment. Cimetidine, which in two of three studies had not reached statistically significant differences (Dyck et al., 1978; Ciclitera et al., 1977), was associated with 80 percent healing in their patients, but the "effective" carbenoxolone with only 30 percent!

Conclusion

Overall response to therapy that aims at neutralizing or eliminating acid is generally better than that of placebo, but the 22 percent failure rate even in Peterson's study of high dose antacids, as well as the high healing rate from placebo in many studies, emphasizes that many factors besides the amount of acid in the stomach must play a role in this disorder and in its natural history. Clearly, further study is needed. It is noteworthy that in the study by Sturdevant et al. of pain relief in patients with duodenal ulcers, two out of twelve originally enrolled patients had to be dismissed from analysis; one became pain free after selection but before receiving the study drug, and the other became pain free after receiving only one dose of the study drug, which happened to be placebo! In Doll's study on the treatment of gastric ulcer with carbenoxolone and estrogens, 102 patients were referred for the study, but

56 were considered unsuitable, 20 of them because their crater had already healed.

It may be that the Heisenberg principle, which suggests that the observer always affects the results, will make such studies of ulcer healing impossible to complete, for as long as there is an observer, he will have an effect. Certainly nothing can be more intrusive into the clinical experimental setting than the physician and his endoscope, which is, after all, the common denominator of all recent studies. Morrissey has commented on therapy: "The choice and timing of these maneuvers is a complex art involving a variety of pharmacological, surgical, dietary, psychological, and social manipulations." In modern medicine, these last mentioned factors in the placebo effect of therapy have been neglected (Benson and Epstein, 1975) in favor of more suitably elegant pharmacologic means.

This review is not meant to suggest that antacids should not be used, but it is meant simply to reassure the clinician that no antacid is obviously and unmistakably the best antacid, at least thus far, and that the case for using large amounts of antacids in the treatment of ulcer disease is not as strong as concluded by the mathematically minded researchers. Neither intensive antacid programs nor other drugs studied thus far have proved to be strikingly better than placebos in the relief of pain or in the induction of healing, despite some exceptions. The variations noted thus far in the often impressive response to placebo therapy, which sometimes have made therapeutic results statistically insignificant, seem to suggest that perhaps what we need are more effective and harmless placebos!

Obviously, use of antacids should continue, as there is a place for *them* as symptom *relievers*, although it is evident that placebos are symptomatically as good as antacids for the average duodenal ulcer patient or for the patient with dyspepsia, without regard to their neutralizing capacity. Antacids may promote healing, but studies comparing high and low dose antacid therapies still seem indicated. It seems prudent to regard tolerance, palatability, cost, and the absence of significant side effects as attributes equally important as neutralizing capacity. The old advice, that the physician learn to use one antacid that makes the bowels move and one that constipates, and one that lies somewhere in between, still has its place.

References

Abercrombie, J.: Pathological and practical researches on the diseases of the stomach, the intestinal canal, the liver and other viscera of the body. Philadelphia, Lea and Blanchard, 1845.

Alfrey, A.C., LeGendre, G.R., and Kaehny, W.D.: The dialysis encephalopathy syndrome. Possible aluminum intoxication. N. Engl. J. Med. 294:184–188, 1976.

Ambre, J.J., and Fischer, L.J.: Effect of coadministration of aluminum and magnesium hydroxides on absorption of anticoagulants in man. Clin. Pharmacol. Ther. 14:231–237, 1973.

Amure, B.O.: Anticholinergic drugs in the management of duodenal ulcer. Practitioner 195:335–339, 1965.

Amure, B.O.: Clinical study of duogastrone in the treatment of duodenal ulcers. Gut 11:171–175, 1970.

Bader, J.P., et al.: Treatment of gastric ulcer by cimetidine. A multicentre trial. In Burland, W.L., and Simkins, M.A., eds., Cimetidine: proceedings of the second international symposium on histamine H_2-receptor antagonists, Amsterdam-Oxford, Excerpta Medica, 1977.

Bank, S., Barbezat, G.O., Novis, B.H., Ou Tim, L., Odes, H.S., Helman, C., Narunsky, L., Duys, P.J., and Marks, I.N.: Histamine H_2-receptor antagonists in the treatment of duodenal ulcers. S. Afr. Med J. 50:1781–1785, 1976.

Bank, S., Marks, I.N., Palmer, P.E.S., Groll, A., and van Eldik, E.: A trial of carbenoxolone sodium in the treatment of gastric ulceration. S. Afr. Med. J. 41:297–300, 1967.

Bardhan, K.D., et al.: The effect of cimetidine on duodenal ulceration. An interim report of a multicentre double-blind trial. In Burland, W.L., and Simkins, M.A., eds., Cimetidine: proceedings of the second international symposium on histamine H_2-receptor antagonists, Amsterdam-Oxford, Excerpta Medica, 1977.

Barreras, R.F.: Calcium and gastric secretion. Gastroenterology 64:1168–1184, 1973.

Baume, P.E., and Hunt J.H.: Failure of potent antacid therapy to hasten healing in chronic gastric ulcers. Australas. Ann. Med. 18:113–116, 1969.

Benson, H., and Epstein, M.D.: The placebo effect. A neglected asset in the care of patients. JAMA 232:1225–1227, 1975.

Binder, H.J., Cocco, A., Crossley, R.J., Finkelstein, W., Font, R., Friedman, G., Groarke, J., Hughes, W., Johnson, A.F., McGuigan, J.E., Summers, R., Vlahcevic, R., Wilson, E.C., and Winship, D.H.: Cimetidine in the treatment of duodenal ulcer. Gastroenterology 74:380–388, 1978.

Blackwood, W.S., Maudgal, D.P., Pickard, R.G., Lawrence, D., and Northfield, T.C.: Cimetidine in duodenal ulcer. Controlled trial. Lancet ii:174–176, 1976.

Blaug, S.M., and Gross, M.R.: In vitro adsorption of some anticholinergic drugs by various antacids. J. Pharm. Sci. 54:289–294, 1965.

Bodemar, G., and Walan, A.: Cimetidine in the treatment of active duodenal and prepyloric ulcers. Lancet ii:161–164, 1976.

Brown, D.D., and Juhl, R.P.: Decreased bioavailability of digoxin due to antacids and kaolin-pectin. N. Engl. J. Med. 295:1034–1037, 1976.

Brown, P., Salmon, P.R., Thien-Htut, and Read, A.E.: Double-blind trial of carbenoxolone sodium capsules in duodenal ulcer therapy, based on endoscopic diagnosis and follow-up. Br. Med. J. 3:661–664, 1972.

Butler, M.L., and Gersh, H.: Antacid vs placebo in hospitalized gastric ulcer patients: a controlled therapeutic study. Am. J. Dig. Dis. 20:803–807, 1975.

Celestin, L.R., et al.: A multicentre trial. Treatment of duodenal ulcer by metiamide. Lancet ii:779–781, 1975.

Ciclitera, P.J., Machell, R.J., Farthing, M.J., Dick, A.P., and Hunter, J.: A controlled trial of cimetidine in the treatment of gastric ulcer. In Burland, W.L., and Simkins, M.A., eds., Cimetidine: proceedings of the second international symposium on histamine H_2-receptor antagonists, Amsterdam-Oxford, Excerpta Medica, 1977.

Clemens, J.D., and Feinstein, A.R.: Calcium carbonate and constipation: a historical review of medical mythopoeia. Gastroenterology 72:957–961, 1977.

Cliff, J.M., and Milton-Thompson, G.J.: A double-blind trial of carbenoxolone sodium capsules in the treatment of duodenal ulcer. Gut 11:167–170, 1970.

Cocking, J.B., and MacCaig, J.N.: Effect of low dosage of carbenoxolone sodium on gastric ulcer healing and acid secretion. Gut 10:219–225, 1969.

Craig, O., Hunt, T., Kimerling, J.J., and Parke, D.V.: Carbenoxolone in the treatment of duodenal ulcer. Practitioner 199:109–111, 1967.

Crapper, D.R., Krishnan, S.S., and Quittkot, S.: Aluminum, neurofibrillary degeneration and Alzheimer's disease. Brain 99:67–80, 1976.

Davies, W.A., and Reed, P.I.: Controlled trial of duogastrone in duodenal ulcer. Gut 18:78–83, 1977.

Doll, R., Hill, I.D., and Hutton, C.F.: Treatment of gastric ulcer with carbenoxolone sodium and oestrogens. Gut 6:19–24, 1965.

Doll, R., Hill, I.D., Hutton, C., and Underwood, D.J.: Clinical trial of triterpenoid liquorice compound in gastric and duodenal ulcer. Lancet ii:793–796, 1962.

Doll, R., Price, A.V., Pygott, F., and Sanderson, P.H.: Continuous intragastric milk drip in treatment of uncomplicated gastric ulcer. Lancet i:70–73, 1956.

Doll, R., and Pygott, F.: Factors influencing the rate of healing of gastric ulcers. Admission to hospital, phenobarbitone, and ascorbic Acid. Lancet i:171–175, 1952.

Dyck, W.P., Belsito, A., Fleshler, B., Liebermann, T.R., Dickinson, P.B., and Wood, J.M.: Cimetidine and placebo in the treatment of benign gastric ulcer. Gastroenterology 74:410–415, 1978.

Englert, E., Freston, J.W., Graham, D.Y., Findelstein, W., Kruss, D.M., Priest, R.J., Raskin, J.B., Rhodes, J.B., Rogers, A.I., Wenger, J., Wilcox, L.L., and Crossley, R.J.: Cimetidine, antacid and hospitalization in the treatment of benign gastric ulcer. Gastroenterology 74:416–425, 1978.

Eshelman, F., Sanzari, N., and DeFelice, S.: "Placebo" responsiveness of peptic ulcers. Gastroenterology 74:159, 1978.

Feldman, H., and Gilat, T.: A trial of deglycyrrhizinated liquorice in the treatment of duodenal ulcer. Gut 12:449–451, 1971.

Flood, C.A., and Mullins, C.R.: Treatment of peptic ulcer by means of injections. Am. J. Dig. Dis. 3:303–305, 1936.

Fordtran, J.S.: Acid rebound. N. Engl. J. Med. 279:900–905, 1968.

Fordtran, J.S., and Collyns, J.A.H.: Antacid pharmacology in duodenal ulcer. Effect of antacids on postcibal gastric acidity and peptic activity. N. Engl. J. Med. 274:921–927, 1966.

Fordtran, J.S., Morawski, S.G., and Richardson, C.T.: In vivo and in vitro evaluation of liquid antacids. N. Engl. J. Med. 288:923–928, 1973.

Friedlander, P.H.: Ambulatory treatment of duodenal ulcers. Effects of fruit juice, olive oil, hexamethonium and methantheline. Lancet i:386–390, 1954.

Gill, A.M.: Pain and the healing of peptic ulcers. Lancet i:291, 1947.

Gillespie, G., Gray, G.R., Smith, I.S., Mackenzie, I., and Crean, G.P.: Short-term and maintenance cimetidine treatment in severe duodenal ulceration. In Burland, W.L., and Simkins, M.A., eds., Cimetidine: proceedings of the second international symposium on histamine H_2-receptor antagonists, Amsterdam-Oxford, Excerpta Medica, 1977.

Gray, G.R., Mackenzie, I., Smith, I.S., Crean, G.P., and Gillespie, G.: Oral cimetidine in severe duodenal ulceration. A double-blind controlled trial. Lancet i:4–7, 1977.

Hampel, K.E., Billich, C., Dannenmeier, H.D., Fintelmann, V., Fischer, R., Schmid, E., Treske, U., and Walz, A.: Therapie des ulcus ventriculi et duodeni mit carbenoxolon-natrium (Doppelblindversuch). Munch. Med. Wochenschr. 114:925–929, 1972.

Harvey, S.C.: Gastric antacids and digestants. In Goodman, L.S., and Gilman, A., *The Pharmacological Basis of Therapeutics*, New York, Macmillan Publishing Co., Inc., 1975.

Hetzel, D.J., Hansky, J., Sherman, D.J.C., Korman, M.G., Hecker, R., Taggert, G.J., Jackson, R., and Gabb, B.W.: Cimetidine treatment of duodenal ulceration. Short term clinical trial and maintenance study. Gastroenterology 74:389–392, 1978.

Hollander, D., and Harlan, J.: Antacids vs placebos in peptic ulcer therapy. A controlled double-blind investigation. JAMA 226:1181–1185, 1973.

Horwich, L., and Galloway, R.: Treatment of gastric ulceration with carbenoxolone sodium: clinical and radiological evaluation. Br. Med. J. 2:1274–1277, 1965.

Hunt, T., et al.: A multicentre trial. Carbenoxolone in the treatment of duodenal ulcer. Br. J. Clin. Pract. 27:50–55, 1973.

Hunt, R.H., Vincent, S.H., Milton-Thompson, G.J., Pounder, R.E., Taylor, R., Misiewicz, J.J., Golding, P.L., and Colin-Jones, D.G.: Short communication: cimetidine in the treatment of gastric ulcer. In Burland, W.L., and Simkins, M.A., eds., Cimetidine: proceedings of the second international symposium on histamine H_2-receptor antagonists, Amsterdam-Oxford, Excerpta Medica, 1977.

Hurwitz, A., Robinson, R.G., Vats, T.S., Whittier, F.C., and Herrin, W.F.: Effects of antacids on gastric emptying. Gastroenterology 71:268–273, 1976.

Ippoliti, A.F., Sturdevant, R.A.L., Isenberg, J.I., et al.: Cimetidine versus intensive antacid therapy for duodenal ulcer: a mulitcenter trial. Gastroenterology 74(suppl):393–395, 1978.

Isenberg, J.I., Best, W.P., Gillespie, G., Gillies, R.R., Ippoliti, A.F., McGuigan, J.E., Rubin, C.E., Shearman, D.J.C., and Winship, D.H.: Round table discussion on duodenal ulcer. Gastroenterology 74:407–409, 1978.

Kaehny, W.D., Hegg, A.P., and Alfrey, A.C.: Gastrointestinal absorption of aluminum from aluminum-containing antacids. N. Engl. J. Med. 296:1389–1390, 1977.

Kaye, M.D., Rhodes, J., Beck P., Sweetnam, P.M., Davies, G.T., and Evans, K.T.: a controlled trial of glycopyrronium and 1-hyoscyamine in the long-term treatment of duodenal ulcer. Gut 11:559–566, 1970.

Khalil, S.A.H.: The uptake of digoxin and digitoxin by some antacids. J. Pharm. Pharmacol. 26:961–967, 1974.

Kothari, M.L., and Kothari, J.M.: The illogic of peptic ulcer. Postgrad. Med. 23:1–9, 1977.
Kothari, M.L., and Kothari, J.M.: The logic of dyspeptic ulcer. Postgrad. Med. 23:53–63, 1977.
Landecker, K.D., McCallum, E.M., Fevre, D.I., Green, P.H.R., Kasumi, A., and Piper, D.W.: Effect of sodium amylosulfate (depepsen) on the healing of duodenal ulcer. Gastroenterology 71:723–725, 1976.
Lawrence J.S.: Dietetic and other methods in the treatment of peptic ulcer. Lancet i:482–485, 1952.
Lennard-Jones, J.E.: Experimental and clinical observations on poldine in treatment of duodenal ulcer. Br. Med. J. 1:1071–1076, 1961.
Levant, J.A., Walsh, J.H., and Isenberg, J.I.: Stimulation of gastric secretion and gastrin release by single oral doses of calcium carbonate in man. N. Engl. J. Med. 289:555–558, 1973.
Littman, A.: Reactive and nonreactive aluminum hydroxide gels. Dose-response relationships in vivo. Gastroenterology 52:948–951, 1967.
Littman, A., Welch, R., Fruin, R.C., and Aronson, A.R.: Controlled trials of aluminum hydroxide gels for peptic ulcer. Gastroenterology 73:6–10, 1977.
Lotz, M., Zisman, E., and Bartter, F.C.: Evidence for a phosphorus-depletion syndrome in man. N. Engl. J. Med. 278:409–415, 1968.
Melrose, A.G., and Pinkerton, I.W.: Clinical evaluation of poldine methosulphate. Br. Med. J. 1:1076–1078, 1961.
Montgomery, R.D., Lawrence, I.H., Manton, D.J. Mendl, K., and Rowe, P.: A controlled trial of carbenoxolone sodium capsules in the treatment of duodenal ulcer. Gut 9:704–706, 1968.
Morrissey, J.F., and Barreras, R.F.: Drug therapy. Antacid therapy. N. Engl. J. Med. 290:550–554, 1974.
Myhill, J., and Piper, W.: Antacid therapy of peptic ulcer. I, A mathematical definition of an adequate dose. Gut 5:581–585, 1964.
Nagy, G.S.: Evaluation of carbenoxolone sodium in the treatment of duodenal ulcer. Gastroenterology 74:7–10, 1978.
Nitter, L., Haraldsson, A., Holck, P., Hoy, Chr., Menthe-Kaas, J., Myrhol, K., and Paulsen, W.: The effect of trimipramine on the healing of peptic ulcer. A double-blind study. Multicentre investigation. Scand. J. Gastroenterol. 12:(Suppl) 43:39–41, 1977.
Northfield, T.C., and Blackwood, W.S.: Short communication: controlled clinical trial of cimetidine for duodenal ulcer. In Burland, W.L., and Simkins, M.A., eds., Cimetidine: proceedings of the second international symposium on histamine H_2-receptor antagonists, Amsterdam-Oxford, Excerpta Medica, 1977.
Peterson, W.L., Sturdevant, R.A.L., Frankl, H.D., Richardson, C.T., Isenberg, J.I., Elashoff, J.D., Sones, J.Q., Gross, R.A., McCallum, R.W., and Fordtran, J.S.: Healing of duodenal ulcer with an antacid regimen. N. Engl. J. Med. 297:341–345, 1977.
Piper, D.W.: Antacid and anticholinergic drug therapy of peptic ulcer. Gastroenterology 52:1009–1018, 1967.
Piper, D.W., and Fenton, B.H.: Antacid therapy of peptic ulcer. II, An evaluation of antacids in vitro. Gut 5:585–589, 1964.
Pounder, R.E., Williams, J.G., Milton-Thompson, G.J., and Misiewicz, J.J.: Relief of duodenal ulcer symptoms by oral metiamide. Br. Med. J. 2:307–309, 1975.
Sahel, J., et al.: An endoscopic controlled trial. Carbenoxolone sodium capsules in the treatment of duodenal ulcer. Gut 18: 717–720, 1977.
Salmon, P.R., Brown, P., Htut, T., and Read, A.E.: Endoscopic examination of the duodenal bulb: clinical evaluation of forward- and side-viewing fibreoptic systems in 200 cases. Gut 13:170–175, 1972.
Salmon, P.R., Brown, P., Williams, R., and Read A.E.: Evaluation of colloidal bismuth (De-Nol) in the treatment of duodenal ulcer employing endoscopic selection and follow up. Gut 15:189–193, 1974.
Scheurer, U., Witzel, L., Halter, F., Hans-Martin, K., Huber, R., and Galeazzi, R.: Gastric and duodenal ulcer healing under placebo treatment. Gastroenterology 72:838–841, 1977.
Segre, E.J., Sevelius, H., and Varady, J.: Effects of antacids on naproxen absorption. N. Engl. J. Med. 291:582–583, 1974.
Semb, L.S., Berstad, A., Myren, J., Foss, J. Chr., Carlsen, E., and Kruse-Jensen, A.: A double-blind multicentre comparative study of cimetidine and placebo in short-term treatment of active duodenal ulceration. In Burland, W.L., and Simkins, M.A., eds., Cimetidine: proceedings of the second international symposium on histamine H_2-receptor antagonists, Amsterdam-Oxford, Excerpta Medica, 1977.
Sturdevant, R.A.L., Isenberg, J.I., Secreist, D., and Ansfield, J.: Antacid and placebo produced similar pain relief in duodenal ulcer patients. Gastroenterology 72:1–5, 1977.

Trevino, H., Anderson, J., Davey, P.H., and Henley, K.S.: The effect of glycopyrrolate on the course of symptomatic duodenal ulcer. Am. J. Dig. Dis. 12:983–987, 1967.

Turpie, A.G.G., Runcie, J., and Thomson, T.J.: Clinical trial of deglycyrrhizinized liquorice in gastric ulcer. Gut 10:299–302, 1969.

Turpie, A.G.G., and Thomson, T.J.: Carbenoxolone sodium in the treatment of gastric ulcer with special reference to side-effects. Gut 5:591–594, 1965.

Villalobos, J.J., Kershenobich, D., and Ramirez Mata, M.: Antiacido adicionado a leche semidescremade en el tratamiento de la ulcera duodenal. Rev. Invest. Clin. 22:183–190, 1970.

Waisbren, B.A., and Hueckel, J.S.: Reduced absorption of aureomycin caused by aluminum hydroxide gel (Amphojel). Proc. Soc. Exp. Biol. Med. 73:73–74, 1950.

Wetterhus, S., Aubert, E., Berg, C.E., Bjerkeset, T., Halvorsen, L., Hovdenak, N., Myren, J., Roland, M., Sigstad, H., and Guldahl, M.: The effect of trimipramine (Surmontil) on symptoms and healing of peptic ulcer. A double-blind study. Scand. J. Gastroenterol. 12(Suppl) 43:33–38, 1977.

Wormsley, K.G.: The pathophysiology of duodenal ulceration. Gut 15:59–81, 1974.

11

Should Foods Be Fortified with Iron?

William H. Crosby, M.D.

American lads and lasses are all pale. . . . All this comes from those damnable hot-air pipes with which every tenement in America is infested.

Anthony Trollope, *North America*

She was dreadfully anaemic and suffered from the dyspepsia which accompanies that ailing.

W. Somerset Maugham, *Of Human Bondage*

She never told her love,
But let concealment, like a worm i' the bud
Feed on her damask cheek: She pined in thought,
And with a green and yellow melancholy
She sat like patience on a monument,
Smiling at grief.

Shakespeare, *Twelfth Night*

Introduction

The controversy about the addition of iron to food is well presented by Dr. Crosby. Proponents of routinely adding iron to flour argue that iron deficiency is a serious nutritional problem in the United States, and that it can be effectively and safely prevented by fortifying flour with iron.

Crosby rebuts by pointing out that iron deficiency usually results from blood loss, not malnutrition; that it makes little sense to fortify everyone's diet to remedy anemia that may afflict 1 percent of the population; that the proposed method for providing extra iron to the population is of dubious efficacy; and that excess iron is hardly nontoxic.

Legal moves to fortify flour with iron began in 1970 with the Bakers' and Millers' petition. A preliminary decision by the FDA Commissioner in 1973 to mandate such fortification was withdrawn in 1974 and laid to final rest in the Federal Register as of Nov. 27, 1978, by another FDA Commissioner.

This story is made even more fantastic by the fact that the fortification policy was backed by the AMA Council on Foods, the American Society for Clinical Nutrition, the American Dietetic Association, and the Food and Nutrition Board of the National Research Council! In 1978, former FDA Commissioner A.M. Schmidt publicly applauded his successor Donald Kennedy for reversing the order Schmidt had signed.

It is of interest that a recent editorial in the British Medical Journal (1978)* argues that the time honored habit of prescribing iron supplements for all pregnant women has little merit.

LOUIS LASAGNA, M.D.

*Editorial: Do all pregnant women need iron? Br. Med. J. 2:1317, 1978.

Should Foods Be Fortified with Iron?

William H. Crosby, M.D.
Scripps Clinic and Research Foundation, La Jolla, California

Iron is different from other foods. Excess iron in the body cannot be metabolized like vitamins or excreted like other nutrient metals. In the body, excess iron is toxic and can cause lethal disease. Further, a natural impediment to absorption of iron causes wide variation in the ability to absorb iron. Blood loss is the factor that causes the greatest variation of this absorptive ability. Iron deficiency rarely results from malnutrition; blood loss is actually the most common cause.

In this tangled paragraph, I have presented the complexity of a problem for which a simple, unwise solution has been proposed: that iron deficiency in the U.S. population be repaired by requiring that a large amount of iron be added to all bread and flour. Proponents of this flour fortification proposal (FFP) maintain:

1. That iron deficiency is a serious nutritional problem in the U.S.
2. That the fortification of flour can prevent iron deficiency.
3. That fortification of flour is without danger.

Members of the nutritionist-industrial complex who originated the FFP believe these truths to be self-evident (AMA Council on Foods and Nutrition, 1972). When challenged, they were unable to provide any substantial evidence to support their contentions. Committees and workshops generated "informed opinions," but no scientific data (Goldsmith, 1971; Enloe, 1972; Waddell et al., 1972a). In this vacuum, the proposal has finally expired (Kennedy, 1977). Iron deficiency and iron overload are the Scylla and Charybdis of the FFP. Efficacy of the program requires that it prevent iron-deficiency anemia in the target population. Safety of the program requires that it be harmless. First of all, however, it is necessary to demonstrate a need for FFP. Is nutritional iron deficiency so serious a problem in the U.S. as to require a major modification of the national diet?

Iron Metabolism

Iron is an essential constituent of every living cell. It is present in enzymes of intermediary metabolism and is the oxygen-binding locus of cellular pigments that hold and transport oxygen. Most of the body's iron is invested in hemoglobin. Thus, much iron is lost when blood is shed; 1 ml of red cells contains 1 mg of iron. By contrast, 1 kg of intestinal epithelial cells contains 1 mg of iron. The shedding of epithelial cells from the skin, the gut, the bladder, and the lungs removes about 1 mg of iron per day from the body, an "obligatory" metabolic loss. This loss must be offset by absorption of dietary iron. Loss of blood may impose a further requirement for replacement. Normal menstruation, for example, increases average requirements by about 1 mg per day. Greater blood loss can cause iron deficiency.

As much as 1 g of storage iron is normally present in the body. Physiologically uncommitted iron is invested in the storage protein, ferritin, from which it can be withdrawn when requirement for iron exceeds absorption. Partial depletion of normal storage iron may be called the mildest state of iron deficiency.

The balance of iron between the body and its environment is controlled by a unique mechanism. Because there is no normal excretion of excess iron, the balance is maintained by controlling absorption of dietary iron. When the body loses 1 mg of iron, the intestine permits 1 mg to be absorbed; a loss of 3 mg is offset by absorption of 3 mg. Incompetence of this control permits unneeded iron to enter the body. The excess, which cannot be excreted, is placed in storage. Accumulating iron insidiously damages the organs in which it is deposited, resulting in cirrhosis of the liver, diabetes, heart disease, arthritis, impotence, and sterility. This disease (or group or diseases) is called *hemochromatosis*.

Iron deficiency and iron storage disease are the medical problems that must be taken into account in attempting to resolve the risk-benefit ratio of the FFP.

Fortified Flour in the U.S.

Mandated iron fortification in the U.S. began during World War II, when the War Food Administration required that all bakers' bread be fortified with niacin, riboflavin, thiamine, calcium, and iron (Wilder, 1956). The stipulated level of iron was 13 to 16.5 mg per pound of flour and 8 to 12.5 mg per pound of bread. These quantities were intended to approximate the amount of iron removed during milling. The enrichment program played an important role in the disappearance of beriberi and pellagra, but the effect on iron deficiency remains uncertain. First, we have no information on the incidence of iron deficiency prior to or after beginning the program. Second, the sort of iron added to the flour was biologically inert. Absorbable forms of iron such as ferrous sulfate cause flour to become rancid; reduced iron, a black powder, discolors white flour. Although the regulations stipulate that the added iron must be "harmless and assimilable," the Food and Drug Administration (FDA) permitted the use of iron pyrophosphate and iron orthophosphate on the grounds that although only a small fraction could be absorbed, it satisfied the FDA's requirement (nutritionally worthless but legally assimilable). This was a commercially helpful oversight because these iron phosphate compounds do not react with flour and they are white.

The Flour Fortification Proposal of the 1970s went far beyond the intent of the 1940 mandate to restore the nutritive value of milled flour. On April 1, 1970, the American Bakers Association and the Millers' National Federation petitioned the FDA to require the addition of about 50 mg of iron per pound of flour, thereby increasing the dose to about 400 percent of the presently required 13 mg (Duggan, 1970):

1. The petitioners propose that iron (Fe) be required at a level of not less than 50 milligrams and not more than 60 milligrams per pound of enriched flour and enriched self-rising flour, and

2. They propose that iron (Fe) be required at a level of not less than 32 milligrams and not more than 38 milligrams per pound of enriched bread and enriched rolls.

Grounds given in support of the proposed amendments are that: (1) Iron is presently a required nutrient in the above-identified foods and may be added only in forms that are harmless and assimilable; (2) substantial agreement has been reached among nutritional and medical authorities regarding the need for the addition of larger amounts of iron to the American dietary; (3) circumstances required for the endorsement of the addition of nutrients to foods by the joint statement of the Council on Foods and Nutrition of the American Medical Association and the Food and Nutrition Board of the National Academy of Sciences—National Research Council are all met with respect to the increased level of iron proposed to be added to flour and bakery products by the petitioners; (4) further enrichment of flour and bread would provide a convenient and practical way to increase iron intake of the American population; and (5) "the proposed increased levels of iron would be adequate to furnish the levels of iron now recommended for all segments of the American population without creating any safety hazard" for those segments of the population whose iron requirements are met by the present levels of fortificiation.

This proposal provoked the FFP controversy. It was modified by the FDA on December 3, 1971, and it was promulgated in a tentative order on October 15, 1973, in a long document that contained a defense of FFP (Schmidt, 1973) and was notable for its incompetence (Crosby, 1975). On February 11, 1974, the Commissioner stayed the regulation and ordered a public hearing to be held in April. The hearing examiner voted in favor of the order, but the Commissioner, who considered the evidence to be more important than the judge's opinion, finally concluded that the FFP should not be approved (Kennedy, 1977). "In this case, the Commissioner had the luxury of not making a decision—that is, the weight of evidence didn't support the regulation, and so he withdrew it" (Schmidt, 1978).

Basic Problems of the FFP

During the seven years of contention, extending from publication of the Bakers' and Millers' petition in 1971 until the Commissioner's withdrawal of the FFP in 1978, four problems of fundamental importance were defined: iron in the American diet, iron deficiency in the American population, efficacy of the FFP, and safety of the FFP.

Iron in American Food

In its deliberations regarding iron, the Food and Nutrition Board of the National Research Council (NRC) traditionally has been more intent upon the food than the folk. One of the Board's responsibilities has been to divine and recommend a daily allowance (RDA) for each nutrient, including, of course, iron. Initially, the RDA for iron was 10 mg; later, it was increased to 15 mg, and 10 years ago it was increased yet again to 18 mg. These changes were not provoked by any deterioration of American citizenry—the Board had no data on this issue. Nor was it based upon any substantial evidence of lowered quality of the American diet. It was suspected that we were using less iron cookware and therefore eating less iron, and that by improving the cleanliness of food handling, a considerable amount of dirt iron was denied us, to say nothing of the unsavory iron removed from water supplies (Butterworth, 1972). (Iron in the earth, mostly oxides and carbonates, is unabsorbable. We eat our peck of dirt with no threat of iron-storage disease.) This escalation of iron requirement was, in fact, a paper transaction, but with each spiral, the reportable quality of the Amercian diet grew worse and worse. In the midst of the FFP confrontation, the media in Washington, D.C. were handed a story: 95 percent of American women eat an iron-deficient diet. This revelation was based on a diet survey plus the magic RDA, yet the same HANES survey (Abraham et al., 1974) demonstrated that less than 2 percent of U.S. women are iron deficient. The diet purportedly deficient in iron evidently provided adequately for 98 percent.

For years, the fortification of flour that was mandated in 1943 was nullified by using iron phosphate compounds that are unabsorbable. Recently, that has changed; technical improvements have made the iron phosphates obsolete (Waddell, 1973). For example, ferrous iron is now added to flour when it is being mixed to make bread. The shelf life of bread is so brief that rancidity is no problem. Carbonyl iron is a finely particulate, metallic iron that is not reactive in flour but is as nutritionally effective as ferrous sulfate (Sacks and Houchin, 1978).

Changing from the inert iron phosphates to these efficacious forms of iron has the effect of adding 13 mg of iron per pound of flour. This modification, mandated in the 1940s but implemented only in the 1970s, may have some effect upon iron deficiency in the population.

The food industry is also making an effort to modify our diet. Iron is on the list of food additives that are generally regarded as safe (the GRAS list). Any quantity of iron is permitted to be added to food. (The controversy concerns iron that is required to be added.) Voluntary fortification of foods is gradually increasing the iron in our diet. In 1977, the FDA estimated that 25 percent of American dietary iron is additive iron (Forbes, 1977). Does iron belong on the GRAS list?

Iron Deficiency in the U.S.

Iron deficiency can exist at many levels of severity. In the ideal state of iron repletion, all physiologic requirements for iron have been fulfilled and iron in the uncommitted stores is at an optimal level.

Suppose a person with a normal iron balance takes himself to a blood bank and donates a unit of blood. During those 10 minutes of donation, he becomes iron deficient, losing 250 mg of iron in 500 ml of blood. The marrow reacts to make more red cells, iron for the red cells is withdrawn from the stores, and the intestine, informed of the deficiency, admits more dietary iron. Within three weeks, the red cell mass will be restored. Within three months, the iron deficiency will be repaired.

Consider a young woman who habitually has copious menstruation, losing each month 150 ml of blood containing 60 mg of iron. Each day, she absorbs 3 mg of iron, thereby restoring the menstrual loss plus the obligatory loss. Her iron stores, however, remain empty, and she has a mild anemia. Women with less menstrual loss may have low iron stores but no anemia. They resemble the blood donor.

A man with a hiatus hernia loses 1 ml of red cells per hour. He digests the blood and absorbs from this and from his diet about 6 mg of iron per day. The decrement is 15 to 20 mg per day. In two months, his iron stores are emptied. In two months more, he develops moderate anemia, and in another two months, severe anemia.

These are three levels of iron deficiency, arbitrarily selected (the spectrum extends across all three). Defining iron deficiency can be a slippery problem because of the effort to equate *deficiency* with *disease*. It is obvious that a post-donation blood donor is not diseased, nor is a woman diseased at the end of a normal menstrual period. At what point along the spectrum of severity is deficiency equivalent to disease? In the U.S., no important attempt has been made to establish this critical clinical information.

Such a study was performed superbly by Elwood, an epidemiologist who examined thousands of young women in the villages of Wales. Each experiment was controlled either by dividing the women into two comparable groups or by examining each woman repeatedly, before and after the repair of iron-deficiency anemia. Subjective evidence was collected by questionnaires; objective evidence was obtained by fitness testing and hemoglobin measurements. Elwood's astonishing results demonstrated no statistically significant symptomatic or physical deficits unless the level of hemoglobin was of the order of 8 g/dl or less (Elwood, 1973). This is not to say that some people are not uncomfortable or physically below par with a hemoglobin of 10 g. But the numbers of such people in Elwood's sample were so few as not to be perceived among the hundreds tested.

Surveys of iron deficiency in the U.S. have not attempted any scientific correlation. Instead, the surveyors have sought out evidence of deficiency and presented that as evidence of endemic disease, requiring bureaucratic action to correct it. The Ten-State Nutrition Survey 1968–1970 (1972) is a case in point. It was undertaken to demonstrate the nutritional status of people with low incomes (thus, the 32,000 subjects of the survey did not represent a cross section of American citizenry). In the analysis of anemia and iron deficiency, an attempt was made to have Art improve upon Nature. This is described in the Report:

> The Ten-State Nutrition Survey standards are slightly higher than those recommended by the World Health Organization Scientific Group on Nutritional Anemias. Applying WHO Standards to the Ten-State Survey population would reduce the prevalence of 'deficient' and 'low' hemoglobin values in males by one half (DHEW, 1972).

In the analysis of the survey, all anemia was interpreted to represent iron deficiency. Thus, by fiddling with the normal values for hemoglobin, it was possible to "increase" the rate of iron deficiency perceived in the population, which, of course, emphasized our need for the FFP. Tampering with the standards produced another astonishing statistic: 22 percent of the men were declared to have iron-deficiency anemia. Because iron-deficiency anemia is relatively rare in American men of any economic status, this ridiculous result should have indicated to the analysts that they had a serious problem, but the embarrassing figures were published anyway.

The FDA Commissioner, in finally rejecting the FFP, commented upon the nutritional surveys purporting to demonstrate a serious problem of iron deficiency in the U.S.:

> The Ten-State survey is a case in point. This study admittedly shows a high prevalence of anemia among lower income people but not necessarily iron-deficiency anemia. Indeed, some studies show that some anemia can be cured with a well-balanced diet with or without iron fortification. The figures from the Ten-State survey are based upon hemoglobin tests; these are indicators of iron concentration in blood, but low hemoglobin may result from causes other than iron deficiency.
>
> Serum iron test results have not always correlated well with results of hemoglobin tests. For example, in that small fraction of samples of the Ten-State survey wherein serum iron tests were used, only a small number of people with the lowest hemoglobin levels also had low serum iron levels. This lack of correlation with hemoglobin tests also extends to the transferrin saturation test. In the Ten-State survey, the results of transferrin saturation tests in the one state in which they were performed were similar to results in the serum iron tests in relation to hemoglobin concentration. This cautions against facile equation of 'anemia' with 'iron-deficiency anemia.' Also, the finding by the Ten-State survey of a large number of iron-deficient males does not correlate well with the results of other studies, giving rise to further questions as to the significance of the findings of this survey.
>
> The HANES study also showed a high incidence of anemia but did not prove that the incidence was caused by iron deficiency. See affidavit of Dr. Maxwell Wintrobe.
>
> The Commissioner concludes that, whereas available data show that there is a need for additional iron for two well-defined groups (preschool infants and pregnant women), the need has not been proven to be as great or as general as the proponents of the amendments have argued (Kennedy, 1977).

The Commissioner also noted that "there are

at least 2.5 million women in the United States with iron-deficiency anemia." These millions of women are the target population of the FFP. Although 2.5 million is an enormous number, it represents only 1 percent of our population. Does it make sense to fortify everyone's diet in order to reach the tiny percentage with a deficiency that may or may not represent a disease? And by using a nutritional device that may or may not be effective? It seems reasonable to suggest that these young women are not iron deficient because their diets are malnutritious. Their proportion does not vary significantly among the poor and nonpoor, the white and nonwhite (Abraham et al., 1974). Experience indicates that as a group, the iron-deficient young women are the copious menstruators. Aside from the special situations of growth and pregnancy, iron deficiency invariably means blood loss.

Efficacy of Flour Fortification

The intention of the FFP was to prevent iron deficiency. Therapeutic iron certainly cures iron-deficiency anemia. It is also well established that iron-fortified milk formulas can prevent iron-deficiency anemia in infants. Yet, the proponents of the FFP had not put to test their hypothesis that adding 40 to 60 mg of iron to a pound of flour will reduce the incidence of iron deficiency in a population that uses the flour. Elwood has done the experiment in Wales and found that the groups of women who had eaten fortified bread for nine months showed no decrease in the rate of iron deficiency (Elwood et al., 1971). Although Elwood was criticized for not having used enough iron, the proponents of FFP in this country did nothing and were content to perform an uncontrolled experiment upon the entire population.

It is known that in the laboratory, an iron-deficient woman does absorb more iron from a single challenge dose of a bioavailable iron than does a normal, iron-replete woman. Why, then, is such experimental evidence not adequate as a test of efficacy for the fortification program? There are several cogent reasons:

1. No person can be surrogate for a population. Individuals vary in ways that we do not understand.

2. A single-shot experiment in a laboratory does not represent what happens in daily living. Bread is eaten with other foods, some of which facilitate absorption of food iron (ascorbic acid, alcohol, methionine, fructose) and some of which inhibit iron absorption (tea, corn, phytates, egg).

3. Some women eat little or no bread.

4. Some women supplement their diets with iron-containing tonics and tablets.

Only a carefully designed and executed pilot study conducted on a significantly large population over an extended time could demonstrate the efficacy of the fortification proposal. The results of such a study have only now been published (Bazzano et al., 1978):

> Anemia due to iron-deficiency is common in menstruating females and rapidly growing children. In order to test the efficacy of various levels of iron-enrichment of flour-based products in these two groups, a controlled study (in a school setting) and a free-living study were conducted in Hammond, Louisiana. The total population studied consisted of 230 women with sub-optimal hematological values and 700 children. Those parameters measured were hemoglobin, hematocrit, serum Fe, TIBC, % saturation, folate and serum ferritin levels. In the free-living study, no differences in hematology in adult women and their children could be detected after one year of consumption of iron-enriched sliced bread providing double and six-times the levels of iron presently contained in enriched bread. In the controlled school study, all flour-based products were enriched with iron to levels providing 3 and 6 mg additional iron per day. These products were consumed by the children aged 5–9 years for 4 months at school breakfast and lunch. There were significant mean changes in hemoglobin levels in the groups consuming the iron-fortified products and these positive changes correlated well with their levels of consumption. The control group demonstrated no significant mean change in hemoglobin over the time period studied.

Again, a comment from the Commissioner of the FDA:

> The commissioner concludes that there are far better ways of reaching those persons in need of additional iron than through fortification of bread. Bread is not particularly effective as a supplement to the diet of women of child-bearing age and preschool children, the groups most in need for additional iron. Surely, it would be more effective to reach people in need, once these people have been identified, by directing educational programs to them, by improving their overall diet, and by encouraging their use of foods naturally high in iron or foods specially designed for them. Additional fortification of bread, which would subject the entire population, including those involuntarily exposed, to increased dietary iron, would seem to be an inefficient and—in light of unresolved safety questions—a possibly more dangerous approach to take (Kennedy, 1977).

Safety of Iron Fortification

Hemochromatosis was mentioned earlier as a genetically determined disorder of the small intestine that results in the absorption of dietary iron that the body does not need. Because no normal excretory mechanism exists for iron, unneeded iron is put into storage in the liver, pancreas, pituitary, and heart muscle tissues. The accumulated pigment gradually brings about disability of these organs. Hemochromatosis is a serious disease; before we knew how to treat it, average survival after diagnosis was four to five years.

No one knows how many people have hemochromatosis. A review of autopsies in the early 1950s indicated a rate of 1 per 7000 in the U.S. (Finch and Finch, 1955). Among the Bantu tribe of South Africa, whose dietary intake of iron is about 100 mg per day, the rate at autopsy is greater than 1 per 100 (Bothwell and Bradlow, 1960). It has been estimated that in the U.S., the gene frequency for hemochromatosis may be about 1 in 50 (Scheinberg, 1973, 1974, 1975). Expression of the gene as disease may depend upon inheritance from both parents or upon environmental stress—for example, the dose of iron in the diet.

Proponents of the fortification proposal had not taken into account the possibility of increased risk to the carriers of this gene with or without overt disease or to people with other iron-storage diseases such as thalassemia and sickle cell anemia. When the possibility was brought to attention, it was not taken seriously. It was argued that patients with hemochromatosis are too few to merit concern when compared with the millions who are iron deficient (Butterworth, 1972; Goldsmith, 1973). This attitude rejects the evidence that the degree of iron deficiency correctable by FFP is harmless, whereas hemochromatosis is lethal. It was argued that such patients should avoid iron-fortified flour, ignoring the fact that the patient with hemochromatosis is unaware that he has the disease until it has injured him.

In the autumn of 1971, the FDA contracted with the Federation of American Societies for Experimental Biology to devise an experiment that would demonstrate whether iron accumulates in healthy men with diets that included fortified flour. Protocols for the experiment, recommended by FASEB's expert committee, indicated that it would take years to provide significant data (Waddell et al., 1972a). The experiments were never done.

In Sweden, 30 years ago, the government mandated a program for iron fortification of the national diet. Between 40 and 50 percent of the iron in the food in Sweden is fortification iron. Average intake of dietary iron in Sweden is 19 mg per day (Olsson et al., 1978). Thus, the Swedes have, in fact, achieved the daily allowance recommended for the U.S. by the Food and Nutrition Board of the National Academy of Sciences. What have 30 years of high-level fortification accomplished in Sweden? Recently, there has been some diminution of iron-deficiency anemia among Swedish women, but Hallberg (1977), the country's foremost authority on iron metabolism, believes that the change has been accomplished by voluntary dosing with supplemental iron tonics and tablets.

In 1975, Olsson, a physician working in a remote district of Sweden with a population of 130,000, noted that he had encountered five new cases of hemochromatosis in two years. Because this seemed high to him, he undertook a survey in one of the villages. All citizens aged 30 through 39 were enrolled (approximately 200 men and 200 women). Serum iron tests were done on everyone; 16 men and 10 women proved to have abnormally high values. Several months later, the serum iron tests were repeated. This time, the 10 women were normal, but 9 of the men again had abnormally high values. These men were then injected with a test dose of desferrioxamine, and four of them excreted in their urine abnormally large amounts of iron—substantial evidence of inceased stores of tissue iron. Liver biopsy demonstrated excessive storage iron in all four, diagnostic of "preclinical" hemochromatosis (Olsson et al., 1978). This is not a large enough sample to achieve statistical stability, but Olsson's entire experience does suggest that the Swedes have done on a national scale the experiment recommended by FASEB to the FDA (Waddell et al., 1972a). Increasing the iron load in the diet may increase the incidence of iron-storage disease, contrary to the informed opinion of FASEB's expert committee (Waddell et al., 1972b).

The FDA Commissioner, in rejecting the FFP, commented:

> In balancing benefits against risks, the defenselessness of those potentially at risk from iron overage due to involuntary exposure must be weighed heavily in view of the availability of an alternative strategy: selective targeting of those in need.
>
> The Commissioner concludes that, on the present

record, the increased iron levels should not be approved, since, among other things, the burden of proving them safe has not been satisfied. Better data must be obtained before what amounts to an uncontrolled study on the United States population is attempted (Kennedy, 1977).

Another problem with hemochromatosis, one that the FDA has not yet taken into account, is the carcinogenicity of excess storage iron. It is known that hemochromatosis causes cirrhosis of the liver. It is also known that cirrhosis is a precancerous lesion. In hemochromatosis, the connection is not debatable. Malignant hepatoma is the most common cause of death in people with clinically evident hemochromatosis (Bomford et al., 1975). Excess iron in this situation must be regarded as a carcinogen. It is a subtle problem: does a normal nutrient known to be carcinogenic fall within the scope of the Delaney Clause as a food additive? Because iron is known to be a carcinogen in man, should not its addition to food be prohibited (Crosby, 1977)?

Conclusion

On April 1, 1970, the American Bakers Association and the Millers' National Federation petitioned the Food and Drug Administration to raise the standard of enriched bread and flour by tripling the amount of iron in the staples. In so doing, they thought they were responding to public demand and the scientific community's concern over anemia. Instead, they stirred up a hornet's nest of controversy between several leading nutritionists and most hematologists. The dispute has now come to an abrupt conclusion. The FDA rejected the proposed super-enrichment in one of the bluntest rebukes the Federal government has ever handed a group of scientists.

In its decision, the FDA stated that the recommendation was based on faulty scientific evidence, that the need for more iron has not been established, that enrichment has not been shown to be a useful remedy for anemia, and that even if it were, doubling or tripling the amount of iron in foodstuffs might do more harm than good. . . .

Not only has the iron enrichment proposal produced one of the greatest nutrition debates in recent times, the move has had another effect. In their attempt to greatly alter the amount of a specific nutrient in an enriched food, the Millers and Bakers may, without intending to do so, prompt a reexamination of all food enrichment. . . . Should confidence in the efficacy and safety of nutrient enrichment of staple foodstuffs be weakened, there'll be a whole new ball game in nutrition science and dietetics. The effect on food processing and marketing will also be far reaching. The rejection of the iron proposal may be the prologue of a new drama in nutrition (Enloe, 1978).

On August 13, 1978, the Commissioner of Food and Drugs finally withdrew the order that would have mandated an increase of iron fortification of bread and flour (Kennedy, 1978):

Although currently available data show that there is a need for increased iron for 1 to 2 percent of the population, there is a question whether surveys or studies show it to be greater than that . . . .

There is insufficient evidence that the augmentation in iron-fortified bread would ameliorate the condition of those who need additional iron . . . .

There are no adequate studies showing the safety of the increased levels of iron in bread, especially with reference to hemochromatosis and thalassemia. Therefore, the proponents of the augmentation have failed to sustain their burden of proof . . . .

Because of the findings and conclusions above, the augmentation of iron fortification of bread, as set forth in the stayed provisions of the regulation, should not be approved . . . .

This order is effective November 27, 1978.

Donald Kennedy
Commissioner of Food and Drugs

References

Abraham, S., Lowenstein, F.W., and Johnson, C.L.: *Preliminary Fhndings of the First Health and Nutrition Examination Survey, United States, 1971 to 1972.* Rockville, MD. Office of Information, National Center for Health Statistics, 1974.

AMA Council on Foods and Nutrition: Iron in enriched wheat flour, farina, bread, buns and rolls. JAMA 220:855, 1972.

Bazzano, G., Trosclair, G., Carlisle, J., Weiss, R., and Carter, J.: The effect of iron fortification of flour-based products on hematology in two study groups. Clin. Res. 26:283A, 1978.

Bomford, A., Walker, R.J., and Williams, R.: Treatment of iron overload including results in a personal series of 85 patients with idiopathic haemochromatosis. In Kief, H., *Iron Metabolism and its Disorders,* New York, American Elsevier, 1975.

Bothwell, T.H., and Bradlow, B.A.: Siderosis in the Bantu. A combined histopathological and chemical study. Arch. Pathol. 70:279, 1960.

Butterworth, C.E.: Iron "undercontamination." JAMA 220:581, 1972.

Crosby, W.H.: Bureaucratic clout, and a parable: the iron-enrichment-now brouhaha. JAMA 228:1651, 231:1054, 1975.

Crosby, W.H.: Current concepts in nutrition. Who needs iron? N. Engl. J. Med. 297:1238, 1977.

Duggan, R.E.: Cereal flours and related products. Proposal to increase required maximum and minimum iron levels. Federal Register 35:5412, 1970.

Elwood, P.C.: Evaluation of the clinical importance of anemia. Am. J. Clin. Nutr. 26:958, 1973.

Elwood, P.C., Waters, W.E., and Sweetman, P.: The haematinic effect of iron in flour. Clin. Sci. 40:31, 1971.

Enloe, C.F.: The experts debate. The added enrichment of bread and flour with iron. Nutrition Today 7:4, 1972.

Enloe, C.F.: Anatomy of a decision. Nutrition Today 15:6, 1978.

Finch, S.C., and Finch, C.A.: Idiopathic hemochromatosis, an iron storage disease. Medicine (Baltimore) 34:381, 1955.

Forbes, A.L.: Personal communication. April 8, 1977.

Goldsmith, G.A., Chairman, Committee on Iron Nutritional Deficiency: Extent and Meanings of Iron Deficiency in the U.S. Summary Proceedings of a Workshop, March 8–9, 1971. Washington, Food and Nutrition Board, NAS-NRC, 1971.

Goldsmith, G.A.: Fortification of flour and bread with iron. JAMA 233:322, 224:400, 1973.

Hallberg, Leif: Reduced prevalence of iron deficiency in Swedish women. Läkartidningen 74:1722, 1977.

Kennedy, D.: Iron fortification of flour and bread. Federal Register 42:59513, 1977.

Kennedy, D.: Iron fortification of flour and bread; findings of fact, conclusions, and final order. Federal Register 43:38575, 1978.

Olsson, K.S., Heedman, P.A., and Stangård, F.: Preclinical hemochromatosis in a population on a high-iron-fortified diet. JAMA 239:1999–2000, 1978.

Sacks, P.V., and Houchin, D.N.: Comparative bioavailability of elemental iron powders for repair of iron deficiency anemia in rats. Studies of efficacy and toxicity of carbonyl iron. Am. J. Clin. Nutr. 31:566–571, 1978.

Scheinberg, I.H.: The genetics of hemochromatosis. Arch. Intern. Med. 132:126, 1973, 133:1072, 1974, 135:1269, 1975.

Schmidt, A.M.: Enriched flour, enriched self-rising flour, and enriched bread. Federal Register 38:28558, October 1973.

Schmidt, A.M.: By bread alone. Nutrition Today 13:11, 1978.

Ten-State Nutrition Survey 1968–1970, Vol. 4, Biochemical. Publication (HSM) 72-8132. Atlanta, U.S. Department of Health, Education and Welfare, Center for Disease Control, 1972.

Waddell, J.: *The Bioavailability of Iron Sources and Their Utilization in Food Enrichment.* Bethesda, Life Sciences Research Office FASEB, 1973.

Waddell, J., Sassoon, H.F., Carr, C.J., and Fisher, K.D.: *Clinical Research Protocols to Elucidate the Possible Hazards of Increased Iron Enrichment of Cereal Products.* Bethesda, Life Sciences Research Office FASEB, 1972a.

Waddell, J., Sassoon, H.F., Fisher, K.D., and Carr, C.J.: *A Review of the Significance of Dietary Iron on Iron Storage Phenomena.* Bethesda, Life Sciences Research Office FASEB, 1972b.

Wilder, R.M.: A brief history of the enrichment of flour and bread. JAMA 162:1539, 1956.

12

How Should Sore Throats Be Treated?

My sore throats, you know, are always worse than anybody's.

Jane Austen, *Persuasion*

There are sure to be two prescriptions diametrically opposite. Stuff a cold and starve a cold are but two ways.

Henry Thoreau, *A Week on the Concord and Merrimack Rivers*

If you think that you have caught a cold, call in a good doctor. Call in three good doctors and play bridge.

Robert Benchley, *From Bed to Worse*

Introduction

The long-standing controversy about how to treat sore throats continues. Academicians and infectious disease experts tend to favor taking throat cultures in patients with this complaint, waiting for the results, and treating only those whose throat cultures grow out beta hemolytic streptococci. Many practitioners regard this approach as unrealistically pedantic, and they believe that it is easier, cheaper, and generally better for the health of patients to overtreat some (or even many) patients in order to treat properly (and early) those who will benefit from antibiotics.

Dr. Breese is a distinguished pediatrician who has many years of experience in treating children with sore throats. He and his associates, by a combined approach that utilizes history, physical examination, epidemiologic information, and laboratory data, have honed their diagnostic skills to a fine edge. They seem to be correct in diagnosing streptococcal etiology at least 75 percent of the time, and if the cultures disagree with the rest of the data, they quite properly ignore the laboratory. Breese's philosophy is middle-of-the-road, eschewing both the "treat 'em all" and the "treat hardly any" schools. Of particular interest to the reader should be his discussion of the data concerning the risks of rheumatic fever and penicillin toxicity and the frequency of the carrier state.

Hurtado and Greenlick look at the issue from the viewpoint of the professional health standard evaluator. Their approach is primarily an empirical one that examines objective data on what doctors are actually seeing and doing in practice and what happens to their patients. The authors observe that the percentages of false positives and false negatives in throat cultures are disturbingly high in some studies.

The data presented by Hurtado and Greenlick are derived from a large, prepaid group practice involving both pediatricians and internists. The majority of cases of upper respiratory infection seen were uncomplicated at the time of the first visit. The low yield of positive throat cultures in both children and adults raises doubts in their minds about the wisdom of routine throat cultures, especially in view of the cost. In the practice studied, antibiotics were used sparingly, with little in the way of subsequent complications.

Patterns of culture data and antibiotic treatment were quite different in the patients suspected of having streptococcal sore throats. Throat culture reports did not seem to have a great impact on the course of treatment once antibiotics had been started, and the authors rightly wonder why cultures are being ordered in what seems to be a ritualistic fashion. Few complications of infection or therapy were observed.

Tompkins, in the third contribution, recommends a management strategy for sore throats based on a cost-effectiveness analysis that takes account of individual cost and disease as well as the prevalence of streptococcal infection in a given community at any given time. He concludes that different strategies will be most cost-effective in different situations, but that a "decision-tree" can be devised that will allow rapid identification and treatment of patients at high risk for streptococcal infection, as well as identification of those who will not benefit sufficiently from treatment to justify any diagnostic evaluation.

All three papers agree that the doctor's diagnostic and therapeutic approach should be determined by facts and therapeutic outcome rather than by dogma and habit.

LOUIS LASAGNA, M.D.

How Should One Treat Sore Throats?

Burtis B. Breese, M.D.
Islamorada, Fla.

Sore throats caused by beta hemolytic streptococci (BHS) should be treated with appropriate antibiotics, and all other sore throats should be treated only symptomatically (excluding such uncommon ones as those resulting from diphtheria, tuberculosis, syphilis, and neoplasms).

There are several reasons for this recommended approach. Proper antibiotic therapy of sore throats due to BHS will (1) cure the acute sore throat, (2) prevent most complications, including rheumatic fever, and (3) render the patient noncontagious. Antibiotic therapy of other types of sore throat is (1) ineffectual (2) expensive, and (3) often associated with undesirable side effects (Denny et al., 1950; Stollerman, 1954; Breese and Disney, 1958; Caldwell and Cluff, 1974; Bass et al., 1976; Arndt and Hershel, 1976).

Such a therapeutic program requires that the clinician be able to distinguish sore throats caused by BHS from those caused by a large array of other agents, notably viral. Furthermore, it is desirable that methods for such differentiation be accurate, prompt, inexpensive, and readily available.

Unfortunately, there are no ways to fulfull all these diagnostic and therapeutic requirements. Thus, the practitioner may have to treat an ailment that he is not able to diagnose correctly and that, if untreated, may lead to disaster (e.g., severe rheumatic fever), but if treated, may result in an even more catastrophic end (anaphylactic death). In between are a variety of less compelling reasons for or against specific antibiotic therapy. Under these circumstances, controversy surrounding treatment of sore throats is inevitable.

Current Therapeutic Regimens

General agreement on the broad objectives and means of treatment of sore throat exists. The controversy focuses on the particular methods of attaining these objectives. The three basic approaches and their underlying philosophies are as follows.

Treat All Sore Throats with Antibiotics (Usually Penicillin) when There Is Any Reasonable Possibility that BHS Is the Etiologic Agent. Bacteriologic confirmation, although possibly of interest, may be omitted or deemed unimportant in deciding when an antimicrobial should be used. By such universal antibiotic management, although it is often not necessary, practically all streptococcal sore throats will be treated and cured at low cost. Complications, including rheumatic fever, will be prevented.

Proponents of this approach—the play-it-safe therapeutic school—present the following arguments:

1. Almost any group A BHS sore throat may lead to complications, most important of which is rheumatic fever. Penicillin treatment prevents this complication (Denny et al., 1950).

2. Antibiotic therapy is such a safe procedure (Caldwell and Cluff, 1974; Arndt and Hershel, 1976) that it is better to use it, although it is often unnecessary, than to risk streptococcal complications.

3. Clinical differentiation of BHS sore throat from nonstreptococcal sore throat is reasonably accurate without culture confirmation.

4. Taking cultures for BHS is impractical in many circumstances because of lack of facilities. When they are available, they are often inconvenient; the reporting is slow and the procedure

can be unduly expensive.

5. Cultures frequently miss BHS present in patients' throats (false negatives).

6. Penicillin treatment of all suspected sore throats without culture confirmation is the most cost-effective means of rheumatic fever prevention.

In opposition and in rebuttal to these six points, consider these points:

1. It is questionable whether all cases of group A streptococcal pharyngitis can lead to complications, including rheumatic fever. Even if they can, the risk is not great. Although shortly after World War II, it was demonstrated that approximately 3 percent of untreated patients with epidemic streptococcal pharyngitis seen at Fort Warren developed rheumatic fever, regardless of the M type responsible (Denny et al., 1950), this high incidence has not been observed in civilians since. In a clinic population in Chicago, the incidence was approximately one tenth of that in Fort Warren (Siegel et al., 1961). In relatively affluent populations, as exemplified by my patient groups in Rochester, N.Y., it is probably even less, despite the fact that streptococcal pharyngitis is exceedingly common and frequently unwittingly untreated. The reason for this almost complete disappearance of rheumatic fever in such populations is not clear, but whatever the cause, failure to treat streptococcal pharyngitis today carries less risk to the patient than it did in the past.

2. Antibiotic therapy, although relatively safe, is by no means always innocuous, especially if wantonly and uncritically administered. Major deleterious effects are possible, such as sensitization, which may cause allergic reactions ranging from mild urticaria to anaphylactic death. Such sensitization usually precludes the drug's further use in that patient. A sensitization to penicillin creates a double jeopardy: loss of a superior drug for future treatment and danger of severe reaction if it is inadvertently administered. Development of resistant strains of bacteria in the host or in the population to which he belongs has also occurred with antibiotic therapy, as has suppression of normal bacterial protective flora (Crowe et al., 1973; Hahn, 1973; Caldwell and Cluff, 1974; Brande, 1976; Sparling et al., 1977).

3. Clinical diagnosis of streptococcal pharyngitis without bacteriologic aid is not accurate.

Given only the symptoms of sore throat and a good look at the pharynx, even the astute clinician's diagnostic choice between a streptococcal and nonstreptococcal pharyngitis is often no better than the choice that might be made by tossing a coin. As one increases the number of selected parameters upon which to base a presumptive diagnosis of a streptococcal sore throat, accuracy increases up to the point beyond which the procedure becomes unwieldy. But even then, we found, in an unpublished study based on reports from over three dozen offices, that most physicians were able to predict the results of throat cultures no better than 60 percent of the time.

Many years ago, my associate Dr. Frank Disney and I, using throat cultures for BHS as our criterion, concluded that we could diagnose streptococcal sore throat from other etiologic data on clinical grounds in about 75 percent of those suspected of such illness (Breese and Disney, 1954). Today, although on occasion and in selected groups we have reached 85 percent accuracy, 75 percent still remains a very satisfactory figure for a correct tentative diagnosis, and, in order to reach this degree of accuracy, we and others (Stillerman and Bernstein, 1961; Randolph et al., 1970) have used a constellation of symptoms, physical signs, and laboratory and epidemiologic data to aid diagnosis.

I have recently condensed these into a nine-point scoring system that has proved clinically useful (Breese, 1977). Randolph has devised a similar score card (Randolph et al., 1970). However, even though 75 percent is a respectable figure, 25 percent is too large a margin of error for a final diagnosis upon which critical therapy may be based. Consequently, throat cultures for BHS have justifiably been used to assure more specific diagnosis in millions of patients with sore throats.

4. The belief that taking of cultures for BHS is impractical and therefore a good reason for not utilizing bacteriologic confirmation of tentative diagnoses is incorrect. The varied reasons given for this belief, including lack of facilities for processing specimens, difficulty in transporting specimens, delay in reporting, and high cost and incovenience, have not proved valid in practice. Most of these do not exist, and none is insurmountable. On the contrary, facilities for processing such specimens are widely available in public health or private laboratories, or they can be set up in the doctor's own office.

For those cultures processed locally, throat swabs may be delivered directly or through the mail. In either case, using special envelopes for transport, survival of streptococci is excellent (Redys et al. 1968). Cotton swabs allowed to dry in ordinary pill envelopes provide a cheap and effective transport method (Breese, 1965).

When the number of cultures warrant it (roughly 25 a week), I favor doing one's own streptococcal bacteriology. In addition to solving transport problems, this method has the advantages of rapid determination of results and reasonable cost (not more than three dollars per culture) (Breese, 1969).

For those who wish to "do their own thing" and yet avoid even the simple steps of plating swabs by conventional methods, kits for identification of group A BHS may be purchased. Except for the increased cost and the difficulty entailed in estimating the number of streptococci found (because of the selective media used and other characteristics favoring growth, even a few BHS may grow with undue profusion), these kits are highly practical and result in few false negative results (Randolph et al., 1976).

The experience of our own small pediatric group attests further to the practicality of simple streptococcal bacteriologic tests. During the past 33 years, we have processed approximately one quarter million cultures for BHS. In 1969, I reported this experience favorably (Breese, 1969) and have had no reason to change this opinion since. Thus, the argument that culturing patients for BHS is impractical is specious.

5. The contention that such bacteriologic study involves unacceptable errors is misleading. Although Mondzak observed that practitioners' bacteriologic tests frequently failed to come up with positive cultures (Mondzac, 1967), others have found such studies satisfactory (Rosenstein et al., 1970). In our practice, we estimate the amount of false negative cultures at approximately 8 percent, most resulting from missing small numbers of streptococci in carriers, a point usually of little clinical significance (Breese, 1969). With the use of the highly sensitive kits, even these errors can be eliminated. Randolph found that with little training, nonprofessional members of his own family could perform accurate bacteriologic tests using one such kit (Detekta). In his practice, use of the kit resulted in not missing a single case of streptococcal pharyngitis that required treatment (Randolph et al., 1976).

6. The argument that universal treatment of sore throats without culture confirmation is the most cost-effective method of rheumatic fever control and should therefore be used is dangerous and untenable. Even if it were so (which I doubt), it is a broad invitation to the overuse of antibiotics (already a malignant ailment of too many therapists), with the aforementioned possible adverse consequences. Furthermore, it could encourage treatment without diagnosis even where diagnosis is possible.

Thus, in consideration of these six arguments against the indiscriminate use of antibiotics in sore throats of undetermined etiology, I believe that the "treat 'em all" approach should not be used.

Treat with Penicillin Only Those Sore Throats in which the Severity of the Infection or the Nature of the Causative Streptococcus Suggests a High Risk of Complications, Particularly Rheumatic Fever. With this plan, the severe sore throat patient will receive adequate treatment and complications will be prevented. The much larger group of patients who have benign sore throats, although they may be streptococcal, will be spared the adverse effects of antibiotic therapy.

The arguments for this "cautious treatment" approach are as follows:

1. The risk of nontreatment is not great.
2. Antibiotic therapy is not always innocuous, and its risk may exceed that of nontreatment.

In rebuttal, one must consider the following arguments:

1. Although the risk of complications, including rheumatic fever, is not great, such complications are preventable by proper therapy of recognized cases of streptococcal pharyngitis. Even mild streptococcal sore throats may lead to complications. At present, there is no way in which the clinician can determine in advance which cases or which strains of streptococci may lead to such results. He is therefore obligated to treat all cases of streptococcal pharyngitis with antibiotics. (The same does not apply to BHS carriers.)
2. Although antibiotic therapy, like any good treatment, carries some risk, it is minimal. No fatal reactions followed over one million injected doses of benzathine penicillin (Stollerman, 1975). Skin reactions (mostly urticarial) occurred in approximately 1 percent of penicillin-treated patients in my pediatric group (Breese, 1977). Nor has the use of penicillin for treatment of streptococcal pharyngitis led to widespread streptococcal resistance or failure of immunity to BHS to develop with advancing age.

Therefore, a regimen based on treatment of only severe cases of streptococcal pharyngitis is not warranted.

Finally, after consideration and negation of

the two extreme treatment regimens ("treat 'em all" and "treat hardly any"), we are left with the middle-of-the-road approach, which I advocate.

Treat All Sore Throats in Which There Is Good Evidence (Preferably Microbiologic) of Group A BHS Etiology, Regardless of Severity. By so doing, these patients' sore throats will be cured, and complications, including rheumatic fever, will be prevented. The clinician can thus achieve the best balance in preventing both streptococcal complications and the adverse effects of antibiotic therapy. This requires, as outlined in my initial answer, that sore throats caused by BHS be treated with antibiotics, primarily penicillin, and that other sore throats should receive only symptomatic therapy.

The problem with implementation of this solution is that determination of causality is not always easy, largely because of throat carriers of beta hemolytic streptococci in most populations. Thus, the isolation of these organisms from the pharynx of a sore throat patient does not prove that they are the responsible agents, and this may present a thorny diagnostic problem. The two most important factors in its solution are (1) the frequency of carriers in the population from which the patient is drawn and (2) the clinical picture presented by the patient. Streptococcal antibody assays, although of value retrospectively, are not helpful during the acute disease.

The frequency of the carrier state has been reported to be as high as 60 percent in some epidemiologic studies in which repeated cultures are taken on the same individuals and highly sensitive bacteriologic methods are utilized for their detection (Zanen et al., 1959). A large proportion of streptococci occur in small numbers or may not be group A, and many are of no clinical importance.

In contrast, in our pediatric practice and in similar practices where only single diagnostic specimens are obtained and the bacteriologic methods are not highly sensitive, the carrier rate for BHS is no more than 5 percent, and the number of those carrying group A in moderate or larger quantities (as usually seen in acute streptococcal pharyngitis) is considerably less than that. These differences can be attributed partly to bacteriologic and sampling techniques and partly to true differences in the carrier rates found in a public school and that of a private office population. (The former are often heavily weighted with the underprivileged and different from those found in the private practice sample.)

Whatever the cause of these varying carrier rates, the higher the rate, the lower the diagnostic value of a positive culture in an individual from that population.

In the clinical picture, the carrier state by definition causes neither abnormal signs nor symptoms, whereas the disease state is associated with either or both.

Kaplan and his associates, in a study made in the emergency department at a St. Paul hospital, found that a large proportion of patients with positive BHS cultures treated there (mostly with antibiotics) failed to show a streptococcal antibody response. They concluded that many of these patients were carriers who were unnecessarily treated (Kaplan et al., 1971).

This report, wrongly interpreted, has been extremely damaging to the gospel of the importance and validity of using throat cultures as a mainstay in diagnosis. Dr. Roth, a house officer, remarked plaintively during a journal club meeting in which he received this report, "Now I have no way of knowing the way to treat a sore throat."

Cheer up, Dr. Roth, and continue to take throat cultures. Surely Dr. Kaplan and his associates do so also. Furthermore, they use the results of such cultures as an aid in deciding when antibiotics should be used in the treatment of sore throats. Although other factors may have played a more important part in the failure of antibody response than the authors contend, certainly many did not respond because they were, in fact, carriers of BHS with viral ailments. The message I derive from their presentation is not that cultures are of little value but that they are only a single factor in the diagnostic process.

However, in this St. Paul population, the carrier rate was high and thus was the source of much more confusion and overtreatment than in our own pediatric patients. Here, since at most only 5 percent of normal patients carry BHS in their throats, this would be the maximal overtreatment error if used as the sole criterion for antibiotic treatment.

Conclusion

In making a decision about proper treatment, culture results should not be the only criterion. As mentioned, the clinical picture presented by the patient is of utmost diagnostic value. Whether based on the clinician's value judgment of symptoms, signs, and other factors or on some diagnostic gimmick such as a score card, the clinical picture should carry equal weight with the culture results. In patients in whom the clinical picture and the culture results are not compatible, the clinician must still make a diagnosis upon which to base his therapy. For example, if the culture is positive and the febrile sore throat patient has respiratory symptoms such as cough and hoarseness with a normal white blood count, most likely he is a carrier with a viral illness. On the other hand, if the patient has a clinical picture highly suggestive of streptococcal pharyngitis, particularly with a high white blood count, but with no streptococci in this throat culture, the possibility of a falsely negative culture should be considered. In either case, the wisest course to follow is a therapeutic trial using oral penicillin. If the patient is markedly improved within 36 hours (usually sooner), the drug should be continued for 10 days; if not, it may be discontinued.

Thus, although therapeutic controversy in the treatment of sore throat exists, I believe that every effort should be made to determine the etiology of sore throats. Those caused by beta hemolytic streptococci should be treated with penicillin and others should be treated only symptomatically.

References

American Heart Association Committee Report: Prevention of rheumatic fever. Circulation 55:1, 1977.

Arndt, K.A., and Hershel, J.: Rates of cutaneous reactions to drugs. A report from the Boston collaborative drug surveillance program. JAMA 263:918, 1976.

Bass, J.N., Crest, F.W., Knowles, C.R., and Onufer, C.N.: Streptococcal pharyngitis in children. JAMA 235:1112, 1976.

Breese, B.B.: The use of cotton tipped swabs as a simple method of transporting cultures of beta hemolytic streptococci. Pediatrics 36:599, 1965.

Breese, B.B.: Culturing beta hemolytic streptococci in pediatric practice—observations after twenty years. J. Pediatr. 75:164, 1969.

Breese, B.B.: A simple score card for the tentative diagnosis of streptococcal pharyngitis. Am. J. Dis. Child. 131:514, 1977.

Breese, B.B., and Disney, F.A.: The accuracy of diagnosis of beta hemolytic streptococcal infections on clinical grounds. J. Pediatr. 44:670, 1954.

Breese, B.B., and Disney, F.A.: Penicillin in the treatment of streptococcal infections. A comparison of effectiveness of five different oral and one parenteral form. N. Engl. J. Med. 259:57, 1958.

Breese, B.B., Disney, F.A., and Talpey, N.B.: The incidence of beta hemolytic streptococcal illness in a private pediatric practice, Part II. Pediatrics 38:278, 1966.

Breese, B.B., Disney, F.A., Talpey, N.B., and Green, J.I.: Beta hemolytic streptococcal infection. The clinical and epidemiologic importance of the number of organisms found in cultures. Am. J. Dis. Child. 119:17, 1970.

Breese, B.B., and Hall, C.B.: *Beta Hemolytic Streptococcal Infections*. Boston, Houghton Mifflin, 1977.

Caldwell, J.R., and Cluff, L.E.: Adverse reactions to antimicrobial agents. JAMA 230:77, 1974.

Crowe, C.C., Saunders, W.E., Jr., and Longley, S.: Bacterial interference. II, Role of normal throat flora in prevention of colonization by group A streptococcus. J. Infect. Dis. 128:527, 1973.

Denny, F.W., Jr., Wannamaker, L.W., Brink, N.R., Rammelkamp, C.H., Jr., and Coster, E.A.: Prevention of rheumatic fever. Treatment of the preceding streptococcic infection. JAMA 143:151, 1950.

Hahn, F.E., ed.: Acquired resistance of microorganisms to chemotherapeutic drugs. Antibiot. Chemother. 20, 1976.

Kaplan, E.L., Top, F.H., Duddy, B.A., and Wannamaker, L.W.: Diagnosis of streptococcal pharyngitis—differentiation of active infection from the carrier state in the symptomatic child. J. Infect. Dis. 123:490, 1971.

Mondzac, A.M.: Throat culture processing in the office—a warning. JAMA 200:1132, 1967.

Rammehamp, C.H., Jr.: Epidemiology of streptococcal infections. Harvey Lecture Series 51:113–142, 1955–56.

Randolph, M.F., Redys, J.J., and Hibbard, E.W.: Streptococcal pharyngitis. I, Correlation of cultures and clinical criteria. Del. Med. J. 42:29, 1970.

Randolph, M.F., Redys, J.J., and Morris, K.E.: Streptococcal pharyngitis: evaluation of a new diagnostic kit for clinic and office use. Am. J. Dis. Child. 130:171, 1976.

Redys, J.J., Hibbard, E., and Bonman, E.K.: Improved dry swab transportation for streptococcal cultures. Public Health Rep. 83:143, 1968.

Rosenstein, B.J., Markowitz, M., and Sordis, L.: Accuracy of throat cultures processed in physicians' offices. J. Pediatr. 76:606, 1970.

Siegel, A.C., Johnson, E.E., and Stollerman, G.H.: Controlled studies of streptococcal pharyngitis in a pediatric population. I, Factors related to the attack rate of rheumatic fever. N. Engl. J. Med. 265:559, 1961.

Sparling, P.F., Holmes, K.K., Weisner, P.J., and Priziss, M.: Summary of the problem of penicillin-resistant gonococci. J. Infect. Dis. 135:865, 1977.

Stillerman, M., and Bernstein, S.H.: Streptococcal pharyngitis: evaluation of clinical syndromes in diagnosis. Am. J. Dis. Child. 101:476, 1961.

Stollerman, G.H.: The use of antibiotics for the prevention of rheumatic fever. Am. J. Med. 17:757, 1954.

Stollerman, G.H.: *Rheumatic Fever and Streptococcal Infection*. New York, Grune and Stratton, 1975.

Tompkins, R.K., Burnes, D.C., and Cable, W.E.: An analysis of the cost-effectiveness of pharyngitis management and acute rheumatic fever prevention. Ann. Intern. Med. 86:481, 1977.

Zanen, H.C., Ganor, S., and Van Toorn, M.: A continuous study of hemolytic streptococci in throats of normal children, adults and aged men. Am. J. Hygiene 69:265–273, 1959.

What Should Be the Standard Approach to Diagnosis and Treatment of Common, Acute Respiratory Infections and Streptococcal Sore Throats in Outpatients?*

Arnold V. Hurtado, M.D.
Merwyn R. Greenlick, Ph.D.
Kaiser-Permanente Medical Care Program, Portland, Oregon

The quality of medical care is under ever increasing scrutiny. Whereas studies of the quality of care within a hospital setting are not uncommon (Brook et al., 1977), studies of the quality of care in other settings have been limited. There are several reasons for this. The initial concern of the Professional Standards Review Organizations (PSRO) was directed at care provided in the hospital because of the considerable cost of that care. In addition, the processes and outcomes of care are much easier to measure in the hospital setting than in other settings because the style of care in a hospital can be readily delineated. Laboratory and x-ray procedures, which are performed far more frequently in hospital than in ambulatory care settings, and outcomes, such as length of stay, mortality, complications, and duration of disability are easily documented and measured, and they are more definite than those in an ambulatory care setting, where illness is generally less severe.

Any evaluation of office practice should include assessment of how effectively and efficiently resources are used (Freeborn and Greenlick, 1973). There is an increasing awareness that an adequate assessment of the quality of care must take into account the outcome of the treatment (Brook, 1974), and must include both the costs and the complications of therapy. We can no longer afford to ignore the fact that treatments of even the simplest illnesses must have a rationale if costly laboratory and treatment procedures are to be recommended.

---

*This chapter was stimulated by a study conducted by J. David Bristow, M.D., while at the Kaiser-Permanente Health Services Research Center, Portland, Oregon, during a sabbatical leave from his chairmanship of the Department of Medicine at the University of Oregon Health Sciences Center in 1976. Dr. Bristow is now with the Cardiology Section of the Veterans Administration Hospital in San Francisco.

Phyllis Turner, technical editor, and Dan Azevedo, director of computer operations of the Health Services Research Center, both contributed heavily to this chapter. Acknowledgment must also be extended to Jerry M. Slepack, M.D., internist of Northwest Permanente, for his review and comments.

Problems in Establishing Recommended Standards

As an illustration of the problem, especially of the aspects differentiating academic and clinical views of establishing "standards" of practice, this essay deals with such an analysis of two common, acute, "minor" illnesses seen in the primary care office of a prepaid group practice. The study required a large population with enough cases of illness to validate analysis (Greenlick et al., 1968). In the medical care system from which the study was derived, acute upper respiratory infection (URI) and streptococcal pharyngitis (streptococcal sore throat or ST) were, respectively, the first and third most common acute illnesses seen by pediatricians and internists. These illnesses were studied because some of the laboratory and treatment considerations are similar for both conditions. URI represented 5 percent of all visits to the internists and 10 percent of all visits to pediatricians. ST represented 1 percent of all visits to internists and 4 percent of all visits to pediatricians. Although these are certainly common ailments, they have not been subject to the rigorous studies of management and outcome that their frequencies would warrant. Considering the ubiquitousness of these diseases, any major differences between academic recommendations and the practice of clinicians should be resolved because of their widespread medical and economic impact.

Upper Respiratory Infection

URI, the most common illness seen in primary office practice, is usually considered in standard textbooks as requiring only supportive therapy. A popular textbook on infectious disease states:

> At present there are no antimicrobial drugs of practical effectiveness in man against the virus responsible for the common cold; hence, the use of these drugs is not recommended—routine antibacterial chemoprophylaxis selects resistant bacterial strains and does not prevent suppurative complications (Beeson and McDermott, 1975).

The same recommendation is found in another textbook, *Current Therapy 1976:*

> Antimicrobial agents should not be used during the acute phase of viral respiratory disease. These agents have no antiviral effect and in all probability do not prevent the uncommon case of secondary bacterial infection. Moreover, if secondary bacterial disease develops during their use, it is usually with a resistant organism. In addition, the use of antimicrobials may result in toxic effects or may sensitize the individual to a valuable therapeutic agent. Demanding patients will usually accept the judgment of a thoughtful physician in this regard (Couch, 1976).

These recommendations were openly contested in 1976, when the Medical Tribune, a widely read medical newsletter, published a series of articles and letters on the use of antibiotics for the common cold. The series was initiated by Dr. Lasagna, in whose opinion many patients who saw a physician for a "cold" were suffering some complication, and he suggested that these complications are amenable to treatment with antibiotics. In response, the Medical Tribune "received the largest outpouring of letters in its history."

Lasagna responded to this reaction by indicating that the majority of doctors who wrote were essentially in agreement with his earlier comments. A number of physicians commented that "over the years they had learned from sad experience that treating such patients with studied neglect did not work whereas antibiotics frequently did seem to halt the process." Lasagna noted that a minority of physicians took an opposing point of view, feeling that their practices were "full of demanding neurotics who wanted antibiotics for simple viral infections that could never be expected to respond to any presently available antibiotics." In a subsequent interview in the same publication (1976), Dr. Eugene Stead stated, "If you really look at what happens in day-to-day medical practice, most antibiotics are given empirically. Diseases like mastoiditis have disappeared, not because of the intelligent or scientific use of antibiotics, but because general practitioners gave them en masse."

The foregoing comments and most other available information concerning the use of antibiotics in treating the common cold are based on the unsubstantiated impressions of the commenting physician. It would seem that objective data might dehorn the dilemma of the proper treatment for the common cold. Several questions need to be answered. What percentage of the cases of URI seen in an office practice are, indeed, uncomplicated? What percentage of the cases of uncomplicated URI seen by primary care physicians actually receive antibiotics? How many cases of uncomplicated URI do not receive antibiotics and later develop bacterial complications? Further, how often do complications result from the use of antibiotics among patients who received antibiotics for uncomplicated URI?

Another problem that deserves exploration is the use of the laboratory for cases of URI. Laboratory usage in medical care has shown a steady increase in recent years (Freeborn et al., 1972). In this study, we found that the predominant laboratory procedure ordered in cases of URI was the throat culture. Because of the cost of this procedure, we were interested in the value of throat cultures in the management and outcome of URI.

Streptococcal Pharyngitis

Among the number of current recommendations for treating ST is that the throat be cultured and that chemotherapy be delayed until the result of the culture is obtained. Typical of the recommendations found in the academic literature is that in *Current Therapy 1976:*

> Patients in our practice all have throat cultures taken prior to instituting antibiotic therapy. If the culture is positive for Group A streptococci, the patients are notified to return to the clinic to receive appropriate therapy within 24 to 48 hours after the throat culture has been taken, or a prescription is called to the pharmacy. This approach minimizes unnecessary use of antibiotics in patients who have viral upper respiratory illness (Dudding, 1976).

Recently, an article by Wannamaker (1976) condemned the use of antibiotic treatment for a presumed streptococcal sore throat before a positive throat culture has been confirmed.

Such recommendations are not universal, however, and some data concerning streptococcal pharyngitis would appear to negate them. The number of false negatives in subsequently proven cases of streptococcal pharyngitis is estimated conservatively to be 20 percent (Rosenstein, Markowitz, and Gordis, 1970; Battle and Glasgow, 1971) and as high as 29 to 64 percent in some studies (Mondzac, 1967). On the other hand, positive Group A beta-hemolytic streptococcus cultures can be obtained from 11 to 24 percent of school children who are otherwise asymptomatic (Peter and Smith, 1977). An editorial emphasizing the common prevalence of Group A beta-hemolytic streptococcus in children stresses the fact that "a viral infection in a child who happens to be a streptococcal carrier creates a complex diagnostic problem to which there is no simple answer" (Quinn, 1974).

Another argument against these recommendations is that the delay of treatment for streptococcal pharyngitis could prolong symptoms, although this, too, is open to controversy. Many physicians feel strongly that early treatment will reduce the duration of illness (Merenstein and Rogers, 1974); others feel that a 24-hour delay of treatment does not significantly alter the effectiveness of the treatment (Schroeder, Schliftman, and Piemme, 1974).

Discussing the cost effectiveness of taking active measures to prevent rheumatic fever, Burns, Cable, and Tompkins (1975) have indicated that the most economic method is to treat all sore throats with penicillin without bothering to wait for the results of the throat culture, or indeed without taking a throat culture at all.

In light of these data and opinions, it is not surprising that some authorities have reservations about the currently accepted academic norms for the treatment of streptococcal pharyngitis. As stated in an editorial in the British Medical Journal (1972):

> Despite the massive effort devoted to the study of streptococcal infection, particularly in America, the last word has yet to be written on the utility of swabbing sore throats and giving the patients penicillin. But in the meantime, doctors should critically examine their traditional approach to this common affliction.

What appears to be a simple recommendation of withholding antibiotic treatment until the result of the throat culture is available is not universally accepted. Therefore, the experience of primary care clinicians who deal with the run-of-the-mill cases of ST should be of interest.

Treatment Patterns for URI and ST

Methods

The data for this study were obtained from the Oregon Region of the Kaiser-Permanente Medical Care Program, which is a prepaid group practice providing medical care services to an enrolled membership of more than 200,000 people in the metropolitan area of Portland, Oregon. The study period for the analysis is January 1972 through June 1973. During that period, primary medical care for members under 16 years of age was provided by board-trained pediatricians; those over 16 years of age received care from board-trained internists and physician assistants supervised by the internists. Most of the services for the health plan members in the study period were provided by a group of physicians using a single hospital and providing office care in a number of outpatient facilities located throughout the city.

Since 1965, the Kaiser-Permanente Health Services Research Center has been conducting an ongoing study of the utilization of ambulatory medical care. The population for this study is a 5 percent random sample of all families subscribing to the medical care program (Greenlick et al., 1968). As part of the continuing utilization study, all medical care contacts of the sample population are recorded by specially trained medical records technicians. Information on these contacts describes the nature of the contact, the service provided, the presenting symptoms, and the clinical diagnoses.

Because for this analysis, we were interested in determining the usual patterns of treatments, we accepted the clinical diagnoses of URI that were made at the time of the first visit, even if subsequent observation occasionally suggested a different illness to have been present. Similarly, we accepted clinical impressions of streptococcal pharyngitis, even if throat cultures had not yet or did not subsequently substantiate the presence of Group A beta-hemolytic streptococcus.

Both URI and ST have some similar complicating bacterial illnesses, such as otitis media. We are differentiating between the cases for which no complicating illnesses were recorded in the medical record at the time the patient first contacted the physician and the cases for which a complicating illness was recorded after the first contact. This distinction serves a useful purpose in that a complication of URI, such as otitis media, occurring before the treatment was started could not be attributed to improper management, whereas an otitis media developing after a clinical evaluation had been made might have been avoided by appropriate therapy.

Although there were 1573 episodes of URI in the study population during the 18-month study period, the analysis deals mainly with the subgroup of 1194 episodes in which there were no complicating illnesses at the time of the first clinical visit. Thus, 76 percent of cases of URI seen had no complicating illness when first seen by a clinician, and treatment of this subgroup can more confidently be attributed to the presumed viral infection rather than to any bacterial complicating illness. The fact that 76 percent of cases of URI had no complicating illness at the time of the first office visit conflicts with the previous statements suggesting that most cases of URI seen in the office do have a complicating illness (Conn, 1976).

RESULTS

Acute Upper Respiratory Infection (URI)

A high frequency of URI was seen in the age group 0 to 4 years. Within that age group, physicians treated URIs at the rate of 437 episodes per 1000 people per year (see Table 12–1). That was five times the treatment rate among older age groups. Office visits were limited to one per episode in more than 83 percent of the episodes of URI.

The most common laboratory study for initially uncomplicated URI was the throat cul-

Table 12–1. *Number of Episodes of Acute Upper Respiratory Infection and Streptococcal Sore Throat by Age and per 1000 Member Years, 1/72–6/73*

		URI		ST	
Age	Number of Person Years Eligibility	Number of Episodes	Episodes per 1000 Member Years	Number of Episodes	Episodes per 1000 Member Years
0–4	1228	537	437	61	50
5–14	2712	245	90	226	83
15+	8931	791	88	192	21

ture, ordered by pediatricians in 17 percent of the episodes, by internists in 32 percent, and by physician assistants in 45 percent. The use of throat cultures varied from zero to 80 percent among the internists.

Pediatricians had the highest yield of positive throat cultures (18 percent), physician assistants the next highest (12 percent), and internists the lowest (7 percent). The 18 percent yield of positive cultures obtained by the pediatricians was in the range of the 10 to 20 percent streptococcus carrier rate reported for all children (Peter and Smith, 1977). The even lower percentage of positive cultures found in the adult population seems to bring into open doubt the validity of taking automatic throat cultures in cases of typical, uncomplicated URI. Further, such practice is not without important cost implications. The charge for a throat culture in the United States is approximately half the charge for an office visit. The rate of positive cultures is so low that physicians should be encouraged to have fairly clear indications before doing a throat culture in completely typical cases of URI.

As might be expected, common treatment for uncomplicated URI is the use of antitussives-expectorants. Of particular interest was the use of antibiotics in cases diagnosed as uncomplicated URI (Table 12–2). We found an insignificant use of antibiotics among the pediatric population (about 1 percent), and an approximate 6 percent use in patients over the age of 16 treated by internists or physician assistants. In contrast to the arguments of primary care physicians who, in the recent literature, defended the use of antibiotics as a prophylaxis against complications of URI, we found such use negligible.

In this medical care program, when complications did occur, patients almost invariably returned to one of the group practice clinicians for continued care. Thus, we were able to document complications, including drug reactions. Outcomes of treatment of initially uncomplicated URI are shown in Table 12–3. Evidence shows that very little complicating illness developed after the first visit, despite the minimal use of antibiotics. In fact, the rate of complications was less than 4 percent, and otitis media was the major cause. The incidence of complications from the use of antibiotics was also not very high; only 2 minor complications in 43 cases treated with antibiotics.

Because the use of antibiotics for both adults and children was very slight and the incidence of complications was very low, the effectiveness of antibiotics in preventing complications is difficult to evaluate. Under ordinary circumstances, however, there appears to be little compelling reason to use antibiotics in uncomplicated URI.

Streptococcal Pharyngitis (ST)

In 18 months, clinicians made a presumptive diagnosis of ST at the time of the first visit in 479 cases. The incidence was far greater among children than among adults (Table 12–1). In the age group 5 to 14, incidence was even greater, with 83 episodes per 1000 patient years. Among those over 15 years of age, incidence dropped to 21 episodes per 1000 patient years. After the age of 45, ST was very uncommon.

A throat culture was obtained by pediatricians 79 percent of the time, by internists 88 percent, and by physician assistants 100 percent (Table 12–4). A positive culture for Group A beta-hemolytic streptococcus was found in 81 percent of the pediatricians' cultures, in 67 percent of the internists' cultures, and in 56 percent of the physician assistants' cultures.

Table 12–2. *Antibiotic Treatment for Episodes of Upper Respiratory Infection Without Complicating Illness at Time of First Office Visit (by Specialty of Physician)*

		Antibiotic Ordered	
Specialty of Physician	Number of Cases	Number	Percent
Internal Medicine	460	28	6.1
Pediatrics	589	8	1.2
Physician assistant	145	7	5.4

Table 12-3. *Complicating Illnesses Related to Acute Upper Respiratory Infection by Age of Patient*

Complicating Illness	Percentage by Age of Patient			
	0–4 Years	5–14 Years	15+ Years	Total (N=1194)
Otitis Media	3.4	2.4	0.9	2.0
Streptococcal sore throat	0.2	—	—	0.1
Pneumonia	0.6	—	0.6	0.5
Bronchitis-tonsillitis	1.1	—	1.3	1.0
Adverse effect of antibiotics	—	—	0.2	0.2

° Antibiotics were received by 264 cases of the 1194 cases of URI with complicating illness.

When we looked at the treatment of the cases of presumed streptococcal pharyngitis, the reason for obtaining throat cultures in a number of circumstances was not completely clear. Pediatricians tended to treat with antibiotics in about half their cases at the time of the patient's first visit (Table 12–5). In 39 percent of their cases, pediatricians withheld antibiotic treatment until the throat culture results were known. Patients over 15 years of age, treated by internists and physician assistants, were even more likely to receive treatment at the first visit (76 percent). In only 13 percent of adult cases was treatment delayed until the results of the culture were available, and in 11 percent of cases, no therapy at all was documented.

One may wonder why internists use antibiotics at the time of the first patient contact as commonly as they appeared to do in this study, in view of the frequent recommendation that treatment be delayed until the results of the throat culture are known (Conn, 1976; Wannamaker, 1976). Neither the department of internal medicine nor the department of pediatrics had a policy designed to influence the decision to treat or not to treat before the culture report was available. Of course, informal peer review pressure may have had some influence. During informal discussions, clinicians offered a number of explanations to account for their decisions to start antibiotic therapy at the time of the first visit. One explanation was a desire to initiate medication while the patient was available in the office. Often, a

Table 12-4. *Use and Results of Throat Cultures in the Treatment of Streptococcal Sore Throat (by Specialty of Physician)*

Specialty	Number of Episodes	Episodes Cultured	Percent Cultured	Number of Cultures Positive°	Percent of Cultures Positive°
Internal Medicine	138	121	87.7	81	66.9
Pediatrics	292	231	79.1	187	81.0
Physician assistant	46	46	100.0	26	56.5
Other	3	2	66.7	2	100.0

° For Group A beta streptococci.

Table 12-5. *Relation of Throat Culture to Antibiotic Treatment for Streptococcal Sore Throat (by Age of Patient)*

Antibiotic Treatment	Percent by Age of Patient			
	0–4 Years	5–14 Years	15+ Years	Total
* Cultured, not treated	14	10	11	11
Treatment and culture at first visit	23	30	67	43
Treatment without culture at first visit	24	17	9	15
Treatment after culture results known	39	43	13	31
Total	100	100	100	100

* All were cultured. Cultures were positive in 8 of 52 cases in this category.

patient could not be tracked down after the results of a positive throat culture were available.

Further, if the clinician had confidence in his judgment, he wished to begin relief of symptoms as soon as possible, particularly since it is possible that early treatment more rapidly decreases symptoms (Merenstein and Rogers, 1974). Concern for early treatment had priority over concern about possible complications from the use of antibiotics. Still another explanation was that the clinician doubted the significance of negative throat culture in the face of a clinical impression that streptococcus was present, since negative throat cultures can be expected in at least 20 percent of cases of actual streptococcal infection (Rosenstein, Markowitz, and Gordis, 1970; Battle and Glasgow, 1971). It is also possible that the clinician allowed the expectations of either patient or family to influence his decision to treat a symptomatic individual brought in for medical care.

In reviewing the charts of all patients in this study, we found that once treatment was started, it was not usually discontinued, regardless of which primary care physician was treating the patient. When antibiotic treatment is to be started at the time of the first visit and is not to be stopped regardless of the results of the throat culture, the rationale for using this laboratory procedure is not very clear. Here again, it appears that the throat culture is often being done ritualistically, with little effect on initial or subsequent treatment. As we have already noted, the costs of throat cultures are not insignificant and frequently may represent a waste of money.

Complications of ST and its Treatment. Complications resulting from the episodes of ST in our study were extremely uncommon; they occurred in only 3 of the 479 episodes and 2 of those were in patients awaiting a culture report before receiving antibiotic therapy. We found no cases of rheumatic fever resulting from ST. In fact, there were no cases of acute rheumatic fever in the entire 5 percent sample (containing 9000 persons) during the 18 months of the study.

Complications from antibiotics were also surprisingly infrequent—only 3 cases of a minor nature in the 429 ST patients who received antibiotic therapy. Two of those complications were gastrointestinal upset; the third case was a rash. This low incidence of complication of antibiotic treatment is an important consideration and may be an additional explanation for the usual tendency of internists to treat before the report of a throat culture is available.

Conclusion

Upper respiratory infections (URI) presented to the primary care clinician in this study without significant associated illness over 76 percent of the time. These uncomplicated URIs were rarely treated with antibiotics. Despite this, even in the age group having the highest incidence of URI with complicating illness present at the time of the first visit (0 to 4 years of age), the incidence of new complications was extremely low, never exceeding 5 percent. Complications occurring after the first office visit were usually otitis media. Pneumonia occurred in less than 1 percent of all such initially uncomplicated URIs. Relatively few cases of uncomplicated URI's received antibiotics at the time of their contact with the clinician (less than 4 percent).

Laboratory studies in cases presumed to be URIs were predominantly throat cultures. These were done in 17 percent of the cases seen by the pediatrician and 32 percent of those seen by internists. The incidence of throat cultures positive for Group A beta-hemolytic streptococci was 18 percent in pediatric patients and 7 percent in patients seen by the internists. The yield of positive cultures, therefore, was little different from that seen in an asymptomatic pediatric population.

Clinicians usually ordered a throat culture for cases of presumed streptococcal pharyngitis. In this series, antibiotic treatment was delayed until results of the throat culture were available in only13 percent of the cases seen by internists or physician assistants and in 39 percent of the cases seen by pediatricians. Once started, antibiotic treatment was not usually discontinued, even when the throat culture was subsequently reported to be negative. Complications of streptococcal pharyngitis or antibiotics were rarely encountered in this series.

These data present the usual care of URI and streptococcal pharyngitis seen by this sample of primary care clinicians and show, as well, the outcome of that care. It is our hope that this information will contribute to the development of a more rational approach to the treatment of these two common illnesses so often seen in office practice. At least three of the usual recommendations should be reconsidered:

1. Throat culture in cases of uncomplicated URI may be a wasteful procedure that has little clinical value. This procedure should be done only in cases of suspected bacterial pharyngitis.

2. Antibiotic treatment for cases of URI uncomplicated with any other illness at the time of the first visit is of little value because these cases seldom develop complications. Complications from antibiotics, as well as the cost, should be considered in the decision to use this medication in simple cases of URI.

3. The value of throat cultures when antibiotics are given at the time the patient with presumed streptococcal pharyngitis is first seen by the clinician is open to question, as such therapy, once initiated, is not usually stopped even after the throat culture is reported to be negative.

References

Ambulatory Health Care Newsletter. 1:1, 1977.

Battle, C.U., and Glasgow, L.A.: Reliability of bacteriologic identification of β-hemolytic streptococci in private offices. Am. J. Dis. Child. 122:134, 1971.

Beeson, P.B., and McDermott, W.: *Textbook of Medicine,* Vol. II. Philadelphia, W.B. Saunders Co., 1975.

Br. Med. J. 3:132, 1972.

Brook, R.H.: Quality assurance: the state of the art. Hosp. Med. Staff 3:15, 1974.

Brook, R.H., Davies-Avery, A., Greenfield, S., Harris, L.J., Lelah, T., Solomon, N.E., and Ware, J.E., Jr.: Assessing the quality of medical care using outcome measures: an overview method. Med. Care 15 (Supplement):1, 1977.

Burns, D.C., Cable, W.E., and Tompkins, R.E.: The cost-effectiveness of acute rheumatic fever prevention, abstracted. Clin. Res. 23:441, 1975.

Couch, R.B., Viral respiratory infections. In Conn, H.F., *Current Therapy 1976,* Philadelphia, W.B. Saunders Co., 1976.

Department of Health, Education and Welfare: Chapter VII, PSRO health care review responsibility. In *PSRO Program Manual.* Washington, D.C., U.S. Government Printing Office, 1974.

Dudding, B.A.: Streptococcal pharyngitis. In Conn, H.F., *Current Therapy 1976,* Philadelphia, W.B. Saunders Co., 1976.

Freeborn, D.K., Baer, D., Greenlick, M.R., and Bailey, J.W.: Determinants of medical care utilization: physicians' use of laboratory services. Am. J. Public Health, 62:846, 1972.

Freeborn, D.K., and Greenlick, M.R.: Evaluation of the performance of ambulatory systems: research requirements and opportunities. Med. Care 11 (Supplement):68, 1973.

Goran, M.J., Roberts, J.S., Kellogg, M., Fielding, J., and Jessee, W.: The PSRO review system. Med. Care. 13 (Supplement):1, 1975.

Greenlick, M.R., Hurtado, A.V., Pope, C.R., Saward, E.W., and Yoshioka, S.S.: Determinants of medical care utilization. Health Serv. Res. 3:296, 1968.

Lasagna, L.: An open letter on colds and antibiotics. Med. Trib. 17:1, Nov. 10, 1976.

Lasagna, L.: An open letter on colds and antibiotics, part II. Med. Trib. 17:1, Nov. 17, 1976.

Medical Tribune: Internist OKs empiric use of antibiotics, interview with Dr. Stead. 17:1, Nov. 24, 1976.

Merenstein, J.H., and Rogers, K.D.: Streptococcal pharyngitis: early treatment and management by nurse practitioners. JAMA 227:1278, 1974.

Mondzac, A.M.: Throat culture processing in the office—a warning. JAMA 200:1132, 1967.

Peter, G., and Smith, A.L.: Group A streptococcal infections of the skin and pharynx (second of two parts). N. Engl. J. Med. 297:365, 1977.

Quinn, R.W.: The positive throat culture—what does it mean? South. Med. J. 67:1009, 1974.

Rosenstein, B.J., Markowitz, M., and Gordis, L.: Accuracy of throat cultures processed in physicians' offices. J. Pediatr. 76:606, 1970.

Schroeder, S.A., Schliftman, A., and Piemme, T.E.: Variation amoung physicians in use of laboratory tests: relation to quality of care. Med. Care 12:709, 1974.

Starfield, B., and Scheff, D.: Effectiveness of pediatric care: the relationship between processes and outcome. Pediatrics 49:547, 1972.

Wannamaker, L.W.: A penicillin shot without culturing the child's throat. JAMA 235:913, 1976.

A Management Strategy for Sore Throat Based on Cost-Effectiveness Analysis

Richard K. Tompkins, M.D.[*]
United States Public Health Service Hospital, Seattle

Evaluating and treating patients with pharyngitis is a common, routine activity for all providers of primary medical services. Sore throat is the third most common symptom that causes patients to visit a physician's office (lower extremity and back pain rank first and second), and in 1975, it was responsible for an estimated 15.3 million office visits (National Center for Health Statistics, 1977). The effort and resources devoted to pharyngitis management are concerned with one objective: to diagnose and treat patients with group A streptococcal infections. This illness has been shown to be a predisposing factor for acute rheumatic fever (ARF) and acute glomerulonephritis, and it is one cause of severe local infection (e.g., peritonsillar abscess). Prompt treatment can prevent most of its complications and limit its spread.

The throat culture is the only diagnostic test that can distinguish accurately between streptococcal and other forms of pharyngitis. Currently accepted medical care standards recommend culturing all patients with sore throats and treating with penicillin those whose cultures are positive for group A streptococci (Kaplan et al., 1977). This straightforward approach, however, is often not used in practice, is unrealistic in many medical care settings, and is not necessarily the most cost-effective strategy for most patient populations. In actuality, therefore, patients with pharyngitis are evaluated and treated in many different ways, and because the disease is so prevalent, the medical decisions have enormous impact:

1. Pharyngitis and respiratory tract illness in general are major determinants of antimicrobial use.

2. Large sums of money are spent on pharyngitis management: a minimal estimate of annual medical care costs is about $300 million (Tompkins et al., 1977a).

3. Pharyngitis management not only costs dollars but also consumes valuable human resources. Patient time is lost seeking care, provider time that might be used in addressing other health problems goes into pharyngitis management, microbiology laboratories or office technicians must process large numbers of throat cultures, and clerical personnel have to handle the throat culture paperwork and inform patients of throat culture results.

I shall review the major issues concerning pharyngitis evaluation and management from both a medical and cost-effectiveness viewpoint. A specific clinical strategy for management will be presented, which may help physicians to standardize their approach to the sore throat patient with the knowledge that they are maximizing medical effectiveness and minimizing costs.

[*] The opinions expressed herein are exclusively those of the author and not of either the Department of Health, Education and Welfare or the University of Washington.

Identifying the Patient Infected with Streptococci

The throat culture is a sensitive test (Kaplan, 1972) that, when performed properly, will identify about 90 percent of patients with group A streptococci in their pharynx (streptococcal-positive). In nonepidemic situations, these patients constitute about 10 percent of all adult patients with sore throats (Tompkins et al., 1977b) and about 35 percent of children. However, fewer than 50 percent of patients with positive cultures are actually infected with streptococci and are at any risk of developing complications. Noninfected patients will not benefit from antibiotic treatment, nor do they spread infection; most are probably chronic carriers with some other cause for their symptoms (Kaplan, 1971; Wannamaker, 1976; Stollerman, 1975).

Although the throat culture will miss only 10 percent of streptococcal-positive patients, epidemiologic data suggest that subclinical infections—in individuals who do not come to the attention of a physician—may account for many of the true streptococcal infections (Markowitz and Gordis, 1972). Some of these people undoubtedly are infected by contact with symptomatic individuals, as is suggested by the streptococcal-positive throat cultures in up to 25 percent of family contacts of infected children (James et al., 1960; Levine et al., 1966). Thus, a physician who treats patients with penicillin only on the basis of a positive throat culture will miss at least 10 percent of the symptomatic, streptococcal-positive patients as well as all the asymptomatic infected patients, an unknown proportion of whom are at risk for ARF development. Furthermore, 50 to 60 percent of the streptococcal-positive antibiotic-treated patients will not be infected and will not benefit from such therapy. Additionally, because 24 to 48 hours are needed before throat culture results are available, treatment will not be given early enough to reduce the patient's symptoms (Merenstein and Rogers, 1974) or to decrease the chance of spreading the disease to family members (Breese and Disney, 1956), and some streptococcal-positive patients will be lost to follow-up and not be treated at all (Glass and Cohen, 1977). Thus, it is clear that the diagnostic and therapeutic strategy currently recommended by most authorities fails to identify and treat many streptococcal-infected patients, does little for the patient's symptoms, is not optimal in preventing spread of the disease, and consumes significant resources.

Efficacy and Toxicity of Treatment

Penicillin (oral or intramuscular), erythromycin, and lincomycin are effective in eradicating pharyngeal group A streptococci (Stollerman, 1975). Presumably, therefore, any of these antibiotics will also prevent associated complications. Spread of infection to family contacts can be decreased by penicillin treatment of the sicker patients within 48 hours of symptom onset (Breese and Disney, 1956). Early treatment (within 24 hours) also diminishes symptom duration and morbidity for some patients (Merenstein and Rogers, 1974). Most importantly, however, intramuscular penicillin has been shown to be effective in preventing primary acute rheumatic fever (acute glomerulonephritis probably is not prevented by treatment).

On the negative side, penicillin treatment carries with it the risk of allergic reactions, some of which may be serious (Tompkins et al., 1977a). Published figures for allergic reaction rates to benzathine and oral penicillin vary from 0.55 percent (oral penicillin G, 0.5 gm daily) to 5.20 percent (benzathine penicillin, 1.2 million units IM given to adults). The best estimate—based on data from very large patient populations with good follow-up—is that a person without a penicillin allergy history has less than 1 chance in 100 (0.94 percent) of reacting to intramuscular benzathine penicillin and, at most, a 0.55 percent chance when oral penicillin is used. Benzathine penicillin results in at least 2.5 times as many serious reactions (predominantly serum sickness) as does oral penicillin. Death from benzathine penicillin allergy, however, is an extremely unusual event (Frank et al., (1965); there were *no* deaths when 315,000 military recruits were given intramuscular benzathine penicillin to prevent streptococcal epidemics.

PRIMARY ACUTE RHEUMATIC FEVER PREVENTION

Penicillin treatment is very effective in preventing ARF in patients with streptococcal pharyngitis. The probability of a patient with untreated streptococcal pharyngitis developing ARF is 2.90 percent in streptococcal epidemics (Wannamaker et al., 1951) and 0.64 percent in the endemic situation (Siegel et al., 1961). Intramuscular penicillin treatment reduces the probabilities tenfold. Of patients who develop ARF and receive optimal medical management, only 3.90 percent will develop severe rheumatic heart disease within 8 years (Wood et al., 1964). Therefore, the chance, under endemic circumstances, that a child with untreated streptococcal positive pharyngitis will develop significant rheumatic heart disease is 1.5×10^{-4}.* These probabilities, derived from clinical data collected in the early 1950s and 1960s, are the basis for the current treatment standards.

Epidemiologic data (Markowitz and Gordis, 1972) collected in the mid-1960s show a decrease in the prevalence of rheumatic heart disease over the prior 20 years. The incidence and severity of primary acute rheumatic fever may have decreased, but the available data are inconclusive. A change in ARF epidemiology could be due to many different factors, including better recognition and treatment of streptococcal infections, fewer epidemics, and better living and health conditions nationally. The possibility also exists that the rheumatogenic capability of group A streptococci may have decreased (Bisno et al., 1977), thus lowering the ARF probability in patients with untreated streptococcal pharyngitis. The varying ARF prevalence in different geographic regions at different times of the year also suggests that rheumatogenicity may vary among streptococcal strains. Unfortunately, reliable data are not available either to support these hypotheses or to allow a recalculation of the probability of ARF. The conscientious physician, eager to prevent ARF in his patient with pharyngitis and anxious not to treat patients who do not need antibiotics, is thus caught in a dilemma. The only controlled studies of ARF prevention mandate penicillin therapy for streptococcal-positive pharyngitis, but low ARF prevalence rates, undoubtedly influenced by success in treating streptococcal disease, raise the possibility that medical care costs are higher than can be justified by potential benefits.

*Probability of being infected (0.59) × probability of ARF (0.0064) × probability of ARF leading to RHD (0.039) = 1.47×10^{-4}.

Cost-Effective Pharyngitis Management

The foregoing discussion has highlighted some of the complexities that must be considered when deciding how to manage a patient with a sore throat. Because of these, and because the prevalence of pharyngitis is so high and its economic impact so large, decision analysis was used to study the cost effectiveness of alternative ways to manage pharyngitis and to prevent acute rheumatic fever (Tompkins et al., 1977a). Published data were used to calculate values and probabilities, and the costs and medical efficacy of the three following pharyngitis management strategies were compared (Figure 12–1):

A. Culturing all patients and treating with penicillin those whose throat cultures are positive for group A streptococci.

B. Treating all patients with penicillin without taking a throat culture.

Figure 12-1.

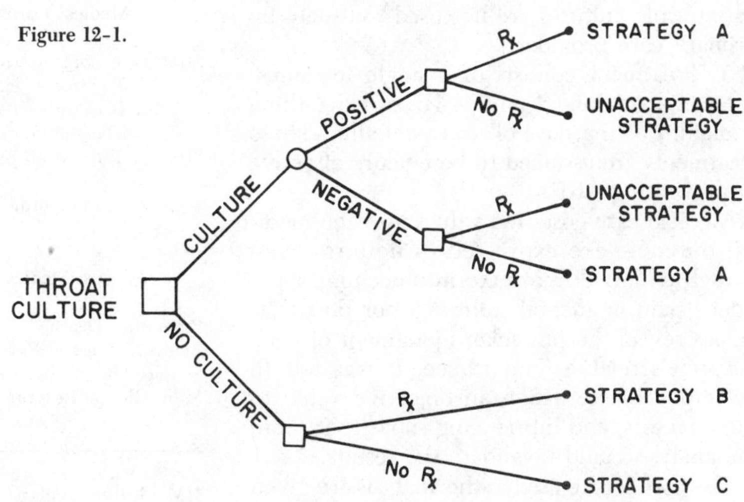

C. Neither culturing nor treating any patients.

An analysis was done for both epidemic and endemic situations and for both intramuscular and oral penicillin treatment. The results of the analysis can be used to select other cost-effective approaches to pharyngitis management that attempt to make an early penicillin treatment decision without awaiting throat culture results.

Details of the Analysis

The decision trees, the analytic methods, and the calculation of the probabilities and costs have been published and will not be repeated. In order to understand the results, however, it is important to know the assumptions on which the analysis was based.

Adverse medical outcomes considered in the decision trees included acute rheumatic fever, death from an allergic reaction, nonfatal serious allergic reactions to penicillin (anaphylaxis and serum sickness), and mild penicillin allergies (principally urticaria). In performing the analysis and in suggesting alternative approaches to pharyngitis management, the following assumptions were made about the patient populations:

1. No patient has had a prior attack of rheumatic fever.
2. No patient has a history of penicillin allergy.
3. Within each patient population, there are carriers (i.e., not infected) of group A streptococci, as well as patients with streptococcal pharyngitis.
4. A single throat culture is used in strategy A (multiple cultures are not used routinely by primary care providers).
5. Treatment consists of a single intramuscular injection of 1.2 million IUs of benzathine penicillin or ten days of oral penicillin. These treatments are assumed to be equally effective in preventing ARF.

Medical care costs and values for each medical outcome are expressed in dollars—even though dollars do not take into account a patient's pain or mental suffering, nor do dollar values reveal the physician's judgment of each outcome's relative importance. It was felt to be impossible to assign an objective value to these factors, and introducing subjectivity into the analysis could invalidate the results.

The cost figures used in the analysis are given in Table 12–6. Charges for throat cultures, office visits, and penicillin are derived from the rates charged in 1974 by a prepaid group clinic in southern New Hampshire, where most patients with sore throats are managed by physician's assistants. These charges are probably no higher than those in most other primary care facilities; indeed, a survey of hospital-based laboratories in Seattle indicated that the average 1977 throat culture charge was $6.00. Increasing unit costs, especially for throat cultures, will be shown to have a profound effect on the cost effectiveness of treatment.

Analysis Results

Analyses were done separately for epidemic and endemic streptococcal pharyngitis. In the epidemic situation, it was shown that early treatment without relying on throat culture results (strategy B) is least costly and most effective medically. Since this strategy has been used for years in the armed forces to control streptococcal epidemics (Frank et al., 1965; Schneider et al., 1964; Seal et al., 1954), there appears to be little controversy in these recom-

Table 12–6. *Cost Figures Used in Analyses*

Unit Costs (in Dollars)	
Throat Culture	2.00
Oral or Benzathine Penicillin	3.00
Patient Time per Office Visit	4.50
Diagnostic Office Visit	10.00
Therapy Only Office Visit	4.00
Daily cost of Hospitalization	94.00
Medical Care Strategy Costs (in Dollars)	
Strategy A (culture, treat positives)	
No Treatment (culture negative patients)	16.50
IM Benzathine Penicillin*	28.00
Oral Penicillin	19.50
Strategy B (treat all patients, oral or IM penicillin)	17.50
Strategy C (no culture or treatment)	14.50
Adverse Medical Outcome Costs (in Dollars)	
Premature Death	72,000.00
Acute Rheumatic Fever	10,560.00
Serious Allergic Reaction	826.00
Mild Allergic Reaction	15.00

*IM = Intramuscular

mendations. For the endemic situation, the principal population was that described by Siegel, Johnson, and Stollerman (1961). These patients were predominantly middle-class children of Chicago, who were seen for their pharyngitis in a university outpatient clinic.

The results for this endemic population are in Table 12–7. The data show that ARF prevention is cost effective: the total predicted cost per patient is higher for strategy C (no antibiotic treatment) than for either strategy A or B, both of which include penicillin therapy. The data also indicate that strategy B is the most effective medically and costs less per patient, particularly with optimal oral penicillin therapy, than either of the other strategies. However, the cost difference between strategy A and strategy B is less than 10 percent of the total predicted cost, and the incidence of serious penicillin reactions in strategy B is more than twice that in strategy A. Although the ARF cases prevented by either antibiotic treatment strategy are few (approximately 2 per 1000 patients), there is a considerable saving in the predicted adverse outcome cost (allergies plus ARF). When oral penicillin and strategy B are used, the adverse outcome costs are 13 percent of those incurred with strategy C and 63 percent of those with strategy A.

Total predicted cost per patient for any treatment strategy varies in direct proportion to the prevalence of streptococcal infection, which is indirectly measured by determining the incidence of streptococcal-positive patients (positive throat culture rate) in any population. This direct relationship between per patient costs and positive throat culture rates (Figure 12–2) reflects the rise in ARF cases with increasing numbers of infected patients. The data on which Figure 12–2 is based are from an analysis of eight different endemic situations that involved both adult and pediatric patients. The point at which the curves for each strategy intersect denote equivalent cost effectiveness. For instance, strategies A and B are equally cost effective in a patient population with a streptococcal-positive rate of 0.20. When the incidence is higher, strategy B (treat all patients) is more cost effective. Likewise, when the rate falls below 0.07, the no treatment strategy (C) is preferable. Thus, knowing that a patient population's streptococcal-positive rate—which can be assessed by clinical criteria alone—is likely to fall below 0.07 or to rise above 0.20

Table 12-7. *Endemic Situation: Effectiveness of Alternative Treatment Strategies*

	Predicted Cases per 1000 Sore Throat Patients		
	(A) CULTURE TREAT	(B) TREAT ALL	(C) NO TREATMENT
Acute Rheumatic Fever	0.33	0.17	1.75
IM Benzathine Penicillin:°			
Serious Allergy	2.6	6.4	0.00
Mild Allergy	1.2	3.0	0.00
Total Predicted Cost/Patient	$26.97	$24.90	$32.94
Allergic Reaction Cost	2.27	5.56	0.00
ARF Cost°	3.50	1.84	18.44
Patient Time Cost	6.34	4.50	4.50
Medical Care Cost	14.86	13.00	10.00
Oral Penicillin:			
Serious Allergy	0.10	0.25	0.00
Mild Allergy	2.10	5.20	0.00
Total Predicted Cost/Patient	$21.42	$19.84	$32.94
Allergic Reaction Cost	.20	.50	0.00
ARF Cost°	3.50	1.84	18.44
Patient Time Cost	4.50	4.50	4.50
Medical Care Cost	13.22	13.00	10.00

° IM = Intramuscular; ARF = Acute Rheumatic Fever

Data for analysis obtained from Siegel et al. (1961).

Figure 12-2.

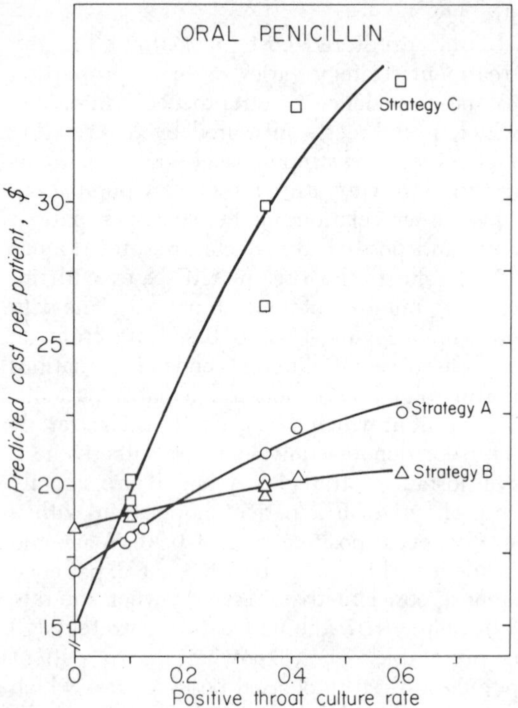

allows a treatment decision to be made for an individual patient within the population.

Throat culture cost is another important variable that must be considered. If it is higher than the $2.00 used in this analysis, the cost difference between strategies A and B is magnified. Since all patients managed by strategy A (culture, treat positives) receive a throat culture, the predicted cost per patient for this strategy varies directly with the throat culture cost, whereas total costs of strategy B (treat all) and strategy C (no culture or treatment) are not affected. Raising the cost to $4.00 per culture makes strategy A more costly than strategy B at all streptococcal-positive rates.

Another important variable in determining the relative cost effectiveness of the three strategies is the probability of an allergic reaction occurring with benzathine penicillin treatment. When oral penicillin can be used effectively, the probability of allergic reaction is so low that it has no significant effect on the predicted cost per patient.

The analysis illustrates an important principle: cost-effective medical care for some illnesses does not always require the most powerful diagnostic test available in the physician's armamentarium. Lower diagnostic accuracy may be quite acceptable when disease incidence is low, the chance of morbidity is minimal, and treatment carries little risk for the patient. If the accuracy in determining a patient's chance of having pharyngitis does not require the diagnostic power provided by the throat culture, clinical criteria alone (i.e., history and physical examination) may be used to select patients with a defined chance of having streptococcal-positive pharyngitis. Knowing the probability that a patient will be streptococcal-positive usually is sufficient to allow a penicillin treatment decision, if the throat culture cost is known and if the cost-effectiveness analysis discussed above is accepted as valid.

Treatment Decisions Based on Clinical Guidelines

Clinical characteristics of patients with streptococcal positive and negative pharyngitis have been compared in several different pediatric and adult populations. The incidence of positive throat cultures is highest in school-aged children and lowest in patients under 6 or over 35 years old. Among adults, women with sore throats are at least twice as likely as men to be streptococcal-positive; about 80 percent of women who are positive will be between the ages of 18 and 35.

Table 12-8 presents data that characterize some history and physical examination findings (attributes) useful for identifying streptococcal-positive patients. It is clear that none of the attributes by itself is satisfactory. Those that are adequately sensitive (e.g., age, pharyngeal erythema, cervical adenitis) lack specificity, and, if used by themselves to determine treatment, would cause one to treat 70 percent of the patients inappropriately. Conversely, attributes that are most specific (e.g., recent streptococcal exposure, fever of 38.3°C or greater) are not adequately sensitive and, if used alone, would miss many streptococcal-positive patients. None of the attributes has a predictive value very much above the streptococcal prevalence of the original population (15 percent), indicating that they are not very useful for selecting streptococcal-positive patients. Additionally, some attributes are not reproducible*, such as "history of streptococcal exposure" and

* Interphysician agreement is expressed by the kappa (k) statistic, which varies between −1 for complete disagreement and +1 for perfect agreement. Zero indicates random agreement.

Table 12-8. *Clinical Predictors of Streptococcal-Positive Patients*[*]

	Sensitivity	Specificity	Positive Value	Overall Accuracy	Inter-MD Agreement (kappa)[†]
Random Choice	0.50	0.50	0.15	0.50	0.00
Female	0.84	0.38	0.20	0.45	1.00
Age <35 years	0.94	0.18	0.17	0.30	1.00
Streptococcal exposure (recent)	0.25	0.88	0.27	0.78	0.12
Absence of cough	0.83	0.48	0.22	0.53	0.87
Absence of rhinorrhea	0.73	0.48	0.20	0.52	0.75
Fever ≥38.3°C	0.17	0.94	0.33	0.82	0.94
Pharyngeal erythema	0.98	0.16	0.17	0.28	0.36
Pharyngeal exudate	0.47	0.79	0.29	0.74	0.36
Enlarged/tender cervical nodes	0.94	0.27	0.19	0.37	0.02

[*] Data on adult patients calculated from Walsh et al. (1975). The streptococcal positive prevalence rate in this patient population was 0.15. Similar data were calculated from Breese and Disney (1954) and Stillerman and Bernstein (1961), who dealt with children. Data from all three patient groups fit on the identical ROC curve.

[†] Kappa values: complete agreement = +1.0; complete disagreement = −1.0; zero values = agreement due to chance. Data from Wood et al. (1978).

"enlarged or tender cervical nodes"; important throat abnormalities are also not very reproducible, although physicians do agree significantly more than by chance alone. Combining attributes into decision rules or algorithms (Walsh et al., 1975) can overcome some of the deficiencies noted above—that is, an acceptable sensitivity can be maintained while increasing specificity, predictive value, and overall accuracy. Treatment decisions based on combinations of attributes can be at least 70 percent as accurate as basing treatment on throat cultures results.

Noteworthy is the potential utility of gram stain examination of a pharyngeal swab. Crawford, Brancato, and Holmes (1979) have developed and evaluated an easily performed, reproducible (kappa = 0.68), inexpensive (about $2.00) diagnostic test, the results of which can be available within minutes. A penicillin treatment decision based on the pharyngeal gram stain is superior to decision rules based only on historical and physical exam criteria; its use results in few streptococcal-negative patients receiving antibiotics (specificity = 0.96). When used jointly with appropriate clinical criteria for patient selection, it should permit early penicillin treatment for most streptococcal-positive patients at a cost per patient well below that of the throat culture. If these results are confirmed, the pharyngeal swab gram stain may simplify medical management of sore throat patients.

Clinical strategies also have the potential for reducing the number of patients needing contact with a medical care provider. For instance, Honikman and Massell (1971) showed that 81 percent of streptococcal-positive children had pure or predominant sore throat and a temperature above 37°C, or they had fever of 38.3°C (101° F) or greater with or without other symptoms. The remaining patients had only a 3 percent chance of being streptococcal-positive, and, furthermore, they constituted 70 percent of the entire population. Based on the cost-effectiveness analysis, this group of children would not benefit enough from treatment to warrant the expense and risk of medical evaluation or intervention. Adequate telephone triage could prevent these children and their families from making an unnecessary office visit. Walsh et al. (1975) demonstrated a similar situation in an adult population: 33 percent of patients with sore throats lacked a history of streptococcal exposure, had a cough, and their oral temperature was less than 37.8°C (100° F). These patients had only a 5 percent risk of being streptococcal-positive, which is not high enough to warrant medical evaluation.

Thus, the objectives of a medical strategy for sore throat management should be:

1. To identify and treat properly those patients who are at sufficient risk of being streptococcal-positive to justify treatment on a cost-effectiveness basis.

2. To make a treatment decision as soon after illness onset as possible, preferably within 48 hours. (Realistically, this means at the patient's initial contact with the medical care system.)

3. To identify those patients who will not benefit from treatment sufficiently to justify any diagnostic evaluation.

Decision Tree

Figure 12–3 presents a decision tree for adults with sore throats that will accomplish all three objectives. In one population of 1338 adults seen in a New Hampshire clinic (Tompkins et al., 1977b), these rules would have correctly treated 81 percent of the patients, with a sensitivity of 0.86 and a specificity of 0.80. If these same adult patients had telephoned before coming to the clinic, the decision tree rules could have permitted a treatment decision for 51 percent of them without a clinic visit. Of the patients with streptococcal pharyngitis, 74 percent would have received antibiotic treatment on the same day; only 32 percent of all patients would have required a throat culture. Because of potential differences between patient populations, this strategy's efficacy should be validated prospectively (before being implemented in other clinical sites) by obtaining throat cultures on the initial 300 to 400 patients. This will permit calculation of the popula-

Figure 12-3.

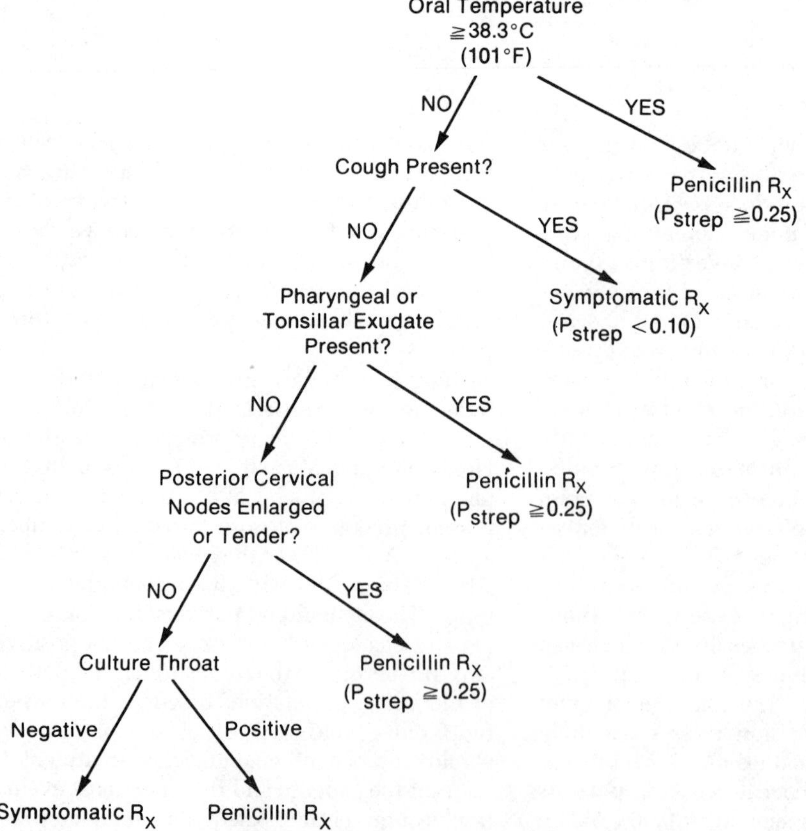

tion-specific sensitivity, specificity, and overall accuracy, as well as the predicted positive throat culture rate (P_{strep}) for each endpoint in the decision tree. If an endpoint's (P_{strep}) falls within the expected range (see Figure 12–3), and the throat culture costs at least $2.00, the recommended decisions are cost-effective. Should the pharyngeal gram stain be available and its use be routine and accurate, it could replace the throat culture and also refine penicillin treatment decisions, with improvement in treatment accuracy and treatment of more patients at the initial office visit. Sore throat patients may need to be evaluated for other treatable disease not addressed by this decision tree, such as otitis media, sinusitis, and pneumonia. Algorithms that give decision rules for all adult respiratory illness patients have been defined and evaluated (Greenfield et al., 1974; Wood et al., 1978), but their content is beyond this discussion.

Conclusion

This recommended approach to pharyngitis management differs substantially from generally recommended methods. Results of a formal cost-effectiveness analysis have been used to select decision rules for treating individual patients with acute pharyngitis. In order to do this, several major assumptions were made:

1. *The cost-effectiveness analysis is accurate.* This implies accepting, within measurable limits, the probabilities, values, and decision trees used in the analysis. It could be argued that there is too much uncertainty in the data on which the analysis was based to justify accepting the results. Granted that uncertainties do exist, the data are still the basis for all clinicians' decisions about pharyngitis management. By performing formal decision analyses, uncertainties were made explicit—it was shown where the results are likely to be affected by variances in probabilities and values, and the critical elements needed for a management decision were identified.

2. *The published data used for the cost-effectiveness analysis are applicable to patient populations that a practicing physician may encounter.* Because the conclusions were consistent when clinical data collected by several investigators were analyzed, it is likely that the results also apply to other populations.

3. *Cost should be a factor in medical decision-making.* In many respects, this contradicts traditional medical teaching, which, in the past, has demanded that the physician do as much as possible for his patient without considering the cost of his actions. In a society with unlimited resources for medical care, this philosophy might be appropriate. Reality, however, dictates a different approach. The clinician must explore ways to optimize benefits for his patients and still reduce medical care costs. Interestingly, these two goals are not incompatible (Enthoven, 1978). For instance, the cheapest approach to pharyngitis management is also most effective medically in preventing acute rheumatic fever, relieving symptoms and preventing disease spread.

Is this approach to pharyngitis management really that different from established practice? Regardless of the recommendations about throat culture use, most practitioners probably use decision rules quite similar to those presented here. Their reasons for modifying what some authorities recommend as optimal medical care are probably similar to those presented: practitioners recognize that a same-day penicillin treatment decision is efficient, effective, and not dangerous. The cost-effectiveness analysis and the definition of explicit decision rules for pharyngitis management provide a solid, objective basis for an already widespread practice.

Table 12–9. *Definition of Terms*

Clinical Decisions	Throat Culture Results		
	Positive	Negative	Total
Positive	a	b	c
Negative	d	e	f
Total	g	h	i

GLOSSARY (See Table 12–9 for reference)

Sensitivity: the proportion of streptococcal-positive patients correctly identified by a diagnostic strategy (a/g).

Specificity: the proportion of streptococcal-negative patients correctly identified (e/h).

Overall Accuracy: the proportion of patients correctly identified as either streptococcal-positive or negative (a + e/i).

Predicted Positive Culture Rate: the proportion of patients selected by a diagnostic strategy as "streptococcal-positive" who actually have group A streptococci on their throat culture. That is, the probability that the selected patients will have a positive culture (P_{Strep}); also known as the *positive predictive value* (a/c).

References

Bisno, A.L., Pearce, I.A., and Stollerman, G.H.: Streptococcal infections that fail to cause recurrences of rheumatic fever. J. Infect. Dis. 136:278, 1977.

Breese, B.B., and Disney, F.A.: Factors influencing the spread of beta-hemolytic streptococcal infections within the family group. Pediatrics 17:834, 1956.

Breese, B.B., and Disney, F.A.: The accuracy of diagnosis of beta streptococcal infections in clinical grounds. J. Pediatr. 44:670, 1954.

Commission on Acute Respiratory Diseases: Role of β-hemolytic streptococci in common respiratory diseases. Am. J. Public Health 35:675–682, 1945.

Commission on Acute Respiratory Diseases: The role of Lancefield groups of beta-hemolytic streptococci in respiratory infections. N. Engl. J. Med. 236:157, 1946.

Crawford, G., Brancato, F., and Holmes, K.K.: Streptococcal pharyngitis: diagnosis by gram-stain. Ann. Int. Med. In press, 1979.

Denny, F.W., Wannamaker, L.W., Brink, W.R., et al.: Prevention of rheumatic fever. JAMA 143:151, 1950.

Enthoven, A.C.: Shattuck Lecture—Cutting cost without cutting the quality of care. N. Engl. J. Med. 298:1229, 1978.

Forsyth, R.A.: Selective utilization of clinical diagnosis in treatment of pharyngitis. J. Fam. Pract. 2:173, 1975.

Frank, P.F., Stollerman, G.H., and Miller, L.F.: Protection of a military population from rheumatic fever. JAMA 193:775, 1965.

Glass, R.I., and Cohen, M.: Treatment of streptococcal pharyngitis at initial presentation: a probabilistic model for rational decision making. Clin. Res. 25:459A, 1977.

Greenfield, S., Brass, F.E., McCraith, D.L., et al.: An upper respiratory complaint protocol for physician extenders. Arch. Int. Med. 133:294, 1974.

Honikman, L.H., and Massell, B.F.: Guidelines for the selective use of throat cultures in the diagnosis of streptococcal respiratory infections. Pediatrics 48:573, 1971.

James, W.E.S., Badger, G.F., and Dingle, J.H.: A study of illness in a group of Cleveland families. XIX, The epidemiology of the acquisition of group A streptococci and of associated illnesses. N. Engl. J. Med. 262:687, 1960.

Kaplan, E.L., Bisno, A., Derrick, W., et al.: Prevention of rheumatic fever. Circulation 55:1, 1977.

Kaplan, E.L., Top, F.H., Jr., Dudding, B.A., et al.: Diagnosis of streptococcal pharyngitis: differentiation of active infection from the carrier state in the symptomatic child. J. Infect. Dis. 123:490, 1971.

Kaplan, E.L.: Unsolved problems in diagnosis and epidemiology of streptococcal infection. In Wannamaker, L.L., and Matsen, J.M., eds., *Streptococci and Streptococcal Disease,* New York, Academic Press, 1972.

Komaroff, A.L.: A management strategy for sore throat. JAMA 239:1429, 1978.

Levine, J.I., Chapman, S.S., Guerra, V., et al.: Studies on the transmission within families of group A hemolytic streptococci. J. Lab. Clin. Med. 67:483, 1966.

Markowitz, M., and Gordis, L.: *Rheumatic Fever,* 2nd ed., Philadelphia, W.B. Saunders Co., 1972.

Merenstein, J.H., and Rogers, K.D.: Streptococcal pharyngitis: early treatment and management by nurse practitioners. JAMA 227:1278, 1974.

National Center for Health Statistics: Ambulatory medical care modified in physicians' offices: United States, 1975. Advanced Data, No. 12, October 12, 1977.

Rantz, L.A., Boisvert, P.J., and Spink, W.W.: Hemolytic streptococcic and nonstreptococcic diseases of the respiratory tract. Arch. Intern. Med. 78:369, 1946.

Schneider, W.F., Chapman, S., Schulz, V.B., et al.: Prevention of streptococcal pharyngitis among military personnel and their civilian dependents by mass prophylaxis. N. Engl. J. Med. 270:1205, 1964.

Seal, J.R., Mogabgab, Friou, G.J., et al.: Penicillin prophylaxis of epidemic streptococcal infections. II, The effects of small and large doses of oral penicillin on epidemic streptococcal infections and on carriers of group A streptococci. J. Lab. Clin. Med. 44:832, 1954.

Siegel, A.C., Johnson, E.E., and Stollerman, G.H.: Controlled studies of streptococcal pharyngitis in a pediatric population. 1, factors related to the attack role of rheumatic fever. N. Engl. J. Med. 265:559, 1961.

Stillerman, M., and Bernstein, S.H.: Streptococcal pharyngitis: evaluation of clinical syndromes in diagnosis. Am. J. Dis. Child. 101:476, 1961.

Stollerman, G.H.: *Rheumatic Fever and Streptococcal Infection.* New York, Grune and Stratton, 1975.

Tompkins, R.K., Burnes, D.C., and Cable, W.E.: An analysis of the cost-effectiveness of pharyngitis management and acute rheumatic fever prevention. Ann. Int. Med. 86:481, 1977a.

Tompkins, R.K., Wood, R.W., Wolcott, B.W., and Walsh, B.T.: The effectiveness and cost of acute upper respiratory illness medical care provided by physicians and algorithm-assisted physicians' assistants. Med. Care 15:991, 1977b.

Valkenburg, H.A., Goslings, W.R.O., Bots, A.W., et al.: Attack rate of streptococcal pharyngitis, rheumatic fever and glomerulonephritis in the general population. II, The epidemiology of streptococcal pharyngitis in one village during a two-year period. N. Engl. J. Med. 268:694, 1963.

Walsh, B.T., Bookheim, W.W., Johnson, R.C., and Tompkins, R.K.: Recognition of streptococcal pharyngitis in adults. Arch. Int. Med. 135:1493, 1975.

Wannamaker, L.W.: A penicillin shot without culturing the child's throat. JAMA 235:913, 1976.

Wannamaker, L.W., Rammelkamp, C.H., Jr., Denny, F.W., et al.: Prophylaxis of acute rheumatic fever by treatment of the preceding streptococcal infection with various amounts of depot penicillin. Am. J. Med. 10:673, 1951.

Wood, H.F., Feinstein, A.R., Taranta, A., et al.: Rheumatic fever in children and adolescents. A long-term epidemiologic study of subsequent prophylaxis, streptococcal infections and clinical regimens in preventing streptococcal infections and rheumatic recurrences. Ann. Intern. Med. 60 (suppl 5):31, 1964.

Wood, R.W., Diehr, P., Wolcott, B.W., Slay, L., and Tompkins, R.K.: Reproducibility of clinical data and decisions in the management of upper respiratory illnesses: a double-blind comparison of physicians and non-physician providers. Med. Care. In press, 1978.

Wood, R.W., Tompkins, R.K., and Wolcott, B.W.: Unpublished data, 1978.

13

Which Is Better in Preventing Influenza—Amantadine or Vaccine?

. . . what wastes and deserts of the soul a slight attack of influenza brings to view . . .

Virginia Woolf, *The Moment and Other Essays*

There remains an epidemical distemper, called by the genteel name of l'influenza. *It is a little fever, of which scarcely any body dies . . .*

Lord Chesterfield

During the first great epidemic of influenza toward the end of the nineteenth century a London evening paper sent round a journalist-patient to all the great consultants of that day. . . . The case was the same; but the prescriptions were different, and so was the advice.

George Bernard Shaw, Preface to *The Doctor's Dilemma*

Introduction

The recent swine flu fiasco illustrated many of the problems society and science face in dealing with influenza: the difficulty in predicting epidemics, the lead time required to produce vaccine, the risks from the vaccine itself, the sharp disagreement among experts, and the logistic problems in vaccinating large numbers of people.

Fox admits that flu epidemics cannot be prevented completely, but he points out that vaccine or amantadine can prevent 60 to 80 percent of cases, and that the prophylactic effects of vaccine and drug are additive. He believes that annual vaccination is important for maintenance of a continuing state of immunity, in view of the unpredictability of epidemics. Allergic reactions to vaccines have been the main problem in the past, but recently it has become apparent that a rare complication of flu vaccines, the Guillain-Barré syndrome, can be fatal. Fox argues that the risk of this reaction is far outweighed by the risks of influenza, although fatalities are rare with the latter. He sees no role for amantadine on a populationwide basis because of its side effects and cost, but he does advocate selective use for certain individuals.

Douglas believes that amantadine has been unfairly neglected for a variety of reasons, which he describes cogently. Despite some side effects that are a nuisance, the overall safety of this unusual drug has been well established by its extensive use in parkinsonian patients, the other population for which its use is widely recognized.

The original approval of amantadine as a prophylactic against influenza A has now been extended to include its use in therapy once influenza has developed. Douglas believes that amantadine not only can prevent or treat simple influenza but may prevent or treat pneumonic complications thereof. He recommends that prophylaxis with amantadine be tried only in specific situations, not as a replacement for mass vaccination. In contrast, however, he believes that the drug deserves wider therapeutic use.

Sabin, one of the world's most distinguished virologists, finds the evidence on the efficacy of amantadine as either prophylactic *or* treatment underwhelming. Most importantly, he emphasizes the inevitable disappointment in store for those who intend to prevent what is called "influenza" with either vaccine or amantadine. Sabin's point is that 90 percent of clinical "influenza" is not associated with epidemics or even with the known major influenza viruses. A sobering thought!

Louis Lasagna, M.D.

Which Is Better in Preventing Flu Epidemics—Amantadine or Vaccine?

John P. Fox, M.D., Ph.D.
University of Washington, Seattle

The term *flu epidemic* properly refers to outbreaks of disease due to either type A or type B influenza virus. Although both these viruses cause clinically indistinguishable illnesses, type A epidemics are more frequent and cause greater excess mortality than those of type B. Further, since type B infections are unaffected by amantadine, the question can refer only to type A flu epidemics. Even with this qualification, however, the question cannot be answered as phrased, since there is no realistic way to prevent epidemics. The most one can hope to accomplish is to *protect* individuals against infection. Whether vaccine or amantadine (or a combination) is more appropriate must be determined for each individual in light of certain considerations.

Antigenic Character of Type A Influenza Virus

All type A strains possess identical internal antigens (ribonucleoprotein and matrix protein), but they may differ in their external hemagglutinin (H) and neuraminidase (N) antigens, which are of protective significance. Antibodies to H (hemagglutinin-inhibiting or HI) neutralize the virus and protect against infection, whereas antineuraminidase (NA) inhibits release of virus from infected cells and may help limit clinical response to infection. Both H and N are unstable antigens and commonly undergo variation, which may be complete and abrupt *(antigenic shift)*, or gradual *(antigenic drift)*.

Since 1933, when influenza virus was first isolated from man, three well documented shifts have occurred: in 1957 (Asian flu), in 1968 (Hong Kong flu), and (provisionally) in 1977 (Russian flu). Solid seroarcheologic evidence indicates that a shift also occurred in 1918. All these shifts involved the H, but—at least in 1968—they did not involve the N. This is particularly significant, since immunity induced by infection with the previous variant is ineffective against the new variant. This explains why each of these shifts resulted in worldwide epidemics *(pandemics)*.

Subtypes of H and N are designated numerically. Recent consensus holds that from 1918 to 1957, there was only one H subtype (now designated as H1) rather than three (heretofore designated as Hsw1, H0, and H1). Thus, three subtypes of H and two of N have been identified on "human" type A influenza viruses. These serve to describe variants representing antigenic shifts as follows:

1918	H1N1	Spanish flu
1957	H2N2	Asian flu
1968	H3N2	Hong Kong flu
1977	H1N1	Russian flu

Inclusion of H1N1 in 1977 is provisional, since it is not yet clear whether the prior variant has been replaced. H1N1 virus spread across Russia and China in 1977 and was widely disseminated in other countries, including the United States, in early 1978. However, as of July, 1978, H3N2 strains (1) have reappeared in both China and Russia, (2) were among the latest 1978 isolates recovered in the U.S., and (3) coexist with H1N1 strains in South America. Because of this, vaccine produced for use in the fall of 1978 included two type A antigens (A/Texas-H3N2 and A/USSR-H1N1) as well as B/Hong Kong.

Although both surface antigens undergo drift during the period of prevalence of a major variant, change in H is more important than change in N, since HI antibody relates directly to protection against infection. Although the degree of change from one year to the next is usually small, the cumulative change over several years may be substantial. It is associated with decreased effectiveness of homologous (to the variant) immunity, especially that induced by prior vaccine but, over longer time, also that resulting from prior infection. Thus, in 1947, the prevalent type A virus was sufficiently changed so that it overcame immunity induced by prior infection as well as by vaccine, which had proved highly effective in 1943.

Epidemiologic Considerations

It is convenient to think of the behavior of type A influenza virus in terms of cycles reflecting the periods of introduction and subsequent persistence of major antigenic variants. During the introductory phase, the rapid worldwide spread of the new variant results in major epidemics with little regard to season, and typically affects a wide age spectrum of the population (because H1N1 virus reappeared after only 20 years, the 1977–1978 epidemics of Russian flu have been largely restricted to people under 25). Since neither the antigenic character of the new variant nor the precise time and place of its emergence can be predicted, vaccine cannot be produced and stockpiled in advance. Although the worldwide influenza surveillance by the World Health Oranization (WHO) provides an effective means for recognizing the emergence of new variants, their spread is so rapid that the initial epidemic wave will have occurred in most regions before significant amounts of appropriate vaccine can be made available.

Because the introduction of new variants is usually completed within a year, the great bulk of disease occurs during the interpandemic interval (9 to 38 years), during which time certain characteristics of influenza virus are sufficiently established to be useful in orienting preventive efforts.

One important aspect is *seasonality*. Influenza outbreaks typically occur in the winter, usually peaking in January or February in the northern hemisphere. This means that vaccine is most appropriately given there in the fall. Unfortunately, prediction of epidemic years is so unreliable that annual vaccination is necessary for maximal preventive effect. As an example, the A/Victoria epidemic in 1976 in Houston, Texas, was the sixth H3N2 epidemic in that city since the original A/Hong Kong variant appeared in 1968.

Influenza viruses are spread via airborne droplets of respiratory secretion. Since the virus is relatively labile, transmission is favored by close contact, especially indoors. Although such contact can occur in many settings in the community (e.g., public transit vehicles, stores, movies, etc.), an additional requirement for active transmission is the availability of "susceptibles." Because susceptibility is inversely related to age, settings that bring young people—especially young children—together (day care centers, schools, movies) play key roles in the spread of influenza viruses. Also, the presence of such young people as potential introducers of infection into families increases the risk to older members.

The foregoing helps to define the individual risk of exposure and infection in epidemic situations. For young people, the risk is high because of their probable lack of immunity and their association with equally susceptible peers. Overall risk of infection for older people is lower because they are more likely to be immune (especially later in the interpandemic period). However, for those who may be nonimmune, risk increases with exposure to young people.

Although epidemic years cannot be predicted reliably in advance, influenza surveillance maintained internationally by WHO and in the United States by the Center for Disease Control (CDC) insures that epidemics are recognized as they arise and that their spread is followed. Thus, most of the country has sufficient warning that an epidemic is imminent to put local health authorities on the alert. Several nonvirologic indices (e.g., school or industrial absenteeism, emergency room visits) may signal arrival of an epidemic locally, but the earliest (and most certain) signal is the isolation of influenza virus as the result of systematic cultures of patients (preferably children) with acute febrile respiratory illness.

Evolution of local epidemics is usually so rapid that by the time the signal has been perceived, use of vaccine is of little value, and prevention depends chiefly on avoiding or minimizing exposure. Because of a low level of virus shedding and the absence of cough, subclinical infections are unimportant as sources of infection. Since effective sources are people with symptomatic infection, these sources are potentially recognizable. During epidemics (but not at other times), a high proportion of influenza-like illness is indeed due to influenza virus, a fact that has important implications for the management of patients and recently exposed people.

Influenza Vaccine

In 1943, the recently developed type A influenza vaccine was tested among U.S. military personnel and found to be 70 percent effective. The initial vaccine was a relatively crude product, consisting essentially of formalin-killed virus obtained from the allantoic fluid of infected chick embryos, which was partially purified and then concentrated by adsorption onto and elution from chick embryo red cells. As vaccine was introduced into civilian use, undesirable reactogenicity (especially in children) was reported, and vaccine efficacy was questioned. The relation of efficacy to the changing antigenic character of type A influenza virus was first recognized, as already noted, in 1947.

The history of the further evolution of influenza vaccine and of federal involvement, through the Bureau of Biologics (BOB) and the Food and Drug Administration (FDA), in setting standards of safety and potency and in dictating vaccine formulation is fascinating but not relevant to our present interest. The important point is that early in each year, formulation of vaccine for the coming season (what strains to include as antigens and in what amounts) is determined by the BOB. This decision represents an educated guess (based on knowledge concerning type A strains circulating in the U.S. and elsewhere) as to the antigenic character of the strains that will be active in the next season and against which vaccine-induced immunity is desired. The BOB decision is binding on all U.S. manufacturers of vaccine.

Influenza vaccines now available in the United States are still produced from formalin-inactivated influenza viruses grown in the allantoic sac of developing chick embryos. Although each of the four current vaccine manufacturers employs its own distinctive production methods, the products of two companies—Merck Sharpe and Dohme and Connaught Laboratories (formerly Merrell-National)—contain intact virions (whole virus vaccine), whereas the other two—Parke, Davis and Company and Wyeth Laboratories—employ procedures intended to disrupt the viral particles (subunit vaccine).

Clinical Data

The long-standing dispute over the relative advantages and disadvantages of these two types of vaccine was largely resolved in the course of the federally sponsored nationwide clinical trials of A/New Jersey/76 (H1N1) vaccine (against "swine flu") that were conducted in the summer of 1976. The results of these dose-response trials have been reported in great detail in the December, 1977 Supplement to volume 136 of the *Journal of Infectious Diseases*, but the important features can be stated briefly. First, based on prior experience with H1N1 strains, the trial population could be divided into unprimed (people under age 24, lacking prior experience) and primed (aged 24 and older) subjects. In the latter, good HI antibody response to A/New Jersey antigen was readily elicited by small doses of either type of vaccine. Systemic reactions occurred chiefly in those recipients of larger doses of whole virus vaccines who had low or absent titers of HI antibody to the A/New Jersey virus.

In the younger, unprimed population, immunogenicity and reactogenicity were closely and directly related. In all age groups studied, all doses of subunit vaccines tested were devoid of significant reactogenicity, but no single dose was acceptably immunogenic. Conversely, although whole virus vaccines proved to be immunogenic, their reactogenicity was a major restricting factor. In young adults (17 to 24 years), doses with acceptably low reactogenicity induced marginally acceptable immune response. However, in children aged 10 and younger, all immunogenic doses induced unacceptably frequent and severe reactions. Fortunately, the results of further trials indicated that good immune response could be induced in children as young as six months old without significant reactions when two doses of subunit vaccine were given, separated by an interval of at least one month. Further, children as young as three years old could receive the same doses recommended for adults.

The advent of A/USSR (H1N1) virus as a new major variant strain has led to a smaller scale repetition of the 1976 clinical dose-response trials of vaccines containing the new Russian flu antigen. Since early results of these trials generally conform to those obtained with the swine flu vaccine, the situation with respect to the use of influenza vaccine in the United States during interpandemic intervals can be summarized as follows.

Interpandemic Use of Vaccine

Single nonreactogenic doses of both types of vaccines elicit excellent antibody response in immunologically primed people (response to the Russian flu antigen in the recent vaccine trials identified primed people as those born before 1953). Although no single dose of vaccine of either type was both adequately immunogenic and acceptably nonreactogenic in unprimed people, good response can be obtained with a regimen of two nonreactogenic doses of either type of vaccine (for children under age 13, only subunit vaccine is recommended). Thus, given periodic revision of vaccine formulation to include the most recently prevalent type A strains, it is possible to induce and to maintain in any given individual reasonably protective (70 to 80 percent) levels of immunity by annual or biennial vaccination, using single doses after the priming series. Since vaccines usually are bivalent, they also induce protection against type B influenza. The continuing state of immunity is important in view of the unpredictability of epidemics.

In deciding whether to use influenza vaccine, one additional factor must be considered: a possibly increased potential for developing Guillain-Barré Syndrome (GBS). This condition has a low annual incidence in the United States (about 6 per 1,000,000). GBS causes weakness and paralysis that usually (in 85 percent of cases) disappear within a few weeks, but may persist (in 10 percent) or be fatal (in 5 percent). The intensive postvaccination surveillance that accompanied the swine flu vaccination program in the fall of 1976 led to the recognition that GBS was occurring among vaccinees during the first two months postvaccination with a frequency (about 1 per 100,000) some ten times that expected (about 1 per 1,000,000). Since this possible association was widely publicized, it is very probable that GBS was more completely recognized among vaccinees than among the general population and, hence, that the estimate of vaccine-related risk errs on the high side. Although swine flu vaccination undoubtedly did increase the risk of GBS, the correlation was so small that it would have escaped detection except for three factors: (1) the age of the vaccinees, (2) the large number of vaccinees, and (3) the unusually close surveillance. Indeed, other immunizations may well carry a similar but as yet unrecognized risk.

In the absence of contrary data, one must accept 1 in 100,000 as the conservative measure of the incidence of GBS associated not only with swine flu vaccine but also with inactivated influenza vaccines in general. To set this estimate in perspective, however, one should recall that the risk of influenza illness in epidemics is about 20 percent (20,000 per 100,000), and that of fatal influenza is about 0.2 percent (200 per 100,000). Further, the risk of fatal GBS (1 per 2,000,000 vaccinations) is about the same as the annual risk of being killed by lightning and 400 times less than the risk of dying in an accident.

Amantadine

Amantadine (Symmetrel) is one of the few drugs possessing a well documented antiviral effect. This action is very specific, as it is directed against type A influenza viruses only and not against type B. Although developed as an antiviral agent, amantadine was licensed originally for the treatment of parkinsonism. Patients with the latter disease receive the drug daily over long periods, and the absence of serious side effects in these patients is reassuring as to its safety. However, the doses employed in influenza trials (100 mg twice daily) do cause such side effects as insomnia, dizziness, confusion, and nausea in 3 to 7 percent of recipients. In patients with normal renal function, these manifestations are rapidly and completely reversed when the drug is discontinued. Because the drug is eliminated in the urine, its use is contraindicated in patients with impaired renal function.

Amantadine has been tested in clinical trials for both therapeutic and prophylactic effect. When given soon after onset of illness, some reduction in duration and in peak of fever has been observed. When administration is begun before challenge or natural exposure, 60 to 80 percent of the illness expected is prevented, and illness that does occur is less severe. Also, the prophylactic effects of amantadine and of vaccine are additive.

Amantadine has one important advantage over vaccine in that its effectiveness is unrelated to abrupt or gradual changes in the antigenic character of type A influenza viruses. However, continued administration is required to maintain prophylactic efficacy. Because of its relatively high cost and the frequency of annoying side effects, widespread use of amantadine for the duration of the usual epidemic (three to six weeks) is not feasible. Nonetheless, when influenza is epidemic in a community, selective use of amantadine may be considered in at least two situations.

Usage

In one situation, prophylaxis begins when the epidemic is recognized, and it continues until termination of the epidemic. Such prophylaxis might be regarded as generally beneficial, but it is particularly appropriate when special reasons exist for preventing influenza in certain individuals. These include people with essential occupations (police, medical care personnel) and those with conditions associated with unusually severe and possibly fatal influenza (various chronic debilitating illnesses, ages 65 years and older). These same individuals probably will have been vaccinated already and thus will be receiving maximum feasible protection.

In the second situation, prophylaxis begins shortly after probable exposure has occurred and continues for a few days only (until termination of exposure). Exposure would be defined as *close contact with influenza-like illness*, which, in epidemic periods, has a high probability of being caused by influenza viruses. Patients presenting with such illness would constitute possible index cases who, along with their contacts, would be given amantadine. The rationale for treating the index case is that it may reduce virus shedding (and, therefore, infectivity) and also beneficially modify the illness. Appropriate settings for such postexposure prophylaxis include institutions (closed populations), hospital wards, and family units. Results of studies performed under field conditions suggest that such prophylaxis affords about 50 percent protection against infection and over 60 percent protection against clinical disease. In a placebo-controlled trial of amantadine in family contacts (10 days of treatment), 60 percent protection against infection and 80 percent against illness were demonstrated.

Conclusion

Although flu epidemics (due to type A influenza virus) cannot be prevented, use of vaccine or amantadine or both can afford significant protection to individuals. Under optimal conditions, each is 60 to 80 percent effective in preventing illness, and their prophylactic effects are additive.

One problem with vaccines is the unstable, antigenic character of type A influenza virus. To be maximally effective, vaccines must be produced from virus closely related antigenically to the epidemic challenge strains. Existing vaccine becomes useless in the face of pandemic disease marking the appearance of a new major variant, and effective vaccine, containing the new variant antigen, is not widely available before the flu has become pandemic. During the interpandemic period, the variant undergoes gradual antigenic drift, which requires periodic alteration of vaccine formulation to include the most recently prevalent type A strains. Given such alteration, reasonably protective levels of immunity can be induced and maintained in any given individual by annual vaccination, preferably in the fall. Since vaccines are bivalent, they also induce protection against influenza B. The continuing state of immunity is important, since epidemics are hard to predict.

Another problem with vaccines is their adverse effects. One constraint on vaccine use, systemic reactogenicity (especially in children), has been removed by the demonstration that subunit vaccines are nonreactogenic, although two doses are required to elicit good response in unprimed individuals. However, a new constraint emerged in the fall of 1976, when swine flu vaccination was associated with a small increased risk of Guillain-Barré syndrome (about 1 in 100,000).

Amantadine has an important advantage over vaccines in that changes in the antigenic character of type A virus do not alter its prophylactic effectiveness. Because of its relatively high cost and the occurrence of minor but disagreeable side effects in 3 to 7 percent of recipients, it is not appropriate for use on a widespread basis for the period needed to block an epidemic (three to six weeks). However, selective use does deserve consideration during an epidemic. Continuing prophylaxis can be given to those for whom prevention of influenza is of special importance, because they have essential occupations, or have conditions predisposing them to serious or fatal disease. Also, close contacts of new cases (in families, on hospital wards, in closed institutions) are logical candidates for prophylaxis while close exposure continues.

References

Beveridge, W.I.B.: *Influenza, The Last Great Plague.* New York, Neale Watson Academic Publications, Inc., 1977.

Boffey, P.M.: Guillian-Barré: rare disease paralyzes swine flu campaign. Science 195:155, 1977.

Couch, R.B., and Jackson, G.G.: Antiviral agents in influenza–summary of influenza workshop VIII. J. Infect. Dis. 134:516, 1976.

Fox, J.P., and Kilbourne, E.D.: Epidemiology of influenza–summary of influenza workshop IV. J. Infect. Dis. 128:361, 1973.

Galbraith, A. W., Oxford, J. S., Schild, G.C., and Watson, G. I.: Protective effect of 1-adamantanamine hydrochloride on influenza A2 infections in the family environment. A controlled double-blind study. Lancet 2:1026, 1969.

Glezen, W.P., and Couch, R.B.: Interpandemic influenza in the Houston area, 1974–1976. N. Engl. J. Med. 298:587, 1978.

Kilbourne, E.D., Chanock, R.M., Choppin, P.W., Davenport, F.M., Fox, J.P., Gregg, M.B., Jackson, G.G., and Parkman, P.D.: Influenza vaccines–summary of influenza workshop V. J. Infect. Dis. 129:750, 1974.

Osborne, J., ed.: *History, Science, and Politics. Influenza in America 1918–1976.* New York, Neale Watson Academic Publications, Inc., 1977.

Parkman, P.D., Galasso, G.J., Top, F.H., Jr., and Noble, G.R.: Summary of clinical trials of influenza vaccines. J. Infect. Dis. 134:100, 1976.

Schoenbaum, S.C.: Vaccination for influenza–any alternatives? N. Engl. J. Med. 298:621, 1978.

Amantadine: Should It Be Used as an Antiviral?

R. Gordon Douglas, Jr., M.D.
University of Rochester School of Medicine

Amantadine became the first antiviral available for systemic use in the United States when it was licensed by the Food and Drug Administration (FDA) in 1966 for the prophylaxis of Asian influenza (H2N2). Despite the historical importance of this event, the compound was not commonly used for prevention of influenza for several reasons, and interest in its antiviral activity declined. A second indication for the drug (treatment of Parkinson's disease) was discovered, and amantadine has been widely prescribed for this purpose. However, in the last few years, there has been a resurgence of interest in amantadine as an antiviral because inactivated vaccines leave much to be desired for prevention of influenza, and because the public has consequently become disenchanted with such vaccines. The emphasis has been on defining specific prophylactic indications for which amantadine should be utilized, and on pinpointing its therapeutic benefits.

In this essay, I examine the reasons for the failure of the medical profession to use amantadine as an antiviral in the past, briefly review the data base concerning amantadine, assess the risks of influenza, and recommend the use of amantadine in certain situations. For the interested reader, several detailed reviews of amantadine, including basic and clinical studies, are available (Stalder, 1977; Richman and Oxman, 1978; Douglas, 1979).

Lack of Widespread Use of Amantadine as an Antiviral

Sabin Editorial

In June, 1967, Dr. Albert Sabin published a special communication in the *Journal of the American Medical Association* (JAMA), in which he concluded that amantadine should not be used as a prophylactic against Asian influenza infections (Sabin, 1967). He cited a number of reasons for this recommendation, including (1) limited demonstrated prophylactic effectiveness, (2) lack of resources to make a laboratory diagnosis of influenza A infection in most clinical situations, (3) low likelihood of effect on epidemic when drug is begun because most people would have already contracted influenza, (4) occurrence of undesirable side effects, (5) possible emergence of drug-resistant virus populations, and (6) lack of studies in people exposed to natural influenza as compared with volunteers exposed to experimental infection. This editorial had an enormous impact because of the reputation of the author and the validity of what he said. Many physicians took Dr. Sabin's advice and did not prescribe amantadine. In addition, several other factors contributed to the failure to use amantadine as a preventative in patients exposed to influenza.

Reluctance of Physicians to Accept a Prophylactic Antiviral

In the mid-1960s, most physicians were skeptical of antivirals. They had been taught in medical school and in continuing education programs that antibiotics don't work in viral infections, and since there was no precedent for an antiviral chemotherapeutic agent (except for topical idoxuridine in herpes simplex virus keratitis), they were not prepared to accept an antiviral. This background was coupled with the concept that the drug had to be administered *before* infection was contracted.

Prophylaxis was not a totally new concept, but then-current prophylactic regimens were either short term (e.g., sulfa drugs versus meningococcal infection) or designed to forestall a disease with severe, characteristic, and well recognized consequences (e.g., penicillin to prevent rheumatic fever). To provide protection against influenza, a drug would have to be administered for at least five or six weeks, and severe sequelae to influenza infection are infrequent. In addition, prevention of a disease that ordinarily was self-limited was a new concept.

Side Effects of Amantadine

The question of side effects was raised by Dr. Sabin's article and probably by most discerning physicians. Although no serious organ toxicity was recognized at that time, minor central nervous system side effects were noted in 4 to 27 percent of patients (Sabin, 1967). In attempting to prevent a predominantly self-limited disease, which might affect 5 to 30 percent of the population, large numbers of people would be treated with drug unnecessarily even in the event of a substantial outbreak of influenza, since they would not be expected to contract influenza. For example, to prevent influenza in 100 people, assuming a 70 percent protective efficacy of amantadine and a 10 percent attack rate, the drug would have to be administered to 1428 people. Assuming a 0.1 percent mortality rate in such an epidemic, 14,285 individuals would have to be treated to prevent one death. Thus, even side effects that occur at low incidence became significant. It became essential to develop data to assure physicians that amantadine was safe.

Uncharacteristic Disease

Another major problem with the use of amantadine as an antiviral involves the difficulty of making a clinical diagnosis of influenza. Influenza does not have a single or characteristic manifestation as does poliomyelitis or chicken pox. The most characteristic clinical symptom of an influenza A virus infection is a three-day illness in which fever, headache, muscle aches, and cough are present (Douglas, 1975). Common, but less frequent, manifestations are sore throat, runny nose, and photophobia. Gastrointestinal symptoms occur in less than 10 percent of patients. Some individuals may have common cold-like symptoms, afebrile pharyngitis, tracheobronchitis, or subclinical infections. A small number of cases may develop pneumonia as a result of viral invasion of the lung or secondary bacterial infection or a combination of the two. Thus, influenza A virus infection has a number of clinical manifestations, all of which, including the so-called *influenza syndrome*, can be produced by infection with other respiratory viruses such as rhinovirus, coronavirus, adenovirus, respiratory syncytial virus, or parainfluenza virus. In addition, all the clinical manifestations can be produced by influenza B virus infection not only endemically but also epidemically. Finally, many other infections and even noninfectious diseases result in influenza-like syndromes with fever, headache, and muscle aches; some are even associated with cough.

Perhaps the biggest area of confusion involves gastrointestinal (GI) "flu." As noted, studies of people with naturally acquired or experimentally induced influenza reveal a low incidence of GI symptoms, and yet both lay and professional personnel continue to believe that influenza virus produces gastroenteritis (Douglas, 1975). Recent studies have shown a diverse etiology for the gastroenteritis syndrome, including noninvasive toxin-producing bacteria, invasive bacteria, parasites, rotaviruses, and parvoviruses (Hornick, 1978; Blacklow et al., 1978).

This lack of definition of a specific illness creates problems for acceptance of both amantadine and influenza vaccines. If doctors or patients are not convinced of what they are trying to prevent, they will be reluctant to use a drug.

Virologic Diagnosis

When amantadine was introduced, viral diagnosis was difficult, as few hospital laboratories performed viral isolations. Serologic confirmation of viral infection could be obtained through state health laboratories or laboratories at the Center for Disease Control (CDC), but such determinations required convalescent sera and took days to weeks for results to be returned; thus, they were of little help. Physicians depended on epidemiologic information given to them by local or state health officials, which was derived from surveillance programs, to determine if influenza was present in a community. Once such a determination was made, patients fitting a description compatible with one of the influenza syndromes could be reasonably expected to have influenza. Prophylaxis for unaffected persons could thereafter be initiated.

FDA Approval

The final deterrent to use of amantadine as an antiviral was a legal one. With the advent of the major antigenic shift that occurred with the appearance of influenza A/Hong Kong/68 H3N2 virus and the related H3N2 strains that appeared subsequently, amantadine became a licensed antiviral for a disease that didn't exist—that is, H2N2 strains of influenza, which disappeared after 1967. This fact obviously discouraged use, as the drug could not be advertised or otherwise promoted for the then relevant influenza H3N2 infections. In 1976, however, the license was changed to include all influenza A strains, and to include relief of symptoms (i.e., therapy) as well as prophylaxis.

Current Knowledge Concerning Amantadine

Since its introduction, amantadine has been subjected to a number of additional studies, including investigations into its action and *in vitro* antiviral activity, as well as its prophylactic and therapeutic effect in animals and humans.

Basic Properties and Pharmacokinetics

Amantadine is a white crystalline substance of unusual chemical structure (Figure 13–1); it is supplied as the hydrochloride. Research has shown that it does not block attachment of virus but interferes reversibly with an unknown event that occurs immediately following virus infection (Skehel et al., 1977).

Amantadine is readily absorbed from the gastrointestinal tract. It is not metabolized and has a half-life of 12 to 24 hours in humans, and more than 90 percent of it is excreted in the urine. Peak blood levels of 0.3 to 0.6 μg/ml are attained three to four hours after ingestion of doses of 2.5 to 5.0 mg/kg in normal adults (Bleidner et al., 1965). Levels in respiratory secretions are about one tenth as high (Smith et al., 1967). In the mouse lung, 15- to 50-fold or greater concentrations are found, but whether such tissue concentrations occur in humans is unknown.

Side Effects

Side effects are dose-related and, with few exceptions, are limited to the central nervous system. Since amantadine has been widely used for treatment of Parkinson's disease since 1970, a great deal of information is now available concerning its side effects. No serious renal, hepatic, or bone marrow toxicity has been reported, despite administration of over one million patient doses. However, a few cases of heart failure in patients with preexisting heart disease who were taking amantadine have been documented.

The most frequent side effects are minor, reversible central nervous system symptoms such as insomnia, nervousness, and difficulty in concentrating. Peckinpaugh et al. (1970) compared objective and subjective physical and psychologic abnormalities of 71 navy recruits receiving 200 mg of amantadine per day with the findings in a similar population receiving placebos. In no instance was it necessary to discontinue treatment because of adverse drug effect. There were some minor side effects:

Figure 13-1. The chemical structure of amantadine.

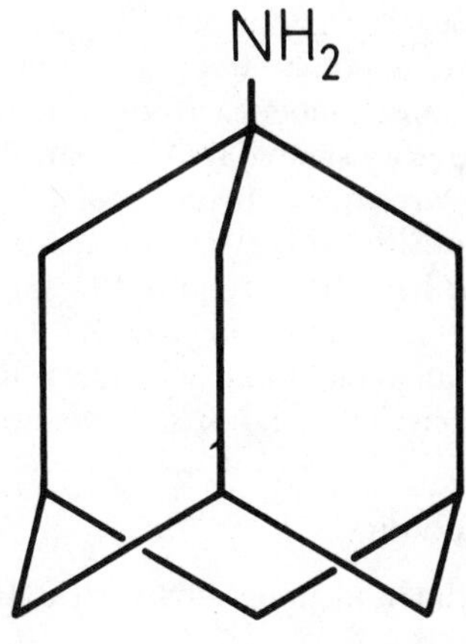

frequency of urination, impaired spatial perception and sense of adaptability, and prolonged reaction time. Among 709 young adults in another placebo-controlled study, symptoms were no more frequent in the amantadine group than in the placebo group (Kitamoto, 1971).

Among 430 older people with Parkinson's disease, 20 percent complained of confusion, nervousness, dizziness, or insomnia when taking amantadine. Most patients continued the drug for more than one year; only 6 percent discontinued the drug or reduced the dosage (Schwab et al., 1972).

It is clear that drug may accumulate in individuals with impaired renal function: hence, the frequency and severity of central nervous system complaints are increased in such patients. Finally, teratogenicity has been described in rats receiving 50 mg per kg, contraindicating the use of the drug in pregnancy.

In Vitro *Studies*

A number of studies in cell cultures and in embryonated hens' eggs have indicated substantial reduction of replication of influenza A virus by small quantities of amantadine (0.1 to 1.0 μg per ml) (Grunert and Hoffman, 1977; Hayden and Douglas, 1977). Most of the early studies used reduction in hemagglutinin production as an endpoint, but more recent studies have used plaque reduction assays as well. All influenza A viruses tested, including strains belonging to Hsw1N1, H0N1, and H1N1 subtypes, as well as H3N2 and H2N2, are sensitive. A/PR8/34 H0N1 is relatively resistant, but it is a multiply passaged laboratory strain. Influenza viruses can be readily made resistant *in vitro* by passaging virus in the presence of amantadine, but resistant strains have not been isolated from people treated with amantadine. Although activity is optimal against influenza A viruses, it is not limited to this virus type. Activity against influenza B virus, influenza C virus, respiratory syncytial virus, parainfluenza, and other viruses has been reported; in such studies, considerably greater quantities of amantadine have been required to show effect than is the case for influenza A. Thus, it is unlikely that amantadine will have any clinically useful activity against such viruses.

Animal Studies

In experimental infections with influenza A virus in mice and other animals, both prophylactic and therapeutic effects have been observed (Grunert et al., 1965). For prophylaxis, only one or a few doses of drug were necessary to achieve effect, whereas for therapy, repeated dosing was required. In general, therapy could be delayed until 72 to 96 hours after inoculation and still demonstrate effectiveness. Beneficial effect could be observed on survival rates as well as on pulmonary virus titers and other manifestations of infection. In a few studies, no effect of amantadine could be measured. In some studies, administration of amantadine by aerosol or intranasal routes resulted in enhanced efficacy as compared with oral ingestion or intraperitoneal injection (Walker et al., 1976; Fenton et al., 1977).

Human Studies: Prophylaxis

Nine of ten reported placebo-controlled double-blind studies of the prophylactic effect of amantadine against challenge in volunteers with an influenza A virus resulted in at least a 50 percent reduction in occurrence of illness (Hoffman, 1973). A variety of strains of H2N2 and H3N2 viruses were used. For example, Togo et al. (1968), as shown in Figure 13–2, demonstrated a 62 percent reduction in occurrence of febrile illness in volunteers challenged with influenza A "Asian" H2N2 virus who were pretreated with amantadine as compared with those pretreated with placebo. In most of these studies, amantadine also reduced antibody responses to influenza A virus, not because of any immunosuppressive effect of amantadine but rather because of its effect in preventing or diminishing virus replication.

Similarly, 14 of 15 reported studies of the prophylactic effect of amantadine in naturally occurring H2N2 or H3N2 influenza have shown an effect (Hoffman, 1973). Most of these studies showed a reduced frequency of symptoms, whereas some showed only their reduced severity. In extensive studies in Russia, protective efficacies of 68 to 80 percent were observed (Smorodintsev et al., 1970).

Another selected aspect of amantadine prophylaxis has been demonstrated by O'Donoghue et al. (1973). These authors studied the prophylactic efficacy of amantadine in hospitalized patients during an outbreak of nosocomial A H3N2 infection in 1971-72. As shown in Table 13–1, the frequency of occurrence of clinical influenza, as well as influenza infection con-

Figure 13-2. Effect of amantadine on prevention of experimental influenza A H2N2 infection. Figure shows distribution of clinical responses for amantadine-treated and placebo-treated subjects.

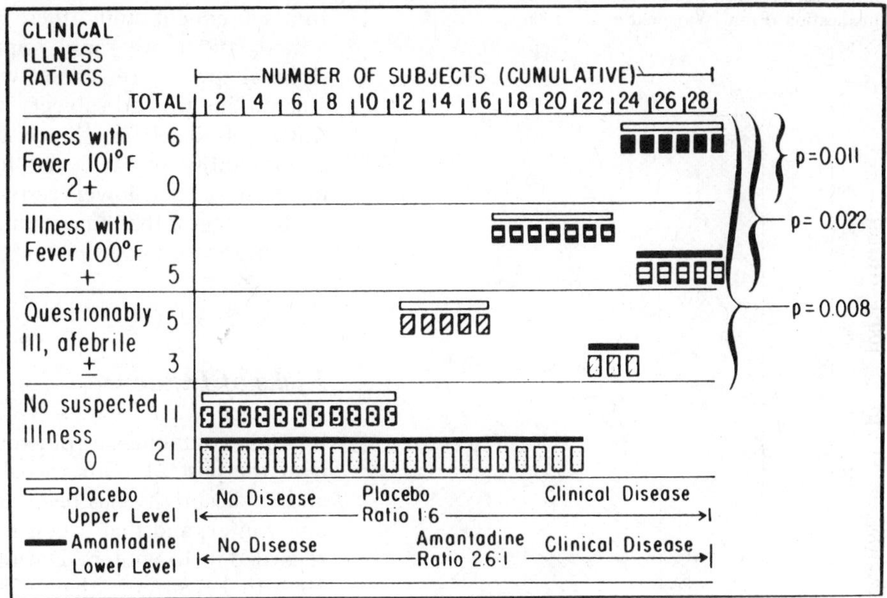

firmed by serology or virus isolation, was reduced.

Human Studies: Treatment

Therapeutic effects of amantadine have not been proved in experimental influenza A infections in volunteers. Perhaps this is due to the mildness of illness in most such recipients of intranasal influenza virus (Douglas, 1975).

Table 13-1. *Prophylaxis of Hospital-Acquired Influenza A (H3N2) Infection Among Amantadine-Treated and Untreated Patients*

Hospital-Acquired Influenza A	Amantadine-Treated	Untreated
Clinical	0/50°	7/61°
Subclinical	2/50	5/61
Total	2/50†	12/61†

° $p<0.02$ (χ^2 analysis)

† $p<0.05$ (χ^2 analysis)

From O'Donoghue et al.: Prevention of nosocomial Influenza Infections with Amantadine, 1973.

On the other hand, 16 placebo-controlled double-blind studies have documented therapeutic effects of amantadine in natural influenza A virus infections due to a variety of strains of H3N2, H2N2, and H1N1 viruses (Hoffman, 1973; Van Voris et al., 1978). For example, Wingfield et al. (1969) demonstrated more rapid defervescence of fever among subjects receiving amantadine than among those treated with placebo in an outbreak of influenza A/Virginia/1/68 H2N2 infection (Figure 13–3). The mean time of defervescence of fever to below 100°F was 23 hours as compared with 45 hours for subjects receiving placebo. Other signs and symptoms paralleled the fever response. Similar results—that is, an approximately 50 percent reduction in duration of the more severe signs and symptoms of influenza—have been documented. Many of the same findings have been observed in children (Galbraith et al., 1973).

In contrast to the data from the prophylactic studies, serum antibody responses are not lower in the amantadine subjects than those in placebo subjects, again attesting to the lack of immunosuppression by amantadine. Studies of virus isolates usually have not revealed significant differences between the two groups, but two instances in which quantitative studies of virus shedding were performed showed that a more rapid decline in virus titers occurred among those treated with amantadine as compared

Figure 13-3. Effect of amantadine HCl and rimantadine HCl administered to humans with naturally occurring influenza infection on the duration of fever after start of medication (From Wingfield et al., 1969).

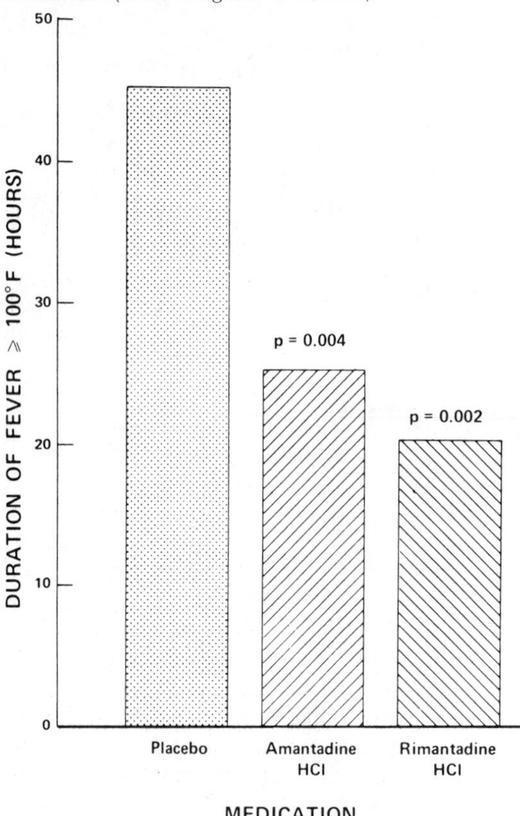

with the controls (Knight et al., 1970; Van Voris et al., 1978).

It should be emphasized that all these therapeutic studies have been performed in patients with uncomplicated, nonpneumonic influenza. Controlled prospective studies have not been performed in patients with influenza virus pneumonia, although favorable anecdotal experience has been reported (Couch and Jackson, 1976). Furthermore, it has not been shown that amantadine treatment of uncomplicated cases prevents pneumonic complications. Obviously, there is need for further study in these situations.

Recently, studies have focused on changes in pulmonary function that occur in uncomplicated influenza and that persist for several weeks after acute influenza: abnormalities in gas exchange, diffusion, pulmonary mechanics as measured by spirometry, and peripheral airways. Little et al. (1976) described accelerated improvement in abnormal helium-oxygen flow rates indicative of peripheral airway resistance in amantadine-treated subjects as compared with subjects who received placebo in an outbreak of A/Port Chalmers/73 H2N2 infection. In a subsequent study, these results were confirmed, and more rapid improvement of peripheral airway resistance was noted among amantadine-treated subjects in additional tests (Little et al., 1978). Since these physiologic abnormalities are believed to represent viral invasion of the lower respiratory tract, the studies suggest that amantadine might be effective in preventing pulmonary complications of influenza.

Risks of Influenza

Studies of influenza epidemics and pandemics over the past 21 years reveal that influenza A and/or B activity has been detected in all but one winter, and that excess mortality has been recorded in 15 winters. During the period from 1968 to 1978, more than 150,000 people died from influenza in the U.S. (Center for Disease Control, 1978).

Moderate interpandemic outbreaks of influenza result in infection in 5 to 30 percent of a given population. Outbreaks may be smaller or larger, particularly in certain defined populations such as institutionalized people or children. Also, in the event of pandemic influenza, a greater proportion of individuals may be infected. Of those infected, approximately 10 percent will have some form of pulmonary complication; i.e., tracheobronchitis and/or pneumonia. Not all such patients will require hospitalization. The rate of pulmonary complications is very low in children (perhaps 1 or 2 percent), and much higher in elderly people or people with chronic diseases, despite a lower attack rate for infection in the elderly than in children. Overall mortality rate for people with influenza has been calculated to be about 0.1 percent. Thus, during an epidemic with a 20 percent attack rate, overall risk of dying from influenza is about 1 in 5000. Many others will be hospitalized, and the majority of those infected will have disabling, albeit self-limited, infections.

Recommendations for Use of Amantadine

It is apparent from the foregoing discussion that a great deal of additional information has accumulated since 1966 concerning the prophylactic and therapeutic efficacy of amantadine against a number of different influenza A subtypes and strains. In addition, as a result of the widespread use of amantadine in Parkinson's disease (according to the manufacturer, over 1,000,000 patient doses have been given), a substantial safety record has been accumulated. Based on this information, the physician is in a much better position to judge benefit-risk ratios when assessing the need for amantadine in a given patient or situation.

This accumulation of data is propitious, since it comes at a time when the concept of antivirals is well accepted (e.g., ara-A for herpes simplex encephalitis and herpes zoster), and when parenteral inactivated vaccines for influenza are less well accepted than formerly, a result of the National Immunization Program against swine influenza.

Antiviral chemotherapy should be directed toward two goals: (1) prevention and treatment of uncomplicated influenza and (2) prevention and treatment of pneumonic complications.

Nonpneumonic influenza merits consideration of chemoprophylaxis and chemotherapy because of its tremendous impact on school and industrial absenteeism, not to mention personal discomfort. Pneumonic influenza, with its resultant mortality, is an obvious target for antiviral chemoprophylaxis and chemotherapy.

Prophylaxis

Vaccination with inactivated virus preparations remains, and will remain for a number of years, the mainstay of influenza prevention. Recently, the incomplete efficacy and the potential hazard of those preparations have been well publicized, and such vaccines are usually reserved for groups at high risk: the elderly and the chronically ill. The only life-threatening risk from influenza vaccination is Guillain-Barré Syndrome (GBS). It occurred once in every 100,000 vaccinations in the swine flu vaccination program, and 5 percent of those infected died. Thus, the incidence of death from influenza vaccination is 1 in 2,000,000 immunizations, and that from influenza in a moderate outbreak is 1 in 5000, yielding a benefit-risk ratio of 400 to 1 in favor of vaccinations. This ratio should be lowered by the efficacy of the vaccine, which is about 70 percent. Although deaths have not been documented in association with amantadine, the drug has not been tested acutely in large numbers of subjects as influenza vaccines have been; therefore, it is not possible to estimate this risk. Occurrence of minor side effects in large numbers of subjects given amantadine prophylactically has been discussed previously, and this is an obvious disadvantage of chemoprophylaxis. Other disadvantages of mass prophylaxis with amantadine include compliance (necessity of daily medication for five to six weeks), requirement of an excellent surveillance system to detect the onset of epidemics, lack of activity against influenza B virus, possibility of occurrence of resistance to amantadine, and cost ($0.25 per 100 mg tablet or $21.00 for a course of prophylaxis versus average cost to patient of $5.00 to $10.00 for vaccination).

For these reasons, I recommend using amantadine for prophylaxis only in a few specific situations, and not as a replacement for mass vaccination. First, people in the high risk categories for immunization against influenza (elderly and chronically ill) who cannot receive vaccine because it isn't available or for whom it is contraindicated owing to egg allergy are candidates for amantadine chemoprophylaxis. In addition, individuals with renal disease accompanied by azotemia and those with cancer or who are receiving immunosuppressive therapy may not respond to vaccine and should be better protected by amantadine. In such cases, amantadine should be used alone or as an adjunct to vaccination. Dosage should be modified for people with altered renal function. In the hospital setting, amantadine may be given to patients and staff to prevent or to abort an epidemic. Finally, since the effect of amantadine is additive to the immune response to vaccination, individuals who require maximal protection may be given both vaccine and amantadine.

Therapy

Although I recommend only limited use of amantadine as a preventative in influenza, I believe that the drug should be much more widely used for influenza therapy and feel the existing data strongly support this view. Treatment of nonpneumonic influenza is desired by many physicians and patients. Witness the tremendous use of over-the-counter preparations, abuse of antibiotics for these illnesses, and numbers of physician visits occasioned by influenza. The goal is relief of symptoms and faster return to school or gainful employment. Certainly, it is better to administer a drug shown to reduce duration of illness by 50 percent than to give an antibiotic that is not beneficial and may induce resistance in bacterial flora, resulting in an infection that is difficult to treat with antibiotics should suprainfection occur. The absence of serious toxicity from amantadine is an important consideration.

Minor side effects in amantadine therapy are inconsequential, since it has been shown that total symptoms due to influenza and drug are significantly reduced in amantadine-treated as compared with placebo-treated subjects. In addition, as opposed to the use of chemoprophylaxis, one is not administering drug to uninfected people. Thus, the benefit-risk ratio is highly favorable to treatment. I recommend 200 mg p.o. stat, and 100 mg b.i.d. for a total of five days for patients with influenza-like illness and temperatures over 100°F that occur in the winter and at a time when the Center for Disease Control or the state or local health department has reported influenza in or near the community. In this setting, specific virologic diagnosis is not required for every patient.

Suggestive evidence has been cited to indicate that such treatment may, in addition, prevent pulmonary complications of influenza. Once such complications occur, the available data do not suggest benefit from amantadine. However, since there is no other effective therapy for influenza virus pneumonia or mixed virus and bacterial pneumonia, I suggest treating such patients with amantadine, 3 to 5 mg per kg per day for 10 days. Unfortunately, the only available preparation is an oral tablet; thus, amantadine must be swallowed by the patient or given by nasogastric tube.

Conclusion

The preceding recommendations do not imply that amantadine will solve all our problems with influenza. We need additional studies concerning the therapeutic effectiveness of amantadine in influenza viral pneumonia, prevention of pneumonia by treating elderly patients who have uncomplicated influenza, the proper dosage to be used for treatment, the role of aerosol administration, and so on. In addition, further studies of rimantadine, and perhaps other related compounds, in a search for drugs with enhanced effectiveness and decreased side effects, should be undertaken.

References

Blacklow, N.R., Schreiber, D.S., and Trier, J.S.: Viral enteritis. In Weinstein, L., and Fields, B.N., *Seminars in Infectious Disease,* New York, Stratton Intercontinental Medical Book Corporation, 1978.

Bleidner, W. E., Harmon, J.B., Hewes, W.E., Lynes, T.E., and Hermann, E.C.: Absorption, distribution and excretion of amantadine hydrochloride. J. Pharmacol. Exp. Ther. 150:484, 1965.

Center for Disease Control: Morbidity and mortality weekly report. Influenza vaccine—preliminary statement. 27:205. Atlanta, U.S. Department of Health, Education and Welfare, 1978.

Couch, R.B., and Jackson, G.G.: Antiviral agent in influenza—summary of a workshop VIII. J. Infect. Dis. 134:516–527, 1976.

Douglas, R.G., Jr.: Influenza in man. In Kilbourne, E.D., *The Influenza Viruses and Influenza,* New York, Academic Press, 1975.

Douglas, R.G., Jr.: Viral respiratory diseases. In Galasso, G., Morgan, T.C., and Buchanan, R.D.: *Antiviral Agents and Viral Diseases of Man,* New York, Raven Press, 1979.

Fenton, R.J., Bessell, C., Spilling, C.R., and Potter, C.W.: The effects of peroral or local aerosol administration of 1-aminoadamantane hydrochloride (amantadine hydrochloride) on influenza infections of the ferret. J. Antimicrob. Chemother. 3:463, 1977.

Galbraith, A.W., Schild, G.S., Potter, C.W., and Watson, G.I.: The therapeutic effect of amantadine in influenza occurring during the winter of 1971-72 assessed by double-blind study. J. R. Coll. Gen. Pract. 23:34, 1973.

Grunert, R.R., and Hoffmann, C.E.: Sensitivity of influenza A/New Jersey/8/76 (Hsw1N1) virus to amantadine HCl. J. Infect. Dis. 136:297, 1977.

Grunert, R. R., McGahen, J.W., and Davies, W.L.: The *in vivo* antiviral activity of 1-adamantanamine (amantadine) I. Prophylactic and therapeutic activity against influenza viruses. Virology 26:262, 1965.

Hayden, F.G., and Douglas, R.G., Jr.: Unpublished observations, 1977.

Hoffman, C.E.: Amantadine HCl and related compounds. In Carter, W.A., *Selective Inhibitors of Viral Functions.* Cleveland, Chemical Rubber Co. Press, 1973.

Hornick, R.B.: Bacterial infections of the intestine. In Weinstein, L., and Fields, B.N., *Seminars in Infectious Diseases.* New York, Stratton Intercontinental Medical Book Corporation, 1978.

Kitamoto, O.: Therapeutic effectiveness of amantadine hydrochloride in naturally occurring Hong Kong influenza—double blind studies. Jpn. J. Tuberc. Chest Dis. 17:1, 1971.

Knight, V., Fedson, D., Baldini, J., Douglas, R.G., Jr., and Couch, R.B.: Amantadine therapy of epidemic influenza A2 (Hong Kong). Infect. Immun. 1:200, 1970.

Little, J.W., Hall, W.J., Douglas, R.G., Jr., Hyde, R.W., and Speers, D.M.: Amantadine effect on peripheral airways abnormalities in influenza. A study in 15 students with natural influenza A infection. Ann. Int. Med. 85:177, 1976.

Little, J.W., Hall, W.J., Douglas, R.G., Jr., Mudholkar, G.S., Speers, D.M., and Patel, K.: Airway hyperreactivity and peripheral airway dysfunction in influenza A infection. Am. Rev. Respir. Dis. 118:295–303, 1978.

O'Donoghue, J.M., Ray, C.G., Terry, D.W., Jr., and Beaty, H.N.: Prevention of nosocomial influenza infections with amantadine. Am. J. Epidemiol. 97:276, 1973.

Peckinpaugh, R.O., Askin, F.B., Pierce, W.E., Edwards, E.A., Johnson, D.P., and Jackson, G.G.: Field studies with amantadine: acceptability and protection. Ann. NY Acad. Sci. 173:62, 1970.

Richman, D.D., and Oxman, M.N.: Antiviral agents. In Weinstein, L., and Fields, B.N., *Seminars in Infectious Disease.* New York, Stratton Intercontinental Medical Book Corporation, 1978.

Sabin,A.B.: Amantadine hydrochloride: analysis of data related to its proposed use for prevention of A2 influenza virus disease in human beings. JAMA, 200:943–950, 1967.

Schwab, R.S., Poskanzer, D.C., England, A.C., and Young, R.R.: Amantadine in Parkinson's disease. JAMA 222:792, 1972.

Skehel, J.J., Hay, A.J., and Armstrong, J.A.: On the mechanism of inhibition of influenza virus replication by amantadine hydrochloride. J. Gen. Virol. 38:97–110, 1977.

Smith, C.B., Purcell, R.H., and Chanock, R.M.: Effect of amantadine hydrochloride on parainfluenza type 1 virus infections in adult volunteers. Am. Rev. Respir. Dis. 95:689, 1967.

Smorodintsev, A.A., Karpuchin, G.I., Zlydnikov, D.M., Malysheva, A.M., Shvetsova, E.G., Burov, S.A., Shramtsova, L.M., Romanov, Y.A., Taros, L.Y., Ivannikov, Y.G., and Novoselov, S.D.: The prospect of amantadine for prevention of influenza A2 in humans (Effectiveness of amantadine during influenza A2/Hong Kong epidemic in January–February, 1969, in Leningrad). Ann. NY Acad. Sci. 173:44, 1970.

Stalder, H.: Antiviral therapy. Yale J. Biol. Med. 50:507, 1977.

Togo, Y., Hornick, R.B., and Dawkins, A.T., Jr.: Studies on induced influenza in Man: I. Double-blind studies designed to assess prophylactic efficacy of amantadine hydrochloride against A2/Rockville/1/65 strain. JAMA 203:1089, 1968.

Van Voris, L.P., Hayden, F.G., Betts, R:F., Douglas, R.G., Jr., and Christmas, W.A.: Oral amantadine (A) and rimantadine (R) therapy of natural influenza A/USSR/77 H1N1. 18th Interscience Conference on Antimicrobial Agents and Chemotherapy. Atlanta, Oct. 1978.

Walker, J.S., Stephen, E.L., and Spertzel, R.O.: Small-particle aerosols of antiviral compounds in treatment of type A influenza pneumonia in mice. J. Infect. Dis. 133S:A140–A144, 1976.

Wingfield, W.L., Pollack, D., and Grunert, R.R.: Therapeutic efficacy of amantadine HCl and rimantadine HCl in naturally occurring influenza A2 respiratory illness in man. 281:579, 1969.

Amantadine and Influenza: Evaluation of Conflicting Reports*

Albert B. Sabin, M.D.
Medical University of South Carolina, Charleston

In an editorial entitled "Sensitivity of Influenza A Virus to Amantadine," Jackson (1977) posed the question: "Can [the drug] get wider circulation, without its advocates being overly enthusiastic about the likelihood of a successful performance?" He then said that "further evaluation of amantadine must come from its use by a large enough number of physicians and in a variety of conditions to determine the practical effects in the prophylaxis and treatment of influenza A." I cannot understand how the uncontrolled extensive use of amantadine by physicians in at best only suspect cases of influenza A virus disease can provide further scientifically valid evaluation beyond what the controlled tests under actual conditions of proposed use that I called for twelve years ago (Sabin, 1967) have established to date. Valid studies performed during the past decade showing a lack of effectiveness of amantadine in experimentally infected volunteers and in people with naturally acquired infection have been discounted without explanation by amantadine advocates (Jackson, 1976, 1977; Couch, 1977). Accordingly, the most recent Food and Drug Administration (FDA) approval of amantadine for prophylaxis and therapy of acute respiratory illness suspected of being caused by *present and future* influenza A viruses (Couch, 1977) is, in my judgment, not justified by the existing data.

FDA approval of amantadine for such viruses is related to the following evaluation:

> Field trials to test the susceptibility of the Hong Kong (H3N2) virus and some of its variants during epidemics of influenza in different countries showed prophylaxis by amantadine to be as effective as it was against the earlier H2N2 subtype (Jackson et al., 1971; Oker-Blom et al., 1970; Smorodincev et al., 1970a). *In vitro* measurements and mouse protection tests were proper indicators of the sensitivity of the viral strain in naturally occurring disease; no resistant strains have been recognized in man (Jackson, 1976).

Others have evaluated the available data differently in regard to both prophylaxis and therapy. In their recent book on influenza, Stuart-Harris and Schild (1976) concluded:

> In view of the somewhat conflicting evidence of the activity of amantadine as a prophylactic, it is hardly surprising that the drug has not won favour for large-scale administration to man during epidemics ... yet the lack of consistent and rapid defervescence in the above therapeutic trials affords little support for the wider use of amantadine in the therapy of influenza.

My purposes here are (1) to examine some of the "conflicting evidence" of the past decade to determine if there may not be a more scientific way to resolve the conflicts of "evidence" than by the number of publications pro and con and (2) to point out the expected inadequacy of even a highly effective antiinfluenza A virus drug (which amantadine is not claimed by anyone to be) in the control of the massive annual incidence of severe illness associated

*This paper is a version of material that originally appeared in the Journal of Infectious Diseases, Vol. 138, Oct. 1978, pp. 557–566.

with the clinical syndrome of influenza, but which is mostly not caused by influenza A viruses. Exceptions occur for short periods in a given geographic region during the infrequent worldwide epidemics caused by totally new antigenic types of influenza A virus. An analysis of amantadine effectiveness must deal separately with (1) studies on properly matched, isolated volunteers of known immune status experimentally infected with known strains of influenza A virus that can multiply sufficiently to produce significant febrile illness in 30 to 50 percent of placebo controls and (2) properly monitored field trials in which illness caused by laboratory-confirmed natural infections with different strains of influenza A virus are compared with the total amount of comparable respiratory illness caused by other agents.

Tests in Experimentally Infected Volunteers

Using the same H2N2 influenza A virus strain of moderate virulence for experimental infection of nonimmune volunteers, two separate groups of investigators (Togo et al., 1968; Bloomfield et al., 1970) reported that amantadine resulted in marked protection against clinical illness without prevention of infection, although the antibody titers following infection were distinctly lower in the amantadine-treated than in the placebo-treated volunteers. These results were in striking contrast to the completely negative results with another H2N2 strain of influenza A virus obtained in an equally excellent study reported earlier by Tyrrell, Bynoe, and Hoorn (1965).

The report of Smorodintsev et al. (1970) that amantadine was "51 percent effective in preventing the development of artificially induced A2 influenza [H2N2 attenuated vaccine strains] and 73 percent to 92 percent effective in preventing the more severe form of A2 influenza" with a "2-fold drop in the frequency and intensity of the immune response" is difficult to interpret. The very small number of nonimmune volunteers, the rarity of clinically significant illness among them, and the absence of isolation all cast considerable doubt on the interpretation of this study by the authors and others.

Smorodintsev et al. (1970) also tested an H3N2 Hong Kong/68 strain, sensitive to amantadine *in vitro*, in volunteers of unreported immune status. Again, contrary to the results of the studies on volunteers infected with pre-Hong Kong influenza A viruses (Tyrrell et al., 1965; Togo et al., 1968; Bloomfield et al., 1970), there was only a 24 percent serologic response in the amantadine group compared with 88 percent in the placebo group. Severe influenza was reported in only 1 of 17 in the amantadine group compared with 8 of 16 in the placebo group. Likar (1970) reported different results in a study in Yugoslavia on 141 steel workers. Partly attenuated Hong Kong influenza A virus was given intranasally as an aerosol spray. There was no statistically significant difference in the incidence of clinical symptoms. Cohen et al. (1976) gave an H3N2, 1974 influenza A virus by nasal instillation and by pharyngeal spray to volunteers with negligible serum neutralizing antibody titers. Although amantadine diminished the development of moderate and severe illness, the difference between the combined clinical scores in the two groups was not statistically significant. Serum antibody developed in 8 of the 10 amantadine volunteers, but the titers were significantly lower than those in the placebo volunteers. There was no significant difference in the frequency or duration of excretion of virus.

In summary, the tests on volunteers experimentally infected with influenza A viruses that were highly sensitive to amantadine in laboratory tests have shown a reduction in incidence of significant clinical illness without preventing infection when one strain was used (Togo et al., 1968; Bloomfield et al., 1970) but no effect with another strain (Tyrrell et al., 1965). In two (Likar, 1970; Cohen et al., 1976) of three volunteer studies with different H3N2 strains, amantadine showed no significant effect. These data do not support the conclusion of consistency in studies on volunteers or the claim that laboratory tests can predict the effectiveness of amantadine against influenza A virus infections and illness in experimentally infected volunteers (Jackson, 1977).

Tests Under Natural Conditions of Infection

A study of 794 prisoners in Pennsylvania (Wendel et al., 1966) suffered from three deficiencies: (1) 90 percent of the volunteers already had significant antibody titers for the current strain of influenza A virus; (2) the study was begun after about 50 cases of acute respiratory illness of undefined etiology had occurred in the institution, and the total number of illnesses during the study period was very small, especially so for those associated with infection by influenza A virus; and (3) the smaller number of illnesses observed in the amantadine-treated group applied also for those illnesses that were not associated with influenza A virus infection. A study on 676 prisoners in California (Harris et al., 1966) showed no effect of amantadine either on total respiratory illness or on serologically confirmed influenza A virus illness.

A limited study in Sweden (Callmander and Hellgren, 1968) on adults in various occupations in an open community during a period of influenza A virus (Leningrad strain) activity yielded few definitive data, except that the number of people who were troubled by various respiratory signs and symptoms was the same in both groups, although twice as many had cough in the placebo group as in the amantadine group—and the cough was less severe in the amantadine group.

An excellently designed and implemented double-blind trial carried out in a family environment in Britain in 1967, at a time when H2N2 influenza A virus was active, showed a definite protective effect of amantadine in reducing both clinical influenza (defined as *cough accompanied by fever of 37.8°C or more*) and infection (Galbraith et al., 1970). Two hundred and eight people living in 52 households in which one member developed clinical influenza were carefully studied both clinically and serologically. Only 35 of the 52 clinically diagnosed patients had serologic evidence of infection with influenza A virus. Serologically confirmed cases of influenza A virus illness were subsequently found in 12 of 90 placebo-treated contacts and in none of 91 amantadine-treated contacts. Six other cases of clinical influenza, which were not confirmed serologically or which lacked paired sera, were equally distributed between the two groups.

However, in another excellent study by the same group of investigators (Galbraith et al., 1969), carried out in Britain during the initial A/Hong Kong/68 virus epidemic in January–March 1969, no protective effect of amantadine was demonstrated. Despite the first appearance of this pandemic (Hong Kong) influenza virus in the communities, only 36 of the 58 index cases with a clinical diagnosis of influenza could be serologically confirmed, indicating that influenza caused by other agents was occurring at the same time. Among the contacts of the confirmed index cases, clinical influenza occurred equally frequently in amantadine- and placebo-treated subjects. Among the contacts of the unconfirmed cases, the incidence of clinical influenza was slightly lower than among the contacts of the confirmed cases. The total influenza A virus infection rate (clinical and subclinical) was significantly lower among the contacts of the unconfirmed cases, but among 130 contacts from both groups with paired sera, 26 percent of those on placebo and 36 percent of those on amantadine showed evidence of infection. Since the number of people with little or no antibody at the beginning of the second trial was much higher than in the first trial, the authors were inclined to explain the discrepant results of the two trials on the assumption that amantadine is ineffective in individuals without antibody for the infecting virus, because the influenza A strains during both outbreaks were equally sensitive to amantadine in tissue culture. However, the carefully controlled studies on antibody negative volunteers, in which amantadine reduced the incidence of illness but not of infection following experimental infection, and my analysis of their own data on the incidence of infection among those with low initial hemagglutination inhibition (HAI) titers in the two trials do not support their explanation. It appears rather either that amantadine behaves differently against different influenza strains under natural conditions of infection or that it has no effect on the infection rate with any strain in people without antibody. Whether or not amantadine can reduce the incidence of illness as well as of infection caused by different strains of influenza virus in individuals with higher initial titers of HAI antibody cannot be determined from the British field trials because the number of subjects with antibody against the Hong Kong virus was too small.

A number of other field trials during the A/Hong Kong pandemic period, not as well controlled as the above British studies, do not permit more definitive conclusions on the effect of amantadine in reducing the amount of illness, despite the larger numbers involved.

In contradistinction to the negative or equivocal results in five different trials, Nafta et al. (1970) reported that in a double-blind trial during A/Hong Kong epidemic in Romania, amantadine completely prevented influenza A virus clinical disease and reduced the total infection rate by half; i.e., 10.5 percent amantadine versus 20.5 percent placebo.

The only field trial in the U.S. during the A/Hong Kong pandemic period was carried out on 2650 naval recruits (Peckingpaugh et al., 1970). There was no statistically significant difference between the amantadine-treated and placebo-treated recruits as regards the different types of illness or the incidence of infection with influenza A virus, which was low (6 percent) in both groups.

A study on 111 hospitalized patients was carried out in a medical center in Seattle, Washington, after a sharp outbreak of illness associated with influenza A virus had occurred in the community and after 30 percent of the medical house staff and nursing personnel were absent from work because of respiratory illness (O'Donoghue et al., 1973). The total influenza A virus infection rate was 20 percent in the placebo patients versus 4 percent in the amantadine patients. Since the results of this small study resemble only those reported from Romania (Nafta et al., 1970) and are different from all the other trials under natural conditions of infection, it would have been desirable to repeat such tests in other hospital settings to determine if these unusual findings are indeed reproducible, especially in patients without preexisting antibody.

The conflicting data on the effect of amantadine on experimental and natural infections of human beings with different strains of influenza A virus that are sensitive to this drug in laboratory tests cannot be reconciled, nor can scientific validity be achieved by an indiscriminate pooling of some positive results and by a disregard of negative results in carefully controlled studies. The summary of a recent workshop on antiviral agents in influenza (Couch and Jackson, 1976) contained the following statement:

> The sum total of the experience with controlled studies included well over 1,000 individuals who received artificial challenge and more than 20,000 persons who were exposed naturally to influenza. Various degrees of protection were reported, but the overall results provided by the studies under field conditions suggest that amantadine provides about 50 percent protection against influenzal infection and > 60% protection against illness. These studies established that amantadine is an effective prophylactic agent for influenza caused by the type A viruses but that it has no effect against type B infection.

This evaluation of the available data and of the conclusions that can be drawn from them is in accord neither with the data that I have summarized here nor with the conclusions that have been drawn from them by other investigators (Tyrrell et al., 1965; Harris et al., 1966; Callmander and Hellgren, 1968; Togo et al., 1968; Galbraith et al., 1969; Bloomfield et al., 1970; Likar, 1970; Cohen et al., 1976). The same comment applies to the following recent statement by Jackson (1977): "Investigations with amantadine in volunteers and field trials have *consistently* [my emphasis] established a prophylactic effect at a level between 50% and 70% in the prevention of infection and at a level of 70%–100% in the prevention of clinical influenza."

Amantadine Therapy for Influenza

Many careful double-blind placebo-controlled studies (Wingfield et al., 1969; Togo et al., 1970; Knight et al., 1970; Galbraith et al., 1971) have shown that amantadine therapy started soon after the onset of naturally occurring influenza shortened the duration of fever in laboratory-confirmed influenza A illnesses. The study on a large number of influenza A virus illnesses in family practice (Galbraith et al., 1971) showed more rapid defervescence without any difference in the duration of symptoms in the amantadine-treated patients, but no mention was made of what was found in the 30 patients on whom serologic tests showed no evidence of infection with influenza A virus. In a 1973–74 study done by Galbraith (cited as a personal communication by Stuart-Harris and Schild, 1976) during a mixed outbreak of influenza A and influenza B, the more rapid defervescence associated with amantadine therapy was observed in those subjects who were subsequently confirmed as having been infected with influenza A virus, but not in those infected with influenza B virus. Controlled studies on meaningfully large numbers of amantadine-treated and placebo-treated patients exhibiting the clinically indistinguishable syndrome of influenza that is not caused by influenza viruses are needed to indicate whether amantadine may have a pharmacologic effect on the course of this particular syndrome that is not related to its action on influenza A virus. Controlled studies are also needed to answer the question whether aspirin, not necessarily related to its antipyretic properties, might prove to be as effective as amantadine, which is not antipyretic against endotoxin-induced fever in rats but has other pharmacologic properties (Vernier et al., 1969). The interesting studies of Little et al. (1976) on pulmonary expiratory flow volumes in naturally occurring "nonpneumonic" influenza A virus illness in eight amantadine-treated and seven placebo-treated students need to be repeated not only on larger numbers of people of different ages but also with the additional control groups mentioned above before one can conclude that amantadine "significantly accelerates the resolution of peripheral airways dysfunction" in influenza A virus disease (Little et al., 1976). No significant effect of large doses of amantadine (400 to 550 mg per day) was observed in 11 patients with "pure influenza pneumonia" (Couch and Jackson, 1976). During a recent workshop on antiviral agents in influenza, "no unanimity of opinion emerged regarding the therapeutic use of amantadine" (Couch and Jackson, 1976).

Limitations of Any Specific Antiinfluenza Drug in the Prevention of Clinical Influenza, a Disease of Multiple Etiology

It is essential to differentiate between the disease that has been called *influenza* for centuries and the diseases caused by the influenza viruses. Natural infection of human beings with influenza viruses gives rise to a spectrum of manifestations ranging from no illness to mild, afebrile upper respiratory (i.e., above the larynx) with or without lower respiratory (i.e., larynx, trachea, bronchi, bronchioles) disease, febrile upper respiratory disease of varying severity with or without generalized malaise, febrile lower respiratory disease with varying degrees of systemic illness, and occasionally pneumonia. The disease called *influenza* is properly limited to an acute febrile respiratory illness that includes cough, with generalized malaise of varying severity, and has a multiple etiology in the same way that the clinically defined syndromes of pneumonia, encephalitis, etc., have multiple etiologies. Without special viral laboratory tests, the influenza that is caused by the influenza viruses cannot be distinguished by clinical criteria or simple routine clinical laboratory tests from the influenza caused by a host of other respiratory tract pathogens, most of them still unidentified.

Since the discovery of the influenza viruses, the continuing enormous health problem of influenza has been equated by virologists and public health officials with the recurrent epidemics of influenza caused by constantly changing antigenic variants of predominantly influenza A virus. It is true that influenza epidemics are caused only by influenza viruses, but it is not true that most of the clinical influenza problem is associated with epidemics. Recently, I documented the enormity of disabling morbidity of what I would call endemic or interepidemic influenza, approximately 90 percent of which is *not* caused by influenza A or B viruses, and most of which cannot be accounted for by presently known viruses and mycoplasma (Sabin, 1977, 1978). Thus, during the period of July 1, 1973, to June 30, 1974, when there was no national influenza virus epidemic in the U.S., the Health Interview Survey (HIS) data of the National Center for Health Statistics (NCHS) showed a total of 61,841,000 episodes of clinical influenza severe enough to send people to bed for an average of 3.6 days; i.e., a total of 223 million days of bed disability, in addition to a total of 146 million days of bed disability attributable to upper respiratory illness. Viral isolation tests on 6841 people with "influenza" illness during this period yielded only 2.3 percent influenza A and 7.4 percent influenza B viruses, whereas serologic tests on paired sera from 6532 patients yielded 2.8 percent positives for influenza A and 9.5 percent positives for influenza B (Influenza Surveillance Report, 1976). I found that the peak seasonal incidence of endemic influenza, unlike the upper respiratory illnesses in the HIS data, was during January, February, and March, the same as during most of the influenza A virus epidemic years. The unpublished HIS data for respiratory illnesses during the most recent nonepidemic year of July 1, 1976, to June 30, 1977, show (1) 65,232,000 illnesses with an average of 3.1 days of bed disability per illness for influenza, (2) 65,543,000 illnesses with an average of 2.6 days for upper respiratory, and (3) 1,844,000 illnesses with an average of 15.8 days per illness for pneumonia. Total mortality (based on death certificates) for this period was only 862 for influenza and 48,708 for all pneumonias for the entire U.S., the lowest for any preceding nonepidemic year (personal communication from Mr. Ronald W. Wilson, Chief, Health Status and Demographic Analysis Branch, NCHS, Hyattsville, Maryland). During the recent influenza A virus epidemic years, there has been a 6 to 9 percent rise in combined influenza and upper respiratory bed disability over the preceding nonepidemic year; i.e., 390 million in 1974-75 and 401 million in 1975-76 as compared with 369 million in 1973-74. Influenza mortality per million total population rose from 9 in 1973-74 to 24 and 36 in 1974-75 and 1975-76, respectively; pneumonia mortality per million total population fell slightly from 258 during the nonepidemic year of 1973-74 to 251 and 252 during the epidemic years of 1974-75 and 1975-76, respectively. Mortality rates from heart disease; bronchitis, emphysema, and asthma; diabetes mellitus; chronic nephritis; leukemia; and respiratory tuberculosis have been falling or not rising in the U.S. since 1972 without reference to influenza virus epidemics (Sabin, 1977, 1978). During the recent influenza virus epidemics, approximately 80 percent of the total influenza was still not accounted for by infection with the influenza viruses.

Conclusion

Data on the amantadine prophylactic studies in various countries during the initial A/Hong Kong pandemic virus outbreaks show how often clinically diagnosed influenza was not confirmed as having been caused by influenza A virus, even during brief periods of very sharp outbreaks. In my judgment, therefore, even very extensive use of a drug that would be highly effective against both influenza A and B viruses could not be expected to have a significant impact on the massive total influenza disease problem and its significant disabling morbidity.

References

Bloomfield, S.S., Gaffney, T.E., and Schniff, G.M.: A design for the evaluation of antiviral drugs in human influenza. Am. J. Epidemiol. 91:568–574, 1970.

Callmander, E., and Hellgren, L.: Amantadine hydrochloride as a prophylactic in respiratory infections; a double-blind investigation of its clinical use and serology. J. Clin. Pharmacol. 8:186–189, 1968.

Cohen, A., Tago, Y., Khakoo, R., Waldman, R., and Sigel, M.: Comparative clinical and laboratory evaluation of prophylactic capacity of ribavirin, amantadine hydrochloride, and placebo in induced human influenza type A. J. Infect. Dis. 133 (Supplement): A114–A120, 1976.

Couch, R.B.: An assessment of amantadine for influenza. Infect. Dis. 7:4, 16, 32, 1977.

Couch, R.B., and Jackson, G.G.: Antiviral agents in influenza—summary of influenza workshop VIII. J. Infect. Dis. 134:516–527, 1976.

Galbraith, A.W., Oxford, J.S., Schild, C.G., and Watson, G.I.: Study of 1-adamantanamine hydrochloride used prophylactically during the Hong Kong influenza epidemic in the family environment. Bull. WHO. 41:677–682, 1969.

Galbraith, A.W., Oxford, J.S., Schild, C.G., and Watson, G.I.: Protective effect of aminoadamantane in influenza A2 infections in the family environment. Ann. NY Acad. Sci. 173:29–43, 1970.

Galbraith, A.W., Oxford, J.S., Schild, G.C., Potter, C.W., and Watson, G.I.: Therapeutic effect of 1-adamantanamine hydrochloride in naturally occurring influenza A_2/Hong Kong infection. Lancet 2:113–115, 1971.

Harris, B., Keating, W.C., Jr., and Iezzoni, D.G.: Report to clinical evaluation section. Delaware, E.I. DuPont de Nemours Company, 1966.

Influenza Surveillance Report No. 90, 1973-1974 and 1974-1975. Atlanta, Center for Disease Control, 1976.

Jackson G.G.: Chemoprophylaxis and chemotherapy. In Selby, P., ed., *Virus, Vaccines and Strategy*, London and New York, Academic Press, 1976.

Jackson, G.G.: Sensitivity of influenza A virus to amantadine. J. Infect. Dis. 136:301–302, 1977.

Knight, V., Fedson, D., Baldini, J., Douglas, R.G., and Couch, R.B.: Amantadine therapy of epidemic influenza A_2 (Hong Kong). Infect. Immun. 1:200–204, 1970.

Likar, M.: Effectiveness of amantadine in protecting vaccinated volunteers from an attenuated strain of influenza A_2/Hong Kong virus. Ann. NY Acad. Sci. 173:108–112, 1970.

Little, J.W., Hall, W.J., Douglas, F.G., Jr., Hyde, R.W., and Speers, D.M.: Amantadine effect on peripheral airways abnormalities in influenza. Ann. Intern. Med. 85:177–182, 1976.

Nafta, I., Turcanu, A.G., Braun, I., Companetz, W., Simionescu, A., Birt, E., and Florea, V.: Administration of amantadine for the prevention of Hong Kong influenza. Bull. WHO 42:423–427, 1970.

O'Donoghue, J.M., Ray, C.G., Terry, D.W., Jr., and Beaty, H.N.: Prevention of nosocomial influenza infection with amantadine. Am. J. Epidemiol. 97:276–282, 1973.

Peckingpaugh, R.O., Askin, F.B., Pierce, W.E., Edwards, E.A., Johnson, D.P., and Jackson, G.G.: Field studies with amantadine: acceptability and protection. Ann. NY Acad. Sci. 173:62–73, 1970.

Sabin, A.B.: Amantadine hydrochloride: analysis of data related to its proposed use for prevention of A2 influenza virus disease in human beings. JAMA 200:943–950, 1967.

Sabin, A.B.: Mortality from pneumonia and risk conditions during influenza epidemics; high influenza morbidity during nonepidemic years. JAMA 237:2823–2828, 1977.

Sabin, A.B.: Overview and horizons in prevention of some human infectious diseases by vaccination. Am. J. Clin. Pathol. 70(Supplement):114–127, 1978.

Smorodintsev, A.A., Zlydnikov, D.M., Kiseleva, A.M., Romanov, J.A., Kazantsev, A.P., and Rumovsky, V.I.: Evaluation of amantadine in artificially induced A2 and B influenza. JAMA 213:1448–1454, 1970.

Stuart-Harris, C.H., and Schild, G.C.: *Influenza: The Viruses and the Disease.* Littleton, Mass., Publishing Sciences Group, Inc., 1976.

Togo, Y., Hornick, R.B., and Dawkins, A.T., Jr.: Studies on induced influenza in man. I. Double-blind studies designed to assess prophylactic efficacy of amantadine hydrochloride against A/2 Rockville/1/65 strain. JAMA 203:1089–1094, 1968.

Togo, Y., Hornick, R.B., Felitti, V.J., Kaufman, M.L., Dawkins, A.T., Jr., Kilpe, V.E., and Claghorn, J.L.: Evaluation of therapeutic efficacy of amantadine in patients with naturally occurring A2 influenza. JAMA 211:1149–1156, 1970.

Tyrrell, D.A.J., Bynoe, M.L., and Hoorn, B.: Studies on the antiviral activity of 1-adamantanamine. Br. J. Exp. Path. 46:370–375, 1965.

Vernier, V.G., Harmon, J.B., Stump, J.M., Lynes, T.E., Marvel, J.P., and Smith, D.H.: The toxicologic and pharmacologic properties of amantadine hydrochloride. Toxicol. Appl. Pharmacol. 15:642–665, 1969.

Wendel, H.A., Snyder, M.T., and Pell, S.: Trial of amantadine in epidemic influenza. Clin. Pharmacol. Ther. 7:38–43, 1966.

Wingfield, W.L., Pollack, D., and Grunert, R.R.: Therapeutic efficacy of amantadine HCl and rimantadine HCl in naturally occurring influenza A2 respiratory illness in man. N. Engl. J. Med. 281:579–584, 1969.

14

Should All Mild Hypertension Be Treated?

SHOULD ONE TREAT ALL MILD HYPERTENSION? NO.
John Fry, O.B.E. , M.D., F.R.C.S., F.R.C.G.P.

SHOULD ALL MILD HYPERTENSION BE TREATED? YES.
William B. Kannel, M.D.

Why, universal plodding prisons up
The nimble spirits in the arteries.

Shakespeare, *Love's Labour Lost*

A man is as old as his arteries.

Thomas Sydenham

Of all the ailments which may blow out life's little candle, heart disease is the chief.

William Boyd, *Pathology for the Surgeon*

Introduction

It is common for physicians to be accused of overtreating. One condition that they are often accused of undertreating, however, is hypertension. It is said repeatedly that most high blood pressure is undiagnosed, that the cases that *are* known are often untreated, and that those patients who *are* treated are often poorly treated.

There is little disagreement on the desirability of drug treatment for the more severe degrees of hypertension, but there is controversy about both the danger of mild hypertension and the desirability of treating it. Our two contributors disagree vigorously on this point.

Fry contends, largely on the basis of personal experience, that it is not necessary to treat mild hypertension, especially in the elderly. He does not consider it socially defensible to engage in massive screening campaigns to detect large numbers of people with a "disease" whose prognosis he considers to be often benign. He does not, however, advocate such a philosophy for younger patients, especially males.

Kannel, relying primarily on epidemiologic data, comes down squarely on the other side. He sees no evidence for calling *any* level of high blood pressure benign, and he therefore advocates treating all hypertension, although not necessarily with drugs. Kannel reminds us that risk factors have been identified that suggest strongly that a given level of blood pressure does not carry the same prognosis for everyone, and he suggests that the vigor of the therapeutic approach be conditioned by such knowledge. Risk factors include race, carbohydrate tolerance, blood lipid levels, cigarette smoking, and weight, among others.

Kannel also attacks a series of misconceptions, including the alleged triviality of "labile" hypertension, the belief that systolic hypertension is less important prognostically than diastolic hypertension, the benign course of hypertension in the female, and the importance of renin measurements. Most readers should at the very least be provoked by his account to reexamine some favorite clichés.

Louis Lasagna, M.D.

Should One Treat All Mild Hypertension? No.

John Fry, O.B.E., M.D., F.R.C.S., F.R.C.G.P.
Family Physician, Beckenham, Kent, England

All mild hypertension most definitely need not be treated.

Who am I and on what basis do I make this statement? I am a family physician in Britain, part of the National Health Service, and have been in my practice for 30 years. During this time, we have cared for some 10,000 people. As part of my research, I have been observing and following almost 1000 hypertensive patients. The methods of study are reported in previous papers (Fry, 1974b, 1975a, 1975b).

What I have found it possible to do is to carry out a study of the natural history of hypertension. Since I have never been convinced of the value of treating mild high blood pressure, most of the people I followed up on have been untreated and really do represent the "natural" course of mild hypertension.

What Is High Blood Pressure?

When we take our sphygmomanometers to measure our patients' blood pressures, we seem to believe that we know and understand what the implications of our findings will be. But do we?

If we discover a high blood pressure, we enter an uncertain and unpredictable situation. The causes of high blood pressure still are largely unknown. Secondary hypertension accounts for less than one tenth of all diagnosed cases of high blood pressure; the rest are termed *essential hypertension*. It is this condition that we usually are dealing with, but we are quite uncertain of the probable outcome in each individual patient.

Despite the great amount of research on essential hypertension in hospital clinics and laboratories, we must admit to having very little knowledge of the condition as it exists in the community outside the hospital setting. Certain groups and types of individuals are being defined as "vulnerables" and "at risk," and it is becoming clear that these patients have to be diagnosed early and managed energetically and effectively for the rest of their lives. But what of the others who may not be vulnerable or at risk? The modern challenge to us as clinicians must be to develop a discriminating system of early diagnosis and continuing surveillance and care over many years.

However we try to define *high blood pressure*, it is wrong to accept it as a general disease that has to be treated in all individuals and at all ages. Simple logistics will show how ludicrous such a policy would be. In developed societies such as the U.K., the U.S., and the countries of Western Europe, it is likely that 10 to 15 percent of the population will have sustained blood pressures of 160/100 or higher. In the U.S., this means that there are between 20 and 30 million hypertensives. To have an effective and reliable service to screen, diagnose, assess, treat, manage, support, and provide follow-up for all these hypertensives, about 10 percent of all the available medical and nursing resources, or 25,000 physicians and 100,000 nurses, would be required! Would this be a reasonable expenditure and allocation of these resources?

Clearly a compromise has to be arrived at.

On the one hand, we have to accept that high blood pressure is dangerous in some individuals. In these patients, modern, effective antihypertensive drugs have to be used, although they do cause side effects. We must be prepared to consider also that it may not be necessary, and indeed is not possible, to screen the whole adult population at frequent intervals or to treat and follow up the huge numbers whose blood pressures happen to be above predetermined figures.

There is no single "all or none" answer. We must be prepared to combine the warmth and personal humanity of clinical art with the cold and impersonal brusqueness of medical science.

Incidence of High Blood Pressure

Hypertension is a condition associated with aging; that is, its incidence increases with age (Figure 14–1). It is also more frequent in females.

An important fact is that more than half of all hypertensives are over the age of 60 when the condition is first diagnosed.

Nature of High Blood Pressure

Hypertension in average individuals is less severe and less dramatic than in the selected cases seen in hospital practice. In my own series, 28 percent of hypertensive patients had an initial diastolic blood pressure (DBP) between 100 and 110 mm Hg, 35 percent had a DBP between 110 and 120 mm Hg, and 14 percent had a DBP over 120 mm Hg.

It must not be assumed that high blood pressure, or any level of blood pressure, remains constant and unaltered. In a group of hypertensives that I have followed closely for 15 years, I have found that the DBP fell spontaneously in 30 percent, it remained unchanged in 20 percent, and it increased with time and age in 50 percent. Therefore, there is quite a good possibility that blood pressure may decrease on its own.

Risks of High Blood Pressure

In my long-term follow-up of hypertensive patients, I was not able for ethical reasons to carry out a blind controlled trial using antihypertensive drugs. What I was able to do, however, was to compare the observed mortality rates in hypertensives with those expected for the population as a whole. I was able also to compare the observed rates of complications of strokes or coronary artery disease in hypertensives with those of nonhypertensives in my practice.

In this way, it is possible to obtain some guide to the extra risks, if any, of high blood pressure,

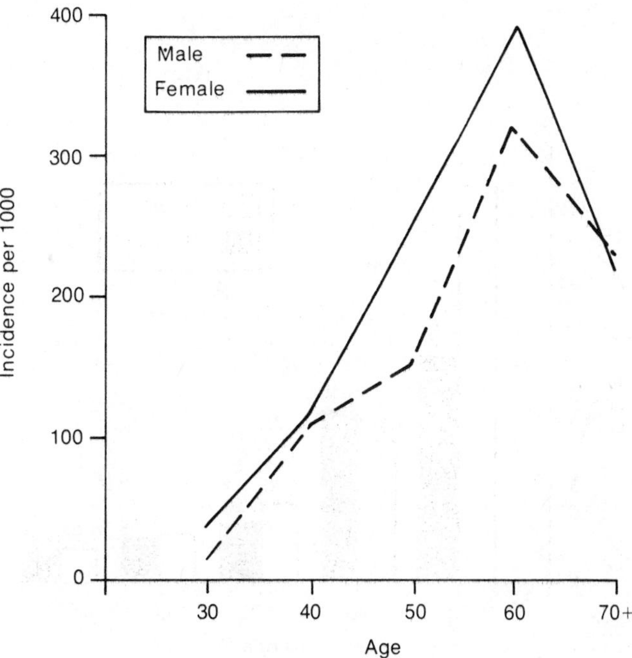

Figure 14-1. Incidence of high blood pressure as a function of age and sex. Adapted from Fry, J.: Update 10:1238-1243, 1975.

and to relate these risks to certain factors.

Mortality Risks in Hypertension

Figure 14–2 shows the observed/expected (O/E) rates of mortality for hypertensives that I have followed. The risk is related closely to the age of diagnosis. Thus, in the 30 to 39 age group, the risk of a hypertensive dying was 7.51 times greater than expected; at 40 to 49, the risk was 4.91 times greater; and at 50 to 59, it was 2.22 times greater. But if the person was 60 years of age or over when first diagnosed as having high blood pressure, the risks of dying were no greater than expected. As noted already, half of all hypertensives are over the age of 60 when first diagnosed. This suggests that in half of all hypertensives, there is no good case to be made for treating them in order to reduce extra mortality risks. When these mortality risks are expressed by sex, it is evident that at all ages, except between 40 and 49, the risks of dying were greater in males than in females (Figure 14–3).

Complications and Deaths from Strokes, Coronary Artery Disease, and Other Causes in Hypertensives

The observed/expected (O/E) incidence of stroke for hypertensives was appreciably larger than that of mortality. Figure 14–4 shows that these extra risks were greater in the younger

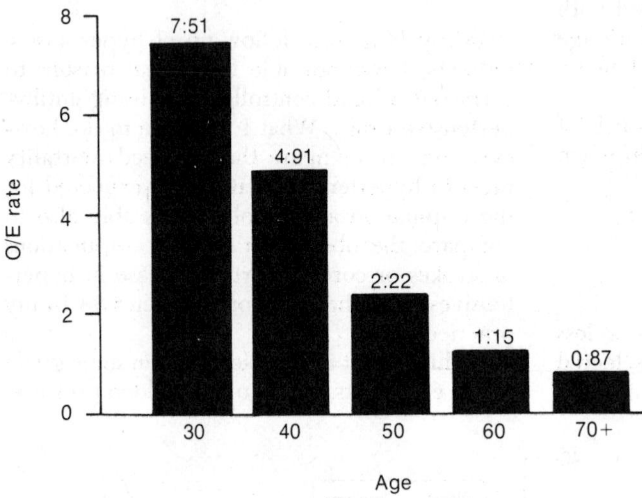

Figure 14-2. Observed/expected mortality ratio in hypertensives. Adapted from Fry, J.: Update 10:1238-1243, 1975.

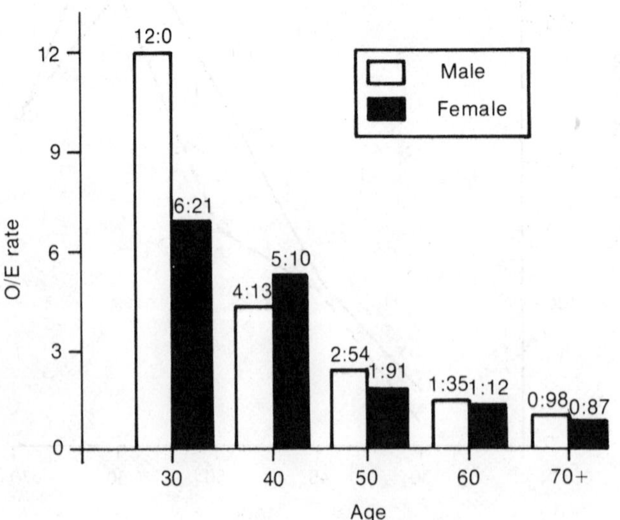

Figure 14-3. Mortality rates in hypertensives: observed/expected ratios in males and females. Adapted from Fry, J.: Update 10:1238-1243, 1975.

hypertensives. Of the 112 strokes observed, 20 were cerebral hemorrhages and 92 were cerebral thromboses (Fry 1975a).

Overall, there were no great differences between the O/E ratios for males and females, but Figure 14–5 shows that in the 40 to 49 age group, the ratio was greater in females, and at 50 to 59, much greater in males.

The overall O/E ratio was 0.95 for coronary artery disease, suggesting that hypertension created no extra risks to its development (Fry 1975a). For males, the O/E ratio was 0.85; for females, it was 2.4. When this is related to age (Figure 14–6), it is seen that only at 40 to 49 was the O/E much above unity, and this was due to a much higher ratio in females (Figure 14–7).

Two other conditions associated with hypertension were specially noted. There were some people (16) in whom renal diseases were found and in whom these may have been an etiologic factor; this represented a rate of only 20 per 1000. It was not possible to compare it with the rate for nonhypertensives in the practice.

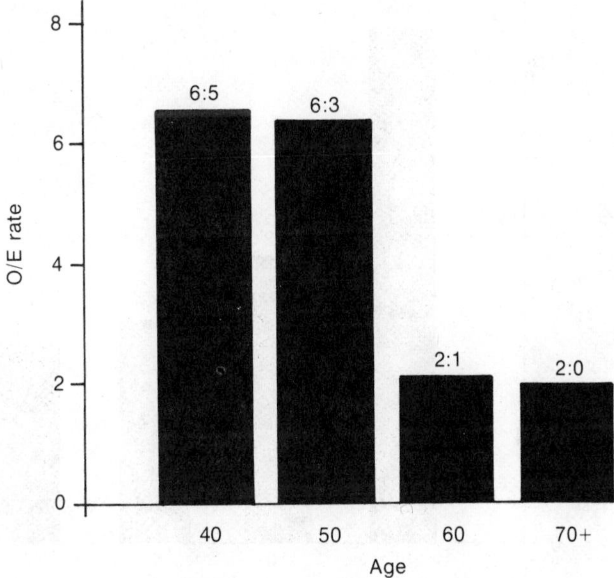

Figure 14–4. Strokes in hypertensives: observed/expected ratios of incidence. Adapted from Fry, J.: Update 10:1238-1243, 1975.

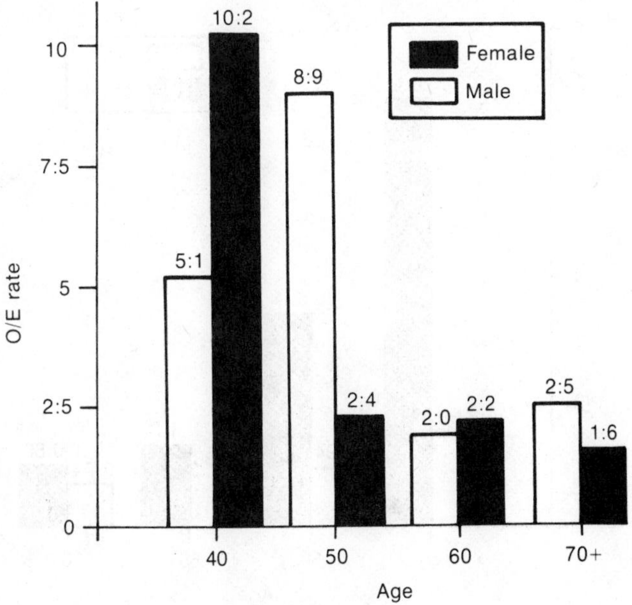

Figure 14–5. Strokes in hypertensives: observed/expected ratios in males and females. Adapted from Fry, J.: Update 1238-1243, 1975.

A surprising correlation was with senile dementia severe enough to require hospitalization. Although the numbers were small (26), there were 21 females. This represented a rate double that for nonhypertensives.

Effects of Diastolic Blood Pressure Levels on Outcome

In hypertension, it is well known that the diastolic blood pressure (DBP) is an important prognostic factor. I found in my series that this was so in general, but the influence of the DBP was more significant in males than in females at all ages. In the patients over 60, there were no relationships between DBP levels and outcomes. DBP levels were of more serious significance in younger and middle-aged hypertensives, particularly in males.

However, most of us in clinical practice will have had the experience of following up patients with high blood pressure, untreated or uncontrollable over many years, who ap-

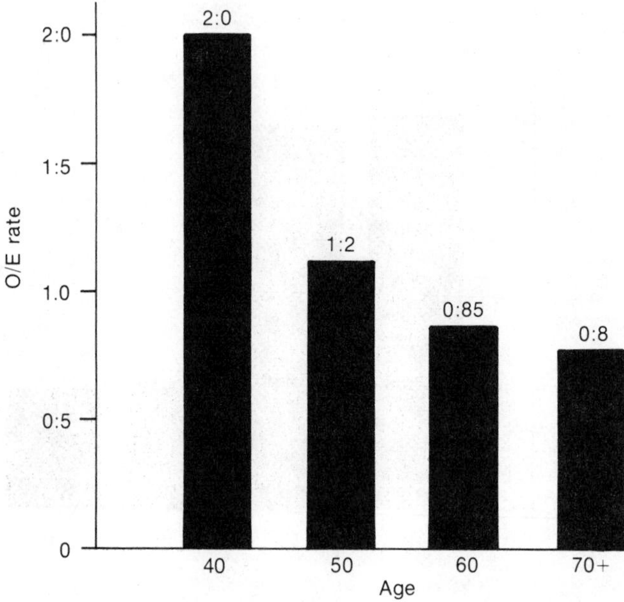

Figure 14-6. Coronary artery disease in hypertensives: observed/expected mortality ratios. Adapted from Fry, J.: Update 1238-1243, 1975.

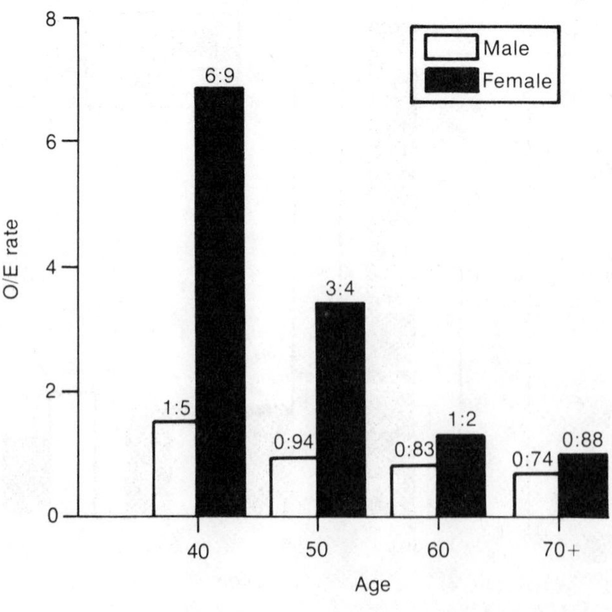

Figure 14-7. Coronary artery disease: observed/expected mortality rates in male and female hypertensives. Adapted from Fry, J.: Update 1238-1243, 1975.

parently come to no great harm. I have followed 87 hypertensives for more than 15 years. They had DBPs over 120 mm Hg at first diagnosis and were subsequently untreated (Fry 1975b). At follow-up 15 to 25 years later, 78 percent were alive—58 percent of whom had no complications. Female hypertensives outnumbered males by 2.5:1, and many of them were overweight. There is a well recognized group of plump female hypertensives whose high blood pressure does not appear to shorten their lives or add to complications.

Implications

In trying to work out a reasonable and sensible policy for management of mild hypertension, we have to take into account factors other than pure science, technology, and facts produced from academic, hospital-based units.

Most mild hypertensives will be diagnosed and managed in the community outside the hospital setting. Such patients will be treated by general practitioners, family physicians, and internists. But what is *mild* hypertension? Presumably, it is blood pressure below certain levels of readings on the sphygmomanometer. Is it reasonable to base the diagnosis only on these figures? I have shown that there are other factors that are related to prognosis, such as age and sex, and there are still others.

Faced with a condition that is likely eventually to affect one fourth or one third of all adults aged 40 and over, can mild hypertension be considered a "disease"? We have to decide on a policy that takes into account the following:

1. Most hypertensives are "mild" in regard to DBP levels; i.e., levels under 120 mm Hg.
2. Most hypertensives are over 60 when first diagnosed.
3. More hypertensives are female than male.
4. Most hypertensives are "primary" and "essential," with no known underlying causes.
5. The prognosis is good in patients over 60 and better in females than in males.
6. The prognosis is poor in those under 60, in males, in those with a family history of sudden death, and in those with sustained DBP above 120 mm Hg.

Conclusion

It is reasonable to conclude that we should maximize our efforts at treating high blood pressure, be it mild or severe, in the following directions.

We should *not* try to detect the existence of high blood pressure through mass screening of all adults. Certainly, in a good health care system, there should be continuity of care by personal primary physicians for all people. These physicians should aim to record blood pressures on an ongoing basis every 3 to 5 years (Miall and Chinn, 1974). In this way, groups and individuals at risk will be picked out for special, more intensive observation.

Certainly, we should endeavor to define and to treat high blood pressure at all levels in young men and to a lesser degree in young women. We should be wary of subjecting our older citizens (those over 60) to senseless and unpleasant therapy with diuretics and antihypertensives for many years, producing unpleasant side effects. It is often found that their blood pressures are lower when they are taken off therapy, as I have found when such patients have moved into my district. These patients are usually in better health without therapy and their blood pressures are no higher.

My plea is for more common sense and uncommon sensibility in the management of mild hypertension. We must regard each hypertensive as an individual case, taking into account various risk and nonrisk factors. In this way, we shall discover, I am sure, that many people with mild hypertension should be selectively nontreated.

References

Fry, J.: *Profiles of Disease.* Churchill Livingstone, Edinburgh, 1966.
Fry, J.: *Common Diseases.* MTP Press Ltd., Lancaster, 1974a.
Fry, J.: Natural history of hypertension, a case for selective non-treatment. Lancet 2:431, 1974b.
Fry, J.: Deaths and complications from hypertension. J. R. Coll. Gen. Pract. 25:489–494, 1975a.
Fry, J.: Long-surviving hypertension—a 15 year followup. J. R. Coll. Gen. Pract. 25:481–486, 1975b.
Miall, W.E., and Chinn, S.: Screening for hypertension: some epidemiological observations. Br. Med. J. 3:595–600, 1974.

Should All Mild Hypertension Be Treated? Yes.

William B. Kannel, M.D.
Boston University School of Medicine

Data from more than two decades of prospective epidemiologic studies of the natural history of hypertension strongly support the contention that all hypertension—systolic or diastolic, labile or fixed, casual or basal, mild or severe—should be treated. However, not all patients with hypertension require antihypertensive *drug* therapy. Such epidemiologic data have indicated that hypertension is one ingredient of a multifactorial complex that contributes to the incidence of cardiovascular disease (McGee, 1973; Kannel et al., 1976). It thus follows that the treatment required is not necessarily antihypertensive drug therapy alone. Reduction of risk factors should replace or supplement drug therapy in some patients. Evidence to support this concept is substantial.

Incidence

Hypertension afflicts about one in every five adults (Table 14–1). This high prevalence indicates the need for a public health approach. Without organized help from the community, physicians could hardly cope effectively with such numbers of hypertensive patients. Both the hypertensive (who is a candidate for cardiovascular catastrophe) and his physician will need considerable assistance if this problem is to be brought under control.

Hazards of Untreated Hypertension

Primary or essential hypertension has, in the past, been unjustifiably labeled "benign hypertension." This appellation was arrived at because accelerated or "malignant" hypertension was used as the standard of comparison. When the fate of those with essential hypertension is (more appropriately) compared with that of the general population (normotensives), the true gravity of hypertension as a factor in morbidity and mortality emerges. Hypertensives have double the overall mortality and triple the cardiovascular mortality of normotensives of the same age and sex (Kannel et al., 1976). By this standard, hypertension can hardly be considered benign, even though it may take decades for the sequelae to appear. Thus, failure to treat hypertension cannot be justified on the grounds that it is a benign condition from which treatment may be withheld until symptoms appear.

Essential hypertension, or elevated blood pressure of unknown cause, is a common and powerful contributor to cardiovascular disease. This can be judged from examining the regression of incidence of cardiovascular disease in relation to blood pressure (Table 14–2). Because the coefficients have been standardized to compensate for the different units of measurement, their size can be directly compared. Clearly, by this yardstick, blood pressure ranks at the top of the list of major risk factors. Although the cardiovascular sequelae may not appear for a decade or more, compared with normotensives, hypertensives develop twice as much occlusive peripheral arterial disease, a threefold excess of coronary heart disease, four times as much cardiac failure, and a sevenfold excess of stroke (Figure 14–8). Since the average male has one chance in three of suffering a major cardiovascular catastrophe before reaching age 60, this constitutes a serious hazard. The attributable risk of hypertension is so large as to warrant a significant effort, and even some inconvenience, at controlling the condition. The benefits of managing hypertension are considerable.

Current Treatment

Physician treatment of hypertensives is not completely effective. With the introduction of effective antihypertensive agents into the Fra-

Table 14-1. *Percent Prevalence of Selected "Risk Factors" in the United States.*

Sex	Age	Inactivity	Obesity	Hyper-tension	Cigarette Smoking	Diabetes	Hyperchol-esterolemia	ECG-LVH°
Men	35–44	12.1	12.5	13.5	48.6	1.1	20.2	2.9
	45–54	16.9	14.7	18.3	43.1	1.1	25.7	4.8
	55–64	21.0	12.5	22.3	37.4	3.3	23.5	10.1
	65–74	27.1	12.7	27.1	22.8†	3.2	21.6	7.1
Women	35–44	13.3	20.1	8.5	38.8	0.8	12.9	0.9
	45–54	19.3	24.2	18.2	36.1	2.9	28.0	3.6
	55–64	30.8	30.9	31.2	24.2	3.2	49.7	4.1
	65–74	39.0	27.2	47.6	10.2†	6.1	51.0	9.6

° Framingham, Mass.

† 65 and over

Definitions: Inactivity—average oxygen consumption less than .30 liter per minute (1954–58); obesity—weight 20 percent or more above median (1960–62); hypertension—blood pressure at least 160/90 (1960–62); cigarette smoking—refers to current habits (1970); diabetes—medically treated (1960–62); hypercholesterolemia—serum cholesterol at least 260 mg percent (1960–62); ECG-LVH—electrocardiographic pattern (1948–53).

Table 14-2. *Regression of Cardiovascular Incidence and Specified Risk Factors*

Cardiovascular Risk Factors	Standardized Regression Coefficients: Cardiovascular Morbidity		Cardiovascular Mortality	
	Men	Women	Men	Women
Systolic Blood Pressure	.405°	.475°	.367°	.486°
Diastolic Blood Pressure	.317°	.393°	–.245°	.300°
Serum Cholesterol	.236°	.255°	.062†	.190°
Relative Weight	.156°	.219°	–.115†	.106†
Vital Capacity/Height	–.180°	–.330°	–.365°	–.610°
Blood Glucose	.124°	.232°	.189°	.258°
Heart Rate	.144°	.058†	.313°	.219°
Cigarettes	.198°	.029†	.197°	.148†
Physical Activity‡	–.200°	.003†	–.260°	–.154†

° P=<.01

† Not significant

‡ Follow-up from 4th biennial exam only.

From Framingham Study, 20-year Follow-up, Men and Women 45 to 74.

Figure 14-8.

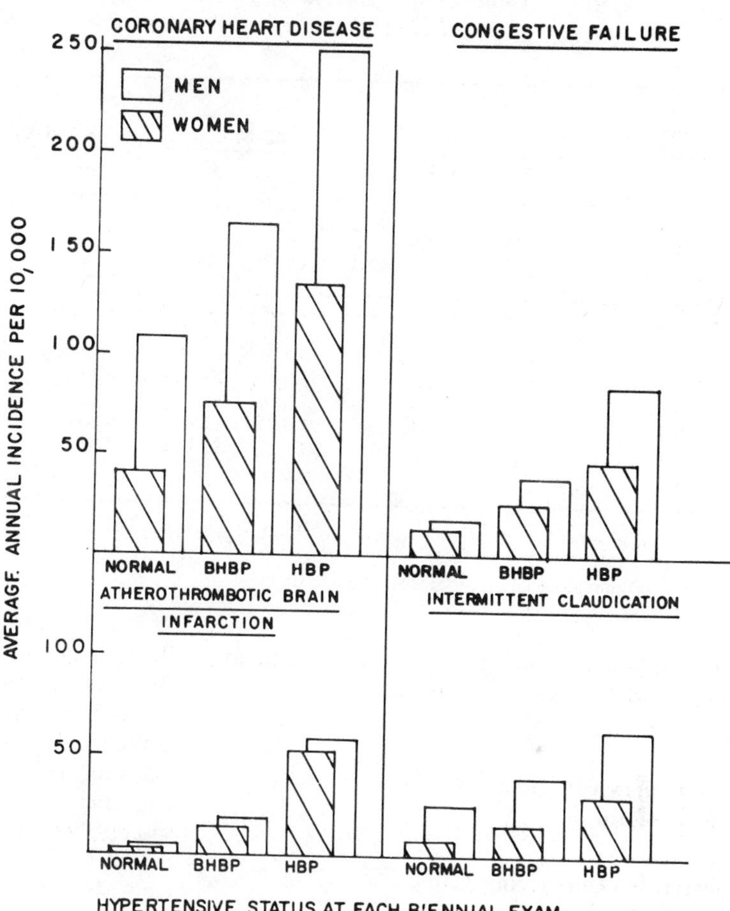

mingham cohort trial, there was a significant reduction in the prevalence of hypertension in the population (Kannel, 1976). Also, the blood pressure of offspring of the cohort was found to be lower than that of their parents at the same age two decades earlier.

However, the prevalence of hypertension has remained high. This is attributable to the difficulties in maintaining adherence to prescribed treatment, and to what appears to be gross undertreatment of hypertension. Even at 200 mm Hg systolic blood pressure, less than half the Framingham cohort received treatment. At borderline pressures, the proportion of subjects who received treatment ranged from only 2 to 11 percent. The group receiving treatment in this blood pressure range does not seem to vary with age, but women uniformly appear to receive more treatment than men at all ages (Table 14–3).

Clinical Misconceptions

A number of misconceptions about hypertension and its treatment have resulted in undertreatment. Most physicians have been taught that it is necessary to judge which hypertensives require treatment. In this context, it is alleged that the young are more in need than the elderly and that the male is in more danger than the female. Labile hypertension is decreed less serious than fixed hypertension, and diastolic elevations are deemed more ominous than systolic ones. Casual pressure elevations are considered misleading, and basal elevations are viewed as the only sound basis for judging the need for treatment. It is often considered safe to await evidence of target organ involvement before initiating treatment. Some consider it wise to withhold treatment until a thorough work-up for secondary hypertension can be

Table 14-3. *Percent of Patients at Specified Borderline and High Pressures on Antihypertensive Drugs*

Systolic Blood Pressure*	35–44		45–54		55–64		65–74	
	M	F	M	F	M	F	M	F
140–149	2.3	3.5	2.2	5.3	2.5	5.9	1.7	6.0
150–159	7.8	10.5	5.7	10.8	7.1	6.4	7.0	8.0
160–169	10.4	10.7	8.3	14.8	8.6	11.6	7.0	9.5
170–179	12.5	22.2	18.9	20.8	15.4	16.3	14.8	16.1
180–189	23.1	22.2	27.3	31.4	23.8	17.5	14.3	20.3
190–199	25.0	40.0	26.9	33.3	30.6	40.9	17.4	26.9
200+	40.0	42.9	27.8	53.3	36.7	39.6	20.8	32.3

* Blood pressure on exam prior to first use of antihypertensive treatment

From Framingham Study, exams 4 through 10.

accomplished. *None of these concepts can be supported by epidemiologic data.*

Factors in the Treatment of Hypertension

Search for Underlying Causes

A routine diagnostic search for elusive causes of hypertension (i.e., to detect secondary hypertension) is impractical because of the low yield and the high prevalence of essential hypertension (Ferguson, 1975; Gifford, 1969). Those in need of extensive diagnostic studies are generally identified by the perceptive physician by distinctive signs and symptoms. In the absence of these indicators, few "curable" hypertensives will be overlooked (Gifford, 1969). Failure to respond to conventional treatment is also a good indication for such diagnostic evaluation.

If we knew the cause of the high prevalence of hypertension in the general population, we might be able to prevent it so that treatment would less often be required. However, although new causes are uncovered each decade, the bulk of hypertension is still of unknown etiology. Close surveillance for development of hypertension is required for (1) those with a positive family history, (2) blacks, (3) the overweight, (4) those who imbibe alcohol, (5) the aged, (6) diabetics, (7) those with gout and kidney ailments, and (8) women taking oral contraceptives (Kannel et al., 1976; Henderson et al., 1974; Biron et al., 1974; Miall et al., 1967; Tobian, 1978). Even spouses of hypertensives merit surveillance because they are at increased risk (Sackett, 1975). However, until the determinants are better understood, we can only monitor susceptibles and treat them as soon as they are detected. Failure to detect some underlying cause is not a justification for delaying treatment.

Age and Sex

Hypertension is a serious threat to life and health in both sexes and at all ages (Table 14–4). There is little evidence to suggest that females tolerate hypertension well. Their relative risk compared with normotensive females is just as great as that for males (Table 14–4). The absolute risk for mortality is lower for female than for male hypertensives, but this statistic also holds for normotensives. For cardiac failure and stroke, even the absolute risk is only a little less in female hypertensives than in their male counterparts (Figure 14–8). There is no valid reason to delay treatment in hypertensive females.

There is also no evidence to support the contention that because blood pressure rises with age, this is an inevitable, innocuous, or compensatory phenomenon designed to maintain perfusion pressure through vessels narrowed by atherosclerosis. Both the absolute and relative risks are as large in the elderly as in the young (Table 14–4). Contrary to other risk factors, regression of incidence of cardiovascular sequelae on blood pressure does not wane with advancing age. There is no good reason to withhold therapy from the elderly hypertensive patient.

Systolic versus Diastolic Pressure

Clinical teaching holds that the cardiovascular consequences of hypertension derive chiefly from the diastolic component of the blood pressure. By dissociating the two components of the pressure, physicians often believe they can more accurately discern true candidates for therapy (Brest and Haddad, 1977; Koch-Weser, 1973). Therapy is often withheld from those whose hypertension is principally systolic in nature. It is claimed that there is no evidence that control of systolic pressure prolongs life, whereas the Veterans Administration (VA) study has demonstrated the efficacy of controlling diastolic pressure (Brest and Haddad, 1977). This is illogical because, by and large, systolic and diastolic pressures are highly correlated. It is thus difficult to dissociate the effects of controlling one from the consequences of controlling the other. If the VA study data were analyzed for efficacy of controlling systolic rather than diastolic pressure, the results would be exactly the same. Even for those with isolated systolic pressure, the need for treatment seems evident. At any age, in either sex, risk in those with "normal" diastolic pressure mounts in proportion to the degree of systolic pressure elevation (Figure 14–9). There is no question that such hypertension carries a high risk (Kannel et al., 1976; Koch-Weser, 1973). This is true even for the disproportionate rise in systolic pressure attributed solely to an inelastic arterial vasculature.

There is no evidence that any component of the blood pressure is more closely linked to risk of cardiovascular disease than is the systolic pressure. In patients with combined systolic and diastolic pressure elevations, systolic pressure would appear to be a better guide to the need for treatment and to the adequacy of treatment than the diastolic pressure. Formal statistical analysis reveals that, if anything, systolic pressure is a more powerful predictor of cardiovascular sequelae than is diastolic pressure (Table 14–5). This applies to borderline elevations as well as to marked rises in pressure.

Table 14–4. *Average Annual Incidence of Cardiovascular Mortality According to Blood Pressure Status*

Blood Pressure Status	Cardivascular Mortality (Rate/1000)					
	45-54		55-64		65-74	
	M	F	M	F	M	F
Normotensive	2.5	0.9	8.4	2.2	9.6	3.8
Borderline	3.8	1.1	10.5	4.5	20.2	9.8
Hypertensive	9.2	4.0	20.6	5.7	24.5	18.6
	Overall Mortality (Rate/1000)					
	45-54		55-64		65-74	
	M	F	M	F	M	F
Normotensive	6.9	4.0	14.7	6.9	23.6	14.5
Borderline	6.9	5.1	15.6	8.1	37.7	17.8
Hypertensive	15.4	8.4	28.6	10.2	42.6	24.7

° Trend not significant at P<.05

From Framingham Study, 20-year Follow-up.

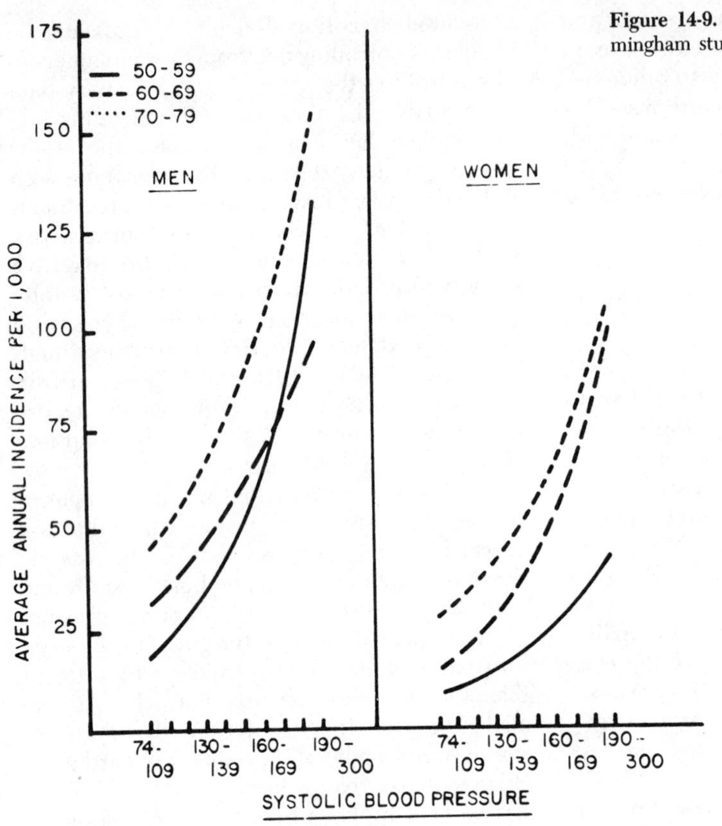

Figure 14-9. Men and women 50-79, Framingham study, 20-year Follow-up.

Table 14-5. *Cardiovascular Morbidity and Mortality According to Systolic versus Diastolic Blood Pressure (Average Standardized Regression Coefficients)*

	Mortality			
	Overall Mortality	Cardiovascular Mortality	Sudden Death	Overall Coronary Heart Disease Mortality
Systolic	.277	.367	.322	.408
Diastolic	.185	.245	.298	.342

	Morbidity			
	Coronary Heart Disease	Cerebrovascular Disease	Congestive Failure	Intermittent Claudication
Systolic	.330	.597	.530	.335
Diastolic	.270	.532	.362	.046

Average standardized coefficients for regression of incidence on systolic versus diastolic blood pressure.

From Framingham Study, 20-year Follow-up, Men 45 to 74.

Labile Hypertension

In judging the need for treatment, it is common practice to disregard "labile" elevations of pressure; only "fixed" hypertension is considered worthy of treatment. Close scrutiny of this concept reveals that it has little substance. For one thing, all hypertension is labile, and this lability increases with age and with the level of blood pressure. Furthermore, there is no evidence to support the contention that lability of pressure is a consistent characteristic of some people. Correlation of lability of pressure, as measured by the standard deviation about the mean of three determinations, is minuscule (r = .07). There is no reason to withhold treatment from people with labile hypertension if the average blood pressure is considered high enough to merit treatment (Gordon et al., 1976).

Categorical Hypertension

Physicians have been taught to deal with hypertension as a categorical entity, as if there were actually some critical value at which "normal" leaves off and "abnormal" begins. An examination of the risk of cardiovascular sequelae according to blood pressure level reveals no indication of such a critical value (Figure 14–10). Risk increases with the blood pressure level, so that on a log scale, for each 10 mm Hg systolic pressure increment, there is a 30 percent increase in risk. This is as true at the lower end of the blood pressure range as at the high end, and it applies even within the borderline range. Consequently, there are no grounds for judging the need for treatment solely on the basis of some critical blood pressure value deemed "hypertensive."

Figure 14-10.

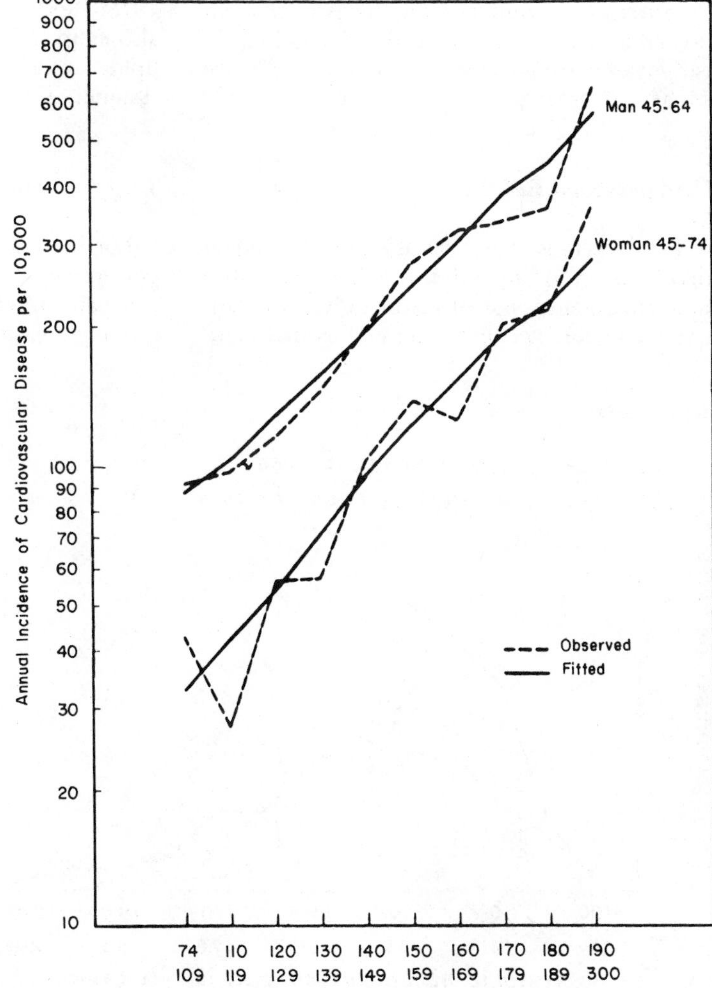

Any discussion of the advisability of treating mild hypertension must come to grips with the considerable problem of defining the condition. A study of the distribution of blood pressure in people who have remained free of cardiovascular disease, as well as those who have developed it, fails to disclose any clear indication of subgroups (Figure 14–11). Although significantly different in mean values, these distributions overlap considerably so that no value, however extreme, clearly discriminates a case from a noncase. Risk simply mounts in relation to the blood pressure level. It is blood pressure that kills, not *hypertension* according to some arbitrary definition.

Any discussion of mild hypertension must be based on arbitrary criteria. That being the case, one might as well use the World Health Organization (WHO) criteria of 140 to 159 over 90 to 94 mm Hg as being definitive of a mild hypertensive pressure. Using these figures as borderline elevations, it is clear that even such pressures can be ominous. On the average, such pressures are associated with a doubling of cardiovascular morbidity and mortality (Figure 14–8).

Cardiovascular Risk Profile

The Veterans Administration study finding that "moderate" hypertensives benefited little from treatment is not surprising, given the failure to take into account other factors that influence risk. Blood pressure is only one aspect of a cardiovascular risk profile. At borderline pressure levels, the risk is not uniform; some people have only a trivial risk, whereas others have a risk that is quite substantial (Figure 14–12). Those in need of treatment can be identified by their cardiovascular risk profile. To treat them all is illogical, since the side effects and inconvenience often outweigh the potential advantages. However, failure to treat those with an ominous cardiovascular profile is also imprudent. There is a clear need to evaluate the efficacy of antihypertensive treatment in borderline hypertensives who have unfavorable cardiovascular risk profiles.

In this borderline group, it is important to recognize that other hygienic measures may be all that are required—for instance, risk can be halved by getting cigarette smokers to quit the habit (Gordon et al., 1974). Weight reductions of 10 percent in the obese can reduce borderline pressures by 6.5 mm Hg (Figure 14–13) (Tobian, 1978; Reisin et al., 1978). Salt restriction may also help, as may a diet that reduces serum lipids, exercise, and reduction of alcohol intake (Kannel et al., 1976; Freis, 1976).

Target Organ Involvement

For both the borderline and the severe hypertensive, it does not appear to be prudent to await target organ involvement before prescribing treatment, even if the hypertension is

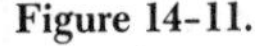
Figure 14-11.

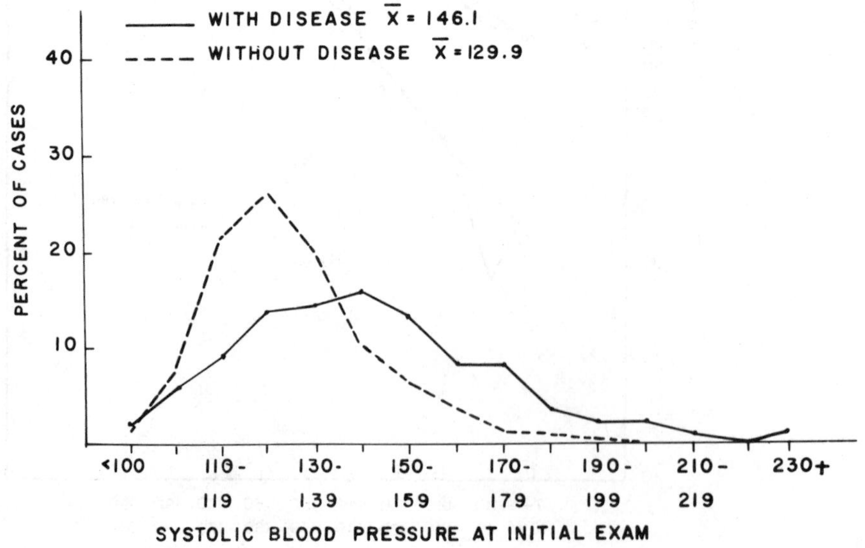

Figure 14-12. From Framingham monograph no. 28.

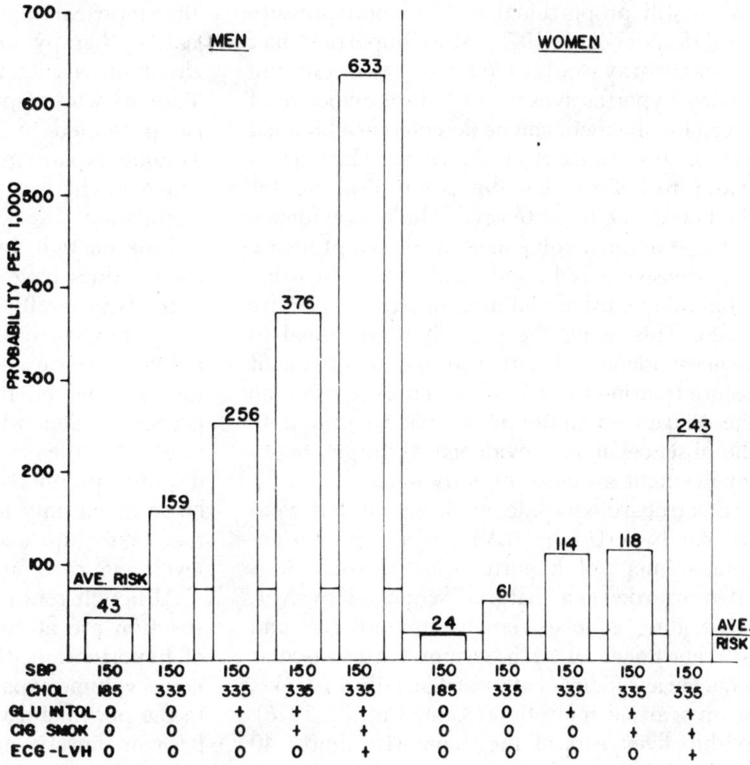

Figure 14-13.

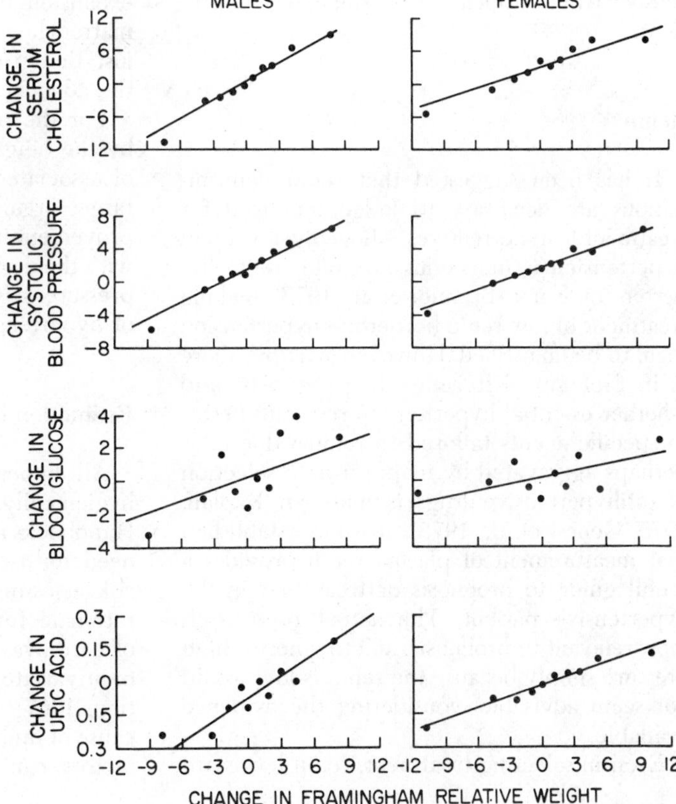

asymptomatic. In the absence of such evidence, risk is still proportional to the blood pressure level (Kannel et al., 1976). More important, half of all cardiovascular catastrophes occurring among hypertensives occur before evidence of organ involvement can be detected in a biennial examination (Kannel et al., 1976). There is no reason to believe that this is not also true for the borderline hypertensive. The first evidence of target organ involvement in an asymptomatic hypertensive may be sudden death, myocardial infarction, cardiac failure, or stroke (Figure 14–8). This being the case, it is irrational to await evidence of target organ involvement before treating hypertension. Trials to examine the efficacy of antihypertensive treatment in the absence of any evidence of target organ involvement are also urgently needed.

Electrocardiographic evidence of left ventricular hypertrophy (LVH) is a common accompaniment of hypertension. As such, it is often regarded as a "natural" sequela. However, this finding is an extremely ominous one and is a harbinger of such serious cardiovascular sequelae as sudden death, cardiac failure, stroke, or myocardial infarction (Kannel et al., 1976). Within five years of the diagnosis, almost 40 percent of men who develop ECG-LVH die. To await this finding before treating a hypertensive would appear to be singularly imprudent.

Renin

It has been suggested that renin determinations are necessary to judge the need for treatment in hypertensives. Allegedly, low renin hypertension is innocuous and high renin hypertension is not (Brunner et al., 1973), making treatment of low renin borderline hypertension seem to be unjustified. However, whether there is in fact any difference in prognosis, and whether essential hypertension responds better to specific agents tailored to renin value or is perhaps aggravated by inappropriate selection of antihypertensive drugs, is unknown (Kaplan, 1975; Genest et al., 1973). It is not established that measurement of plasma renin provides a useful guide to prognosis or treatment in the hypertensive patient. The actual pressure is most relevant to prognosis, and to ignore a high pressure simply because the renin is low would not seem advisable, considering the evidence available.

Even in selecting treatment, renin levels are not too helpful. It is more convenient to use the empirical sequential introduction of combination therapy in order to determine which drugs prove effective for a particular patient. Patients who respond to diuretics alone might be presumed to have low renin values and volume expansion. A response to propranolol alone might be presumed to indicate a high renin state.

True enough, hypertensives with very high renin values have a poor prognosis, but these patients generally have severe hypertension as well. Thus, it is difficult to disentangle the effect of blood pressure level per se on prognosis from the renin effect. It is not clear whether blood pressure is dependent on plasma renin activity or whether the cardiovascular sequelae are. The disputed prognostic implications of renin will be resolved only by a large prospective study that takes into account actual blood pressure level, age, race, and other risk factors.

Although renin and angiotensin II vasoconstriction are at times the predominant causes of hypertension, there may also be a simultaneous volume expansion component and change in the peripheral vasculature. Hence, a vasodilator or diuretic may be needed in addition to a beta blocker. Vasodilators used alone often fail because of the sodium retention and volume expansion they induce. It is not clear that it matters how blood pressure control is achieved, just that prognosis is favorably influenced by the adequacy of blood pressure control.

For the present, physicians are best guided by the height of the blood pressure, the level of associated risk factors, and the evidence of target organ involvement (Figure 14–14). Improvement in most hypertensives correlates best with the degree of success in lowering the blood pressure. Also, the risk is related to the degree of hypertension, whatever its cause.

Estimation of Risk

All hypertensives should be treated—some hygienically, some with antihypertensive drugs. Handbooks are available to assist in judging the need for treatment based on a multifactorial risk assessment (Table 14–6). This provides a rationale for treatment, based on a synthesis of cardiovascular risk factors into a composite multivariate risk score (Veterans Administration, 1967). In this way, those at high risk because of multiple marginal abnormalities of risk factors can be identified for treatment, and

Figure 14-14. From Framingham monograph no. 28.

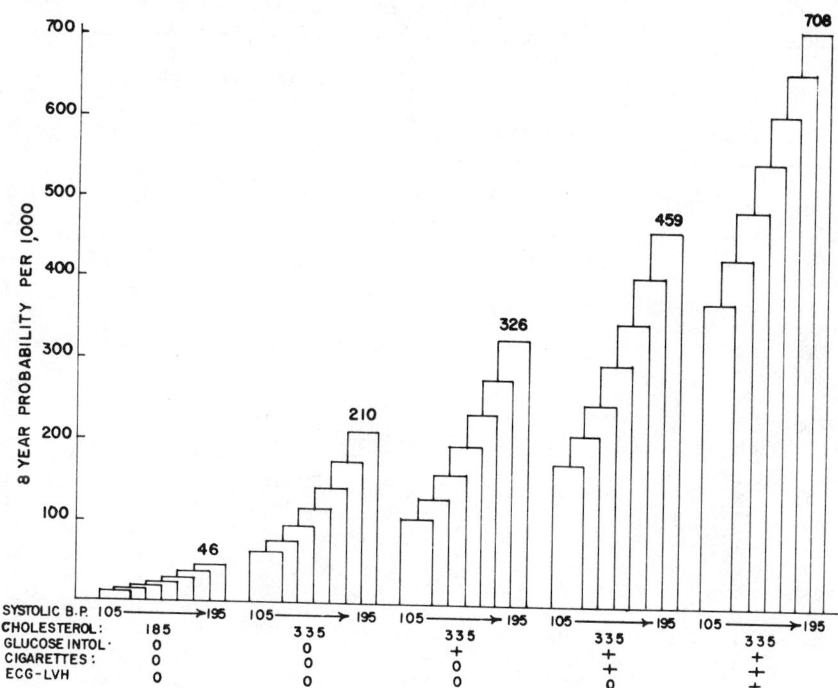

those who (by these criteria) are in little jeopardy may be saved the inconvenience and hazards of inappropriate antihypertensive treatment. This is especially important for the mild hypertensive.

The answer to the question "Should all mild hypertension be treated?" is "Yes." Although this does not mean that all hypertension should be treated with antihypertensive drugs, some patients with mild hypertension should be considered for drug treatment—namely, those with an ominous cardiovascular risk profile. Their risk may be substantial, justifying the side effects, dangers, and inconveniences of drug therapy. Proof of the efficacy of antihypertensive drug therapy for the high risk subgroup of mild hypertensives is urgently needed. The Veterans Administration study's negative findings do not necessarily apply to this highly vulnerable subgroup (Brest and Haddad, 1977; Veterans Administration, 1967).

In general, a sensible approach to the mild hypertensives would be to obtain a cardiovascular risk profile. This requires nothing more than ordinary office procedures and simple laboratory tests (McGee, 1973). For the elderly, the standard risk profile can be substantially improved by obtaining high density lipoprotein cholesterol fractions and using them in a modified risk profile (Table 14–7). For those with a favorable profile according to these criteria, only surveillance is needed, and this only because blood pressure elevation tends to be a progressive disorder. Hence, periodic profiles would be advisable. For those with a poor profile, correction of the other risk factors requiring only hygienic measures would seem to be the first order of business.

Principles of Effective Treatment

Risk can be reduced, at least theoretically, by improving the total profile as well as by reducing the blood pressure. If measures such as salt restriction, dietary modification, weight reduction, exercise programs, and personal hygiene improvement fail, or if the patient will not make the necessary changes, antihypertensive drug therapy should be seriously considered.

Optimal results follow "normalization" of the blood pressure, but even less complete control may be decidedly worthwhile (Taguchi and Freis, 1975), should side effects or inadequate

Table 14-6. *8-Year Probability (Per 100) of Developing Cardiovascular Disease for a 40-Year-Old Man*

LVH-ECG Negative

Does Not Smoke Cigarettes

Glucose Intolerance	Chol \ SBP	105	120	135	150	165	180
Absent	185	1	2	2	2	3	4
	210	2	2	2	3	4	5
	235	2	3	3	4	5	6
	260	3	3	4	5	7	8
	285	4	4	6	7	9	11
	310	5	6	7	9	11	14
	335	6	8	9	12	14	17
Present	185	2	3	3	4	5	7
	210	3	4	4	6	7	9
	235	4	5	6	7	9	11
	260	5	6	8	9	12	14
	285	6	8	10	12	15	18
	310	8	10	13	15	19	22
	335	11	13	16	19	23	28

Smokes Cigarettes

Glucose Intolerance	Chol \ SBP	105	120	135	150	165	180	195
Absent	185	2	3	3	4	5	6	8
	210	3	3	4	5	7	8	10
	235	4	4	6	7	9	11	13
	260	5	6	7	9	11	14	17
	285	6	8	9	12	14	17	21
	310	8	10	12	15	18	22	26
	335	10	13	15	19	23	27	32
Present	185	4	5	6	7	9	11	13
	210	5	6	7	9	11	14	17
	235	6	8	10	12	15	18	21
	260	8	10	12	15	18	22	27
	285	11	13	16	19	23	28	33
	310	13	16	20	24	29	34	39
	335	17	21	25	30	35	40	46

LVH-ECG Positive

Does Not Smoke Cigarettes

Glucose Intolerance	Chol \ SBP	105	120	135	150	165	180
Absent	185	3	4	5	6	8	10
	210	4	5	7	8	10	13
	235	6	7	9	11	13	16
	260	7	9	11	14	17	20
	285	10	12	14	18	21	25
	310	12	15	18	22	26	31
	335	16	19	23	27	32	38
Present	185	6	7	9	11	14	17
	210	8	9	12	14	17	21
	235	10	12	15	18	22	26
	260	13	16	19	23	27	32
	285	16	20	24	28	33	38
	310	20	24	29	34	40	45
	335	25	30	35	41	46	52

Smokes Cigarettes

Glucose Intolerance	Chol \ SBP	105	120	135	150	165	180	195
Absent	185	6	7	9	11	13	16	20
	210	7	9	11	14	17	20	24
	235	9	12	14	17	21	25	30
	260	12	15	18	22	26	31	36
	285	16	19	23	27	32	37	43
	310	20	24	28	33	39	44	50
	335	25	29	34	40	45	51	57
Present	185	10	12	15	18	22	26	31
	210	13	15	19	23	27	32	37
	235	16	19	23	28	33	38	44
	260	20	24	29	34	39	45	51
	285	25	30	35	41	46	52	58
	310	31	36	42	47	53	59	65
	335	37	43	49	55	60	66	71

Average risk for this age group is 4.1 per 100.

patient compliance limit the therapeutic endeavor. Treatment will require exemplary methods in order to elicit long-term adherence. Less complex regimens and a cautious, leisurely introduction to therapy should help, and better follow-up procedures are needed. Most importantly, physicians must be convinced of the need for treatment and must be willing to use community resources to assist in the enterprise. Achievement of a normal blood pressure is not an indication for discontinuing treatment, although dosage can sometimes be safely reduced.

Better methods to persuade asymptomatic hypertensives to continue on antihypertensive medicines are needed. We must also convince their physicians to prescribe these medications more often than they do. Prophylactic treatment of both the mild and severe hypertensive should entail a more comprehensive approach than the simple use of antihypertensive drugs.

Table 14-7. *4-Year Probability (Per 1000) of Developing Coronary Heart Disease According to Lipoproteins and Blood Pressure for a 55-Year-Old Man*

Systolic Blood Pressure: 120

LDL-C / HDL-C	100	120	140	160	180	200	220
25	59	69	80	94	109	126	146
35	40	47	55	65	76	88	103
45	27	32	38	44	52	61	71
55	18	22	26	30	35	42	49
65	12	15	17	20	24	28	33
75	8	10	12	14	16	19	22
85	6	7	8	9	11	13	15

Systolic Blood Pressure: 135

LDL-C / HDL-C	100	120	140	160	180	200	220
25	73	85	99	115	133	153	177
35	50	58	68	80	95	108	126
45	34	40	47	55	64	75	88
55	23	27	32	37	44	52	60
65	15	18	22	25	30	35	41
75	10	12	15	17	20	24	28
85	7	8	10	12	14	16	19

Systolic Blood Pressure: 150

LDL-C / HDL-C	100	120	140	160	180	200	220
25	89	104	121	140	161	185	212
35	62	72	84	98	114	132	153
45	42	49	58	68	79	92	108
55	29	34	40	46	54	64	75
65	19	23	27	32	37	44	51
75	13	15	18	21	25	30	35
85	9	10	12	14	17	20	24

Systolic Blood Pressure: 165

LDL-C / HDL-C	100	120	140	160	180	200	220
25	109	127	147	169	194	222	252
35	76	89	103	120	139	160	184
45	52	61	72	84	97	113	131
55	36	42	49	57	67	79	92
65	24	28	33	39	46	54	63
75	16	19	23	27	31	37	43
85	11	13	15	18	21	25	29

Systolic Blood Pressure: 180

LDL-C / HDL-C	100	120	140	160	180	200	220
25	133	154	177	203	232	263	297
35	93	109	126	146	168	193	220
45	64	75	88	102	119	138	159
55	44	52	61	71	83	97	112
65	30	35	41	49	57	67	78
75	20	24	28	33	39	46	54
85	14	16	19	22	26	31	37

Systolic Blood Pressure: 195

LDL-C / HDL-C	100	120	140	160	180	200	220
25	162	186	212	242	274	309	346
35	114	132	153	176	202	230	261
45	80	93	108	125	145	167	192
55	55	64	75	87	102	118	137
65	37	44	51	60	71	82	96
75	25	30	35	41	48	57	66
85	17	20	24	28	33	39	45

Estimated average probability for this age group is 0.057.

From Framingham Study, 20-Year Follow-up.

Attention to other cardiovascular risk factors is essential, particularly in the mild hypertensive.

Efficacy of Treatment

The value of blood pressure control after the onset of coronary heart disease is even less clear than its efficacy for the prevention of coronary disease. Although the utility of correcting blood pressure after the onset of overt coronary heart disease remains to be clearly demonstrated, the effort seems rational and without great hazard (Humphries, 1977). For those skeptical about the efficacy of controlling blood pressure to prevent initial and recurrent coronary disorders, it must be pointed out that coronary patients are also at high risk for stroke and cardiac failure. These patients have been shown to benefit from blood pressure control (Veterans Administration, 1967). Also, long-term control of blood pressure beginning with treatment of mild hypertension may have an even more beneficial effect in retarding the atherosclerotic process accelerated by hypertension. Short-term therapy restricted to elderly hypertensives, many of whom already have target organ involvement, for short periods—as in the VA antihypertensive trial—may in fact be fruitless. Only long-term control may be effective in retarding the atherosclerotic process leading to coronary heart disease. Blood pressure is clearly a critical factor because lesions seldom occur in low pressure segments of the circulation, despite their being bathed by the same lipid-laden blood (Heath et al., 1960; Burch and DePasquale, 1964; Scott, 1968; Dustan, 1974). If instituted early enough and continued long enough, control of elevated blood pressure could rationally be expected to slow the accelerated pace of atherogenesis. The hazards of isolated systolic hypertension have been clearly established. Also, borderline hypertension associated with a poor cardiovascular risk profile is of ominous import, and treatment by hygienic means is clearly indicated. The efficacy of drug treatment in this circumstance merits study.

Conclusion

Prospective epidemiologic studies demonstrate that blood pressure is a dominant contributor to cardiovascular disease. Its impact is greatest for stroke and cardiac failure and least for peripheral arterial disease. Abnormal blood pressure contributes to the development of every clinical manifestation of coronary disease. The net effect does not wane with advancing age.

Despite the demonstration that treatment prolongs life, much of hypertension goes untreated because of a number of misconceptions. The facts are: (1) treatment based on casual office pressure readings is not ill-advised, (2) the lowest pressure recorded is not a safe basis for deferring treatment if the average pressure is high, (3) risk is just as closely linked to systolic as to diastolic pressure, (4) it is not safe to delay treatment to await evidence of target organ involvement or symptoms, and (5) women do not tolerate hypertension any better than do men.

Whether renin-dependent, volume-dependent, or hyperdynamic varieties of hypertension differ in prognosis or in response to specific therapy is unknown. Host factors associated with hypertension include race, weight, hemoglobin values, pulse, cholesterol values, and other illnesses. Blacks; obese people; people with a high hemoglobin value, rapid pulse, or high cholesterol value; and those with diabetes or gout need close surveillance for development of hypertension.

The determinants of blood pressure in the general population are not well understood. Genetic factors are accorded a major role. Indications of environmental influences include acculturation, secular trends in mortality, water hardness, rudimentary education, salt intake, weight gain, alcohol intake, altitude, and geographic variation. Until we can prevent hypertensive cardiovascular disease by altering its determinants, we can only focus on the high risk candidate for multifactorial intervention aimed at blood pressure control.

All hypertension, even borderline elevations, can be dangerous if associated with a poor risk profile. A risk profile is based on the height of the blood pressure, the number of other risk factors, and the evidence of target organ involvement. Appropriate treatment with hygienic measures and, if necessary, antihypertensive drugs is indicated for the high risk subgroup.

References

Biron, P., Mongeau, J.D., Bertrand, D.: Familial aggregation of blood pressure in adopted and natural children. Circulation (Supplement III) 50:106, 1974.

Brest, A.N., and Haddad, M.: Should systolic hypertension be treated? In Corday, E., *Controversies in Cardiology,* Philadelphia, F.A. Davis Company, 1977.

Brunner, H.R., Sealey, J.E., and Laragh, J.H.: Renin as a risk factor in essential hypertension: more evidence. Am. J. Med. 55:295, 1973.

Burch, G.E., and DePasquale, N.P.: The anomalous left coronary artery. An experiment of nature. Am. J. Med. 37:159, 1964.

Dustan, H.P.: Atherosclerosis complicating chronic hypertension. Circulation 50:871, 1974.

Ferguson, R.K.: Cost and yield of the hypertensive evaluation. Experience of a community-based referral clinic. Ann. Intern. Med. 82:761, 1975.

Freis, E.: Salt, volume and the prevention of hypertension. Circulation 53:589, 1976.

Genest, J., Boucher, R., Kuchel, O., et al.: Renin in hypertension: how important as a risk factor? Can. Med. Assoc. J. 109:475, 1973.

Gifford, R.W., Jr.: Evaluation of the hypertensive patient with emphasis on detecting curable causes. Milbank Memorial Fund Quarterly 47:170, 1969.

Gordon, T., Kannel, W.B., McGee, D., and Dawber, T.R.: Death and coronary attacks in men after giving up cigarette smoking. Lancet 2:1345, 1974.

Gordon, T., Sorlie, P., and Kannel, W.B.: Problems in the assessment of blood pressure. The Framingham Study. Int. J. Epidemiol. 5:327, 1976.

Heath, D., Wood, E.H., Dushane, J.W., and Edwards, J.E.: The relation of age and blood pressure to atheroma in the pulmonary arteries and thoracic aorta in congenital heart disease. Lab. Invest. 9:259, 1960.

Henderson, M., Apostolides, A., Entwisle, G., et al.: A study of hypertension in a black urban community: preliminary epidemiologic findings. Prev. Med. 3:334, 1974.

Humphries, J.O.: Survival after myocardial infarction. Prognosis and management. Mod. Concepts Cardiovasc. Dis. 46:51, 1977.

Kannel, W.B., and Sorlie, P.: Hypertension in Framingham. In Paul, O., *Epidemiology and Control of Hypertension,* Miami, Symposia Specialists, 1976.

Kannel, W.B., Dawber, T.R., Sorlie, P., and Wolf, P.A.: Components of blood pressure and risk of atherothrombotic brain infarction. The Framingham Study. Stroke 7:327, 1976.

Kaplan, N.M.: The prognostic implications of plasma renin in essential hypertension. JAMA 231:167, 1975.

Koch-Weser, J.: The therapeutic challenge of systolic hypertension. N. Engl. J. Med. 289:481, 1973.

McGee, D.: The probability of developing certain cardiovascular diseases in 8 years at specified values of some characteristics. Framingham Study, 18 year follow-up. DHEW Publication No. (NIH) 74:618, 1973.

Miall, W.E., Heneage, P., Khosla, T., et al.: Factors influencing the degree of resemblance in arterial pressure of close relatives. Clin. Sci. 33:271, 1967.

Reisin, E., Abel, R., Modan, M., et al.: Effect of weight loss without salt restriction on the reduction of blood pressure in overweight hypertensive patients. N. Engl. J. Med. 298:1, 1978.

Sackett, D.L.: Study of blood pressure in spouses. In *The Epidemiology of Hypertension,* Second International Symposium, Miami, Symposia Specialists, 1975.

Scott, T.M.: Disease of veins. In Gould, S.E., *Pathology of the Heart and Blood Vessels,* Springfield, Ill., Charles C Thomas, 1968.

Tobian, L.: Hypertension and obesity (editorial). N. Engl. J. Med. 298:46, 1978.

Taguchi, J., and Freis, E.D.: Partial versus complete control of blood pressure in the prevention of hypertensive complications. Circ. Res. (6 Supplement) 36:257, 1975.

Veterans Administration Cooperative Study Group on Antihypertensive Agents: Effects of treatment on morbidity in hypertension: results in patients with diastolic blood pressures averaging 115 through 129 mm Hg. JAMA 202:1028, 1967.

15

Are Aspirin and Related Drugs Useful in Preventing Myocardial Infarction, Strokes, or Venous Thromboembolism?

Prevention *of disease must become the goal of every physician.*

Henry E. Sigerist, *Medicine and Human Welfare*

When meditating over a disease, I never think of finding a remedy for it, but, instead, a means of preventing it.

Louis Pasteur

This apoplexy will certainly be his end.

Shakespeare, *Henry IV, Part II*

Introduction

Prevention of disease usually appeals less to both patients and doctors than does the relief or cure of symptoms. This is especially true if continuous medication is required to prevent a disease that may occur years later.

Nevertheless, there has been considerable interest in the prevention of thromboembolism, since clots and emboli in the venous and arterial parts of the circulation are neither rare nor trivial. As Mustard shows, many investigators have been interested in the effects of drugs on the clotting process in animals exposed to a variety of clot-inducing stresses. The mechanisms involved both in thrombus formation and in modification thereof by drugs are complex and incompletely known. Not surprisingly, in view of the differences between experimental approaches and doses used by various investigators, the literature is inconsistent with respect to the utility of either aspirin or sulfinpyrazone in inhibiting thromboembolism. Nor is it certain whether any effects of these drugs on sudden death are related simply to an impact on thrombosis or embolic showers or to an unrelated effect on cardiac arrhythmias.

Mustard reminds us of the various ways in which clinical trials might arrive at erroneously negative conclusions, but he neglects another extremely important consideration—compliance. For reasons already stated, patients are unlikely to be scrupulously compulsive about their drug regimen in a long-term prophylactic trial. To the extent, therefore, that there is doubt about patient compliance with the experimental treatments, negative results would be less important than would otherwise be the case. In my own view, positive trials in these areas—given all the obstacles to their conduct—should carry more weight than trials that show no difference between treatments. Indeed, one wonders whether a series of trials that show trends (even if not statistically significant) in the same direction should not have meaning for us.

Mustard concludes that (1) both aspirin and sulfinpyrazone inhibit thrombosis in arteriovenous shunts, (2) aspirin may reduce venous thromboembolism and cerebrovascular accidents, and (3) both aspirin and sulfinpyrazone may help patients with coronary artery disease.

Verstraete is less sanguine about these two drugs in most clinical situations in which thromboembolism is a consideration, and he reminds us of some important principles to be considered in investigating antithrombotic effects and in choosing therapies:

1. The many tests available for detecting thrombosis do not measure the same events, and they need not therefore agree with one another.
2. Not all types of surgical procedures produce the same kinds of thromboembolic risks.
3. Physical methods and traditional anticoagulants should not be ignored simply because of current interest in nonsteroidal, antiinflammatory, "antiplatelet" drugs.
4. Combinations of drugs or of drugs and physical methods should be considered, as well as single drugs.

5. Treatments that are useful in one situation or for one group of patients may not be useful in other situations or groups.

Both essays leave the practitioner in a bit of a quandary. There are theoretical and experimental reasons for believing that drugs may be of benefit in a wide variety of clinical disorders in which abnormal clotting in arteries or veins is deleterious. The physician, and the patient at risk, cannot be agnostic. A decision not to use a prophylactic drug is as much a decision as is one to use it. Should one be swayed by positive results of any sort? Should one stick closely to the age, sex, or disease groups for which there is considerable positive evidence (as Verstraete suggests), or should one broaden the indications to other patients as well? Finally, should these decisions be made by physicians, by patients to whom the available data have been explained, or by physician and patient acting in concert?

LOUIS LASAGNA, M.D.

Are Aspirin and Sulfinpyrazone Useful in the Prevention of Myocardial Infarction, Strokes, or Venous Thromboembolism?

J.F. Mustard, M.D., Ph.D.
McMaster University, Ontario, Canada

M.A. Packham, Ph.D.
University of Toronto, Ontario, Canada

Two topics to be reviewed in considering the possible value of aspirin and sulfinpyrazone in the management of the clinical complications of arterial or venous thromboembolism are (1) the basic mechanisms by which these drugs affect thrombus formation or other reactions involved in the clinical complications and (2) the results of the clinical trials in which aspirin and sulfinpyrazone have been used in attempts to modify the conditions in which arterial and venous thrombi are thought to play a part.

Basic Mechanisms

Soon after it was demonstrated that platelets interact with collagen in the subendothelium (Hugues, 1962; Hovig, 1963; Spaet and Zucker, 1964), it was observed that nonsteroidal antiinflammatory drugs and related drugs inhibited collagen-induced platelet aggregation *in vitro* (Packham et al., 1967; Evans et al., 1968; Weiss et al., 1968). Recognition of the central role platelets play in arterial thrombosis (Mustard et al., 1967a) led to speculation that drugs such as aspirin and sulfinpyrazone might be useful in inhibiting the build-up of the platelet component in thrombi. It became apparent quite early in these studies that the effect of aspirin lasted much longer than the effect of other nonsteroidal antiinflammatory drugs (Weiss et al., 1968; O'Brien et al., 1970; Packham and Mustard, 1975). A relatively small dose of aspirin produced prolonged inhibition of collagen-induced platelet aggregation. This long-term effect of aspirin on platelets has been shown to be the result of its irreversible acetylation of platelet cyclooxygenase (Rome et al., 1976). This enzyme converts arachidonic acid to prostaglandin G_2 (PGG_2) and prostaglandin H_2 (PGH_2), which form thromboxane A_2 (TXA_2) (Smith et al., 1977; Samuelsson, 1977). These unstable products cause platelet aggregation. In high concentrations, sulfinpyrazone also inhibits the cyclooxygenase, but this inhibition is reversible (Ali and McDonald, 1977). The relative importance of the arachidonate pathway in thrombus formation is not established.

There are five main steps in arterial thrombus formation (Mustard, 1977): (1) platelet adherence to the damaged vessel wall; (2) release of platelet granule contents including ADP, serotonin, and a factor that is mitogenic for smooth muscle cells; (3) activation of platelet phospholipase A_2, which frees platelet arachidonate for conversion to PGG_2, PGH_2, and TXA_2 and the prostaglandins PGD_2, $PGF_2\alpha$, and PGE_2; (4) platelet shape change and aggregation of other platelets around those platelets adherent to the vessel wall; and (5) activation of the coagulation mechanism by the damaged vessel wall and around the platelet aggregate. Activation of the coagulation mechanism leads to the formation of thrombin, which also induces the platelet release reaction, activation of phospholipase A_2, platelet shape change, and aggregation. The constituents of the exposed subendothelium can also initiate the coagulation pathways leading to thrombin formation. If thrombin forms on the surface of the damaged vessel wall, the thrombin enhances the reactivity of the wall with platelets (Essien et al., 1978).

The constituents in the subendothelium of the normal vessel wall to which platelets adhere are microfibrils, basement membrane, and collagen (Baumgartner et al., 1976). We have no information about platelet adherence to the subendothelial constituents of an atherosclerotic plaque. Aspirin and sulfinpyrazone have little inhibitory effect on platelet adherence to the subendothelial constituents of the normal vessel wall under physiologic conditions (Weiss et al., 1975; Cazenave et al., 1978b). These drugs also do not inhibit the release of granule contents from platelets adherent to collagen (Weiss et al., 1975; Cazenave et al., 1978b), although they do prevent the formation of PGG_2, PGH_2, and TXA_2 (Willis et al., 1974; Roth and Majerus, 1975; Smith et al., 1977; Samuelsson, 1977; Ali and McDonald, 1977). Thus, these drugs inhibit the aggregation and release reaction of platelets not adherent to collagen that is induced by these compounds. The ADP released from platelets adherent to collagen causes nonadherent platelets to change shape and to aggregate. This ADP-induced aggregation is not inhibited by the nonsteroidal antiinflammatory drugs in pharmacologic concentrations.

Thrombin can induce platelet aggregation and the release of granule contents through pathways that are independent of the released ADP and the aggregating agents formed from arachidonate (Kinlough-Rathbone et al., 1977). Thus, aspirin and sulfinpyrazone have only a slight effect on thrombin-induced aggregation and the release of granule contents. Since these drugs do not inhibit all the mechanisms involved in thrombus formation, their inhibitory effects on this process may be limited.

These drugs may affect other systems in addition to the cyclooxygenase. There is one report that sulfinpyrazone protects the endothelium from at least some forms of injury (Harker et al., 1978). Aspirin has been found to diminish the morphologic alterations of the endothelium that can be produced by ischemia (Gertz et al., 1975). Since endothelial injury is responsible for the initiation of most arterial thrombi, drugs that modify this response could be expected to have an effect on thrombosis.

Experimental Thrombosis

Experimental thrombosis has been induced in a wide variety of animals by (1) chemical injury to the lining of the vessel wall, (2) mechanical removal of the endothelium, (3) the use of catheters, (4) intraluminal electrodes, (5) the application of electrical currents to the vessel wall, (6) laser beams, (7) the intravenous infusion of endotoxin, and (8) other methods. It is clear that several mechanisms could be involved in the thrombosis that has been observed with each of these stimuli.

Effect of Aspirin

Peterson and Zucker (1970) found that sodium morrhuate injury to the femoral vein in rabbits, along with some restriction of flow, produced thrombi whose formation could be inhibited by the administration of aspirin. The number of veins with thrombi was reduced by about 50 percent with doses of aspirin ranging between 15 and 100 mg per kg. Danese and associates (1971) observed in dogs that injury to arteries by endarterectomy or by exposure of the endothelium to sulphuric acid caused thrombosis; in the femoral and carotid arteries whose diameter was less than 4 mm, 41 percent of the vessels were occluded. They found that the administration of aspirin (600 mg per day) reduced the incidence of thrombosis by more than 70 percent. Aspirin was shown to inhibit thrombosis in the jugular vein of rats injured by a ruby laser in experiments by Meng and O'Dea (1974). Danese and Haimov (1971) demonstrated that aspirin produced an approximate 50 percent reduction in thrombosis in dogs whose peripheral arteries had been injured by intimectomy. Mayer and Hammond (1973) showed that in dogs, when the vessel wall was damaged with pronase, administration of aspirin decreased the amount of thrombus that formed on the injured area. In another study in dogs by Dyken and his associates (1973), it was found that aspirin inhibited the size of the thrombi that formed following chemical injury to the carotid or femoral arteries, but that aspirin did not inhibit the degree of intimal proliferation. In cats, Piepgras et al. (1976) demonstrated that aspirin did not inhibit thrombotic occlusion of endarterectomized carotid arteries. In earlier experiments, Sheppard (1972) had observed that aspirin did not inhibit platelet adherence to the subendothelium in rabbits. He reported an apparent increase in platelet aggregates on the injured surface. Ts'ao (1970) also observed that aspirin-treated platelets adhered to the subendothelium. Recently, Levison et al. (1977) showed that aspirin did not inhibit the formation of thrombi on damaged aortic valves in rabbits; the mean values for the weights of the thrombi in the aspirin-treated groups were greater than those in the controls, but the difference was not statistically significant. Honour and colleagues (1977) demonstrated that aspirin did not inhibit thrombus formation caused by electrical injury in the pial arteries in rabbits. Spilker and van Balken (1973) reported that aspirin produced extensive thrombus formation in electrically stimulated mesenteric vessels. Arfors et al. (1975) could not show that thrombus formation in veins injured with sodium morrhuate was inhibited by the administration of aspirin. In their study, aspirin was given in a dose of 200 mg per kg of body weight. Bergqvist and Arfors (1976) also found that aspirin did not inhibit the formation of platelet plugs at the ends of transected microcirculatory vessels.

In studies of renal allograft rejection in dogs, Mathew et al. (1971) observed that administration of aspirin significantly reduced the vascular injury and thrombosis response. Winchester and coworkers (1977) have shown that aspirin reduces platelet adsorption on activated charcoal in the hemoperfusion apparatus. Gurewich and Lipinski (1976) could not show an effect of aspirin on the extent of thrombus formation when polyethylene catheters were placed in the lumen of rabbit carotid arteries. However, Kricheff and his colleagues (1973) observed that aspirin reduced the incidence of thrombi on catheters placed in the inferior vena cava of cats by as much as 50 percent. Aspirin was found by Mason and his coworkers (1976) to reduce by about 40 percent, thrombus formation in arteriovenous shunts connected to monkeys. Aspirin treatment of dogs was found by Radegran et al. (1971) to protect them against the platelet-aggregating effect of protamine sulphate. Furlow and Bass (1976) showed that aspirin did not protect rats from arachidonate-induced stroke when arachidonate was injected into the carotid arteries, although Kohler et al. (1976) found that aspirin protected mice from respiratory distress associated with platelet aggregates in the lungs caused by the intravenous infusion of arachidonate. Renaud and Godu (1970) observed that aspirin reduced the size of the thrombi formed in response to the intravenous infusion of endotoxin into rats that had been fed a hyperlipemic diet.

Moschos and associates (1973) could not show that aspirin inhibited thrombus formation when a catheter electrode was placed in the lumen of the coronary artery of dogs. However, it was noted that pretreatment with aspirin resulted in a significant reduction in the emboli in the microcirculation distal to the thrombus. They also noted a significant decrease in the number of deaths due to arrhythmias in the aspirin-treated group. In dogs, platelet aggregation associated with partially obstructed vessels was blocked by the administration of aspirin in experiments done by Folts and coworkers (1976). More recently, Moschos and associates (1978) and Vik-Mo (1977) have found that aspirin can prevent arrhythmias in dogs with myocardial ischemia produced by mechanical occlusion of coronary arteries, even through thrombi and platelet aggregates are not present.

All this evidence shows that aspirin does not completely prevent thrombus formation in experimental animals in response to a variety of types of vessel wall injury. In some experiments, aspirin did not inhibit thrombus formation significantly and, in a few experiments, aspirin appeared to potentiate thrombus formation. The finding that the vessel wall produces PGI_2 (prostacyclin) when cyclooxygenase acts on arachidonic acid (Bunting et al., 1976) may have implications for the inhibition of thrombus formation by aspirin. Aspirin acetylates the cyclooxygenase (Rome et al., 1976) and prevents the production of PGI_2 (Moncada et al., 1977). PGI_2 inhibits platelet aggregation (Bunting et al., 1976; Gorman et al., 1977; Moncada et al., 1977; Weksler et al., 1977) and, since its mechanism of action is similar to that of PGE_1 (Cazenave et al., 1978a,b), which is an inhibitor of platelet adhesion to collagen, it seems likely that PGI_2 would also inhibit platelet adherence at a site of vessel wall injury. Thus, if PGI_2 production by the vessel wall is important in inhibiting thrombus formation, prevention of its production could enhance thrombus formation. Bourgain (1978) has shown that inhibition of PGI_2 formation enhances thrombus formation in the microcirculation. It appears that larger doses of aspirin may be required to inhibit the cyclooxygenase in tissues such as the vessel wall than to inhibit the cyclooxygenase in platelets (Burch et al., 1978). Kelton and associates (1978) have recently observed that large doses of aspirin can significantly enhance thrombus formation in injured jugular veins. Lewis and Westwick (1975) injured the microcirculation of the hamster cheek pouch and found that small doses of aspirin (30 mg per kg) enhanced thrombus formation. Thus, some of the variation in the results of the studies of the effect of aspirin on experimental thrombosis may be attributable to the amounts of aspirin given to the animals as well as to the methods used to produce the injury.

Effect of Sulfinpyrazone

Evidence concerning the effect of sulfinpyrazone in preventing experimental thrombus formation is also inconclusive. Sulfinpyrazone has been found to reduce the extent of platelet accumulation in the vessels of transplanted kidneys or hearts in hyperacute rejection experiments (Sharma et al, 1972, 1973). It also suppresses the thrombocytopenia that occurs during the Arthus reaction (Butler and White, 1975). Tsai et al. (1973) have found that sulfinpyrazone has some protective effect on the development of Forssman shock provoked by intravenous injection into guinea pigs of rabbit antiserum to sheep erythrocyte stroma. Although sulfinpyrazone did not significantly reduce thrombus formation in extracorporeal shunts in rabbits (Mustard et al., 1967b), it did reduce thrombosis in shunts in Rhesus monkeys (Mason et al., 1976). Rüegg (1976) has reported that sulfinpyrazone protected rabbits against sudden death following the infusion of arachidonate, and also that the drug increased fibrinolytic activity. Sulfinpyrazone has been shown to inhibit platelet adherence to cuprophane dialyzer membranes and coated activated charcoal (Winchester et al., 1977). Sulfinpyrazone does not appear to be any better than aspirin in inhibiting experimental thrombosis, although it may be more effective in situations involving immunologic reactions.

There is a difference between aspirin and sulfinpyrazone in their effect on platelet survival. Sulfinpyrazone prolongs shortened platelet survival in man (Smythe et al., 1965; Steele et al., 1975, 1977), whereas aspirin does not (Harker and Slichter, 1972; Genton and Steele, 1977). The recent report of Harker et al. (1978) that sulfinpyrazone protects against endothelial injury and the observation that injury or loss of endothelial cells shortens platelet survival (Ross and Harker, 1976; Harker et al., 1977) may indicate an additional mechanism of sulfinpyrazone. There is no evidence that aspirin protects against endothelial injury.

Clinical Complications of Vascular Disease

Studies of the effects of aspirin or sulfinpyrazone on the clinical complications of vascular disease in man involve three major disorders: (1) venous thrombosis, (2) cerebrovascular disease, and (3) coronary artery disease. Before considering these studies, it is worthwhile to review the criteria involved—both the reasons for the trials and the designs thereof.

A major unsolved problem in venous thromboembolic disease revolves around the relative importance of platelets, blood coagulation, and white blood cells. In some circumstances, platelets do not seem to be important. There is recent evidence that white blood cells may be involved in the initiation of some venous thrombi (Stewart et al., 1974). Following trauma or surgery, white cells adhere to venous endothelium and injure the endothelial cells.

Evidence that atherosclerosis of the major extracranial cerebral arteries is a factor in cerebrovascular disorders is fairly good (Fisher, 1959; Russell, 1961; Gunning et al., 1964). Embolization of the cerebral circulation from mural thrombi in the carotid or vertebral arteries is a major cause of transient attacks of cerebral ischemia. Other mechanisms such as embolization of debris from atherosclerotic plaques can also cause transient attacks (Pfaffenbach and Hollenhorst, 1973). Thromboembolism is a major cause of strokes; other causes include cerebral hemorrhage, which is responsible for less than 20 percent of all strokes (Wolf, 1975).

Atherosclerosis of the coronary arteries appears to be a major factor in myocardial ischemia and infarction, but the role of thrombosis is less clear (Mitchell and Schwartz, 1965; Mustard and Packham, 1969). Although some investigators have suggested that patients who develop full myocardial infarcts develop thrombi after the infarct has occurred (Roberts and Buja, 1972; Erhardt et al., 1973), the bulk of the evidence indicates that the thrombi form at the time of the infarct and that the infarct subtends from the point at which the coronary artery is occluded (Chandler et al., 1974; Ridolfi and Hutchins, 1977; Salimi et al., 1977). A number of mechanisms have been proposed as causes of sudden death from coronary artery disease. These range from abnormal metabolism of the myocardium to transient thromboembolic obstruction of parts of the myocardial microcirculation (Jørgensen et al., 1968; James, 1969). Since about 40 percent of individuals who experience the onset of myocardial ischemia will die in the first 24 hours, and about 60 percent of these will die before they reach a hospital (Bainton and Peterson, 1963; Fulton et al., 1969), the importance of understanding the mechanisms causing sudden death is clear.

When vessel injury causes the formation of thrombi, these are usually mural thrombi that undergo repeated formation and dissolution, and they appear to last as long as the injury site is actively stimulating thrombus formation (Fulton et al., 1953; Baumgartner, 1973). The knowledge that has been developed during the last 20 years has reinforced the point that most thrombi are mural thrombi that give rise to showers of thromboemboli (Mustard et al., 1978). It has been shown in animal experiments that transient platelet aggregates in the coronary microcirculation of pigs and dogs can cause ventricular fibrillation and sudden death as well as focal areas of subendocardial infarction, focal scars, and myofibrillar degeneration (Jørgensen et al., 1967; Robbins et al., 1969; Moore et al, 1976). Individuals who die suddenly from what is considered to be myocardial ischemia show increased numbers of intramyocardial platelet aggregates when compared with individuals killed quickly in accidents (Haerem, 1972, 1974; Frink, 1971). Furthermore, these individuals have areas of subendocardial necrosis and focal myocardial lesions (Haerem, 1975) similar to those produced in the myocardium of dogs with mural thrombi in their coronary arteries (Moore et al., 1976).

Although these observations are compatible with embolization of the microcirculation as a cause of focal myocardial injury and sudden death, the frequency of this as a mechanism causing sudden death in man is not known. In addition, the effects on coronary arteries of substances released or formed by platelets add to the complexity of possible mechanisms. Thromboxane A_2 (which is produced by stimulated platelets) is a powerful stimulus for vasoconstriction (Needleman et al., 1977; Svensson and Fredholm, 1977). Thus, a platelet-rich embolus might also cause constriction at the microcirculatory level. On the other hand, PGI_2, which the vessel wall can form from arachidonic acid or prostaglandin endoperoxides, causes relaxation of arterial smooth muscle cells (Dusting et al., 1977). It is not known which of these mechanisms will predominate under different conditions.

Clinical Trials

At present, the establishment of clinical trials to test the value of drugs that inhibit platelet function in preventing complications of atherosclerosis has to be done with incomplete knowledge of the mechanisms involved and of the actions of the drugs. For example, if aspirin were to have a beneficial effect in a trial involving individuals who had myocardial infarcts, the drug could do so by (1) preventing arrhythmias, (2) preventing formation of thromboxane A_2 and thus preventing vasoconstriction, or (3) inhibiting platelet aggregation, or by any combination of these effects.

If the main effect of aspirin is on thromboembolism, and if thromboembolism only accounts for 30 percent of the deaths, and if the trial is not large enough, the effect of aspirin on this patient subgroup could be missed. Furthermore, if only a subgroup of those with thromboembolism benefits from aspirin (e.g., males but not females), the possibility of showing a beneficial effect will be further reduced. Until patients can be classified more accurately in terms of underlying mechanisms and responsiveness to the effect of the drugs, a sufficient number of patients must be included in clinical trials so that if there is a benefit from the treatment, it can be demonstrated. Furthermore, the subjects must be properly randomized, and the endpoints must be as objective as possible (e.g., death). The methods used to analyze the data must take into account variations in the characteristics of the subjects in the randomized groups that could influence the results. This can be done by using appropriate statistical methods.

Aspirin and Sulfinpyrazone with Arteriovenous Shunts

Both aspirin and sulfinpyrazone have been used in situations in which their effect on thrombus formation could be measured in humans. Aspirin was found to reduce the incidence of closure of arteriovenous fistulae (Brescia-Cimino) during the first 28 postoperative days (Andrassy et al., 1971). In a prospective study, sulfinpyrazone (600 mg daily) significantly reduced thrombus formation in arteriovenous shunts (Kaegi et al., 1974). The effect of the sulfinpyrazone was evident within seven days of the start of therapy and was lost by seven days after therapy was discontinued. Thus, although these drugs do not completely prevent thrombus formation in man, they do inhibit the process, at least in arteriovenous shunts.

Venous Thrombosis

There is extensive literature concerning the use of aspirin in the prevention of venous thromboembolism. Venous thrombi have a large coagulation component, and the contribution of platelets to venous thrombosis is not clear.

In the study of venous thrombosis and pulmonary embolism, one limiting factor in the clinical trials is the endpoint used to assess the effect of drugs. Venography is generally regarded as the most objective endpoint for determining whether a venous thrombus is present. If the patient dies, postmortem examination will confirm whether venous thrombosis or pulmonary embolism had occurred. In one well designed trial, aspirin was found to have no effect on postoperative venous thrombosis when the fibrinogen I-125 method was used to detect the thrombi (Medical Research Council, 1972). A number of other studies (Weber et al., 1971; Salzman et al., 1971; Zekert et al., 1974; Harris et al., 1974; Loew et al., 1974) have shown a trend favoring aspirin, but all these studies have weaknesses in the basic designs of the clinical trials. Claggett et al. (1975) observed that aspirin decreased the incidence of venous thrombosis in surgical patients when compared with a control group given a placebo. In this study, some of the patients originally allocated to the aspirin group were excluded from the calculations because they did not receive aspirin. A recent report indicates that in patients undergoing knee operations, a dose of aspirin of 3.6 g per day was effective in preventing venous thrombosis, whereas a dose of 960 mg per day gave results similar to those for patients given a placebo (McKenna et al., 1976). In six trials in which the diagnosis of deep venous thrombosis following surgery was made on clinical grounds, the four trials conducted with aspirin (Weber et al., 1971; Salzman et al., 1971; Zekert et al., 1974; Loew et al., 1974) showed a significant reduction in clinically detectable venous thrombosis. In the two trials that were performed with dipyridamole, the drug did not have a beneficial effect (Browse and Hall, 1969; Salzman et al., 1971). One has to question whether this difference in clinically detectable thrombosis shown by the effects of aspirin and dipyridamole is related to the ability of aspirin to inhibit cyclooxygenase in cells (Roth and Majerus, 1975) and to prevent the formation of cyclooxygenase-derived products from arachidonic acid. Some of these products contribute to the inflammatory response (Moncada et al., 1973; Kuehl et al., 1977). Suppression of their formation may mask the clinical signs of venous thrombosis.

Zekert et al. (1974) reported that aspirin caused a statistically significant reduction in autopsy-confirmed fatal pulmonary emboli in a study of 240 elderly patients with hip fractures who received either aspirin or a placebo. Recently, Harris and associates (1977) compared aspirin and placebo in patients over the age of 40 undergoing total hip replacement. Phlebography was used for diagnosis. There were significantly fewer thromboembolic episodes in the patients given aspirin (11 of 44) than in the patients receiving the placebo (23 of 51). Unfortunately, 22 patients in the trial withdrew, and the article does not indicate if the withdrawals were evenly divided between the two groups. An interesting observation in this study was that aspirin did not appear to have any beneficial effect for women, although the number of women in the study was small. Schöndorf and associates (1977) compared the effects of subcutaneous heparin and intravenous aspirin in the prevention of venous thrombosis using fibrinogen I-125 to detect the thrombi. Although heparin showed a beneficial effect, aspirin—in the dose used in this study (3.6 g per day)—was not effective in preventing accumulation of fibrinogen I-125. Using the leg-scanning method, Silvergleid and coworkers (1977) could not show that the combination of dipyridamole and aspirin prevented venous thrombosis in patients undergoing hip surgery.

Thus, the value of aspirin for the prevention of venous thrombosis and pulmonary embolism is far from settled. It may well be that in some forms of surgery, aspirin in the correct dose will be effective. However, at present, we do not know (1) which surgical procedures are best suited to aspirin therapy (although hip surgery is a good candidate), (2) which subjects are most likely to respond to aspirin, and (3) the optimal dose of aspirin. The problem of trying to assess the effect of aspirin on venous thrombosis and pulmonary embolism is made more complex by the fact that there are several mechanisms proposed for the initiation of venous thrombi and, in some, platelets play a minor role.

Cerebrovascular Disease

Theoretically, patients with transient attacks of cerebral ischemia or monocular blindness should be ideal subjects for testing whether nonsteroidal antiinflammatory drugs can significantly modify mural arterial thrombi that embolize into the microcirculation. Any compound that inhibits the formation of the thrombi or causes the emboli to break up quickly should reduce the incidence of transient attacks of cerebral ischemia. Treatment should also reduce the incidence of strokes and death in patients in whom thrombosis is the principal cause. Preliminary studies with both aspirin and sulfinpyrazone indicated that these agents might be effective in preventing transient attacks of cerebral ischemia (Harrison et al., 1971; Mundall et al., 1972; Evans, 1973; Dyken et al., 1973). Aspirin has also been examined in a larger study of 178 individuals who had experienced transient ischemic attacks (Fields et al., 1977). In this study, it was found that of a total of 88 patients treated for six months with aspirin, only 15 suffered an unfavorable outcome (death due to cerebral infarction, cardiovascular disease, or intracerebral hemorrhage; nonfatal cerebral infarction, retinal infarction or excessive ratio of transient ischemic attacks). Out of a total of 90 patients in the placebo-treated group, 34 experienced an unfavorable outcome. The difference between the aspirin-treated and placebo-treated groups was statistically significant. Aspirin caused a marked reduction in the number of episodes of transient cerebral ischemia experienced by patients who had had multiple episodes of transient cerebral ischemia before entry into the study. However, the probability of death, nonfatal cerebral infarction, or retinal infarction was not significantly altered by aspirin therapy. A major difficulty in interpreting this study is the fact that multiple analyses were made of the data, which weakens the statistical significance of the tests (Tukey, 1977).

In the Coronary Drug Project aspirin study (Coronary Drug Project Research Group, 1976), strokes and deaths from cerebral vascular accidents (CVA) were equal in the more than 700 patients given aspirin and the more than 700 patients given the placebo. Thus, in this group of patients, aspirin was not found to be effective in prevention of the major complications of cerebrovascular disease.

The effect of aspirin and sulfinpyrazone, singly or in combination, on the occurrence of continuing transient ischemic attacks (TIAs) and on strokes and death was studied in a clinical trial with 585 patients (Canadian Cooperative Study Group, 1978) (Table 15-1). The patients were randomly divided into four groups. Since there was no statistically significant interaction found for aspirin and sulfinpyrazone, comparisons were made between all patients receiving sulfinpyrazone (alone and with acetylsalicylic acid) and all patients not receiving sulfinpyrazone, and between all patients receiving aspirin (alone and with sulfinpyrazone) and all patients not receiving aspirin. Using this analysis, sulfinpyrazone showed no risk reduction (based on

Table 15-1. *Effect of Sulfinpyrazone or Aspirin or Both on Stroke and Death of Patients Who Had Had a Transient Ischemic Attack*

Treatment	Total Number of Patients	First Event	
		Stroke (Mild, Moderate, or Major)	Death
Placebo	138	20	10
Sulfinpyrazone	156	29	9
Aspirin	144	24	5
Sulfinpyrazone + Aspirin	146	14	6

Canadian Cooperative Study Group, 1978.

continuing TIA's, stroke, or death), whereas aspirin showed a 19 percent risk reduction, which was significant at the 0.05 level. If the risk for only strokes and death was considered, aspirin reduced the risk by 31 percent ($P<0.05$), whereas sulfinpyrazone reduced it by 10 percent. An interesting observation in this study was that aspirin appeared not to reduce the risk of stroke or death in women. The risk reduction for men was 48 percent ($P<0.005$). It is possible that in the whole group, the observations obtained with the large number of less responsive patients masked the interaction between the drugs. Although the results from this trial show a beneficial effect for aspirin dependent on the analytic approach used, they do not exclude the possibility that interaction between the drugs may have been a factor in reducing the risk.

Myocardial Infarction

Elwood and associates (1974) found that a single daily dose of aspirin in subjects who had had a myocardial infarction (MI) reduced mortality by 25 percent at 12 months. This reduction was not statistically significant. A problem with this study is that when it was expanded to other trial centers, the period from the time of infarction to admission to the trial was lengthened. Therefore, the original group of patients admitted shortly after myocardial infarction was diluted by a larger group of patients, admitted from other centers, who were several months postinfarction. The greatest effect of aspirin in reducing mortality appeared to be in those subjects admitted to the study soon after their MI, in particular during the initial three months.

The Coronary Drug Project Research Group (1976) studied the effect of aspirin in a group of men who had had an infarct and who had previously been treated with dextrothyroxine or estrogen. Of the 758 men given aspirin, 44 died during the study; 64 of the 771 men given the placebo died in the same period. Twenty of the deaths in the aspirin-treated group were listed as sudden cardiovascular deaths, and twenty-five of the deaths in the placebo group were listed in the same way. In this study, in which the patients had already received previous therapy for a considerable period, overall mortality was 5.8 percent in the aspirin group and 8.3 percent in the placebo group. There was, therefore, a 30 percent benefit from aspirin therapy, although the difference was not statistically significant. It should be pointed out that most of the patients in this study had had their most recent myocardial infarct several years before entry into the trial.

A collaborative Austrian-German study (Breddin et al., 1977) compared the effects of phenprocoumon and aspirin therapy (1.5 g per day). Thirteen of the 317 patients given aspirin died, whereas 22 of the 309 patients given the placebo and 26 of the 320 patients given the oral anticoagulant died.

A recent report has shown that the administration of sulfinpyrazone (200 mg four times per day) to 733 patients, commencing four weeks after a myocardial infarction, produced a 48.5 percent reduction in cardiac deaths when compared with the 742 patients given the placebo (Anturane Reinfarction Trial Research Group, 1978). Sulfinpyrazone produced a 57 percent reduction in sudden cardiac deaths. In this study, all deaths occurring during the first seven days of therapy or during the first seven days after cessation of therapy were excluded. There were seven deaths in the placebo group and seven in the sulfinpyrazone group during the first seven days of therapy. There were nine deaths in the placebo group and nine in the sulfinpyrazone group during the period beginning seven days after cessation of therapy. The original design of the study was to have these deaths excluded from the analysis. The reason for excluding the deaths during the initial seven days of therapy was the same as that in the sulfinpyrazone-aspirin study by the Canadian Cooperative Study Group (1978), since it was believed that sulfinpyrazone administration did not immediately affect platelets and the thrombotic process. If these patients are included in the analysis, the effects of sulfinpyrazone are less impressive. The impact of sulfinpyrazone appears to have been most marked during the first few months. Whether it will have an effect over a longer period is not known at present.

Some concern has been expressed about the possible effect of the differences in the baseline values for arrhythmias between the placebo and sulfinpyrazone groups (Editorial, British Medical Journal, 1978). It should be pointed out that the Cox method of analysis (Cox, 1974) used in the study allows for adjustments in the tests of significance related to variations in baseline data. The unadjusted probability for reduction in overall cardiac mortality in the sulfinpyrazone group was $P=0.011$; for the adjusted values based on the Cox method of analysis, $P=0.018$.

The failure of sulfinpyrazone to have much effect in the patients with transient attacks of cerebral ischemia (Canadian Cooperative Study Group, 1978) raises significant questions as to whether sulfinpyrazone has much effect on carotid artery thrombi and their thromboembolic effects on the cerebral vascular circulation. If sulfinpyrazone were effective in modifying this process, one would have expected a beneficial effect from sulfinpyrazone in the study of strokes by the Canadian Cooperative Study Group (1978). The apparently striking effect of sulfinpyrazone in reducing sudden death in subjects who have had a myocardial infarction could be considered as evidence in favor of mural thrombi and platelet thromboemboli being a factor in causing sudden cardiac death. However, if the process in the coronary arteries is essentially the same as that in the carotid arteries, it would be difficult to explain the effects on the coronary circulation as being due to embolization of mural thrombi, because of the lack of effect of sulfinpyrazone in the stroke study. The action of sulfinpyrazone in influencing sudden cardiac death may be related to some other effect, such as modification of the mechanisms involved in producing cardiac arrhythmias. This could also be a possible effect of aspirin, since, as indicated earlier in the discussion, there is some evidence that aspirin may reduce the incidence of cardiac arrhythmia in animals subjected to experimental ischemia without the presence of thromboemboli (Moschos et al., 1978).

Conclusion

Evidence from the clinical trials concerning the effects of aspirin and sulfinpyrazone in reducing the incidence of clinical complications of atherosclerosis in patients who have already had a complication is far from conclusive. The same is true concerning the effect of these drugs in the prevention of venous thrombosis and pulmonary embolism.

In coronary artery disease, there are some indications that both aspirin and sulfinpyrazone may exert their greatest effect during the first few months after a myocardial infarct.

The results of the stroke studies indicate that some subgroups may be much more responsive to aspirin than the entire patient population characterized by transient attacks of cerebral ischemia. Patients with a history of diabetes or myocardial infarction and female patients show little benefit from aspirin therapy. In the most sensitive subgroup in the stroke study, a combination of aspirin and sulfinpyrazone produced a greater risk reduction than either drug alone. Although aspirin and sulfinpyrazone have similar effects on collagen-induced platelet aggregation, they differ in their effects on platelet survival, and thus they may show some synergistic effects on thromboembolism. Finally, the failure of sulfinpyrazone to influence significantly the outcome in patients with transient cerebral ischemia, compared with its success in reducing the incidence of sudden death in the myocardial infarction study, raises the possibility that the action of sulfinpyrazone in coronary artery disease involves processes other than thromboembolism (e.g., factors responsible for arrhythmia).

Future trials should be done to determine the effects of these drugs on subgroups of patients for which they appear to be most beneficial. Such studies may also help to define the mechanisms involved in the death of patients with cerebrovascular or coronary artery disease.

References

Ali, M., and McDonald, J.W.D.: Effects of sulfinpyrazone on platelet prostaglandin synthesis and platelet release of serotonin. J. Lab. Clin. Med. 89:868–875, 1977.

Andrassy, K., Ritz, E., Schoeffner, W., Hahn, G., and Walter, K.: The influence of acetylsalicylic acid on platelet adhesiveness and thrombotic fistula complications in hemodialysed patients. Klin. Wochenschr. 49:166–167, 1971.

Anturane Reinfarction Trial Research Group: Sulfinpyrazone in the prevention of cardiac death after myocardial infarction. N. Engl. J. Med. 298:289–295, 1978.

Arfors, K.-E., Bergqvist, D., and Tangen, O.: The effect of platelet function inhibitors on experimental venous thrombosis formation in rabbits. Acta. Chir. Scand. 141:40–42, 1975.

Bainton, C.R., and Peterson, D.R.: Deaths from coronary heart disease in persons fifty years of age and younger: a community-wide study. N. Engl. J. Med. 268:569–575, 1963.

Baumgartner, H.R.: The role of blood flow in platelet adhesion, fibrin deposition and formation of mural thrombi. Microvasc. Res. 5:167–179, 1973.

Baumgartner, H.R., Muggli, R., Tschopp, T.B., and Turitto, V.T.: Platelet adhesion, release and aggregation in flowing blood: effects of surface properties and platelet function. Thromb. Haemostas. 35:124–138, 1976.

Bergqvist, D., and Arfors, K.-E.: Haemostasis in the microvasculature of the rabbit mesentery, effects of some pharmacological agents of current interest in haemostasis and thrombosis. Haemostasis 5:74–84, 1976.

Bourgain, R.H.: Inhibition of PGI_2 (prostacyclin) synthesis in the arterial wall enhances the formation of white platelet thrombi in vivo. Haemostasis 7: 252-255, 1978.

Breddin, K., Överla, K., and Walter, E.: German-Austrian multicenter two years prospective study on the prevention of secondary myocardial infarction by ASA in comparison to phenprocoumon and placebo. Thromb. Haemostas. 38:168, 1977.

Browse, N.L., and Hall, J.H.: Effect of dipyridamole on the incidence of clinically detectable deep-vein thrombosis. Lancet 2:718–721, 1969.

Bunting, S., Gryglewski, R., Moncada, S., and Vane, J.R.: Arterial walls generate from prostaglandin endoperoxides a substance (prostaglandin X) which relaxes strips of mesenteric and coeliac arteries and inhibits platelet aggregation. Prostaglandins 12:897–913, 1976.

Burch, J.W., Stanford, N., and Majerus, P.W.: Inhibition of platelet prostaglandin synthetase by oral aspirin. J. Clin. Invest. 61:314–319, 1978.

Butler, K.D., and White, A.M.: The effect of sulphinpyrazone on the thrombocytopenia occurring in the Arthus reaction. Br. J. Pharmacol. 55:256P–257P, 1975.

Canadian Cooperative Study Group: A randomized trial of aspirin and sulfinpyrazone in threatened stroke. N. Engl. J. Med. 299: 53-59, 1978.

Cazenave, J.-P., Packham, M.A., Davies, J.A., Kinlough-Rathbone, R.L., and Mustard, J.F.: Studies of platelet adherence to collagen and the subendothelium. In Day, H.J., Holmsen, H., and Zucker, M.B., *Platelet Function Testing*, DHEW Publication No. (NIH) 78–1087, Washington, D.C., U.S. Government Printing Office, 181-198, 1978a.

Cazenave, J.-P., Packham, M.A., Kinlough-Rathbone, R.L., and Mustard, J.F.: Platelet adherence to the vessel wall and to collagen-coated surfaces. In Day, H.J., Molony, B.A., Nishizawa, E.E., and Rynbrandt, R.H., *Thrombosis: Animal and Clinical Models*, Adv. Exp. Med. Biol. 102: 31-49, 1978b.

Chandler, A.B., Chapman, I., Erhardt, L.R., Roberts, W.C., Schwartz, C.J., Sinapius, D., Spain, D.M., Sherry, S., Ness, P.M., and Simon, T.L.: Coronary thrombosis in myocardial infarction. Report of a workshop on the role of coronary thrombosis in the pathogenesis of acute myocardial infarction. Am. J. Cardiol. 34:823–833, 1974.

Clagett, G.P., Schneider, P., Rosoff, C.B., and Salzman, E.W.: The influence of aspirin on postoperative platelet kinetics and venous thrombosis. Surgery 77:61–74, 1975.

Coronary Drug Project Research Group: Aspirin in coronary heart disease. J. Chronic Dis. 29:625–642, 1976.

Cox, D.R.: Regression models and life-tables. J.R. Stat Soc. (B) 34:187–220, 1974.

Danese, C.A., and Haimov, M.: Inhibition of experimental arterial thrombosis in dogs with platelet-deaggregating agents. Surgery 70:927–934, 1971.

Danese, C.A., Voleti, C.D., and Weiss, H.J.: Protection by aspirin against experimentally induced arterial thrombosis in dogs. Thromb. Diath. Haemorrh. 25:288–296, 1971.

Dusting, G.J., Moncada, S., and Vane, J.R.: Prostacyclin (PGX) is the endogenous metabolite responsible for relaxation of coronary arteries induced by arachidonic acid. Prostaglandins 13:3–15, 1977.

Dyken, M.L., Campbell, R.L., Muller, J., Feuer, H., Horner, T., King, R., Kolar, O., Solow, E., and Jones, F.H.: Effect of aspirin on experimentally induced arterial thrombosis during the healing phase. Stroke 4:387–389, 1973.

Dyken, M.L., Kolar, O.J., and Jones, F.H.: Differences in the occurrence of carotid transient ischemic attacks associated with antiplatelet aggregation therapy. Stroke 4:732–736, 1973.

Editorial: Sulphinpyrazone, cardiac infarction, and the prevention of death: a successful trial or another tribulation? Br. Med. J. 2:941–942, 1978.

Elwood, P.C., Cochrane, A.L., Burr, M.L., Sweetnam, P.M., Williams, G., Welsby, E., Hughes, S.J., and Renton, R.: A randomized controlled trial of acetylsalicylic acid in the secondary prevention of mortality from myocardial infarction. Br. Med. J. 1:436–440, 1974.

Erhardt, L.R., Lundman, T., and Mellstedt, H.: Incorporation of ^{125}I-labelled fibrinogen into coronary arterial thrombi in acute myocardial infarction in man. Lancet 1:387–390, 1973.

Essien, E.M., Cazenave, J.-P., Moore, S., and Mustard, J.F.: Effect of heparin and thrombin on platelet adherence to the surface of rabbit aorta. Thromb. Res. 13: 69-78, 1978.

Evans, G.: Effect of platelet-suppressive agents in the incidence of amaurosis fugax and transient cerebral ischemia. In McDowell, F.H., and Brennan, R.W., *Cerebral Vascular Diseases,* Eighth conference, New York, Grune and Stratton, 297-300, 1973.

Evans, G., Packham, M.A., Nishizawa, E.E., Mustard, J.F., and Murphy, E.A.: The effect of acetylsalicylic acid on platelet function. J. Exp. Med. 128:877–894, 1968.

Fields, W.S., Lemak, N.A., Frankowski, R.F., and Hardy, R.J.: Controlled trial of aspirin in cerebral ischemia. Stroke 8:301–316, 1977.

Fisher, C.M.: Observations of the fundus oculi in transient-monocular blindness. Neurology (Minneap.) 9:333–347, 1959.

Folts, J.D., Crowell, E.B., and Rowe, G.G.: Platelet aggregation in partially obstructed vessels and its elimination with aspirin. Circulation 54:365–370, 1976.

Frink, R.J.: Non-obstructive mural coronary thrombosis in sudden death. In Manning, G.W., and Haust, M.D., *Atherosclerosis. Metabolic, Morphologic and Clinical Aspects,* Adv. Exp. Med. Biol. 82:124–126, 1971.

Fulton, G.P., Akers, R.P., and Lutz, B.R.: White thromboemboli and vascular fragility in hamster cheek pouch after anticoagulants. Blood 8:140–152, 1953.

Fulton, M., Julian, D.G., and Oliver, M.: Sudden death and myocardial infarction. In Bondurant, S., *Research on Acute Myocardial Infarction.* New York, American Heart Association Monograph 27, : IV-182-IV-193, 1969.

Furlow, T.W., and Bass, N.H.: Arachidonate-induced cerebrovascular occlusion in the rat. The role of platelets and aspirin in stroke. Neurology 26:297–304, 1976.

Genton, E., Steele, P.: Platelet survival: value for the diagnosis of thromboembolism and evaluation of anti-thrombotic drugs. In Mills, D.C.B., and Pareti, F.I., *Platelets and Thrombosis,* London, Academic Press, 157–166, 1977.

Gertz, S.D., Rennels, M.L., and Nelson, E.: Endothelial cell ischemic injury: protective effect of heparin or aspirin assessed by scanning electron microscopy. Stroke 6:357–360, 1975.

Gorman, R.R., Bunting, S., and Miller, O.V.: Modulation of human platelet adenylate cyclase by prostacyclin (PGX). Prostaglandins 13:377–388, 1977.

Gunning, A.J., Pickering, G.W., Robb-Smith, A.H.T., and Russell, R.R.: Mural thrombosis of the internal carotid artery and subsequent embolism. Q. J. Med. 33:155–195, 1964.

Gurewich, V., and Lipinski, B.: Evaluation of antithrombotic properties of suloctidil in comparison with aspirin and dipyridamole. Thromb. Res. 9:101–108, 1976.

Haerem, J.W.: Platelet aggregates in intramyocardial vessels of patients dying suddenly and unexpectedly of coronary artery disease. Atherosclerosis 15:199–213, 1972.

Haerem, J.W.: Mural platelet microthrombi and major acute lesions of main epicardial arteries in sudden coronary death. Atherosclerosis 19:529–541, 1974.

Haerem, J.W.: Myocardial lesions in sudden, unexpected coronary death. Am. Heart J. 90:562–568, 1975.

Harker, L.A., and Slichter, S.J.: Platelet and fibrinogen consumption in man. N. Engl. J. Med. 287:999–1005, 1972.

Harker, L.A., Slichter, S.J., and Sauvage, L.R.: Platelet consumption by arterial prostheses: the effects of endothelialization and pharmacologic inhibition of platelet function. Ann. Surg. 186:594–601, 1977.

Harker, L.A., Wall, R.T., Harlan, J.M., and Ross, R.: Sulfinpyrazone prevention of homocysteine-induced endothelial cell injury and arteriosclerosis. Clin. Res. 26:554A, 1978.

Harris, W.H., Salzman, E.W., Athanasoulis, C., Waltman, A.C., Baum, S., and DeSanctis, R.W.: Comparison of warfarin, low-molecular-weight dextran, aspirin, and subcutaneous heparin in prevention of venous thromboembolism following total hip replacement. J. Bone Joint Surg. (Am) 56:1552–1562, 1974.

Harris, W.H., Salzman, E.W., Athanasoulis, C.A., Waltman, A.C., and DeSanctis, R.W.: Aspirin prophylaxis of venous thromboembolism after total hip replacement. N. Engl. J. Med. 297:1246–1249, 1977.

Harrison, M.J.G., Marshall, J., Meadows, J.C., and Russell, R.W.R.: Effect of aspirin in amaurosis fugax. Lancet 2:743–744, 1971.

Honour, A.J., Hockaday, T.D.R., and Mann, J.I.: The synergistic effect of aspirin and dipyridamole upon platelet thrombi in living blood vessels. Br. J. Exp. Pathol. 58:268–272, 1977.

Hovig, T.: Release of a platelet aggregating substance (adenosine diphosphate) from rabbit blood platelets induced by saline "extract" of tendons. Thromb. Diath. Haemorrh. 9:264–278, 1963.

Hugues, J.: Accolement des plaquettes aux structures conjonctives périvasculaires. Thromb. Diath. Haemorrh. 8:241-255, 1962.

James, T.N.: The role of small vessel disease in myocardial infarction. In Bondurant, S., *Research on Acute Myocardial Infarction*, Circulation 39 and 40, Suppl. 4, IV-13–IV-30, 1969.

Jørgensen, L., Haerem, J., Chandler, A.B., and Borchgrevink, C.F.: The pathology of acute coronary death. Acta Anaesthesiol. Scand. (Suppl) 29:193–199, 1968.

Jørgensen, L., Rowsell, H.C., Hovig, T., Glynn, M.F., and Mustard, J.F.: Adenosine diphosphate-induced platelet aggregation and myocardial infarction in swine. Lab. Invest. 17:616–644, 1967.

Kaegi, A., Pineo, G.F., Shimizu, A., Trivedi, H., Hirsh, J., and Gent, M.: Arteriovenous-shunt thrombosis: prevention by sulfinpyrazone. N. Engl. J. Med. 290:304–306, 1974.

Kelton, J., Carter, C., Buchanan, M.R., and Hirsh, J.: Thrombogenic effect of high dose aspirin in injury induced experimental venous thrombosis. Clin. Res. 26:350A, 1978.

Kinlough-Rathbone, R.L., Packham, M.A., Reimers, H.-J., Cazenave, J.-P., and Mustard, J.F.: Mechanisms of platelet shape change, aggregation and release induced by collagen, thrombin or A23,187. J. Lab. Clin. Med. 90:707–719, 1977.

Kohler, C., Wooding, W., and Ellenbogen, L.: Intravenous arachidonate in the mouse: a model for the evaluation of antithrombotic drugs. Thromb. Res. 9:67–80, 1976.

Kricheff, I.I., Zucker, M.B., Tschopp, T.B., and Kolodjiez, A.: Inhibition of thrombosis on vascular catheters in cats. Radiology 106:49–51, 1973.

Kuehl, F.A., Jr., Humes, J.L., Egan, R.W., Ham, E.A., Beveridge, G.C., and Van Arman, C.G.: Role of prostaglandin endoperoxide PGG_2 in inflammatory processes. Nature 265:170–173, 1977.

Levison, M.E., Carrizosa, J., Tanphaichitra, D., Schick, P.K., and Rubin, W.: Effect of aspirin on thrombogenesis and on production of experimental aortic valvular Streptococcus viridans endocarditis in rabbits. Blood 49:645–650, 1977.

Lewis, G.P., and Westwick, J.: The effect of sulphinpyrazone, sodium aspirin and oxprenolol on the formation of arterial platelet thrombi. Br. J. Pharmacol. 55:255P–256P, 1975.

Loew, D., Wellmer, H.-K., Baer, U., Merguet, H., Rumpf, P., Petersen, H., Bromig, G., Persch, W.F., Marx, F.J., on von Bary, S.M.: Postoperative Thromboembolie-prophylaxe mit Acetylsalicylsäure. Dtsch. Med. Wochenschr. 99:565–572, 1974.

Mason, R.G., Wolf, R.H., Zucker, W.H., Shinoda, B.A., and Mohammad, S.F.: Effects of antithrombotic agents evaluated in a nonhuman primate vascular shunt model. Am. J. Pathol. 83:557–568, 1976.

Mathew, T.H., Hogan, G.P., Lewers, D.T., Bauer, H., Maher, J.F., and Schreiner, G.E.: Controlled, double-blind trial of antiplatelet aggregating agents in vascular renal allograft rejection. Transplant Proc. 3:901–904, 1971.

Mayer, J.E., Jr., and Hammond, G.L.: Dipyridamole and aspirin tested against an experimental model of thrombosis. Ann. Surg. 178:108–112, 1973.

McKenna, R., Bachmann, F., Galante, J., Kaushal, S.P., and Meredith, P.: Prospective trial of aspirin and phlebo-dynastat in the prevention of thrombo-embolic disease. Blood 48:977, 1976.

Medical Research Council (Report of the Steering Committee): Effect of aspirin on postoperative venous thrombosis. Lancet 2:441–445, 1972.

Meng, K., and O'Dea, K.: The protective effect of acetylsalicylic acid on laser-induced venous thrombosis in the rat. Naunyn. Schmiedebergs Arch. Pharmacol. 283:379–388, 1974.

Mitchell, J.R.A., and Schwartz, C.J.: *Arterial Disease.* Oxford, Blackwell, 1965.

Moncada, S., Ferreira, S.H., and Vane, J.R.: Prostaglandins, aspirin-like drugs and the oedema of inflammation. Nature 246:217–219, 1973.

Moncada, S., Higgs, E.A., and Vane, J.R.: Human arterial and venous tissues generate prostacyclin (prostaglandin X), a potent inhibitor of platelet aggregation. Lancet 1:18–20, 1977.

Moore, S., Belbeck, L.W., and Evans, G.: Myocardial lesions associated with partial, compared to complete, thrombotic occlusion of a coronary artery. Circulation 54:Suppl. II–202, 1976.

Moschos, C.B., Haider, B., DeLaCruz, C., Jr., Lyons, M.M., and Regan, T.J.: Antiarrhythmic effects of aspirin during nonthrombotic coronary occlusion. Circulation 57:681–684, 1978.

Moschos, C.B., Lahiri, K., Lyons, M.M., Weisse, A.B., Oldewurtel, H.A., and Regan, T.J.: Relation of microcirculatory thrombosis to thrombus in the proximal coronary artery: effect of aspirin, dipyridamole, and thrombosis. Am. Heart J. 86:61–68, 1973.

Mundall, J., Quintero, P., von Kaulla, K., Austin, J., and Harmon, R.: Transient monocular blindness and increased platelet aggregability treated with aspirin. A case report. Neurology 22:280–285, 1972.

Mustard, J.F.: Atherosclerosis, thrombosis and clinical complications. In Mitchell, J.R.A., and Domenet, J.G., *Thromboembolism. A New Approach to Therapy,* New York, Academic Press, 3-25, 1977.

Mustard, J.F., Glynn, M.F., Nishizawa, E.E., and Packham, M.A.: Platelet-surface interactions: relationship to thrombosis and hemostasis. Fed. Proc. 26:106–114, 1967a.

Mustard, J.F., and Packham, M.A.: Platelet function and myocardial infarction. Circulation 39 and 40:Suppl. IV, 20–30, 1969.

Mustard, J.F., Packham, M.A., and Kinlough-Rathbone, R.L.: Platelets and thrombosis in the development of atherosclerosis and its complications. In Day, H.J., Molony, B.A., Nishizawa, E.E., and Rynbrandt, R.H., *Thrombosis: Animal and Clinical Models,* Adv. Exp. Biol. Med., 102:7-30, 1978.

Mustard, J.F., Rowsell, H.C., Smythe, H.A., Senyi, A., and Murphy, E.A.: The effect of sulfinpyrazone on platelet economy and thrombus formation in rabbits. Blood 29:859–866, 1967b.

Needleman, P., Kulkarni, P.S., and Raz, A.: Coronary tone modulation: formation and actions of prostaglandins, endoperoxides and thromboxanes. Science 195:409–412, 1977.

O'Brien, J.R., Finch, W., and Clark, E.: A comparison of an effect of different anti-inflammatory drugs on human platelets. J. Clin. Pathol. 23:522–525, 1970.

Packham, M.A., and Mustard, J.F.: Non-steroidal anti-inflammatory drugs, pyrimido-pyrimidine compounds and tricyclic compounds. Effects on platelet function. In Hirsh, J., Cade, J.F., Gallus, A.S., and Schönbaum, E., *Platelets, Drugs and Thrombosis,* Basel, S. Karger, 111-123, 1975.

Packham, M.A., Warrior, E.S., Glynn, M.F., Senyi, A.S., and Mustard, J.F.: Alteration of the response of platelets to surface stimuli by pyrazole compounds. J. Exp. Med. 126:171–188, 1967.

Peterson, J., and Zucker, M.B.: The effect of adenosine monophosphate, arcaine and anti-inflammatory agents on thrombosis and platelet function in rabbits. Thromb. Diath. Haemorrh. 23:148–158, 1970.

Pfaffenbach, D.D., and Hollenhorst, R.W.: Morbidity and survivorship of patients with embolic cholesterol crystals in the ocular fundus. Am. J. Ophthalmol. 75:66–72, 1973.

Piepgras, D.G., Sundt, T.M., and Didisheim, P.: Effect of anticoagulants and inhibitors of platelet aggregation on thrombotic occlusion of endarterectomized cat carotid arteries. Stroke 7:248–254, 1976.

Radegran, K., Bergentz, S.-E., Lewis, D.H., Ljungqvist, U., and Olsson, P.: Pulmonary effects of induced platelet aggregation. Intravascular obstruction or vasoconstriction? Scand. J. Clin. Lab. Invest. 28:423–427, 1971.

Renaud, S., and Godu, J.: Thrombosis prevention by acetylsalicylic acid in hyperlipemic rats. Can. Med. Assoc. J. 103:1037–1040, 1970.

Ridolfi, R.L., and Hutchins, G.M.: The relationship between coronary artery lesions and myocardial infarcts: ulceration of atherosclerotic plaques precipitating coronary thrombosis. Am. Heart J. 93:468–486, 1977.

Robbins, S.L., Berger, R.L., Suda, Y., and Ryan, T.J.: Myocardial infarction produced by temporary microcoronary occlusion. Circulation Suppl. 3, 40:171, 1969.

Roberts, W.C., and Buja, L.M.: The frequency and significance of coronary arterial thrombi and other observations in fatal acute myocardial infarction: a study of 107 necropsy patients. Am. J. Med. 52:425–443, 1972.

Rome, L.H., Lands, W.E.M., Roth, G.J., and Majerus, P.W.: Aspirin as a quantitative acetylating reagent for the fatty acid oxygenase that forms prostaglandins. Prostaglandins 11:23–30, 1976.

Ross, R., and Harker, L.: Hyperlipidemia and atherosclerosis. Science 193:1094–1100, 1976.

Roth, G.J., and Majerus, P.W.: The mechanism of the effect of aspirin on human platelets. I. Acetylation of a particulate fraction protein. J. Clin. Invest. 56:624–632, 1975.

Rüegg, M.: Antithrombotic effects of sulfinpyrazone in animals: influence on fibrinolysis and sodium arachidonate-induced pulmonary embolism. Pharmacology 14:522–536, 1976.

Russell, R.W.R.: Observations on the retinal blood-vessels in monocular blindness. Lancet 2:1422–1428, 1961.

Salimi, A., Oliver, G.C., Jr., Lee, J., and Sherman, L.A.: Continued incorporation of circulating radiolabeled fibrinogen into preformed coronary artery thrombi. Circulation 56:213–217, 1977.

Salzman, E.W., Harris, W.H., and DeSanctis, R.W.: Reduction in venous thromboembolism by agents affecting platelet function. N. Engl. J. Med. 284:1287–1292, 1971.

Samuelsson, B.: The role of prostaglandin endoperoxides and thromboxanes in human platelets. In Silver, M.J., Smith, J.B., and Kocsis, J.J., *Prostaglandins in Hematology,* New York, Spectrum Publications, Inc. 1977.

Schöndorf, T.H., Weber, U., and Lasch, H.G.: Niedrig dosiertes Heparin und Acetylsalicylsäure nach elektiven Operationen am Hüftgelenk. Dtsch. Med. Wochenschr. 102:1314–1318, 1977.

Sharma, H.M., Moore, S., Merrick, H.W., and Smith, M.R.: Platelets in early hyperacute allograft rejection in kidneys and their modification by sulfinpyrazone (anturan) therapy. An experimental study. Am. J. Pathol. 66:445–460, 1972.

Sharma, H.M., Rosensweig, J., Chatterjee, S., Moore, S., and de Champlain, M.-L.: Platelets in hyperacute rejection of heterotopic cardiac allografts in presensitized dogs. An experimental study. Am. J. Path. 70:155–174, 1973.

Sheppard, B.L.: The effect of acetylsalicylic acid on platelet adhesion in the injured abdominal aorta. Q. J. Exp. Physiol. 57:319–323, 1972.

Silvergleid, A.J., Bernstein, R. Burton, D.S., Tanner, J.B., Silverman, J.F., and Schrier, S.L.: Aspirin-persantin prophylaxis in elective total hip replacement. Thromb. Haemostas. 38:166, 1977.

Smith, J.B., Ingerman, C.M., and Silver, M.J.: Effects of arachidonic acid and some of its metabolites on platelets. In Silver, M.J., Smith, J.B., and Kocsis, J.J., *Prostaglandins in Hematology*, New York, Spectrum Publications Inc., 277-292, 1977.

Smythe, H.A., Ogryzlo, M.A., Murphy, E.A., and Mustard, J.F.: The effect of sulfinpyrazone (Anturan) on platelet economy and blood coagulation in man. Can. Med. Assoc. J. 92:818–821, 1965.

Spaet, T.H., and Zucker, M.B.: Mechanism of platelet plug formation and role of adenosine diphosphate. Am. J. Physiol. 206:1267–1274, 1964.

Spilker, B.A., and van Balken, H.: Formation and embolization of thrombi after electrical stimulation. On the method and evaluation of drugs. Thromb. Diath. Haemorrh. 30:352–362, 1973.

Steele, P., Battock, D., and Genton, E.: Effects of clofibrate and sulfinpyrazone on platelet survival time in coronary artery disease. Circulation 52:473–476, 1975.

Steele, P., Carroll, J., Overfield, D., and Genton, E.: Effect of sulfinpyrazone on platelet survival time in patients with transient cerebral ischemic attacks. Stroke 8:396–398, 1977.

Stewart, G.J., Ritchie, W.G.M., and Lynch, P.R.: Venous endothelial damage produced by massive sticking and emigration of leukocytes. Am. J. Pathol. 74:507–532, 1974.

Svensson, J., and Fredholm, B.B.: Vasoconstrictor effect of thromboxane A_2. Acta Physiol. Scand. 101:366–368, 1977.

Tsai, C.-C., Taichman, N.S., Pulver, W.H., and Schönbaum, E.: Heterophile antibodies and tissue injury. III. A role for platelets in the development of lethal vascular injury during Forssman shock in guinea pigs. Am. J. Pathol. 72:179–200, 1973.

Ts'ao, C.-h.: Ultrastructural study of the effect of aspirin on *in vitro* platelet-collagen interaction and platelet adhesion to injured intima in the rabbit. Am. J. Pathol. 59:327–345, 1970.

Tukey, J.W.: Some thoughts on clinical trials, especially problems of multiplicity. Science 198:679–684, 1977.

Vik-Mo, H.: Effects of acute myocardial ischaemia on platelet aggregation in the coronary sinus and aorta in dogs. Scand. J. Haematol. 19:68–74, 1977.

Weber, W., Wolff, U., and Bromig, G.: Postoperative thromboemboliepropylaxe mit Colfarit. Therap. Berichte 43:229–293, 1971.

Weiss, H.J., Aledort, L.M., and Kochwa, S.: The effects of salicylates on the hemostatic properties of platelets in man. J. Clin. Invest. 47:2169–2180, 1968.

Weiss, H.J., Tschopp, T.B., and Baumgartner, H.R.: Impaired interaction (adhesion-aggregation) of platelets with the subendothelium in storage-pool disease and after aspirin ingestion. A comparison with von Willebrand's disease. N. Engl. J. Med. 293:619–623, 1975.

Weksler, B.B., Marcus, A.J., and Jaffe, E.A.: Synthesis of prostaglandin I_2 (prostacyclin) by cultured human and bovine endothelial cells. Proc. Natl. Acad. Sci. USA. 74:3922–3926, 1977.

Willis, A.L., Vane, F.M., Kuhn, D.C., Scott, C.G., and Petrin, M.: An endoperoxide aggregator (LASS), formed in platelets in response to thrombotic stimuli. Purification, identification and unique biological significance. Prostaglandins 8:453–507, 1974.

Winchester, J.F., Forbes, C.D., Courtney, J.M., Reavey, M., and Prentice, C.R.M.: Effect of sulphinpyrazone and aspirin on platelet adhesion to activated charcoal and dialysis membranes in vitro. Thromb. Res. 11:443–451, 1977.

Wolf, P.A.: Hypertension as a risk factor for stroke. In Whisnant, J.P., and Sandok, B.A., Ninth Princeton Conference on Cerebral Vascular Disease. New York, Grune and Stratton, 9:105–112, 1975.

Zekert, F., Kohn, P., Vormittag, E., Poigenfürst, J., and Thien, M.: Thromboemboliepropylaxe mit Acetylsalicylsäure bei Operationen wegen hüftgelenksnaher Frakturen. Monatsschr. Unfallheilkd., 77:97–110, 1974.

Can Drugs, by Suppressing Some Platelet Functions, Prevent Postoperative Deep Vein Thrombosis and Coronary Heart Disease?

Marc Verstraete, M.D., Ph.D.
University of Leuven, Belgium

Many agents capable of interfering with normal platelet function *in vitro* have been described in recent years; most are nonsteroidal antiinflammatory agents. Not all these compounds have been shown to affect platelet aggregation and adhesiveness in experimental animals, but since animals do not develop spontaneous thrombosis, the relevance of such experiments to clinical medicine is rather tenuous. The only drugs suppressing platelet function that have been evaluated in clinical trials are aspirin, sulfinpyrazone, dipyridamole, hydroxychloroquine, clofibrate, flurbiprofen, and lidocaine, all of which were originally used for other therapeutic purposes. Even today, it is uncertain whether the potential antithrombotic effects of these drugs are due to their impact on platelets or to some other mode of action.

Prevention of Postoperative Deep Vein Thrombosis and Pulmonary Embolism

Incidence and Detection of Deep Vein Thrombosis

Deep vein thrombosis is a frequent, usually insignificant and unrecognized incident of the pre- and postoperative period. Its seriousness lies in the possibility of a rare but potentially fatal sudden pulmonary embolus and in damage to the venous wall with a subsequent postphlebitic syndrome. On the basis of autopsy evidence, thrombosis in lower limb veins and pulmonary emboli are found in 30 to 50 percent of patients dying after surgery. The incidence of deep vein thrombosis as diagnosed by the fibrinogen I-125 technique is around 35 percent in patients over 40 years of age undergoing major (nonorthopedic) operations (Flanc et al., 1968; Lambie et al., 1970; Le Quesne, 1975). The apparent but misleading incidence as assessed during life on the basis of clinical signs is around 2 percent. The diagnosis of venous thrombosis constitutes a perplexing problem, and it is obvious that differences in (1) the methods of determining the presence of thromboembolic phenomena, (2) the patient samples involved, and (3) the type of operation will result in differences in the estimated incidence of postoperative deep vein thrombosis.

Ascending venography has become the diagnostic reference method for detecting deep vein thrombosis (Rabinov and Paulin., 1972; Thomas, 1972). Leg scanning—usually after injection of radioactive fibrinogen and less often of technetium-99m urokinase (Millar and Smith, 1974) or streptokinase (Kempi et al., 1974)—is a sensitive technique for detection of developing calf vein thrombosis (Browse, 1972; Kakkar, 1972). Plethysmography (Wheeler et al., 1974; Hull et al., 1976) and ultrasound (Evans, 1970, 1971; Little, 1971; Strandness et al., 1967, 1972) techniques are more sensitive to proximal venous thrombosis than to calf vein thrombosis (Browse, 1972; Kakkar, 1972). The combination of fibrinogen leg scanning with impedance plethysmography results in a sensitivity of 94 percent and a specificity of 91 percent for calf vein thrombosis or more proximal deep vein thrombosis (Hull et al., 1977).

The highest incidence of deep vein thrombosis seems to be in patients who have undergone orthopedic surgery (particularly total hip replacement). Positive phlebography is obtained in 50 percent of these patient (Fields et al., 1972; Cooke et al., 1977; Stamatakis et al., 1977). In general surgery, a phlebographic diagnosis of deep vein thrombosis is made in 20 percent of patients (Carter et al., 1974; Clagett et al., 1975). The incidence of positive fibrinogen scans in the calf is around 30 percent (Kakkar et al., 1970), but it is considerably less (12 percent) when the Doppler ultrasonic method is applied to assess the pelvic veins (Williams et al., 1973; Bolton and Hoffman, 1975). Puerperal thrombosis of the calf or pelvic veins is a rare event (Jackson, 1973).

Prevention of Deep Vein Thrombosis in Surgical Patients

From the pathogenesis of venous thrombosis, one can predict two types of methods for its prevention: those using physical techniques designed to prevent venous stasis and those designed to prevent the formation of fibrin. Included in the latter approach are agents affecting the interaction of coagulation components with each other and also with the vessel wall.

Simple physical methods of stimulating the venous flow have proved to be effective in the prevention of deep venous thrombosis. At least three prospective, randomized clinical trials with an objective endpoint have shown a significant reduction of deep vein thrombosis in the calf after intermittent electrical stimulation of calf muscles both during surgery and in the postoperative period (Nicolaides et al., 1972; Becker et al., 1973; Browse et al., 1974). Rhythmic calf compression with pneumatic leggings, commencing after the induction of anesthesia and continued for 24 to 48 hours, also appears to be effective, at least in surgical patients without malignant disease (Sabri et al., 1971; Hills et al., 1972; Clarke et al., 1974). Even simple graduated static compression stockings reduce the incidence of calf vein thrombosis (Holford, 1970; Scurr et al., 1977). Usually, these mechanical procedures, which are simple and inexpensive, have been applied only during the operation and not during the postoperative period, which may explain the lower success rate when compared with a more extended prophylaxis with drugs. That these mechanical measures also protect the surgical patients against pulmonary embolism is still to be proven.

Prevention of hypercoagulability can be achieved by the use of oral anticoagulants. Coumarin drugs started before surgery have been shown to diminish markedly the incidence of and mortality from pulmonary embolism, even in patients with fracture of the femur, a group with an unusually high incidence of deep vein thrombosis that is difficult to prevent (Sevitt and Gallagher, 1959). More recently, the prophylactic value of warfarin (in doses aimed at maintaining a thrombotest value of 10 percent) was demonstrated in elderly patients who had sustained a fracture of the femoral neck (Morris and Mitchell, 1976). Anticoagulant treatment was maintained until independent mobility was achieved or for three months, and it resulted in a significant reduction of positive leg scans and the frequency of venous thrombosis found at necropsy.

Surgeons usually dislike oral anticoagulants, however, as they fear serious operative and postoperative bleeding. Prophylaxis of postoperative leg vein thrombosis by low dose heparin (5000 IU administered subcutaneously two hours before and every eight or twelve hours after surgery for six days or until full mobilization) has been studied in a number of prospective, randomized controlled trials having an objective endpoint. It is well accepted that this approach significantly reduces the frequency of deep vein thrombosis and of nonfatal and fatal pulmonary embolism in patients over 40 years of age undergoing major abdominal-thoracic or gynecologic surgery under general anesthesia for more than 30 minutes (Kakkar, 1975). Evidence of the effectiveness of low dose heparin in urologic and orthopedic patients is still lacking, even when the standard dose of heparin is administered every eight hours (Verstraete, 1976b). However, major orthopedic operations are precisely the type of surgery in which the effectiveness of dextran in reducing the incidence of deep venous thrombosis has been most convincingly demonstrated by phlebography. Unless otherwise proven, dextran-70 in an infusion of 500 to 1000 milliliters of a 6 percent solution started before operation and 500 milliliters the following day and the next three alternate days may, at present, be the method of choice for preventing deep venous thrombosis after major orthopedic operations. Whether the protection offered by dextran-70 will also prevent fatal and nonfatal pulmonary embolism in general surgery and in the higher risk groups of orthopedic patients is still an open question, which is being explored in an ongoing multicenter trial (Svensjö, 1977).

Clinical Trials

The obstacle to the universal acceptance of low dose heparin prophylaxis is the fear of hemorrhage; with dextran, certain anaphylactoid reactions and pulmonary edema in elderly patients are feared. Because both heparin in low concentrations (Clayton and Cross, 1963; Mustard and Packham, 1970) and dextran (Bygdeman et al., 1966; Aberg et al., 1977) affect some platelet functions, many compounds with more specific antiaggregating properties *in vitro* have been evaluated in clinical trials conducted with surgical patients.

Important differences exist in the design and execution of these numerous trials, and it would therefore be unfair to give them all the same credence. A critical review limited to prospective, controlled trials conducted with aspirin, dipyridamole, sulfinpyrazone, or hydroxychloroquine was published recently (Verstraete, 1976a), and the major conclusions can be updated as follows:

Individual effects. When the diagnosis of deep venous thrombosis was based on leg scanning and/or phlebography, sulfinpyrazone (0.8 g daily) (Gruber et al., 1977); dipyridamole (0.3 g daily) (Parodi et al., 1973; Wood et al., 1973; Morris and Mitchell, 1977b); or flurbiprofen (0.15 g daily) (Morris and Mitchell, 1977b) used alone did not appear to offer adequate protection to surgical patients.

In discussing the effectiveness of aspirin in the prevention of deep venous thrombosis, one has to distinguish between those trials conducted with a low daily dose (0.6 g) and those conducted with a high dose (1.2 g). O'Brien et al. (1971) were unable to demonstrate a protective effect with either 0.6 g aspirin or three times this daily dose. However, four of five more recent trials, in which a fairly high dose of aspirin (at least 1.2 g) was used, have reported a statistically significant reduction in deep venous thrombosis even in thrombosis-prone orthopedic patients (Harris et al., 1974; Clagett et al., 1975; Harris et al., 1977; Morris and Mitchell, 1977b; McKenna et al., 1978).

Two prospective, randomized trials with the antimalarial agent hydroxychloroquine (0.8 g daily) were conducted in patients undergoing general surgery, and they showed a significant reduction in deep vein thrombosis (Carter et al., 1971, 1974). Methods used in these trials have been criticized (Genton and Steele, 1975); however, using an even lower dose of hydroxychloroquine (0.6 g daily), another group confirmed the initial findings in patients who had either fractures or orthopedic operations involving the skeleton between the knee and the pelvis (Christman et al., 1976). More attention should therefore be given to the antithrombotic potential of this compound.

Lidocaine, administered intravenously in patients undergoing hip surgery, appeared to reduce significantly the incidence of calf and thigh vein thrombosis diagnosed phlebographically (Cooke et al., 1977).

Combined effects. Since drugs that inhibit platelet function differ in their mode of action, the combined use of some of them has been tried. Aspirin acts on platelet adhesion and collagen- and adrenaline-induced aggregation, whereas dipyridamole is effective against ADP-induced aggregation. Aspirin and dipyridamole in combination have been found to be effective in inhibiting the formation of electrically induced thrombi in dogs (Lahiri et al., 1972). This anticipated potentiating effect of aspirin on dipyridamole could also be demonstrated in an *in vivo* model in man. Patients with serious types of thrombotic disease, including those with artificial heart valves, have a short platelet survival; dipyridamole can prolong this survival, but this effect is more marked when dipyridamole is combined with aspirin, although the latter drug does not have the capacity to correct the reduced platelet survival when used alone (Harker et al., 1974).

Five prospective controlled trials with objective postoperative assessment of deep venous thrombosis were performed to evaluate the efficacy of daily intake of aspirin (usually 1 g) and dipyridamole (0.1 g). The results of four trials in general surgery patients revealed that the combination of dipyridamole and aspirin significantly decreases the incidence of postoperative deep vein thrombosis as detected by radioactive fibrinogen leg scanning (O'Sullivan and Vellar, 1972; Parodi et al., 1973; Weiss et al., 1977; Renney et al., 1976). These four trials did not include orthopedic patients. In the fifth trial, done on elderly patients with hip fractures, the combination of dipyridamole (0.3 g daily) and aspirin (0.9 g daily) was tested, and it failed to reveal a significant benefit in the treatment group (Morris and Mitchell, 1977b).

Mechanism of effect. It is not known whether the antithrombotic properties of drugs inhibiting certain platelet functions are due to this described action on platelets or to some other mechanism. It is therefore not surprising that combinations of antiaggregating compounds with heparin, oral anticoagulants, or dextran have been tried.

Although heparin may enhance platelet aggregation (Eika, 1973), its combination with aspirin was revealed to circumvent this untoward effect. It was indeed found that 1.5 g aspirin per day could suppress this undesired heparin effect; moreover, there was a synergistic action of the two drugs on the depression of platelet factor 3 availability (Loew and Vinazzer, 1974). Loew et al. (1977) conducted a double-blind trial on the prevention of thromboembolism using aspirin (1 g daily) or low dose heparin (5000 units subcutaneously every 12 hours) or a combination of the two substances in 177 general surgery patients. Therapy was started on the evening prior to surgery and maintained for one week. Diagnosis of deep vein thrombosis was made with radiofibrinogen leg scanning. The lowest incidence of deep vein thrombosis was in the group of patients treated with aspirin and low dose heparin; the two types of monotherapy each showed a significantly higher incidence of thrombosis. The difference, though not significant, between the two monotherapies was in favor of low dose heparin. This beneficial effect of the low dose heparin and aspirin combination was, however, not confirmed in a randomized trial conducted in patients who had undergone hip replacement (Kher et al., 1977). In this trial a higher dose of heparin (15,000 IU per day) was used (the dose of aspirin being the same as in the previous trial), but a surgical population with a higher thromboembolic risk was being studied.

The combination of dextran and aspirin (1.2 g daily) has also been compared with that of dextran and warfarin in hip replacement patients (Salvati and Lachiencz, 1977). Unfortunately, the diagnosis of deep vein thrombosis was made on clinical grounds only, and the two prophylactic schedules were not compared simultaneously. With these important limitations in mind, it seems that both prophylactic regimens are effective, but the dextran-aspirin combination is somewhat less so than the other one, although it has the advantage of producing fewer wound complications.

Use of Drugs that Inhibit Platelet Function in Coronary Artery Disease

Primary Prevention of Myocardial Infarction in Apparently Healthy and in Aged Individuals

Krasno and Kidera (1972) reported a large, prospective trial with clofibrate (2 g daily) in hyperlipemic men free of coronary heart disease. In the first series, which involved a group of men with an average age of 47.5 years who were followed for 39 months, a reduced incidence of nonfatal myocardial infarction was found in the clofibrate-treated group (1.26 per 1000 a year in 518 patients) when compared with the untreated control group (5.4 per 1000 a year in 550 patients). This difference is not statistically significant. A second series of 2218 younger men (average age 37.5 years) who were free of coronary heart disease and were followed for 32 months had an incidence of nonfatal infarct of 0.63 per 1000 a year in the clofibrate-treated group and of 5.0 per 1000 a year in the untreated group, a difference that is statistically significant ($P<0.01$). However, major deficiencies in trial design and execution of the study prevent an unequivocal interpretation of the data. The World Health Organization (WHO) sponsored a primary prevention, placebo-controlled trial with clofibrate on the incidence of ischemic heart disease in healthy men with a known cholesterol level conducted in Edinburgh, Prague, and Budapest (Heady, 1973).

In total 15,000 men between 30 and 59 years of age without hypertension, diabetes and myocardial infarction were studied for an average of 5.3 years. The treatment group, given 1.6 g clofibrate per day, consisted of a randomly chosen half of the men whose serum cholesterol fell within the upper third of the distribution in some 30,000 volunteers. The other 5,000 men with similar cholesterol concentrations received placebo. The overall lowering of nonfatal ischemic heart disease was 20 percent in the clofibrate group and the benefit was greatest in those with the highest cholesterol and with the greatest reduction. The overall mean decrease in cholesterol was 9 percent in the treatment group. However, the number of deaths and the crude mortality rates from all causes in the clofibrate group were significantly higher than those in the control group, the excess being particularly due to a group of noncardiovascular diseases including malignant neoplasms.

Evidence is also uncertain for aspirin. The Boston Collaborative Drug Surveillance Group (1974) analyzed the use of aspirin in a group of 325 patients having a hospital discharge diagnosis of myocardial infarction and 3807 control patients hospitalized for other illnesses, excluding those for whom aspirin was prescribed or contraindicated. This retrospective study suggested that aspirin may protect against myocardial infarction, since there was a negative association between regular aspirin ingestion and nonfatal myocardial infarction. However, in a placebo-controlled trial carried out in a municipal old-age home and involving 430 elderly people (82 percent were females), there was no evidence of any prophylactic effect of aspirin (1g per day) on the incidence of fatal or nonfatal myocardial infarction after one year of follow-up observation (Heikinheimo and Jarvinen, 1971).

Sulfinpyrazone, the uricosuric agent, also affects a number of platelet reactions. A double-blind study was carried out over four years on 291 institutionalized elderly males allocated at random to receive either sulfinpyrazone (0.6 g per day) or a placebo (Blakely and Gent, 1975). At entry to the trial, more than half these elderly men had clinical signs of atherosclerosis (coronary, cerebral, or peripheral arteries). No statistically significant reduction in mortality could be demonstrated in the sulfinpyrazone-treated patients. The data were then reanalyzed separately for patients with prior myocardial infarction and patients with history of stroke at entry. A further analysis was made of patients who had a history of both infarct and stroke. Either way, patients with a prior history of stroke seemed to be the ones to benefit, but the data were insufficient to assess the question of prophylactic effect in patients with prior myocardial infarction. In this group, there was a favorable mortality trend in the fourth year, but by that time, the number of cases was too small to be meaningful.

The evidence available at present, therefore, does not allow the recommendation of clofibrate, aspirin, or sulfinpyrazone for the primary prevention of myocardial infarction in apparently healthy men or in elderly individuals.

Prevention of a First Myocardial Infarction in Patients with Angina

The Scottish (1971) and Newcastle (1971) trials with clofibrate included patients with symptoms of angina alone, patients who had suffered a myocardial infarction, and those who had had both. In the first trial, 1.6 to 2 g clofibrate was given daily for 6 years, and in the second trial, 1.5 to 2 g clofibrate was given daily for 5 years. In both trials, there was a significant reduction in sudden death and in all deaths in the clofibrate-treated patients who had only angina when admitted to the trial. These results show without doubt that clofibrate caused a reduction of morbidity and mortality in patients with angina alone. Most surprising was the fact that this beneficial effect did not correlate with the initial cholesterol level or its reduction. As clofibrate also affects platelet function, it was suggested that this effect may be related to the clinical gain (Gilbert and Mustard, 1963). Thus, there seems to be reasonable evidence that patients with angina only may benefit from prophylactic treatment with clofibrate. It is necessary to emphasize the importance of proper patient selection when clofibrate is to be used, since it cannot be recommended as a prophylactic agent in patients with a prior infarct, either with or without angina.

Prevention of Recurrent Myocardial Infarction

The Scottish and Newcastle trials (1971) with clofibrate also included patients who had survived more than six weeks after a first myocardial infarction. Only one of these trials revealed a significant reduction in total death rate in this subgroup. In the Scottish trial, there was even the disquieting finding that the death rate for patients admitted with myocardial infarction only was slightly higher in the clofibrate group.

The Coronary Drug Project Research Group

(1975) in the U.S. also failed to show a significantly beneficial effect of clofibrate (1.8 g daily for 5 years) on cause-specific mortality or total mortality (20 percent for clofibrate-treated patients and 20.9 percent for placebo-treated). None of the subgroups of clofibrate-treated patients in this study showed a significantly favorable effect when compared with the control group. On the contrary, a significant excess of arrhythmias, new intermittent claudication, and angina was recorded in the clofibrate-treated group.

The first major double-blind trial of aspirin for the prevention of death after recovery from myocardial infarction was reported by Elwood et al. (1974). Of the 1239 males under the age of 65 years studied after discharge from hospital, half were given a low dose of aspirin (0.3 g daily for 24 months) and half were given a placebo. The final analysis is on 1126 patients. After 24 months, the follow-up revealed that the treated group had a cumulative mortality of 12.2 percent and the control group of 18.5 percent; at no point during the study did the reduction in mortality after intake of aspirin reach a level of statistical significance. An interesting finding, however, was that in the subgroup of men whose infarction occurred less than six weeks before entry into the study, the mortality rate was statistically significantly reduced.

A similar reduction of 30 percent in overall mortality was also observed in a double-blind prospective trial organized by The Coronary Drug Project Group (1976). Over 1500 male survivors of a myocardial infarction were randomly assigned to regimens of 1 g aspirin daily or placebo; an insignificant reduction of the total mortality rate of 8.3 percent in the placebo group compared with 5.8 percent in the aspirin group was observed after an average of 22 months.

A more recent double-blind trial of patients of both sexes with myocardial infarction was set up by Elwood (1977) in South Wales to answer the question of whether administration of a single dose of 300 mg aspirin could reduce immediate mortality. This did not appear to be the case in 1000 patients with subsequent confirmatory evidence of infarction. The second aim of the trial was to evaluate the prophylactic effect of 300 mg aspirin 3 times daily started a few days after infarction and continued for one year. This trial is still in progress.

The preliminary results of a multicenter trial conducted in seven hospitals in Germany and Austria on 946 patients who survived a myocardial infarction for six weeks have recently became available (Asbrand et al., 1979). The patients were allocated at random to regimens of aspirin (1.5 g daily), phenprocoumon, or placebo. After two years' observation, 56.1 percent (531 patients) had no complications, 12.2 percent had to be excluded for technical reasons (e.g., poor cooperation with family physician, myocardial infarction not confirmed), 10.5 percent failed to attend their appointments for follow-up, 1.2 percent had intercurrent diseases, and 6.3 percent dropped out because of side effects (30 aspirin-treated patients, 17 control patients, 13 phenprocoumon-treated patients). Of aspirin-treated patients, 13 of 317 died from a secondary infarction or died suddenly, in comparison with 22 of 309 placebo-treated patients and 26 of 320 phenprocoumon-treated patients. Eleven of 317 aspirin-treated patients survived a secondary myocardial infarction, as did 15 of 309 control patients and 6 of 320 phenprocoumon-treated patients. These differences are not statistically significant.

There is only one prospective clinical trial with dipyridamole (0.4 g daily) in patients with acute myocardial infarction. This short-term trial (one month) provided no evidence of prevention of fatal or nonfatal infarction (Gent et al., 1968).

Sulfinpyrazone, a potent uricosuric agent, was shown in 1960 to lengthen platelet survival and to decrease platelet purnover in gouty patients with various thromboembolic disorders (Smythe et al., 1965). A multicenter double-blind clinical trial has recently been completed that compares the effect of sulfinpyrazone (200 mg four times daily) and placebo on the rates of cardiac mortality in 1475 patients surviving a myocardial infarction (The Anturane Reinfarction Trial Research Group, 1978). To be eligible, the patients, both male and female, had to be between 45 and 70 years of age, and had to have suffered a myocardial infarction 25 to 35 days before enrollment. After an average observation period of 8.6 months, there were 69 deaths of a cardiovascular nature (68 were cardiac and 1 was cerebrovascular). The death rate corrected for exposure time was 9.5 percent in the placebo group and 5.1 percent in the sulfinpyrazone group, which corresponds to a highly significant reduction of 46 percent in overall death rate.

The published prospective trials with clofibrate, aspirin, or dipyridamole in the prevention of recurrent myocardial infarction do not, therefore, reveal a significant reduction of morbidity or mortality. There was a positive trend in some trials that used a higher dose of one of these drugs alone or in combination, and this seems to be confirmed in some reported but as yet unpublished trials. Hopes for secondary prevention have been raised by the multicenter sulfinpyrazone trial, with its impressive reduction in overall death rate. This trial is not yet complete, but its present results suggest that a substantial reduction in reinfarction deaths may now be obtained.

Prevention of Thromboembolism in Patients with Prosthetic Heart Valves

Patients with valvular disease of the heart have a high incidence of thromboembolism, especially if the mitral valve is stenosed. Valvular repair improves heart function, but patients are still susceptible to thromboembolic complications—often for a long time after surgery. Newer materials employed in the more modern prosthetic valves are less frequently associated with systemic emboli than those used previously (Weily et al., 1972), and although platelet turnover is considerably increased in patients with older prosthetic valves, it is not increased, or much less so, with Starr-Edwards or Björk-Shilley valves (Lander et al., 1965). More intensive treatment with oral anticoagulants would probably provide more effective antithrombotic protection, but there would need to be frequent and accurate monitoring of the prothrombin time, and there would probably be a higher incidence of bleeding complications. Another drawback is that oral anticoagulants such as warfarin are thought to be potentially dysmorphogenic in the first weeks of pregnancy, which constitutes a problem in young women with cardiac valve replacement who wish to become pregnant (Warkany, 1975). We cannot avoid the conclusion that, at present, thromboembolism and hemorrhage related to anticoagulants cannot be disregarded as causes of morbidity and mortality in the late follow-up period after prosthetic heart valve replacement.

Sullivan et al. (1968) have shown, in a controlled study of patients with prosthetic heart valves of the older type, that dipyridamole (0.4 g daily) given in addition to oral anticoagulants (warfarin sodium) resulted in greater protection against nonfatal thromboembolism than did anticoagulants alone. The same authors later confirmed their initial findings: 14.3 percent of 84 patients who had prosthetic valves and were on anticoagulants for one year after surgery showed clinical evidence of arterial emboli, compared with 1.3 percent of 79 patients who, in addition to oral anticoagulants, also received daily 0.4 g dipyridamole. There was no difference in mortality between the two groups (Sullivan et al., 1971). In a still not fully reported large-scale trial conducted in France on 385 patients with prosthetic valves, no significant reduction in thromboembolism or overall mortality was observed in patients receiving anticoagulants and 0.375 g dipyridamole daily when compared with patients receiving oral anticoagulants alone (Pell, 1975). There are three other nonrandomized trials with dipyridamole that report a superiority of the combination of oral anticoagulants and dipyridamole over anticoagulants alone (Arrants el al., 1970; Meyer et al., 1971; Rabello et al., 1973).

It also appears that large doses of dipyridamole (0.45 g daily) with aspirin (3 g daily) given over a period of fourteen months can significantly reduce the incidence of thromboembolism after prosthetic valve replacement (Taguchi et al., 1975). In a randomized trial in patients with Starr valves, therapy with the addition of 0.5 g aspirin was significantly more effective than anticoagulants alone (Altman et al., 1976).

In another trial, 153 patients with aortic ball valves received 1 g of aspirin daily in addition to oral coumarin anticoagulants, and they had fewer thromboembolic complications than a control group who received anticoagulants alone (Dale, 1977). Only 1.8 arterial thromboembolic complications occurred in 100 patients per year in the combined treatment group, compared with 9.3 in the control group. In a second study, oral coumarin therapy was gradually withdrawn and the same patients were given only 1 g aspirin daily. Six arterial thromboembolic events occurred in five patients during the following five months, and the investigators terminated this study and returned to the combined prevention scheme.

There is therefore little evidence to suggest that a combination of oral anticoagulants and either dipyridamole or aspirin is significantly more effective in preventing arterial embolism in patients with prosthetic heart valves than anticoagulants alone. The combination with aspirin is associated, however, with a high incidence of bleeding (7 percent according to Altman et al., 1976; 5 percent according to Dale et al., 1975). Aspirin alone does not appear to afford the desired protection. Whether aspirin combined with dipyridamole would be as effective in preventing systemic embolism as oral anticoagulants supplemented with either one of these antiplatelet drugs has still to be demonstrated.

Prevention of Graft Occlusion after Aortocoronary Bypass Surgery

Relief of chest pain after aortocoronary bypass surgery is achieved in 85 to 90 percent of cases. Recurrence of symptoms seems to be associated with coronary bypass closure or progression of the disease. A definite relationship exists between the initial blood flow through the bypass and the closure rate, and the former depends, among other factors, upon the size of the anastomosis and the distal runoff. Another factor could be the adherence of platelets to the graft wall. It is known that platelet survival is shortened in patients with angiographically defined coronary artery disease (Steele and Genton, 1976), and a difference in the mean platelet survival time between patients with and without closure of an aortocoronary bypass graft was also found by the same authors. Attention was therefore directed to the outcome of trials testing the effect of anticoagulants or antiplatelet drugs on long-term graft patency.

In a report published by the Texas Heart Institute, all groups of patients who received (in a nonrandom fashion) dipyridamole, aspirin, or oral coumarin anticoagulant drugs experienced higher survival rates over a 4-year observation period than control groups who did not receive one of these drugs (Hall et al., 1974).

Conclusion

It is appropriate to add a few sobering remarks to the end of this review.

The gross inaccuracy of clinical diagnosis of deep venous thrombosis and the variations in the definition thereof do not permit valid direct comparisons among studies performed by different investigators. Nor do these factors allow reliable conclusions to be drawn from studies in which the diagnosis of deep vein thrombosis is based on clinical signs alone. Therefore, only prospective trials on prophylaxis that include an objective assessment of deep vein thrombosis have been discussed.

It must be pointed out that although ascending phlebography is increasingly considered to be the diagnostic anatomic standard, other unambiguous tests for detection are based on different principles and do not necessarily measure the same event. Transcutaneous Doppler-ultrasound (flow rate) and the less sensitive plethysmographic (resistance of blood flow) techniques mainly detect thrombosis located in deep veins more proximal to the popliteal vein, whereas leg scanning (measuring thrombosis acitivity) is sensitive to thrombosis located in the calf, but only when the fibrin is deposited after injection of the radiolabeled fibrinogen. Owing to high blood background, a thrombosis in the thigh is more difficult to detect. Leg scanning is oversensitive and detects small thrombi in the soleal mass that do not show up with venography; conversely, due to high blood background, a venous thrombosis in the thigh is often missed. The mere presence of radioactive fibrinogen in a limb is not indicative of a developing thrombus per se. Increased capillary permeability, inflammatory changes in the area of the surgical wound, hematomas, and persistence of radioactivity in vessel walls after the release of thrombi previously present within that vascular lumen may all cause accumulation of fibrinogen I-125 (Hladovec et al., 1973; Kerrigan et al., 1974; McKenna et al., 1976). Leg scanning is, however, the only method that can distinguish between an active and an old thrombus. A need still exists for standardization of the fibrinogen uptake scanning before the results of different techniques of prophylaxis can rationally be compared (Roberts, 1975).

The results of one clinical trial conducted in a certain surgical population cannot be applied to other surgical populations, because the stimulus to thrombosis may differ in various clinical circumstances. In most patients undergoing major surgery, thromboembolic events start with a thrombus in the soleal sinusoids and remain localized in the calf; in some patients, the thrombus spreads into the main venous channels in the lower leg, but in a few patients it also spreads to the popliteal, femoral, or even iliac veins. A fragment can become detached from this proximal propagation of thrombus, leading to a pulmonary embolus. In orthopedic surgery, however, and more particularly in total hip replacement, intraoperative distortion of the femoral vein results in local damage and may thus exaggerate the contribution of platelets to femoral vein thrombosis, which is then the first thrombotic event (Harris et al., 1977; Stamatakis et al., 1977). In any patients with previous venous thrombosis, wall damage may still be present—even without direct trauma to the vein.

In addition to the fact that the stimuli to thrombosis may differ, the various drugs grouped together as "platelet-function regulating agents" may have different modes of action. For this reason, also, clinical results in different trials are not necessarily interchangeable.

The antithrombotic potency of the drugs affecting platelet functions is not always the same. A drug that is highly effective in preventing deep venous thrombosis in patients after general thoracoabdominal surgery may be less beneficial in patients with cancer undergoing the same operation, or may even be inadequate in noncancer patients with fractures or patients undergoing orthopedic surgery. Although it is tempting to assume that a drug effective in the last group will also prevent deep vein thrombosis in patients with a lesser thrombogenic potential, clinical judgment has to be used to evaluate the risk benefit ratio of an effective drug regimen in surgical patients less prone to thrombosis.

It is recognized that secondary prevention trials in myocardial infarction require a smaller sample size and are more expedient than primary prevention studies. However, any drug that is effective in a secondary prevention trial has to be tested separately in a primary prevention trial before it can be recommended for use in the larger clinical setting. Some reduction of the sample size of primary prevention trials on myocardial infarction can be made by selecting individuals at risk who are identified by as many determinants as possible, and by confining any clinical recommendations strictly to this subgroup.

Retrospective clinical studies can only be used to formulate hypotheses concerning the prophylactic effect of a given drug, and these hypotheses must then be studied in prospective trials.

Since Virchow, it has been stated that the causes of thrombus formation are changes in the biochemistry of the blood, damage to the lining of the vessel wall, and stasis of the blood. So far, little can be done to measure or control physical damage to the vessel wall in an attempt to prevent thrombus formation.

References

Aberg, M., Hedner, U., and Bergentz, S.E.: The effect of dextran on hemostasis and coagulation with special regard to factor VIII. In Lewis, D.H., and Thorén, L., eds., *Dextran–30 years,* Upsala, Acta Univ. Ups. 3:23, 1977.

Altman, R., Boullon, F., Rouvier, J., Raca, R., de la Fuente, L., and Favaloro, R.: Aspirin and prophylaxis of thromboembolic complications in patients with substitute heart valves. J. Thorac. Cardiovasc. Surg. 72:127, 1976.

Anturane Reinfarction Trial Research Group: Sulfinpyrazone in the prevention of cardiac death after myocardial infarction. N. Engl. J. Med. 298:289, 1978.

Arrants, J.E., Hairston, P., and Lee, W.H., Jr.: Use of dipyridamole (persantine) in preventing thromboembolism following valve replacement. Chest (Abstract) 58:275, 1970.

Asbrand, E., Becker, H.J., Breddin, K., Jaser, W., Lechner, K., Loew, D., Meyer-Hofman, G., Niessner, H., Novotny, C., Pfleiderer, T., Quack, M., Schmutzler, R., Thaler, E., Walter, E., Weber, E., Wolf, H., Ueberla, K., and Wolf, U.: German-Austrian multicenter two years prospective study on the prevention of secondary myocardial infarction by ASA in comparison with phenprocoumon and placebo. In press, 1979.

Becker, J., and Schampi, B.: The incidence of postoperative venous thrombosis of the legs. A comparative study on the prophylactic effect of dextran-70 and electrical calf muscle stimulation. Acta Chir. Scand. 139:357, 1973.

Blakely, J.A., and Gent, M.: Platelets, drugs and longevity in a geriatric population. In Hirsh, Cade, Gallus and Schönbaum, eds., *Platelet, Drugs and Thrombosis,* Basel, Karger, 1975.

Bolton, J.P., and Hoffman, V.J.: Incidence of early post-operative iliofemoral thrombosis. Br. Med. J. i:247, 1975.

Boston Collaborative Drug Surveillance Group: Regular aspirin intake and acute myocardial infarction. Br. Med. J. i:440, 1974.

Browse, N.L.: the I^{125}-fibrinogen uptake test. Arch. Surg. 104:160, 1972.

Browse, N.L., Clemenson, G., and Croft, D.N.: Fibrinogen-detectable thrombosis in the legs and pulmonary embolism. Br. Med. J. 1:603, 1974.

Bygdeman, S., Eliasson, R., and Gullbring, B.: Effect of dextran infusion on the adenosine diphosphate adhesiveness and the spreading capacity of human blood platelets. Thromb. Haemostas. 15:451, 1966.

Carter, A.E., and Eban, R.: Prevention of postoperative deep venous thrombosis in legs by orally administered hydroxychloroquine sulphate. Br. Med. J. 2:94, 1974.

Carter, A.E., Eban, R., and Perrett, R.D.: Prevention of postoperative deep venous thrombosis and pulmonary embolism. Br. Med. J. 1:312, 1971.

Christman, O.D., Snook, G.A., Wilson, T.C., and Short, J.Y.: Prevention of venous thromboembolism by administration of hydroxychloroquine. J. Bone Joint Surg. 58:918, 1976.

Clagett, G.P., Schneider, P., Rosoff, C.B., and Salzman, E.W.: The influence of aspirin on postoperative platelet kinetics and venous thrombosis. Surgery 77:61, 1975.

Clarke, W.B., Prescott, R.J., MacGregor, A.B., and Ruckley, C.B.: Pneumatic compression of the calf and postoperative deep-vein thrombosis. Lancet ii:5, 1974.

Clayton, S., and Cross, M.J.: The aggregation of blood platelets by catecholamines and by thrombin. J. Physiol. 169:82, 1963.

Committee of Principal Investigators: A co-operative trial on the primary prevention of ischaemic heart disease using clofibrate. Report from the Committee of Principal Investigators. Br. Heart J. 40:1069, 1978.

Cooke, E.D., Lloyd, M.J., Bowcock S.A., and Pilcher, M.F.: Intravenous lignocaine in prevention of deep venous thrombosis after elective hip surgery. Lancet ii:797, 1977.

Coronary Drug Project Research Group: Clofibrate and niacin in coronary heart disease. JAMA 27:360, 1975.

Coronary Drug Project Group: Aspirin in coronary heart disease. J. Chron. Dis. 29:625, 1976.

Dale, J.: Prevention of cerebral embolism from prosthetic heart valves with acetylsalicylic acid. Preliminary results reported at the IV Colfarit Symposium. Berlin, 1977.

Dale, J., Myhre, E., Storstein, D., and Stormorken, H.: Proceedings–arterial thromboembolism and prosthetic heart valves. Effect of acetylsalicylic acid. Thromb. Haemostas. 34:587, 1975.

Deykin, D., Cochios, F., Decamp, G., and Lopez, A.: Hepatic removal of activated factor X by the perfused rabbit liver. Am. J. Physiol. 214:414, 1968.

Eika, C.: Anticoagulant and platelet aggregating activities of heparin. Thromb. Res. 2:349, 1973.

Elwood, P.C.: The Cardiff aspirin reinfarction studies. Preliminary findings reported at the IV Colfarit Symposium. Berlin, 1977.

Elwood, P.C., Cochrane, A.L., Burr, M.L., Sweetman, P.M., Williams, G., Welsby, E., Hughes, S.J., and Renton, R.: A randomized controlled trial of acetylsalicylic acid in the secondary prevention of mortality from myocardial infarction. Br. Med. J. 1:436, 1974.

Evans, D.S.: The early diagnosis of deep-vein thrombosis by ultrasound. Br. J. Surg. 57:726, 1970.
Evans, D.S.: The early diagnosis of thromboembolism by ultrasound. Ann. R. Coll. Surg. Engl. 49:225, 1971.
Fields, E.S., Nicolaides, A.N., Kakkar, V.V., and Crellin, R.Q.: Deep-vein thrombosis in patients with fractures of the femoral neck. Br. J. Surg. 59:377, 1972.
Flanc, C., Kakkar, V.V., and Clarke, M.B.: The detection of venous thrombosis of the legs using ^{125}I-labelled fibrinogen. Br. J. Surg. 55:742, 1968.
Gent, A.E., Brook, C.G.D., Foley, T.H., and Miller, T.N.: Dipyridamole: a controlled trial of its effect in acute myocardial infarction. Br. Med. J. ii:366, 1968.
Genton, E., and Steele, P.: Platelets, drugs and heart disease. In Hirsh, Cade, Gallus, and Schönbaum, eds., *Platelets, Drugs and Thrombosis*, Basel, Karger, 1975.
Gilbert, J.B., and Mustard, J.F.: Some effects of atromid on platelet economy and blood coagulation in man. J. Atheroscler. Res. 3:623, 1963.
Gruber, U.F., Buser, J., Frick, J., Loosli, J., Matt, E., and Segesser, D.: Sulfinpyrazone and postoperative deep vein thrombosis. Eur. Surg. Res. 9:303, 1977.
Hall, R.J., Garcia, E., Al-Bassam, M.S., and Dawson, J.T.: Aortocoronary bypass surgery, 1969–1973, review of 2566 patients. Cardiov. Res. Cent. Bull. 1:74, 1974.
Harker, L.A., and Slichter, S.J.: Studies of platelet and fibrinogen kinetics in patients with prosthetic heart valves. N. Engl. J. Med. 183: 1302, 1970.
Harker, L.A., and Slichter, S.J.: Arterial and venous thromboembolism—kinetic characterization and evaluation of therapy. Thromb. Haemostas. 31:188, 1974.
Harris, W.H., Salzman, E.W., Athanasoulis, C., Waltman, A.C., Baum, S., and Desanctis, R.W.: Comparison of warfarin, low-molecular weight dextran, aspirin, and subcutaneous heparin in prevention of venous thromboembolism following total hip replacement. J. Bone Joint Surg. 56:1552, 1974.
Harris, W.H., Salzman, E.W., Athanasoulis, C.A., Waltman, A.C., and Desanctis, R.W.: Aspirin prophylaxis of venous thromboembolism after total hip replacement. N. Engl. J. Med. 297:1246, 1977.
Heady, J.A.: A cooperative trial on the primary prevention of ischaemic heart disease using clofibrate: design, methods and progress. Bull. WHO 48:243, 1973.
Heikinheimo, R., and Jarvinen, K.: Acetylsalicylic acid and arteriosclerotic thromboembolic diseases in the aged. J. Am. Geriatr. Soc. 19:403, 1971.
Hills, N.H., Pflug, J.J., Jejasingh, K., Boardman, L., and Calnan, J.S.: Prevention of deep vein thrombosis by intermittent pneumatic compression of the calf. Br. Med. J. i:131, 1972.
Hladovec, J., Prerousky, I., and Roztocil, K.: The influence of inflammation on the ^{125}I-fibrinogen uptake test in experimental thrombosis. Angiologia 10:93, 1973.
Holford, C.P.: Graded compression for preventing deep venous thrombosis. Br. J. Surg. 63:157, 1970.
Hull, R., Van Aken, W.G., Hirsh, J., Gallus, A.S., Hoicka, G., and Turpie, A.G.G.: Impedance plethysmography using the occlusive cuff technique in the diagnosis of venous thrombosis. Circulation 53:696, 1976.
Hull, R., Hirsh, J., Sackett, D.L., Powers, P., Turpie, A.G.G., and Walker, I.: Combined use of leg scanning and impedance plethysmography in suspected venous thrombosis. An alternative to venography. N. Engl. J. Med. 296:1497, 1977.
Jackson, P.: Puerperal thromboembolic disease in "high risk" cases. Br. Med. J. i:263, 1973.
Kakkar, V.V.: The problems of thrombosis in the deep veins of the leg. Am. R. Coll. Surg. Engl. 45:257, 1969.
Kakkar, V.V., Howe, C.T., Nicolaides, A.N., Renney, J.T.C., and Clarke, M.B.: Deep vein thrombosis of the leg. Am. J. Surg. 120:527, 1970.
Kakkar, V.V.: The diagnosis of deep vein thrombosis using the ^{125}I-fibrinogen test. Arch. Surg. 104:152, 1972.
Kakkar, V.V.: Prevention of fatal postoperative pulmonary embolism by low doses of heparin. An international multicentre trial. Lancet ii:45, 1975.
Kempi, V., Van der Linden, W., and von Schelle, C.: Diagnosis of deep vein thrombosis with 99 m Tc-streptokinase: a clinical comparison with phlebography. Br. Med. J. ii:748, 1974.
Kerrigan, G.N.W., Buchanan, M.R., Cade, J.F., Regoeczi, E., and Hirsh, J.: Investigation of the mechanism of false positive ^{125}I-labelled fibrinogen scans. Br. J. Haematol. 26:469, 1974.
Kher, A., Flicoteaux, H., Jean, N., Blery, M., Judet, T., Honnart, F., and Pasteyer, J.: Combined administration of low dose heparin and aspirin versus low dose heparin alone as prophylaxis of deep vein thrombosis (D.V.T.) after total hip replacement. A preliminary report. Thromb. Haemostas. Abstract 38:197, 1977.
Krasno, L.R., and Kidera, G.J.: Clofibrate in coronary heart disease: effect on morbidity and mortality. JAMA 219:845, 1972.

Lahiri, K., Mosches, C.B., Lyons, M., Oldewurtel, H., and Regan, T.J.: Coronary artery versus microcirculatory thrombosis: effects of aspirin and dipyridamole. Clin. Res. 20:382, 1972.

Lambie, J.M., Mahaffy, R.G., Barber, D.C., Karmody, A.M., Scott, M.M., and Matheson, N.A.: Diagnostic accuracy in venous thrombosis. Br. Med. J. i:142, 1970.

Lander, H., Kinlough, R.L., and Robson, H.N.: Reduced platelet survival in patients with Starr-Edwards prostheses. Br. Med. J. 1:688, 1965.

Le Quesne, L.P.: Diagnosis and prevention of postoperative deep-vein thrombosis. In Creger, W.P., Coggins, C.H., and E.W. Hancock, eds., *Annual Review of Medicine* 26:63, 1975.

Little, J.M.: Venous thrombosis in a surgical ward. Result of a survey using diagnostic ultrasound. Med. J. Aust. 2:561, 1971.

Loew, D., and Vinazzer, H.: Influence of simultaneous administration of low-dose heparin and acetylsalicylic acid on blood coagulation and platelet functions. Haemostasis 3:319, 1974.

Loew, D., Brücke, P., Simma, W., Vinazzer, H., Dienstl, E., and Boehme, K.: Acetylsalicylic acid, low dose heparin, and a combination of both substances in the prevention of postoperative thromboembolism. A double-blind study. Thromb. Res. 11:81, 1977.

McKenna, R., Bachman, F., Kaushal, S., and Galante, J.O.: Thromboembolic disease in patients undergoing total knee replacement. J. Bone Joint Surg. 58:928, 1976.

McKenna, R., Galante, J., Bachman, F., Kaushal, S.P., and Meredith, P.: Thromboembolism after total knee replacement and its prevention by high dose aspirin or intermittent calf compression. A prospective randomised study. In press, 1978.

Meyer, J.S., Charney, J.Z., Rivera, V.M., and Mathew, N.J.: Cerebral embolization; prospective clinical analysis of 42 cases. Stroke 2:541, 1971.

Millar, W.T., and Smith, J.F.B.: Localisation of deep-venous thrombosis using technetium-99m-labelled urokinase. Lancet ii:695, 1974.

Morris, G.K., and Mitchell, J.R.A.: Warfarin sodium in prevention of deep venous thrombosis and pulmonary embolism in patients with fractured neck of femur. Lancet ii:869, 1976.

Morris, G.K., and Mitchell, J.R.A.: Evaluation of ^{125}I-fibrinogen test for venous thrombosis in patients with hip fractures: comparison between isotope scanning and necropsy findings. Br. Med. J. i:264, 1977a.

Morris, G.K., and Mitchell, J.R.A.: Preventing venous thromboembolism in elderly patients with hip fractures: studies of low-dose heparin, dipyridamole, aspirin and flurbiprofen. Br. Med. J. ii:535, 1977b.

Mustard, J.F., and Packham, M.A.: Factors influencing platelet function: adhesion, release and aggregation. Pharmacol. Rev. 22:97, 1970.

Newcastle upon Tyne Physicians: Trial of clofibrate in the treatment of ischemic heart disease. Br. Med. J. 4:767, 1971.

Nicolaides, A.N., Kakkar, V.V., Field, E.S., and Fish, P.: Optimal electrical stimulus for prevention of deep-vein thrombosis. Br. Med. J. iii:756, 1972.

O'Brien, J.R., Tulevski, V.G., and Etherington, M.: Two in vivo studies comparing high and low aspirin dosage. Lancet 2:388, 1971.

O'Sullivan, E.F., and Vellar, I.D.A.: Assessment of the efficacy of antiplatelet drugs in the prevention of postoperative deep vein thrombosis. Washington, D.C., IIIrd Congress International Society of Thrombosis and Haemostasis, p. 438, 1972.

Parodi, J.C., Grandi, A., Font, E., Rotondaro, D., and Manrique, J.: El dipiridamol y el acido acetilsalicilico en la profilaxis de las thrombosis venasas postoperatorias de los miembros inferiores. Dia méd. 44:92, 1973.

Pell, E.: Essai clinique contrôlé du dipyridamole dans le traitement préventif des accidents thromboemboliques chez les porteurs de prothèses valvulaires. Thèse Doct. Méd. Lyon, 1975.

Rabello, C., Rivas, J.A., and Rocha, F.: Estudo da açao de dipiridamol na evoluçao de pacientes submetiodos à substituçao de proteses valvares. Revista Bras. Clin. Terap. 2:95, 1973.

Rabinov, K., and Paulin, S.: Roentgen diagnosis of venous thrombosis in the leg. Arch. Surg. 104:134, 1972.

Renney, J.T.G., O'Sullivan, E.F., and Burke, P.F.: Prevention of postoperative deep vein thrombosis with dipyridamole and aspirin. Br. Med. J. i:992, 1976.

Roberts, V.C.: Fibrinogen uptake scanning for diagnosis of deep vein thrombosis: a plea for standardization. Br. Med. J. 3:455, 1975.

Sabri, S., Roberts, V.C., and Cotton, L.T.: Prevention of early postoperative deep vein thrombosis by passive exercise of leg during surgery. Br. Med. J. 3:82, 1971.

Salvati, E.A., and Lachiewcz, P.: Thromboembolism following total hip-replacement arthroplasty. The efficacy of dextran-aspirin and dextran-warfarin in prophylaxis. J. Bone Joint Surg. 58:921, 1977.

Scottish Society of Physicians: Ischemic heart disease: a secondary prevention trial using clofibrate. Br. Med. J. 2:775, 1971.

Scurr, J.H., Ibrahim, S.Z., Faber, R.G., and Le Quesne, L.P.: The efficacy of graduated compression stockings in the prevention of deep vein thrombosis. Br. J. Surg. 64:371, 1977.

Sevitt, S., and Gallagher, N.: Prevention of venous thrombosis and pulmonary embolism in injured patients. Lancet 2:981, 1959.

Smythe, H.A., Ogryzlo, M.A., Murphy, E.A., and Mustard, J.F.: The effect of sulfinpyrazone (Anturan) on platelet economy and blood coagulation in man. Can. Med. Assoc. J. 92:818, 1965.

Stamatakis, J.D., Kakkar, V.V., Sagar, S., Lawrence, D., Nairin, D., and Bentley, P.G.: Femoral vein thrombosis and total hip replacement. Br. Med. J. ii:223, 1977.

Steele, P.P., and Genton, E.: Correlation of platelet survival time with occlusion of saphenous vein aorto-coronary bypass grafts. Circulation 53:685, 1976.

Strandness, D.E. Jr., Schultz, R.D., Sumner, D.S., and Rushmer, R.F.: Ultrasonic flow detection. Am. J. Surg. 113:311, 1967.

Strandness, D.E., and Sumner, D.S.: Ultrasonic velocity detector in the diagnosis of thrombo-phlebitis. Arch. Surg. 104:180, 1972.

Sullivan, J.M., Harken, D.E., and Gorlin, R.: Pharmacologic control of thromboembolic complications of cardiac-valve replacement. N. Engl. J. Med. 279:576, 1968.

Sullivan, J.M., Harken, D.E., and Gorlin, R.: Pharmacologic control of thromboembolic complications of cardiac-valve replacement. N. Engl. J. Med. 284:1391, 1971.

Svensjö, E.: Is a further trial comparing low dose heparin and dextran needed? In Lewis, D.H., and Thorén, L., eds. *Dextran-30 years,* Upsala, Acta Univ. Ups. 3:71, 1977.

Taguchi, K., Matsumura, H., Washizu, T., Hirao, M., Kato, K., Kato, E., Mochizuki, T., Takamura, K., Mashimo, I., Morifuji, K., Nakagaki, M. and Suma, T.: Effect of athrombogenic therapy, especially high dose therapy of dipyridamole after prosthetic valve replacement. J. Cardiovasc. Surg. 16:8, 1975.

Thomas, M.L.: Phlebography. Arch. Surg. 104:145, 1972.

Verstraete, M.: Are agents affecting platelet functions clinically useful? Am. J. Med. 61:897, 1976a.

Verstraete, M.: The prevention of postoperative deep vein thrombosis and pulmonary embolism with low dose heparin and dextran. Surg. Gynecol. Obstet. 143:981, 1976b.

Warkany, J.: A warfarin embryopathy. Am. J. Dis. Child. 128:424, 1975.

Weily, H.S., Steele, P.P., and Genton, E.: Platelet survival in patients with a Beall valve. Relation to low incidence of thromboembolism. Am. J. Cardiol. 30:229, 1972.

Weiss, V., Jekiel, M., Ritschard, J., and Bouvier, C.A.: Preventive effects of dipyridamole and ASA on postoperative thromboembolic disease in gynaecological surgery. Méd. Hyg. 35:943–944, 1977.

Wheeler, H.B., O'Donnell, J.A., Anderson, F.A., and Benedict, K.: Occlusive impedance phlebography: a diagnostic procedure for venous thrombosis and pulmonary embolism. Prog. Cardiovasc. Dis. 17:199, 1974.

Williams, O.B., McCaffrey, J.F., and Lau, O.J.: Deep vein thrombosis in a Queensland hospital. Br. Med. J. 1:517, 1973.

Wood, E.H., Prentice, C.R.M., McGrouther, A.D., Sinclair, J., and McNicol, G.P.: Trial of aspirin and RA 233 in prevention of post-operative deep vein thrombosis. Thromb. Haemostas. 30:18, 1973.

16

Are Beta Blockers Too Dangerous for General Clinical Use?

Edward D. Frohlich, M.D.

My life is in the hands of any rascal who chooses to annoy and tease me.

John Hunter

I have tremor cordis on me; my heart dances.

Shakespeare, *The Winter's Tale*

The heart is the only organ that takes no rest. That's why it is so good.

Martin H. Fischer

Introduction

Lest the question for this section seem pointless to some readers, the history of propranolol's official acceptance in this country needs to be told. As Dr. Frohlich points out, the FDA initially approved the drug for three indications that are actually the *least* important of all its current uses—cardiac arrhythmia, idiopathic hypertrophic subaortic stenosis, and pheochromocytoma. Much later, it was approved for angina pectoris and finally for hypertension.

Why the delay? The reasons are assuredly multiple, but the worldwide professional acceptance of propranolol for these important indications was clearly paradoxic. At least part of the trouble was caused by an advisory committee to the FDA, which was unconvinced that the putative benefits to angina patients were sufficient to offset the hazards of the drug's use. The leadership in the Bureau of Drugs bravely approved the drug for angina pectoris despite the strong opposition of some of these advisors. The bureau received little credit (Lasagna and Wardell, 1975) and a great deal of abuse from a Congressional subcommittee. Today, propranolol (or later congeners) is used almost routinely before considering coronary bypass surgery in patients with intractable angina pectoris. (Coronary surgery has yet to overcome a certain skepticism about its utility, although its use for this specific indication seems least controversial.)

Furthermore, propranolol and other beta blockers have become increasingly important in controlling hypertension, although the U.S. lags behind some other countries in the degree to which beta blockers have replaced or supplemented other antihypertensive drugs.

As Dr. Frohlich points out, beta blockers are no more "safe" than any other drug. The public and the medical community will never be able to enjoy therapeutic benefit without running some risk of untoward effects. Beta blockers are clearly capable of harm, and it is the job of the physician to use them judiciously, especially in patients in whom the risk of adverse effects is likely to be higher than average.

LOUIS LASAGNA, M.D.

---

1. Lasagna, L., and Wardell, W.M.: The FDA, politics, and the public. JAMA 232:141–143, 1975.

Are Beta Blockers Too Dangerous for General Clinical Use?

Edward D. Frohlich, M.D.
Alton Ochsner Medical Foundation, New Orleans

Adrenergic Receptor Sites: Transmission, Stimulation, and Blockade

Cardiovascular adrenergic receptor sites may be conceptualized as cellular transducers that translate the extracellular neurally mediated message into intracellular biochemical and physiologic events. In the instance of cardiovascular function, these neural impulses are transmitted through postganglionic neural fibers to vascular smooth muscle and myocardium by means of the neurohumoral substance norepinephrine. This neurotransmitter is stored freely or in vesicles in the postganglionic nerve ending. It is released from that nerve ending into the synaptic cleft, a space between the nerve ending and the membrane of the vascular smooth muscle or myocardium. Not all the released norepinephrine interacts with cardiovascular cellular receptor sites; some of the released catecholamine is destroyed in this synaptic space and some is taken up once again for storage (and later release) by the nerve ending. For a detailed discussion on the specifics of catecholamine synthesis, release, uptake, and receptor interaction, the reader is referred to a number of reviews (Wurtman, 1965; Moran, 1967; Cotton, Udenfriend, and Spector, 1972; Patil, Miller, and Trendelenburg, 1974).

Langley (1905) and Dale (1906) envisioned these effector receptor sites as "excitatory" or "inhibitory" areas; Ahlquist (1948) later classified them as alpha- or beta-adrenotropic receptors. Sympathomimetic drugs and naturally occurring adrenergic vasoactive agents, therefore, exert their respective effects on myocardium or vascular smooth muscle by stimulating specific centers in the brain, the autonomic ganglia, postganglionic nerve endings, or adrenergic receptor sites. Conversely, agents that reduce adrenergic function inhibit these anatomic levels of neural transmission and reception. It is therefore actually possible to dissect pharmacologically the adrenergic nervous system at a multiplicity of anatomic levels (Table 16–1). This does not exclude the direct action that other nonadrenergic naturally occurring agents (e.g., glucagon, kinins, vasopressin, histamine, angiotensin II) also have on cardiovascular function. These agents exert their respective actions on myocardial or vascular smooth muscle by stimulating their respective receptor sites.

In general, alpha-adrenergic receptor sites are located primarily on the vascular smooth muscle membrane of arterioles and venules (Nickerson, 1973); only a small number of alpha receptors seem to be present in myocardium (Govier, 1968). In contrast, beta-adrenergic receptor sites are present on vascular smooth muscle membranes, and they are also present as the predominant type of adrenergic receptor in myocardium. When alpha-adrenergic receptor sites

Table 16–1. *Pharmacologic Dissection of Adrenergic Function at a Multiplicity of Anatomic Levels*

Class of Compounds	Site of Action	Generic Name
Central alpha-receptor stimulants	Brainstem	Clonidine; methyldopa
Veratrum alkaloids	Baroreceptor mechanism	Cryptenamine
Ganglion blocking agents	Thoracodorsal ganglia	Trimethaphan
Catecholamine depletors	Postganglionic nerve ending and brain	Rauwolfia alkaloids
	Postganglionic nerve ending	Rauwolfia alkaloids; guanethidine; bethanidine
False neurohumoral transmitters	Peripheral alpha-adrenergic receptors	Methyldopa
Alpha-adrenergic receptor inhibitors	Peripheral alpha-adrenergic receptors	Phentolamine; phenoxybenzamine
Beta-adrenergic receptor inhibitors	Beta-adrenergic receptors	Propranolol (and many others including cardioselective agents, which are undergoing clinical trials)

are stimulated by a "pure" alpha receptor agonist, arteriolar and venular constriction result. Beta receptor stimulation produces arteriolar dilatation (Nickerson, 1973). Questions still exist concerning the magnitude and importance of beta-adrenergic receptor sites on venular smooth muscle. When cardiac beta-adrenergic receptor sites are stimulated, increased myocardial chronotropic, inotropic, and metabolic activity results (Nickerson, 1973). It therefore follows that an agent that specifically inhibits these beta-adrenergic receptor sites should attenuate or prevent the effects of naturally occurring or exogenously administered beta receptor agonists. As a result, the dose-response curve will be shifted to the right (Fig. 16–1). Therefore, beta-adrenergic receptor inhibition will result in a lesser heart rate increase and lesser myocardial contractility and metabolism in proportion to the dosage of the inhibitors.

Adrenergic receptor sites are present not only in cardiovascular tissue but also on cell membranes of other tissues innervated by adrenergic neurons. Thus, stimulation of beta receptor sites on bronchiolar smooth muscle will result in bronchodilation (Innes and Nickerson, 1965). And, although renal vascular smooth muscle contains relatively few beta-adrenergic receptor sites, these receptors have been demonstrated in the kidney in the region of the juxtaglomerular apparatus. When these receptors are stimulated, they effect a release of renin from the kidney (Winer et al., 1971). When beta-adrenergic receptor sites of the gastrointestinal tract are stimulated, motility of intestinal smooth muscle will be decreased.

As indicated, when beta-adrenergic receptor inhibiting drugs are administered, the effects of stimulation will be attenuated in proportion to the dosage of the inhibitor (Figure 16–1). Thus, with respect to the heart, one might anticipate either no increase or even a decrease

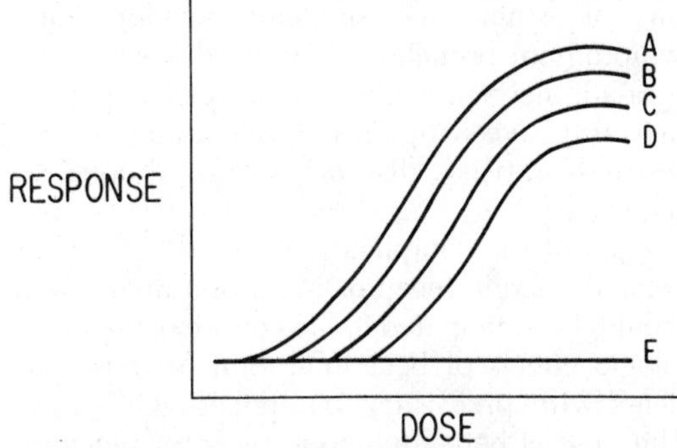

Figure 16–1. Dose-response relationship depicting the effect of stimulation of specific receptors by the specific agonist (A), the progressive inhibition by increasing doses of a specific receptor inhibitor (B, C, D), and finally the effect of total receptor blockade (E).

in myocardial chronotropic, inotropic, and metabolic activity. When beta-adrenergic receptor stimulation of vascular smooth muscle is inhibited, vascular resistance may increase. Inhibition of bronchiolar smooth muscle beta receptor sites will prevent bronchodilation; in fact, actual bronchoconstriction may result (McNeill and Ingram, 1966). Beta inhibition may prevent or inhibit the release from the kidney of renin by the juxtaglomerular apparatus. Inhibition of gastrointestinal beta receptor sites tends to leave parasympathetic activity unopposed, thereby resulting in increased motility.

Adverse Effects

From this general (albeit simplified) but fundamental information concerning the beta-adrenergic receptor sites and the physiologic effects of their stimulation and inhibition, one may anticipate certain adverse effects. For example, following beta adrenergic blockade, the cardiac patient who may already have impaired myocardial function may progress into a state of more severe cardiac decompensation and overt failure. Beta adrenergic inhibition may so impair cardiac rhythmicity and conduction that severe bradycardia or heart block may result. Further, the patient already suffering from a vasospastic disease (e.g., arteriosclerosis obliterans, Raynaud's phenomenon or disease) may, following beta blockade, lose whatever small amount of vasodilation is present so that important nutrition of the peripheral tissues is drastically restricted. As a result, patients with ischemic limb disease may develop more severe pain in cold temperatures, and gangrene may even develop. The individual with preexisting chronic obstructive lung disease or with a history of asthma may suddenly develop acute symptomatic bronchoobstructive disease during beta-adrenergic receptor blockade. The patient may also have symptoms of increased gastrointestinal motility, distention, and abdominal spasm.

Each of the complications or side effects of beta-adrenergic receptor inhibition might (and should) be anticipated if one considers the physiologic effects of beta inhibition in those patients with preexisting complicating diseases. Thus, use of beta-adrenergic receptor blocking drugs in human beings may pose formidable clinical problems and complications: congestive heart failure, heart block, peripheral gangrene, and status asthmaticus, among others. But any potent therapeutic agent with very specific beneficial effects may produce significant deleterious effects. This two-edged sword is a dilemma of modern therapeutics.

Are Beta Blocking Drugs Too Dangerous for Clinical Use?

The question might therefore be posed, "Are any potent and specific drugs without danger?" The answer is obvious; most drugs carry certain inherent dangers with their use. This should not relegate them to disuse. It must be the role and responsibility of the practicing physician to establish in his own mind the risks and the benefits of prescribing these drugs in a particular patient. Having weighed this, a judgment must be made on whether to prescribe the drug.

To use several examples, it is well known that acetylsalicylic acid may provoke peptic ulceration, gastrointestinal hemorrhage, or even laryngeal stridor. Although these complications or side effects are very rare, and although aspirin should not be used indiscriminately, the compound is exceedingly popular for many clinical problems, and it is efficacious, important, and necessary. Antibacterial agents also produce a broad range of clinical side effects. Among these are severe allergic reactions, bone marrow suppression with resulting aplastic anemia and leukopenia, renal impairment, deafness, and the possibility of development of antimicrobial resistance to these agents. Nevertheless, antibiotics have produced a remarkable reduction in the morbidity and mortality from infectious disease, and there is no voice saying that these antibiotic agents are "too dangerous for general clinical use." These drugs must continue to be used broadly throughout the world, but they must be prescribed judiciously.

Similar analogies may be made with drugs that are used for the treatment of anemias. The folic acid in multiple vitamin preparations certainly may mask pernicious anemia, leaving the horrible neural complications uncorrected, and the clinical diagnosis may even remain unrecognized (Frohlich, 1958). As a final example, many drugs that are being used for the treatment of neoplastic diseases may produce severe side effects. Yet, in the instance of severe malignancies, the risks and benefits are weighed, and, in general, specific agents are prescribed for specific neoplasms in order to retard or to palliate them or perhaps even to effect prolonged "cures."

Why should we stop short of these progressive practices in other important areas of medicine by suggesting that drugs that inhibit adrenergic receptor sites are too dangerous for general clinical use? As with any other therapeutic agent, the clinician must anticipate side effects in his patient; he must understand the pathophysiologic alterations produced by the patient's disease; and, having weighed the evidence on both sides, he must decide whether the beta blocking drug should be prescribed for a specific patient. The question is not whether beta blocking drugs are too dangerous for general clinical use but whether beta adrenergic receptor blocking drugs are too dangerous for specific use in specific patients and by certain physicians.

Specificity of Therapy

Selection of many modern drugs not infrequently is based upon the specific action of drugs. Let us pursue this further. Antibiotics are selected on the basis of which organism is most sensitive to the drug. A hematinic is prescribed on the basis of the specific type of anemia encountered: iron for iron-deficiency anemia, vitamin B_6 for a pantothenic-acid-deficiency-induced megaloblastic anemia, folic acid for deficiency that might result from a malabsorption syndrome, and vitamin B_{12} for pernicious anemia. Oncolytic agents are prescribed specifically for particular types of neoplastic disease. Even gastric ulceration and hypersecretion now may be treated specifically with histamine receptor antagonists.

Thus, we must recognize that modern therapy is becoming more specific and more potent. The question of beta blockers being too dangerous for general clinical use becomes inappropriate. More relevant questions might be: "Are beta-adrenergic blocking drugs too dangerous for specific clinical use?" "In whom should these more potent drugs be used?" The answers, to me, are obvious. Beta blocking drugs are not too dangerous for specific use; any physician who has a knowledge of the pathophysiologic alterations in his patient and an understanding of the mechanism of drug action should be able to use these drugs if the clinical situation of his patient indicates their necessity.

A succeeding question might be: "Are potentially severe effects of beta-adrenergic blocking drugs to be anticipated in all patients?" We might expect that anything can happen when a drug is given to a patient; but the individuals who might be thought to suffer side effects from beta-adrenergic blocking therapy are those whose physiologic responses to these drugs will aggravate the underlying pathophysiologic alterations already existing. For example, the patient with borderline cardiac compensation might be expected to develop congestive heart failure when treated with beta-adrenergic blocking therapy. If congestive heart failure is already present, the patient may develop fluid retention and even acute pulmonary edema. If the patient previously had asthma or bronchoobstructive disease, he may be expected to develop an acute episode of bronchial obstruction and asthma during beta-adrenergic blocking therapy. Severe bradycardia or preexisting cardiac conduction abnormalities may be expected to progress to heart block or other conduction abnormalities with beta-blocking therapy. The patient with preexisting peripheral arterial insufficiency may develop further aggravation of the arterial insufficiency—even to the point of gangrene. If these effects can be anticipated, it is perfectly reasonable to suggest that we exclude those patients from consideration for beta-adrenergic blocking therapy and thereby obviate these potential problems.

In our experience, having employed beta-adrenergic receptor blocking drugs for the treatment of patients with hypertension for over 13 years, relatively few side effects have been encountered. We did describe two patients with acute peripheral arterial insufficiency, but these patients were the first to be reported with this adverse effect (Frohlich, Tarazi, and Dustan, 1969a). We might have anticipated this complication had we realized that beta-adrenergically mediated mechanisms were providing the additional degree of vasodilatation necessary for adequate peripheral tissue perfusion in patients with a history of Raynaud's phenomenon.

Specificity of Beta-Adrenergic Receptor Blocking Therapy

Beta-adrenergic blocking drugs thus provide another excellent example of how physicians could select their patients for specific therapy. Indeed, when this cardiovascular therapy was first introduced in the United States, it was approved for three clinical problems: arrhythmia, idiopathic hypertrophic subaortic stenosis, (IHSS), and pheochromocytoma. The rationale for this selection was that inhibition of beta-adrenergic receptor sites would prevent arrhythmias, particularly if they were supraventricular and induced by catecholamines. Beta-adrenergic blocking drugs were also effective in treatment of digitalis-induced arrhythmias. And, because the physiologic abnormality of IHSS can be brought out with isoproterenol or digitalis (both potent inotropic myocardial agents), it was reasoned that beta-adrenergic blocking drugs would prevent enhanced contractility of this ectopic myocardial tissue and thereby relieve left ventricular outflow tract obstruction. The rationale for the use of beta-adrenergic blocking drugs in patients with pheochromocytoma was similarly specific—prevention of arrhythmias produced by excessive amounts of circulating catecholamines.

Within a few years, approval was forthcoming for propranolol's use in the treatment of angina pectoris. The reason for this is also obvious when one thinks of the clinical condition from a pathophysiologic point of view. Patients with chest pain produced by ischemic heart disease may have an increased demand for myocardial oxygen with reduced ability to deliver oxygen to the ischemic myocardial tissue. Beta-adrenergic receptor blocking therapy would reduce heart rate, reduce cardiac output, possibly reduce arterial pressure, lower myocardial oxygen demand by reducing myocardial metabolism, and, consequently, reduce the need for oxygen by the ischemic myocardium. Now beta-adrenergic blocking therapy has become a major adjunct for treatment of patients with ischemic heart disease.

Justification for the use of beta-adrenergic blocking drugs in the treatment of patients with hypertension remains unclear at present. Perhaps this is because the basic mechanism whereby arterial pressure is increased in patients with hypertension is still elusive. Certainly, the antihypertensive mechanisms of beta-adrenergic blocking drugs remain unexplained. Initially, we selected beta-adrenergic blocking therapy for those patients who had a hyperdynamic beta-adrenergic circulatory state (Frohlich, Dustan, and Page, 1966; Frohlich, Tarazi, and Dustan, 1969b). These patients had a hyperkinetic circulation, provocation of their symptoms of cardiac awareness and disability by isoproterenol infusion, and, following beta-adrenergic receptor blockade, remission of these symptoms, reduction of arterial pressure, and normalization of the hyperkinetic circulation. The paradoxic finding was that reduction of arterial pressure in these patients was not associated with a significant reduction in total peripheral resistance (Frohlich, Tarazi, Dustan, and Page, 1968). Thus, following the acute intravenous administration of the beta-adrenergic blocking drug, there was a reduction in cardiac output unassociated with a change in pressure (Ulrych et al., 1968). With prolonged oral antihypertensive therapy, cardiac output remained reduced at approximately the same level, but arterial pressure fell (Frohlich, Tarazi, Dustan, and Page, 1968; Dunn et al., 1978). This might be thought to be associated with a fall in vascular resistance; however, total peripheral resistance was not significantly reduced from pretreatment levels (Frohlich, Tarazi, Dustan, and Page, 1968; Ulrych et al., 1968; Frohlich, Tarazi, and Dustan, 1970; Dunn et al., 1978). This suggested to us some adaptation of the peripheral circulation (Frohlich and Page, 1966; Frohlich, Tarazi, and Dustan, 1970; Frohlich, 1971a; Frohlich, 1971b; Frohlich, 1973). More recently, our studies involving rats with naturally occurring genetic hypertension have shown that certain vascular beds (in skeletal muscle and myocardium) demonstrate remarkable decreases in blood flow and increases in vascular resistance; other circulations (kidney, intestine, brain) demonstrate a negligible change or even increased blood flow after treatment with beta blocking drugs (Nishiyama et al., 1978).

These findings originally suggested to us that other forms of hypertension associated with an increased cardiac output might also be responsive to beta-adrenergic blocking therapy (Frohlich, 1971a; Frohlich, 1972). Patients with borderline (labile) hypertension, mild essential hypertension, and renovascular hypertension demonstrated a significant reduction in arterial pressure with beta-adrenergic blocking therapy (Frohlich, Tarazi, and Dustan, 1970; Frohlich, 1971a; Frohlich, 1971b; Frohlich, 1972; Frohlich, 1973a; Frohlich, 1973b). At the time these clinical observations were reported, we also noted that those patients having the highest cardiac output seemed to have the greatest reduction in arterial pressure with prolonged beta blocking therapy (Frohlich, Tarazi, and Dustan, 1970; Frohlich, 1971; Frohlich, 1973). We also noted that those patients with higher cardiac output levels seemed to have the highest levels of plasma-renin activity (Dustan et al., 1970). Subsequently, Buhler, Laragh, and associates (1972) demonstrated that those patients with the highest plasma-renin activity responded best to beta-adrenergic blocking therapy in reducing arterial pressure.

It seems unlikely, however, that reduction of cardiac output and plasma-renin activity are the sole factors responsible for reducing arterial pressure. Now that there are over 20 beta-adrenergic receptor blocking drugs, we know that some produce greater reduction of cardiac output than others and that some produce greater inhibition of renin release from the kidney than others. Nevertheless, when these agents are compared in the same patient, control of arterial pressure seems to be equivalent.

Another justification for use of beta-adrenergic blocking drugs came with resurgence of vasodilator antihypertensive therapy. Formerly, when vasodilating agents were used, side effects were experienced as a result of the reflexive stimulation of the heart as well as from associated headaches. These symptoms were somewhat attenuated when reserpine was used in conjunction with the vasodilator. However, with the availability of beta-adrenergic blocking drugs, it became possible to use the vasodilating agent to reduce vascular resistance; the beta-adrenergic receptor blocking drug prevented the reflex vasodilator-induced cardiac stimulation but also provided its own intrinsic antihypertensive action (Gilmore et al., 1970; Zacest et al., 1972).

Other antihypertensive mechanisms have been offered to explain the hypertensive action of beta-adrenergic blocking drugs. Among them is the finding that rather than an expansion of intravascular volume associated with pressure reduction, there was an unchanged (or reduced) plasma volume in patients with uncomplicated essential hypertension (Tarazi et al., 1971; Dunn et al., 1978). This might also be explained on the basis of inhibition of renin release and the prevention of the anticipated increase in aldosterone secretion by the adrenal glands in compensation for the pressure reduction. Recent studies with the beta-adrenergic blocking drug timolol indicate that with prolonged treatment, not only are there reduced cardiac output, reduced plasma-renin activity, and reduced plasma volume but there is also reduced aldosterone secretion (Dunn et al., 1978). Further studies are necessary to elucidate the antihypertensive mechanisms of beta blocking drugs. Perhaps with an understanding of these processes, further insight will be available into the pressor mechanisms underlying the hypertensive disease itself.

Conclusion

It is true that beta-adrenergic blocking drugs are potentially dangerous. However, these dangers can be anticipated in most patients. Enlightened physicians are necessary for the proper use of these drugs, but we must ask, "Isn't this what modern medicine is all about?" Although potent drugs are indeed dangerous, they are not too dangerous to use if the practitioner remains well informed, if he prescribes the drug as a specific agent, and if he does not generalize the therapy to an entire population.

References

Ahlquist, R.P.: A study of the adrenotropic receptors. Am. J. Physiol. 153:586, 1948.

Buhler, F.R., Laragh, J.H., Baer, L., Vaughan, E.D., and Brunner, H.R.: Propranolol inhibition of renin secretion; a specific approach to diagnosis and treatment of renin-dependent hypertensive diseases. N. Engl. J. Med. 287:1209, 1972.

Cotton, M. deV., Udenfriend, S., and Spector, S., eds.: Regulation of catecholamine metabolism in the sympathetic nervous system. Pharmacol. Rev. 24:161, 1972.

Dale, H.H.: On some physiological actions of ergot. J. Physiol. 34:163, 1906.

Dunn, F.G., deCarvalho, J.G.R., and Frohlich, E.D.: Hemodynamic, reflexive, and metabolic alterations induced by acute and chronic timolol therapy in hypertensive man. Circulation 57:140, 1978.

Dustan, H.P., Tarazi, R.C., and Frohlich, E.D.: Functional correlates of plasma renin activity in hypertensive patients. Circulation 41:555, 1970.

Frohlich, E.D.: Pernicious anemia masked by a multiple vitamin preparation. N. Engl. J. Med. 259:1221, 1958.

Frohlich, E.D.: Beta-adrenergic blockade in the circulatory regulation of hyperkinetic states. Am. J. Cardiol. 27:195, 1971a.

Frohlich, E.D.: Beta-adrenergic inhibition in hypertension associated with renal arterial disease. In Fisher, J.W., and Cafruny, E.J., eds., *Renal Pharmacology*, New York, Appleton-Century-Crofts, 1971b.

Frohlich, E.D.: Hyperdynamic circulation and hypertension. Postgrad. Med. 52:68, 1972.

Frohlich, E.D.: The use of beta-adrenergic blockade in hypertension. In Onesti, G., Kim, K.E., and Moyer, J.H., eds., *Hypertension: Mechanisms and Management*, New York, Grune & Stratton, Inc., 1973a.

Frohlich, E.D.: Clinical significance of hemodynamic findings in hypertension. Chest 64:94, 1973b.

Frohlich, E.D., Dustan, H.P., and Page, I.H.: Hyperdynamic beta-adrenergic circulatory state. Arch. Intern. Med. 117:614, 1966.

Frohlich, E.D., and Page, I.H.: The clinical meaning of cardiovascular beta-adrenergic receptors. Physiol. Pharmacol. for Physicians 1:No. 11 (Nov), 1966.

Frohlich, E.D., Tarazi, R.C., and Dustan, H.P.: Peripheral arterial insufficiency: a complication of beta-adrenergic blocking therapy. JAMA 208:2471, 1969a.

Frohlich, E.D., Tarazi, R.C., and Dustan, H.P.: Hyperdynamic beta-adrenergic circulatory state: increased beta receptor responsiveness. Arch. Intern. Med. 123:1, 1969b.

Frohlich, E.D., Tarazi, R.C., and Dustan, H.P.: Beta-adrenergic blocking therapy in hypertension: selection of patients. Int. J. Pharm. Therap. Toxicol. 4:151, 1970.

Frohlich, E.D., Tarazi, R.C., and Dustan, H.P.: Use of beta-adrenergic blockade in hypertensive disease. In Kattus, A.A., Ross, G., and Hall, V. eds., Cardiovascular Beta Adrenergic Responses, UCLA Forum in Medical Sciences (Number 13) Los Angeles, University of California Press, 1970.

Frohlich, E.D., Tarazi, R.C., Dustan, H.P., and Page, I.H.: The paradox of beta-adrenergic blockade in hypertension. Circulation 37:417, 1968.

Gilmore, W., Weil, J., and Chidsey, C.: Treatment of essential hypertension with a new vasodilator in combination with beta-adrenergic blockade. N. Engl. J. Med. 282:521, 1970.

Govier, W.C.: Myocardial alpha-adrenergic receptors and their role in the production of a positive inotropic effect by sympathomimetic agents. J. Pharmacol. Exp. Ther. 159:82, 1968.

Innes, J.R., and Nickerson, M.: Drugs acting on postganglionic adrenergic nerve endings and structures innervated by them (sympathomimetic drugs). In Goodman, L.S., and Gilman, A., eds., *The Pharmacological Basis of Therapeutics*, 3rd ed., New York, Macmillan Co., 1965.

Langley, J.N.: On the reaction of cells and of nerve-endings to certain poisons, chiefly as regards the reaction of striated muscles to nicotine and curare. J. Physiol. 33:374, 1905.

McNeill, R.S., and Ingram, C.G.: Effect of propranolol on ventilatory function. Am. J. Cardiol. 18:473, 1966.

Moran, N.C., ed.: New adrenergic blocking drugs: their pharmacological, biochemical and clinical actions. Ann. NY Acad. Sci. 139:541, 1967.

Nickerson, M.: Adrenergic receptors. Circ. Res. 32(I):53, 1973.

Nishiyama, K., Nishiyama, A., Pfeffer, M.A., and Frohlich, E.D.: Systemic and regional flow distribution in normotensive and spontaneously hypertensive young rats subjected to lifetime beta-adrenergic receptor blockade. Blood Vessels 15:333–347, 1978.

Patil, P.N., Miller, D.D., and Trendelenburg, U.: Molecular geometry and adrenergic drug activity. Pharmacol. Rev. 26:323, 1974.

Tarazi, R.C., Frohlich, E.D., and Dustan, H.P.: Plasma volume changes with long-term beta-adrenergic blockade. Am. Heart J. 82:770, 1971.

Ulrych, M., Frohlich, E.D., Dustan, H.P., and Page, I.H.: Immediate hemodynamic effects of beta-adrenergic blockade with propranolol in normotensive and hypertensive man. Circulation 37:411, 1968.

Winer, N., Chokski, D.S., and Walkenhorst, W.G.: Effects of cyclic AMP, sympathomimetic amines, and adrenergic receptor antagonists on renin secretion. Circ. Res. 29:239, 1971.

Wurtman, R.J.: Catecholamines. Boston, Little Brown Co., 1965.

Zacest, R., Gilmore, E., and Koch-Weser, J.: Treatment of essential hypertension with combined vasodilation and beta-adrenergic blockade. N. Engl. J. Med. 286:617, 1972.

17

How Useful Is Drug Therapy for Senile Dementia?

No one is so old as to think he cannot live one more year.

Cicero, *On Old Age*

Tyrawley and I have been dead these two years, but we don't choose to have it known.

Lord Chesterfield

No skill or wit is needed to grow old; the trick is to endure it.

Goethe

It is notorious that the desire to live increases as life itself shortens.

Ramón y Cajal, *Charlas de Café*

Introduction

Dementia is often a diagnosis of despair for both patients and doctors, signifying a future devoid of effective therapy and therefore of hope. Hollister and Shoulson both stress that such a pessimistic attitude is unwarranted for certain dementia-causing diseases, and that a doctor must not fall into the trap of using sloppy and superficial categorization for these disorders. I would tend to agree with Hollister's estimate of the low frequency of remediable dementia, but for each patient in this category, it is terribly important not to overlook such an etiology.

Even when the dementia is not fundamentally reversible, symptomatic therapy is worth trying, a point on which Hollister and Shoulson agree. In regard to specific therapy, however, especially with so-called cerebral vasodilators, there is much controversy in this field. The one remedy for which enough positive evidence exists to have garnered FDA approval (for certain claims in elderly patients) is Hydergine. Average results are modest, and the published data do not allow the reader to judge whether occasional patients experience more significant benefit. Hollister obviously believes that even modest benefits are worth aiming for.

Shoulson urges careful and thorough work-up of dementia patients because he believes that rational therapy is impossible without specific (and accurate) diagnosis. Like Hollister, he would not ignore any rational therapeutic maneuvers that might ameliorate the clinical state.

Where Shoulson parts company with Hollister is on the use of "vasodilators." Specifically, although he is in favor of further assessment of papaverine, he is thoroughly skeptical of the utility of Hydergine. One concludes that Shoulson would never try Hydergine, even if all else had failed.

One last point. I have the disquieting feeling that a lot of institutionalized oldsters are neither "senile" nor "demented," but to a large extent simply elderly and cast off by family, friends, and society. Even where there is deterioration in cerebral functioning, there is often not a great deal to be accomplished with drugs, whereas substantial help might result from human contact. Many of these "patients" are lonely and bored. To them, "attention must be paid," as Willy Loman's wife begged in *Death of a Salesman*. The human contact need not be professional or trained. More important is a willingness to show a sincere interest in the patients. Love and affection and caring might do more than we think.

LOUIS LASAGNA, M.D.

Are Drugs Useful for Treating Senile Dementia?

Leo E. Hollister, M.D.
VA Hospital; Stanford University School of Medicine

Not many drugs are marketed in the United States as treatments for senile dementia, but in some countries, such as West Germany, the market is plentiful. Perhaps the difference exists because the proportion of the population over the age of 65 is only about 11 percent in the United States and probably greater than 15 percent in West Germany. Fortunately, only a minority of the elderly are afflicted with senile dementia. When it occurs, it can be a disaster, both for the patient and his family. The course of illness is usually a long-term decline towards death without dignity.

Importance of Recognizing Treatable Disorders

Most physicians in the United States hold a rather pessimistic view about what can be done for the demented older person. To some extent, this view is warranted. This pessimism should not, however, prejudice the search for remediable causes of the abnormal mental state. A huge list of differential diagnostic possibilities has been proposed. These are broadly categorized into mental symptoms attributable to drugs, including those used socially; endocrinopathies and metabolic disorders; nutritional problems; tumors or trauma; infirmities of the senses; and complications of arteriosclerosis (Hollister, 1975).

Most of these are unlikely possibilities, but they still must be considered. More important is to consider the possibility that the patient may be depressed or may have the late-onset disorder paraphrenia, which resembles schizophrenia. Depression is probably the most common emotional disorder of the elderly and has many easily identifiable causes. Atypical manifestations may include marked social withdrawal, confusion, severe hypochondriasis, delusions of persecution, and hostile behavior. These features may mislead the unwary to think that the patient has an organic brain syndrome rather than true depression.

The yield of remediable disorders among a group of patients thought to have senile dementia is variable, but some have estimated that it may be as high as 35 percent. I suspect that this estimate is high, but even if it were less than 10 percent, the search would be justified.

Pathogenetic Considerations

Contrary to widespread belief, cerebral vascular insufficiency is not the major cause of senile dementia. Senile brain disease, also known by several other terms, including the eponym *Alzheimer's disease*, is either solely responsible or plays the major role in about 70 percent of chronic organic brain syndromes of later life. Cerebral arteriosclerosis is an important factor in less than 15 percent of cases. The remainder are attributable to the consequences of alcohol abuse or to other medical and neurologic diseases.

Brain atrophy may be shown grossly. Microscopically, the hallmarks of senile brain disease are the neurofibrillary tangle and the Alzheimer plaque. Both represent the remains of degenerated neurons, along with aging pigments in the plaque. The cause of these irreversible degenerative changes is unknown, *but it is clear that they are not an inevitable accompaniment of the aging process.* Tenuous evidence suggests a genetic predisposition (Heston and Mastri, 1977). A slow neurotropic virus infection has also been postulated. The main point is that these changes are not directly associated with cerebral arteriosclerosis (although the two conditions may coexist) and are probably not associated directly with ischemia. This consideration bears on pharmacologic approaches to treatment.

Drug Treatment

Treatment of psychoses associated with old age may be directed at the management of certain symptoms (*symptomatic*) or at the presumed cause of the basic pathologic changes (*specific*).

Symptomatic Treatment

Symptomatic treatment includes the use of antipsychotic, antidepressant, and antianxiety drugs. Antipsychotics are probably the most useful. Their main benefits are seen in three areas: (1) restoring a normal sleep-wake cycle, (2) curbing irritable or agitated behavior, and (3) improving self-care. The gains are modest but often clinically valuable. Probably any antipsychotic drug might be used, but thioridazine has been most widely promoted. Some clinicians prefer to take the risk of extrapyramidal reactions and to use small doses of more potent agents such as thiothixene, haloperidol, or fluphenazine. Doses should be the smallest that provide optimal symptomatic control without a disabling parkinsonian syndrome. The goal of treatment is to reduce disturbed behavior to manageable levels, not to immobilize the patient.

Depression may be confounded with or may accompany senile brain disease; in either case, an antidepressant is indicated. Most clinicians prefer one of the tricyclics, despite the risks attendant on their anticholinergic and cardiotoxic actions. The choice of tricyclic is largely empiric. Because both thioridazine and tricyclics have potential cardiotoxicity, these two drugs should not be used in combination.

Anxiety with insomnia in the elderly is best treated with the benzodiazepines. Diazepam is probably the best choice, despite a theoretical advantage for oxazepam, which requires less metabolism. These drugs are best used in single daily doses taken either as needed or in the evening. Flurazepam is still widely used as a hypnotic in the elderly, despite the possible accumulation of long-lived active metabolites over time and reports of occasional behavioral deterioration with the use of benzodiazepines in the elderly.

Specific Treatment

Specific treatment aimed at correcting some postulated cause of senile brain disease includes the use of stimulant or analeptic drugs, cerebral vasodilators, drugs averred to improve brain metabolism, drugs with a variety of special actions, and the experimental precursors of various neurotransmitters.

STIMULANTS. Although stimulants may increase the acquisition of new information in the elderly, no beneficial effects have been proved during chronic treatment. Pentylenetetrazol was widely used in the past but is now considered obsolete. Neither methylphenidate nor magnesium pemoline, among the current stimulants, offers any advantage.

CEREBRAL VASODILATORS. Dilatation of cerebral vessels, even if it could be achieved, would probably not be helpful for the majority of elderly patients with senile brain disease. Because vasodilation is likely to be general rather than selective, one could argue that these drugs might actually divert blood away from the brain.

Three drugs with primary vasodilation as their mode of action have been used in the United States (Yesavage et al., 1978). Cyclandelate has been tested in a number of controlled trials, but results have been controversial. A review of four such trials of cyclandelate concluded that it was no more effective than placebo. One study suggested a slowing of cognitive decline, indicating a possible prophylactic action for cyclandelate.

Papaverine has probably been studied the most, but the majority of controlled trials have been negative, both when it was compared with placebo and with dihydroergotamine mesylate. Papaverine produces enough side effects to suggest that it has some action when given orally, but evidence of clinically important therapeutic effects is lacking.

Cinnarizine, an antihistaminic with vasodilating action, is more popular in Europe than in the United States. Most of the clinical trials have been in patients with diseases other than senile dementia, such as transient ischemic attacks or Meniere's disease. On the whole, one is forced to conclude that not only is the rationale for the use of vasodilators questionable but their efficacy, after many years of use, remains unproven.

Drugs increasing brain metabolism. A number of drugs that were formerly believed to act as cerebral vasodilators are now thought to act by increasing brain metabolism. Increased cerebral blood flow may follow as a consequence of increased carbon dioxide production in the brain. The oldest such drug is Hydergine, a combination of three ergot alkaloids, which has been studied extensively (Gygax et al., 1978). Some 22 controlled comparisons of this drug with placebo or other drugs (most often papaverine) have noted some statistically significant improvement on behavioral or psychologic measures. In addition, the investigator's opinion in 18 of those trials was that the improvement noted was of practical importance. Most of the studies used doses of 3 mg daily, although the current trend is to try higher doses such as 4.5 to 6 mg daily.

A few years ago, I informally reviewed some of the more recent controlled clinical evaluations of Hydergine. The degree of improvement over baseline on the variety of clinical measures used varied from 10 to 20 percent for the groups studied. Thus, even though this was statistically significant the clinical importance of the benefit was somewhat less impressive. Nonetheless, the general consensus seems to be that something positive happens when this drug is used. Most studies have evaluated the drug only over 12-week periods, which may be inadequate for the entire benefits of drug therapy to become evident. A recent study that covered a 26-week period found that most improvement was noted during the latter, rather than the earlier, course of treatment (Gaitz et al., 1977). Thus, not only dose but also duration of treatment may be of importance in producing optimal therapeutic effects.

Nafronyl is a new compound, chemically unrelated to Hydergine, that is also said to act by increasing brain metabolism (Levy and Wallace, 1977). It is marketed in Europe, and most controlled clinical trials comparing the drug to placebo have been favorable. Currently, the drug is under investigation in the United States.

Drugs with special actions. Although almost every vitamin and hormone has been used in the past for treatment of the elderly demented patient, the absence of any proof of efficacy indicates the futility of such treatment. A nostrum called Gerovital H-3 has caught the current fancy. It is procaine in a presumed special pharmaceutical preparation that makes it suitable for intramuscular administration. Since local hydrolysis of procaine given in this fashion is probably complete within minutes, it is difficult to see how very much drug could gain access to the systemic circulation and to the brain. Procaine has been found to inhibit monoamine oxidase weakly, but if that is its only mechanism of action, other drugs are readily available that are more potent, longer lasting, and effective orally. One can't help believing that Gerovital H-3 is only an expensive placebo.

Hyperbaric oxygen has been advocated, again on the familiar but unproven assumption that ischemia and hypoxia are the basis for senile brain disease. A recent controlled trial of this cumbersome and expensive treatment found it to be essentially worthless.

Precursors of neurotransmitters. If monoamine oxidase activity increases in the aging brain, one might expect that a deficiency of biogenic amine neurotransmitters might occur. Further, some cases of Parkinson's disease in which dopamine deficiency is present also have clinical evidence of dementia and pathologic evidence of Alzheimer's disease. Thus, it is tempting to speculate that repletion of dopamine may help patients with senile brain disease. Initial clinical trials with the dopamine precursor, levodopa, have not been very encouraging (Kristensen et al., 1977). The same has been true for more limited trials with the serotonin precursor, 5-hydroxytryptophan.

Involvement of acetylcholine in senile brain disease is somewhat more compelling. Neurochemical evidence suggests that both acetylcholine and choline acetylase are depleted in aging brains. Scopolamine, an anticholinergic drug, is well known to produce delirium, and some aspects of this confusional state resemble those seen in patients with senile brain disease. Scopolamine-induced delirium is reversible with physostigmine, a centrally active cholinesterase inhibitor. This model may be overly simplistic, as the scopolamine-induced changes in thinking are nonspecific, and it is not at all certain that their reversibility in people with normal brains by replenishing acetylcholine can be simulated in demented patients. An initial clinical trial with the presumed acetylcholine precursor, dimethylaminoethanol, produced only slightly encouraging results (Ferris et al., 1977). Clearly, more work is needed in this general area.

Supportive Treatment

Proper psychosocial interventions are not only helpful but obligatory. It is far easier to write off senile patients as dead losses than it is to maintain a supportive and caring environment. Frequent personal contact, expressions of attention, and attempts to keep the patient in touch with the world (perhaps with a discussion of the day's news, alluding frequently to the day of the week, the date, the month, and the year) are ways in which some of the social withdrawal and isolation of these patients can be mitigated. Such care, alas, may tax all the resources of the most dedicated family, and its purchase is terribly dear. Unfortunately, the aims of treatment in most nursing homes are simply to keep the senile patient quiet and dry.

Sources of Negative Bias in Evaluating Drug Treatment

Techniques for evaluating changes induced by drugs or other treatments in the course of senile dementia are still rather poor. Psychometric scales seem to approach the problem at practical levels regarding self-care, behavior, and thinking, yet they have not been fully validated (Shader et al., 1974). More sophisticated approaches, such as formal tests of memory, are even less well validated for an elderly age group. The problem is that one is looking for relatively small changes in a patient with a considerable degree of dysfunction. It is thus not unreasonable that we shall often fail to find such changes, not because they are not there, but because our techniques lack sufficient sensitivity.

Another problem is that senile dementia is progressive and often compounded by other concurrent illnesses. Actually, it may be more reasonable to settle for a delayed progression of the illness than to expect that any current treatment is likely to reverse a substantial portion of established disability. The rate of progression is not the same for every patient, however, and it may be influenced by changing states of physical health or social circumstances.

Virtually all the clinical trials of drug therapy have been conducted over rather brief periods, seldom more than 12 weeks. Such a time period may be inadequate to alter the course of the illness sufficiently so that a difference between treatments could be shown. Relatively short treatment periods favor a positive showing for purely symptomatic treatments; one might reasonably expect that disturbed behavior or depression might improve over a matter of weeks. To reverse established disability in thinking or even to slow the future rate of progression might take much longer.

Many of the studies evaluating such treatments are done with patients who are in mental hospitals or nursing homes. By the time a patient requires this much care, the degree of disability is usually marked and the disease is in an advanced stage. More selective use of patients with early, rather than late, signs of senile dementia might favor the demonstration of therapeutic effects of drugs. No one claims that any of the available drugs will perform miracles, yet we often select patients in whom only a miracle would produce a noticeable degree of improvement.

Experience with many drugs that did not appear to be highly effective when first studied indicates that proper dose of the drug is crucial. A drug may be improperly rejected when it fails to act because the dose was too small. We know little or nothing about the kinetics of drugs of this type; their bioavailability has been open to some question. Compliance with dosage schedules is a major problem in treating the elderly. It is axiomatic that plasma concentrations of drugs vary greatly among different patients, so that if these are at all related to treatment effects, it is mandatory to tailor doses to the needs of individual patients. Yet almost all drug trials testing drugs for senile dementia have used fixed, arbitrary dosage schedules.

What Do Drugs Offer?

Currently available drugs probably do not offer much for treating patients with senile dementia, yet what they do offer should not be discounted. The general clinical belief is that some types of psychotherapeutic drugs, such as antipsychotics, antidepressants, and antianxiety drugs, can provide symptomatic relief for many mental manifestations in old age that may be confounded with senile dementia or that may complicate it. This belief is based on clinical experience more than it is buttressed by controlled clinical trials, yet one feels reasonably secure in recommending use of such drugs for symptomatic treatment. For many patients, such treatment may offer the best chance for improvement.

Specific treatment of senile dementia with drugs aimed at reversing its pathogenesis is much more controversial. At present, only one drug, Hydergine, can be considered for potentially useful treatment. Results in clinical trials of the drug have been neither consistent in the areas of improvement nor tremendously impressive in the degree of improvement. They almost always show some improvement in patients treated with the drug as compared with those treated with a placebo or occasionally with some other vasodilator-type drug. Clinical experience with this drug also produces mixed results, more often disappointing than encouraging. Enough of the latter cases occur, however, to suggest that the treatment may be of real value for some patients.

Conclusion

The question finally comes down to whether one should take a totally pessimistic view of drug treatment of senile dementia or whether one should be more optimistic. A pessimist would either not use any psychotherapeutic drugs at all or would use only those directed at providing symptomatic treatment. An optimist would use symptomatic treatment to the fullest possible extent and then would go a bit further by trying an adequate course of drug aimed at altering the progression of the illness. His optimism would not lead him to expect that a shambling, perplexed oldster would suddenly be transformed into a spry and alert person; rather, he would settle for much less. He would use such drugs as he would any others, increasing the dose until there are either unpleasant side effects or desired beneficial effects. He would not be discouraged too early in treatment, probably settling for no less than three months of treatment and possibly treating for as long as six months before deciding on its value.

Physicians are not expected to cure every patient. They are expected to provide as much as they can for the relief of suffering and disability. Rather than risk doing less than the utmost for the patient with senile dementia, I would choose to be an optimist. I would not deceive myself or the patient about what to expect, nor would I pursue an obviously futile course indefinitely. Meanwhile, I should be most humble about what we know of senile dementia, the final affliction of life for many.

References

Ferris, S.H., Sathananthan, G., Gershon, S., and Clark, C.: Senile dementia: treatment with deanol. J. Am. Geriatr. Soc. 25:241–244, 1977.

Gaitz, C.M., Varner, R.V., and Overall, J.E.: Pharmacotherapy for organic brain syndrome in late life. Arch. Gen. Psychiatry 34:839–845, 1977.

Gygax, P., Wiernspergel, N., Meier-Ruge, W., and Bauman, T.: Effect of papaverine and dihydroergotoxine mesylate on cerebral microflow, EEG, and pO_2 in oligemic hypotension. Gerontology 24 (Supplement 1):14–22, 1978.

Heston, L.L., and Mastri, A.R.: The genetics of Alzheimer's disease: associations with hematologic malignancy and Down's syndrome. Arch. Gen. Psychiatry 34:976–981, 1977.

Hollister, L.E.: Drugs for mental disorders of old age. JAMA 234:195–198, 1975.

Kristensen, V., Olsen, M., and Theilgaard, A.: Levodopa treatment of presenile dementia. Acta psychiatr. Scand. 55:41–51, 1977.

Levy, L.L., and Wallace, J.D.: Cerebral blood flow regulation. II, Vasodilator mechanisms. Stroke 8:189–193, 1977.

Shader, R.I., Harmatz, J.S., and Salzman, C.: A new scale for clinical assessment in geriatric populations: Sandoz Clinical Assessment-Geriatric (SCAG). J. Am. Geriatr. Soc. 22 (Supplement 3):107–113, 1974.

Yesavage, J.A., Tinklenberg, J.R., Berger, P.E., and Hollister, L.E.: Vasodilators in senile dementia: a review of the literature. Arch. Gen. Psychiatry. In press, 1978.

Rational Pharmacotherapy in Dementia: Hazards of "Vasodilator Therapy"

Ira Shoulson, M.D.
University of Rochester School of Medicine and Dentistry

Vasodilator drugs were once advocated for the treatment of cerebral vascular insufficiency. Today, so-called "vasodilator alternatives" are promoted for the therapy of idiopathic cerebral dysfunction. Although drug formulation has changed and ill defined clinical disorders have become further obscured, the essential controversy endures. How useful is vasodilator therapy in cerebral vascular insufficiency? What are the hazards of treating hopeless neuropsychiatric disorders with seemingly innocuous drugs?

In the past five years, there have been noteworthy advances in neuropharmacology and in techniques of neurologic diagnosis. The rational development of levodopa therapy for the treatment of parkinsonism has heightened the standards by which therapeutic strategies are judged. Technical improvement in brain imaging has added considerable precision to neurologic evaluation. The issue of vasoactive drug therapy in idiopathic cerebral dysfunction merits reexamination in light of current knowledge and therapeutic standards.

What Is Idiopathic Cerebral Dysfunction?

Idiopathic cerebral dysfunction may go under the rubric or pseudonym of *cerebral vascular insufficiency, hardening of the arteries, organic brain syndrome, early brain failure, "selected symptoms of the elderly,"* or *dementia.* I prefer the designation *dementia,* since it is the conception least tainted by euphemism and it is the shortest term. Dementia is a symptom complex; it represents a spectrum of neuropsychiatric disorders associated with intellectual failure, and it usually indicates widespread dysfunction of the central nervous system. Signs and symptoms most frequently observed in demented patients reflect impairment of the mental operations of memory, learning, attention, judgment, perception, emotion, and language. Dementia is an exceedingly broad term, since more than one hundred specific and well delineated diseases may produce features of intellectual impairment. The designation *dementia* is analogous to the usage of the terms *congestive heart failure* and *renal failure* in cardiology and nephrology—it carries little diagnostic specificity.

The contention that dementia is caused by a variety of identifiable disorders is supported by Wells' summary of 222 patients with presumably unspecified intellectual failure (Wells, 1977). On the basis of a comprehensive clinical evaluation, a specific diagnosis could be formulated in 97 percent of the surveyed population. In a more recent study by Seltzer and Sherwin, 96 percent of patients with previously unclassified organic brain syndrome were identified as having one or more specific diseases accounting for their mental symptoms (Seltzer and Sherwin, 1978). In these studies, there is some variation in the occurrence of different types of dementing diseases. Different institutional settings and referral patterns may partly account for the variation. Nevertheless, there are remarkable similarities in the surveys. Approximately half the patients with previously unclassified organic brain syndrome were eventually identified as suffering from Alzheimer's-type dementia (ATD). An additional 15 percent of patients had cerebrovascular causes, best designated as Multiinfarct dementia (MID). ATD and MID can be distinguished from other disorders on the basis of clinical and laboratory evaluation (Wells, 1977; Joynt and Shoulson, 1979). Alcoholic, posttraumatic, infectious, space-occupying, genetic, nutritional, metabolic, toxic, and psychiatric causes may alone or in combination produce clinical features of intellectual decline. Space will not be devoted to a discussion of each type of dementia syndrome, but a brief consideration of ATD and MID is warranted.

Alzheimer's Type Dementia (ATD)

ATD is a central nervous system disorder of adulthood; patients develop slow but progressive mental decline with the most prominent features of cognitive dysfunction involving the operations of memory, language, perception, and emotion. The pattern and course of mental impairment are distinctive, in contrast to the vague symptoms attributed to idiopathic cerebral dysfunction. Variable degrees of cortical atrophy and ventricular dilatation are seen on computerized tomography. There is increasing support for the proposition that clinically definable ATD correlates closely with pathologically confirmed Alzheimer's disease (Katzman et al., 1978). Widespread neuron loss and accumulations of tangles and plaques in cortical and limbic regions reflect the pathologic substrate of ATD. Distinctions between senile and presenile dementias are not justified on either clinical or pathologic grounds. Although the incidence of ATD increases rapidly with age, symptoms may appear at any time from the fourth decade to well into the senium.

Multiinfarct Dementia (MID)

MID is the nomenclature that most accurately describes patients with stepwise intellectual deterioration who have suffered repeated cerebral infarctions (Hachinski et al., 1974). In contrast to ATD, onset of MID is typically abrupt, and deterioration is usually fluctuating and stepwise. Hypertension is the major risk factor predisposing an individual to the development of MID. Symptoms and signs reflect the focal nature of localized cerebral injury. Clinical features of MID are distinctive and recognizable (Wells, 1978), and weighted ischemia scores have added quantification to the evaluation process (Hachinski et al., 1975). MID usually results from the incessant ravages of hypertension, with the appearance of multiple lacunar infarcts. A virtually identical decline in intellect may be due to emboli originating from extracranial vessels or from the heart. Cerebral arteriosclerosis or the progressive narrowing of intracerebral arteries is not a typical finding. In most patients with MID, computed tomography shows scattered cerebral radiolucencies reflecting the multiple infarct sites.

Evaluation of the Demented Patient

Specific and accurate diagnosis of the dementias has yielded substantial gains. In the studies reviewing patients with unspecified organic brain syndrome (Wells, 1977; Seltzer and Sherwin, 1978), identification of the causative disease was of therapeutic consequence in more than half the patients. I would contend that a systematic and comprehensive clinical assessment has a salutary influence on all patients and their families. Yet, evaluation of the demented patient is not often accomplished with ease. Incomplete historical information, uncooperative patients, and vague clinical findings present difficult obstacles. However, the skilled and experienced clinician is not deterred by these impediments. Using ineffective vasoactive drugs is a flimsy substitute for obtaining an assiduous history and completing a thorough examination. Patients should not be excluded from indicated laboratory evaluation on the basis of advanced age. The formulation of a specific diagnosis in demented patients is the initial and obligatory step in rational pharmacotherapy.

Rational Pharmacotherapy In Dementia

Just as symptomatic analgesic therapy is not indicated for patients with undiagnosed chest pain, vasodilator drugs should not be administered to patients with idiopathic cerebral dysfunction or to those with other unidentified dementias. Intellectual impairment due to hypothyroidism obviously requires thyroid replacement therapy. Likewise, patients with depressive pseudodementias should be treated specifically with antidepressant therapy. Physicians need not be driven to the necessity of striking out into the dark. Rational pharmacotherapy in dementia is premised on the orderly clarification of symptoms, signs, and laboratory data. The aim is to identify accurately the specific disorder(s) underlying the symptoms. The evaluation process will eventually indicate specific therapy.

ATD

Although the pathogenesis of ATD remains obscure, new knowledge has been generated so that rational approaches can be applied to investigation and patient care. Neurochemical studies from postmortem specimens of patients with ATD point to prominent impairment of central cholinergic neurotransmission. Choline acetyltransferase, the enzyme mediating acetylcholine synthesis, is significantly reduced in Alzheimer's disease (Perry, 1977). The distribution of enzyme reduction corresponds to the major sites of pathologic change. Despite the diminution of choline acetyltransferase, cholinergic receptor binding activity does not decline (Davies and Verth, 1977). This observation suggests that the cholinergic receptors are functionally preserved in ATD, and that precursor or agonist therapy may effectively restore cholinergic neurotransmission and ameliorate symptoms. The recent achievements of dopaminergic therapy in Parkinson's disease are well recognized. A similar therapeutic tactic is being tried in patients with ATD. Admittedly, pharmacologic manipulation of the cholinergic system is more complex than reestablishment of dopaminergic neurotransmission. However, an analytic and well ordered approach to ATD is attended by few risks and great promise.

MID

Selective neurochemical disturbances have not as yet been identified in MID. Nevertheless, such predisposing causes of MID as hypertension and atheromatous embolic disease are well recognized. Once MID is distinguished from organic brain syndrome, focused therapy should be considered in an effort to halt intellectual decline. Antihypertensive therapy, anticoagulants, platelet suppressant drugs, or vascular surgery may improve cognitive performance if early features of MID are recognized. Studies in well defined populations are clearly needed to assess the efficacy of rational therapeutic alternatives. Since cerebral blood flow is reduced in patients with MID (Hachinski et al., 1975), attempts to improve flow with vasodilator drugs should likewise be considered. However, there are limits to the restoration of cerebral blood flow in patients whose vasoregulatory mechanisms are seriously impaired. Cerebral vascular resistance is controlled by a complex interaction of chemical and neurogenic parameters, and the relative contribution of these factors in MID is unknown (Kuschinsky and Wahl, 1978). Application of sophisticated techniques to measure regional blood flow and of computerized analysis will help to clarify the nature and reversibility of impaired cerebral blood flow in MID.

ATD and MID have been discussed in greater detail because they are common causes of dementia that frequently pose diagnostic difficulty. The reader is referred to recent reviews of evaluation and care in the other specific disorders causing dementia (Wells, 1977; Katzman et al., 1978; Joynt and Shoulson, 1979).

Guidelines for Treating Dementia Patients

Although identification of specific causes of dementia will indicate rational therapy, some therapeutic reminders and guidelines prove helpful in the care of all patients with dementia.

1. Patients with intellectual decline usually have other coexistent organic disease. One or more organic disorders may produce symptoms of dementia. Attention to the multiple causes presents a challenge to the clinician, who needs to select appropriate drugs and to avoid unnecessary polypharmacy.

2. Patients with dementia tend to minimize symptoms of intellectual failure. Acute recognition of symptoms is required in formulating therapeutic plans. The failure to elicit or to recognize clinical impairment may result in errors of diagnostic omission. Depressive pseudodementia is a frequently unrecognized source of cognitive impairment.

3. Most patients with dementia have limited perceptual resources and, therefore, are exquisitely sensitive to environmental changes. For example, evening confusion may result from

perceptual inadequacies in failing to appreciate natural alterations. Anticipating the consequences of changing cues helps to minimize the impact of a modified environment. It also follows that patients with dementia appear to improve when the environment is stabilized. Regimentation in a drug investigation produces its own stability, which may partly account for the "continued improvement" found when placebo is substituted for active drug.

4. Elderly individuals, and demented patients in particular, are more susceptible to the adverse effects of drugs. Heightened drug sensitivity warrants consideration in the assessment of therapeutic benefit and risk. A drug that is benign for normal volunteers may produce untoward effects in patients with intellectual problems. Patients with dementia, like children, come to medical attention with nonspecific symptoms of specific diseases. Symptomatic therapy of confusion, anorexia, incontinence, unsteadiness, weakness, dizziness, or agitation leads to a predictably poor outcome. In short, the demented patient should be evaluated with the same attention that is provided to those with intact mental operations.

Proponents of vasodilator therapy for cerebral dysfunction advance the argument that these drugs are devoid of significant toxicity. However, the annals of pharmacology attest to the predictable and recognizable toxicity of genuinely effective drugs. Although vasodilator drugs do not usually produce major side effects, there are hazards of vasodilator therapy that go beyond the usual considerations of risk and benefit.

Hazards of Vasodilator Therapy in Patients with Dementia

In this discussion, "vasodilator therapy" is used in a generic connotation and is not intended to refer to the chemical nature or pharmacologic activity of these compounds. Vasodilator drugs are considered to be those vasoactive agents advocated for the treatment of "selective symptoms of the elderly" that result from cerebrovascular insufficiency or idiopathic cerebral dysfunction. They may be "authentic" vasodilators such as papaverine or "alternatives to vasodilator therapy" such as the dihydrogenated ergot alkaloid (DHEA) compounds. Of the latter, Hydergine is the most widely used. It is recognized that papaverine and DHEA differ substantially in their biologic properties, but the consideration of vasodilator therapy rests on the issues of efficacy and clinical use. The chemistry and pharmacology of these drugs are mere sidelights to the controversy.

The haphazard administration of vasodilator drugs to patients with dementia is contrary to scientific therapeutics. It is this concern that represents the major drawback of vasodilator therapy. There is no compelling scientific evidence to support the claims of those who advocate vasodilator therapy. Methodologic problems in the reports comparing Hydergine with papaverine and with placebo have been examined by other critics (Prien, 1973; Hughes et al., 1976). In the only investigation employing a double-blind crossover design, no significant difference was found between Hydergine and placebo (Rehman, 1973). In the published studies, little care was taken to delineate the type of dementing disease being treated. It is often implied that patients with ATD and MID were evaluated, but diagnostic criteria are rarely mentioned. Certainly, the efficacy of a drug in systemic lupus erythematosus would not be evaluated without taking great pains to define the criteria for diagnosis and for inclusion of subjects in the study. This standard applies even more so to the evaluation of patients with dementia, in whom pathologic verification cannot readily be obtained. The reviewers draw a restrained conclusion that the vasodilator drugs would seem to be of minor value in therapy of dementia.

Failure to characterize neuropsychiatric deficits adequately is a serious problem in the design of the vasodilator studies. The severity or duration of symptoms prior to treatment is rarely mentioned. Poorly defined symptoms such as "bothersomeness, uncooperativeness, or unsociability" are selected for assessment. Substantial variability in drug efficacy is always found. Symptoms of confusion, mood change, or impairment in memory and alertness are not specific. If a vasodilator drug is helpful for confusion, alertness, and depression, why was it not found to be significantly effective in allied symptoms of bothersomeness, uncooperativeness, and unsociability? Something is amiss! When evaluating nonspecific symptoms in unspecified disorders, it is not surprising to discover changes in some features but not in others, regardless of the drug being studied.

The rationale for vasodilator therapy in dementia is based on the assumption that impaired cerebral blood flow relates to the genesis of symptoms. In ATD, cerebral blood flow may be marginally reduced in some patients, but the reduction is in proportion to brain atrophy, and blood flow appears adequate for the demands of cerebral metabolism. In MID, cerebral blood flow is reduced commensurate with the degree of intellectual failure (Hachinski et al., 1975). Papaverine produces a modest increase in cerebral blood flow and a decrease in vascular resistance, whereas Hydergine exerts no consistent effect on these parameters (McHenry, 1972). This observation supports the rationale for an investigation of papaverine as treatment for MID. Surprisingly, there are no reported studies objectively assessing papaverine in a well defined group of patients with MID. It seems unfortunate that the inadequate standards of available vasodilator investigations have helped foster a situation in which a warranted and well-designed vasodilator trial has not been undertaken.

Conclusion

Retardation of drug development and therapeutic investigation may represent an unforeseen hazard of vasodilator therapy. The dearth of effective therapy in dementia should not be disguised by well-intended but unjustifiable claims of drug potency. It is expected that advances in the neural sciences will continue to provide rational approaches to pharmacotherapy. It is hoped that new drugs will be developed and evaluated in an objective and orderly fashion. In promoting drugs for idiopathic cerebral dysfunction, attention may be inadvisably diverted from the bona fide neuropharmacologic effects exerted by papaverine and DHEA. Efforts to explore the therapeutic potential of the vasodilator drugs should not be abandoned. On the other hand, the haphazard use of vasodilator therapy in dementia should be forsaken for intellectual rigor, rational pharmacotherapy, and thoughtful care.

References

Davies, P., and Verth, A.H.: Regional distribution of muscarinic acetylcholine receptor in normal and Alzheimer's type dementia brains. Brain Res. 138:385–392, 1977.

Hachinski, V.C., Lassen, N.A., and Marshall, J.: Multi-infarct dementia. Lancet 2:207–210, 1974.

Hachinski, V.C., et. al.: Cerebral blood flow in dementia. Arch. Neurol. 32:632–637, 1975.

Hughes, J.R., Williams, J.G., and Currier, R.D.: An ergot alkaloid preparation (Hydergine) in the treatment of dementia: critical review of the clinical literature. J. Am. Geriatr. Soc. 34:490–497, 1976.

Joynt, R.J., and Shoulson, I.: Dementia. In Heilman, K.M., *Clinical Neuropsychology*, New York, Oxford University Press, 1979.

Katzman, R., Terry, R.D., and Bick, K.L.: *Alzheimer's Disease: Senile Dementia and Related Disorders.* New York, Raven Press, 1978.

Kuschinsky, W., and Wahl, M.: Local chemical and neurogenic regulation of cerebral vascular resistance. Physiol. Rev. 58:656–689, 1978.

McHenry, L.C.: Cerebral vasodilator therapy in stroke. Stroke 3:686–691, 1972.

Perry, E.K.: Neurotransmitter enzyme abnormalities in senile dementia. J. Neurol. Sci. 34:247–265, 1977.

Prien, R.F.: Chemotherapy in chronic organic brain syndrome—a review of the literature. Psychopharmacal. Bull. 9:5–20, 1973.

Rehman, S.A.: Two trials comparing "Hydergine" with placebo in the treatment of patients suffering from cerebrovascular insufficiency. Curr. Med. Res. Opin. 1:456, 1973.

Seltzer, B., and Sherwin, I.: "Organic brain syndromes": an empirical study and critical review. Am. J. Psychiatry 135:13–21, 1978.

Wells, C.E.: *Dementia,* 2nd edition. Philadelphia, F.A. Davis Company, 1977.

Wells, C.E.: Role of stroke in dementia. Stroke 9:1–3, 1978.

18

Can We Do Without Opium Derivatives?

Thou hast the keys of Paradise, oh, just, subtle, and mighty opium!

De Quincey, *Confessions of an English Opium Eater*

Opium . . . the Creator himself seems to prescribe, for we often see the scarlet poppy growing in the cornfields, as if it were foreseen that wherever there is hunger there must also be pain to be soothed.

Oliver Wendell Holmes, *Medical Essays*

Opium once given is gone beyond your power to recall.

Peter Mere Latham, *General Remarks on the Practice of Medicine*

Introduction

Few areas of medical controversy generate more confusion than the illicit use of medically useful drugs. There is a recurrent temptation to apply sanctions that might make sense for purely illicit drugs but do not make sense for legal medicines. The banning of heroin from legitimate medical prescribing half a century ago in the United States deprived American patients of a useful drug and did little to solve the problem of narcotic abuse.

As Beaver and Brill both point out, the controversy about the need for other opium derivatives in medical practice has also suffered from confusion by extramedical issues such as shortages that might occur in time of national emergency and the diversion of opium to the illegal heroin market.

Beaver pleads that there are compelling reasons why the elimination of opium products would deleteriously affect both medical research and practice. These include the utility of morphine in the treatment of severe pain and acute pulmonary edema, the antitussive and analgesic efficacy of codeine, the antidotal importance of naloxone, and the deficiencies of the synthetic substitutes. Beaver also discusses cogently the special importance of opium derivatives to research in these fields.

Brill counters by pointing to the fact that many doctors seem to use synthetic substitutes quite happily, notably in other countries, but also in the U.S. There is little question that medicine could survive without opium products, although Brill acknowledges that there would be at least some confusion and inferior medical care. He and Beaver independently come to the same conclusion–i.e., that the important question is not "*Could* we do without opium derivatives?" but "*Should* we?" One hopes that future authorities on this problem will be as thoughtful and precise as are our two contributors.

LOUIS LASAGNA, M.D.

Should We Do Without Opium Derivatives?

Henry Brill, M.D.
State University of New York at Stony Brook

Introduction to a Controversy

Experts' answers to this question here and abroad repeatedly have been a firm and unqualified "Yes" within recent years (Eddy, 1973; WHO, 1972). Yet, in 1973, the House of Delegates of the American Medical Association (AMA) stated in a formal resolution that "... opium derivatives are essential in medical practice ... ." Furthermore, on October 18, 1974, the President of the AMA, reacting to a continuing serious depletion of American opium reserve stocks, appealed directly to President Ford for assistance in this matter and reaffirmed the position that "... some opium products are essential in medical practice ... ."

This seems to constitute a total contradiction between two sets of medical authorities. The issue is of more than academic interest because questions about dropping opium-based products (OBP) officially from medical practice in whole or in part have been raised by governmental authorities in Washington repeatedly over the last 30 years. Experience suggests that such long standing and oft repeated questions do not just fade away, and, in this case, they may be expected to recur under conditions of national emergency, preparations for an emergency, or public outcry concerning street use of heroin. Under such conditions, the medical establishment may again be called upon to take a position on this issue. It is the purpose of this paper to explore various aspects of this issue, including its background and the various arguments that have been used by both sides in the debate, and to reexamine certain crucial definitions.

Background

As already mentioned, the question of opium use is not new to officials in Washington. It goes back at least to 1928, when the New York Bureau of Social Hygiene was in the process of persuading the National Research Council (NRC) to accept sponsorship of the Bureau's Committee on Drug Addiction. As an inducement, perhaps, it was proposed that one of the future research directions for the Committee would be "replacement (through chemistry) of all present use of addiction alkaloids by substitutes having no addiction properties" (Eddy, 1973). Obviously, the hope was that chemistry could solve the problems of drug dependence that it had created through its past advances. The idea was based on more than a theoretical construct because, at the time, everyone was much encouraged by the way that cocaine abuse had waned after the introduction of procaine in 1905, and this was the model that the NRC group had in mind.

In any event, the Committee was transferred eventually to the National Research Council, and it became an important quasi-official source of consultation on drug dependence matters for various governmental agencies. In addition, the Committee on Drug Addiction became a major organizing factor for American research in this field. Its first recorded consultation on the medical use of opium derivatives came in 1943, and it had to do with methods that would conserve the stocks of opium that were being depleted because of World War II interference with supplies. Opium alkaloids and derivatives were recognized as essential to medical practice and, after the war, concern about this issue led the government to maintain stockpiles against future contingencies. At the same time, various governmental agencies were continually looking for ways to reduce or even to abolish the need for these drugs, whose supply line was so precarious. This led to correspondence between the NRC Committee on Drug Addiction and Narcotics, later known simply as the Committee on Drug Dependence, and the government. The context of the original discussions seems to have faded in the course of time, but the conclusions apparently left a certain residue in the collective unconscious of the bureaucracy, which may account in part for the way this question has recurred.

A brief chronology of this sequence and of some closely related items may be helpful in understanding the nature of the questions that were posed and what the answers were intended to mean.

A Chronology of Attempts to Replace Opium-Based Products with Synthetics

1928 "Replacement of all present use of addiction alkaloids by substitutes having no addiction properties" is set as a goal for the NRC Committee on Drug Addiction, on the model of procaine as a substitute for cocaine.

1938–40 Pethidine synthesized in Germany and introduced in the U.S.

1941–46 Increasing concern in the U.S. about possible loss of opium supplies (World War II).

1943 The NRC Committee asked about the use of pethidine (Demerol) and desomorphine in an attempt to conserve morphine.

1945 Methadone data brought to the U.S. from Germany.

1947 Munitions Board asks whether any synthetic drugs capable of satisfying an appreciable amount of essential military and civilian requirements in a national emergency exist. The Committee replies that methadone (Amidone) is the most promising of the synthetic drugs.

1951 The NRC Committee, in a review of an Armed Forces Medical Supply List, recommends that half the U.S. stockpile be methadone and half be morphine.

1951 The Munitions Board inquires about the replaceability of opium derivatives. The Committee replies that all uses may be replaced by synthetic substances now known, "... except that a complete answer cannot be given that replacement of codeine for cough is as safe as codeine".

1952 The Munitions Board renews its inquiry, and the Committee reiterates its stand with respect to pain remedies but defers reply pending study of dextromethorphan.

1955 Propoxyphene described as an analgesic (Robbins, see Eddy et al., 1957).

1960 The Division of Health Mobilization of the Public Health Service (PHS) inquires about the stockpiling of opiates. The Committee replies on April 8, 1960, that needs for pain and cough relief can now be met by synthetic substances.

1961 The Committee supplements its previous statement with the proviso that this applies only to conditions of national emergency (Cochin and Harris, 1975).

1968 The Department of Commerce requests advice about stockpiling, and the Committee advises that half the stockpile be made up of 5 synthetics and half of codeine and morphine. An increasing trend toward the use of synthetics is noted, but the importance of physicians' familiarity with a drug is pointed out.

1971 The Drug Enforcement Administration asks the Committee to comment on the effect of removal of opium and its derivatives by substitution of synthetics. The question is referred to the Drug Abuse Council, and a study is set up with the cooperation of the AMA (Cochin and Harris, 1975).

1971 The U.S. proposes to reduce supplies of opium from abroad to control the heroin addiction problem.

1971 Two members of the Committee testify against the proposal.

1972 Opium Pact with Turkey announced.

1972 The World Health Organization (WHO) publishes report (WHO, 1972), with the final conclusion that the natural and semisynthetic opiates may be considered "not indispensable in the practice of modern medicine."

1973 The AMA takes formal notice of the shortage of opium supplies and declares officially that "opium derivatives are still essential to good medical practice."

1973 U.S. releases 58 percent of its stockpile of opium for commercial use as needed.

1974 Turkey sets aside U.S. Opium Pact.

1974 AMA President appeals to President Ford for personal intervention to secure essential supplies of opium for medical purposes.

A Digression on Codeine

As one reviews this chronology and considers the long list of uses of OBPs, it is easy to lose sight of the fact that codeine accounts for no less than 95 percent of the opium used in the U.S. (Mallinckrodt, Merck, and Penick, 1974), and this is essentially the case worldwide. Despite the heavy emphasis on the use of codeine for control of cough, this use is decreasing; in 1974, 25 percent of U.S. codeine was used for that purpose and for 1975, the figure projected was 20 percent. Thus, the use of codeine for analgesia accounts for a growing percentage of total use, which appears to be increasing (U.N., 1972). The U.S. total for codeine rose from 16,582 kgm in 1967 to 35,000 kgm in 1973; processors projected a further jump to 42,500 for 1974. (Mallinckrodt, Merck, and Penick 1974; INCB, 1977). These figures compare with the total U.S. use of morphine, which was 435 kgm in 1971. It thus appears that quantitatively, the problem of OBPs is the need for codeine. All other uses shrink to small dimensions by comparison. Codeine, whether used for pain or for cough, is used predominantly in combination with other medications. Despite such extensive use, it has given rise to only sporadic complaints about abuse. Finally, it appears that the 1973 market stringency of opium supplies noted in the chronology was due at least in part to the upsurge in the use of codeine.

Are Opium Derivatives Essential to Good Medical Practice?

Although most opium is used as codeine (predominantly for analgesia and in combination with other medications), there are other OBPs that, taken as a group, are considered to be essential by almost all physicians. A 1973 survey (Cochin and Harris, 1975) by the American Medical Association showed that only 5 percent of physicians supported the idea of getting along without OBPs, whereas 95 percent opposed it. Another survey (IMS, 1974) done at about the same time gave very similar results. Equally impressive was the reaction of organized medicine in the face of a stringency of supply coupled with an increase in demand in 1973. The AMA House of Delegates voted a resolution on the matter, and the AMA President supported their conclusion that medical practice could not get along without opium derivatives (see chronology). It is to be noted that the AMA cited nine references in support of their position, and that two of these were by scientists who were at that time members of the NRC Committee. Both referred to testimony before the House Select Committee on Crime.

Cochin and Harris confirmed that the attitude of European physicians was quite in line with that of the Americans. The feeling was particularly strong in Britain, where medical opposition had been sufficiently strong to block any efforts to remove even heroin from the list of legal drugs. There is, by and large, an overwhelming consensus among practicing physicians that opium derivatives are essential to good medicine.

Some Flaws in the Consensus

In a society so firmly committed to the adversary system in public affairs, one may be sure that the entire issue of OBPs will be reconsidered if it ever again comes up for discussion, even with a 95 percent consensus of professional opinion against the removal of OBPs. When we examine the figures of the surveys in greater detail, the appearance of unanimity tends to become blurred if not completely lost. This is especially true if we study some of the data on actual usage of these drugs. The AMA survey indicates that 23 percent of physicians never use codeine for mild acute pain, whereas 41 percent use propoxyphene and its combinations most frequently. For severe acute pain, 14 percent never use codeine and 16 percent never use morphine, but 60 percent use meperidine most frequently for this indication. For chronic pain, 14 percent never use codeine and 41 percent never use morphine, whereas 22 percent use meperidine and another 16 percent use pentazocine most frequently. For cough, 57 percent never use codeine alone, 52 percent use codeine combinations most frequently, and 28 percent use dextromethorphan combinations most. Diphenoxylate (as Lomotil) is used for treatment of diarrhea most frequently by 58 percent; only 36 percent use opium preparations more often. Interestingly enough, 46 percent did not use naloxone for narcotic overdose, and only 30 percent used it the most; another 5 percent preferred levallorphan.

Overall judgments are even more confusing. Of physicians surveyed, 22 percent felt that codeine could be dispensed with, 16 percent felt that morphine could be dropped, and over 35 percent judged all other OBPs nonessential. Finally and most surprising is the fact that 36 percent felt that the unavailability of opium and its products would have no effect on quality of care, and only 22 percent stated that this would greatly decrease the quality of care.

Certain market figures seem to reflect the same variability (IMS, 1974). In 1972, OBPs accounted for only 22 percent of pharmacy sales of analgesics and only 20 percent of hospital purchases of such drugs. Even in the case of antitussives, OBPs account for only 47.5 percent of pharmacy sales and 25.8 percent of sales to hospitals. This agrees with the data already noted to the effect that sales of analgesic codeine preparations are about three times as great as sales of codeine antitussives ($258,000,000 compared with $86,000,000).

The variability of practice with respect to use of OBPs and synthetics is not limited to the U.S., although I was unable to find comparable surveys for other countries. Available international data do nevertheless provide some indications of similar situations elsewhere (INCB 1972, 1973, and 1977). The U.N. International Narcotics Control Board lists some 60 drugs controlled as opium-type narcotics (OBPs and synthetics). Of these, Russia seems to use only 7, Holland 18, and the U.S. about 30. International per capita use of medicinal narcotics also varies strikingly; in the case of morphine, it is 0.26 kgm per million of population in Japan, 0.62 kgm in Sweden, and 2.07 kgm in the U.S. During the same year (1971), the corresponding figures for codeine were 133 kgm for Sweden, 209 kgm for U.K., 126 kgm for U.S., 87 kgm for Russia, and 214 kgm for Switzerland. In the case of pethidine (meperidine), we find that use amounts to 52 kgm per million of the population in the U.S., 13 kgm in U.K.,4 kgm in the Netherlands, 19 kgm in Australia, and 0.7 kgm in Japan. Obviously, such figures must be interpreted with caution, but it is still hard to escape the conclusion that much of the variation is not intrinsic to drug actions per se but it reflects variability of medical practices in various parts of the world. This is, of course, confirmed by common experience.

One fact that does stand out in the larger figures is that the long-term trend has been toward the replacement of all OBPs (except codeine) by the use of synthetics. The worldwide use of pethidine rose from 13,758 kgm in 1956 to 20,288 kgm in 1970, whereas during the same period, medical use of morphine fell from 4,377 kgm to 2,474 kgm (U.N., 1972). Worldwide use of codeine has, however, increased from 117,045 kgm in 1967 to 150,290 kgm in 1971. This trend reinforces what we have already seen in the American figures—that the use of OBPs is primarily the use of codeine. The usage volume of other drugs is relatively small, however essential the indications for their administration may be.

Are These the Elements of a Quiescent But Unsettled Controversy?

Although 90 to 95 percent of physicians in the U.S. oppose the removal of OBPs from the pharmacopoeia, the overwhelming consensus appears to be lost as one looks more closely at the data in the polls by the AMA and the IMS and in the actual figures of drug usage. One can anticipate that in the event of renewal of the controversy, the charge will be made that since so many physicians actually find synthetics preferable to OBPs for various individual indications, overall attitude about total removal of OBPs from use is nothing more than a blind resistance to change. However, this would be an unusual charge to be brought against a profession that has been so vigorously criticized for the way in which it has adopted almost a whole new pharmacopoeia of potent new drugs during the last few decades. If the profession is simply resistant to change of its treatment habits, this resistance must be virtually limited to one class of drugs, since little else has remained the same. Yet the statements of the experts both here and abroad will undoubtedly be quoted, even though one can argue that inconsistencies among the various survey findings convey an entirely different message than they seem to—namely, that clinical judgment is essentially holistic and that this aspect is lost in the atomistic approach of a detailed questionnaire, no matter how carefully drawn it may be. One may also raise technical issues with respect to the surveys themselves, yet common experience confirms that there is a very large amount of variability in clinical practice, and there are probably no OBPs that have not been abandoned in favor of synthetics by sizable segments of the medical profession. This leads directly to the question of why all physicians should not do what various groups have done each with a different segment of the OBP, some practicing without use of morphine, others without codeine, etc.

If We Can Get Along Without Opium Derivatives, Should We or Our Patients Have to Do So?

As in so many other controversies, much depends on how one defines the issues and on whether one is asking the proper question. So long as the issue remains "Can we get along without opium derivatives?", it is open to arguments derived from the actual practice of medicine. This may be used to prove the affirmative of the case, and, in addition, we must remember that expert opinion has long held the affirmative to be true. Yet the same expert opinion has held that although it would be technically feasible from the strictly pharmacologic point of view, the actual choice of medication is best determined by many additional factors. When the expert committee was asked about substitution of OBPs by synthetics, it was in the context of a national emergency or preparations for a national emergency. They did not mean to imply that this answer was valid for all conditions of medical practice, and they said so explicitly in January, 1961. Furthermore, two members of this same committee testified against "the feasibility of replacing natural opium products with totally synthetic substances in medical practice" before the Select Committee on Crime of the House of Representatives. This was on April 26, 1971, during a period when national policy was moving toward such a procedure in an effort to control the heroin problem by cutting off production of opium.

The WHO Expert Committee said that "the natural and semisynthetic opiates may be considered not indispensable in the practice of modern medicine" (WHO, 1972). (An interesting and relatively minor exception may possibly be naloxone, which has clear advantages over available existing synthetic antagonists.) The WHO Committee did not say that OBPs were inferior or that the synthetics were preferred, nor did they point to any reason why OBPs should be discarded. In fact, they said specifically that none of the drugs under consideration is ideal in its actions—none is fully effective and none is without its adverse effects—and they called for development of better studies of overall effectiveness of the analgesics and antitussives, as well as increased facilities for such work.

The Burden of Proof

Depending on how one defines the question, the burden of proof falls on opposite sides of this controversy. If one asks what can be done under conditions of national emergency, the burden of proof would seem to fall on those who say that substitution cannot be made. Under certain conditions, it would be far better to have an adequate stockpile of synthetics than to let all drugs of this type run out of supply on the grounds that only the OBPs will serve.

On the other hand, if the question is what should be done under normal conditions of medical practice or whether natural opium products and their derivatives are so unnecessary that they may be discarded for nonemergency reasons, the burden of proof must clearly fall on those who would ask for substitution by synthetics. Up to this time, I know of no good evidence or authoritative opinion that there would be a medical advantage to patients as a result of such a change. In fact, if the proposal were to envision a total withdrawal of OBPs, perhaps abrupt and probably enforced by penalty of prosecution, one could envision a chaotic situation in which physicians would be forced to use medications with which they are not familiar, despite the fact that physicians perform best with drugs that they know well and with ones whose actions and adverse effects are familiar to them through experience. One can anticipate that under circumstances of a forced transition, doctors would soon learn to adapt to drugs whose spectrum of effects is at least quantitatively different—but one can also anticipate that in the course of such a forced transition, the patient would pay a price.

Conclusion

Can we get along without opium derivatives? Everything depends on how we understand the question. This essay describes how the issue first arose and how it changed its significance as circumstances changed over the years. As long ago as 1928, it was proposed that nonaddicting synthetics be developed to replace the opiates, much as cocaine had been replaced by procaine. Then, during World War II, the aim was to conserve stocks of opium by substituting synthetics as far as possible. Finally, the time came when governmental agencies, which were stockpiling opiate-type drugs against possible future national emergencies with a cutoff of overseas supplies, sought advice as to whether we could get along without opium derivatives. At first, the question was answered with a qualified "Yes." Then, by 1960, the qualification was removed and the answer was a full "Yes." I know of no disagreement with these pronouncements, nor with the similar opinion of the WHO Committee in 1972.

When a similar question was raised in 1971, the aim was to substitute synthetics for OBPs to reduce the need for cultivation of opium poppies and in turn to help cut off supplies of the American heroin traffic. At that point, two members of the NRC Committee who had joined in the opinion that we could get along without OBPs testified against the proposed measures to cut opium supplies. Shortly afterward, in 1973–74, a shortage of opium actually did develop in the U.S. for apparently unrelated reasons. Organized medicine reacted vigorously through the AMA, taking the position that opium-based products were essential to good medical practice. Field surveys taken about the same time showed that no less than 95 percent of doctors opposed removal of OBPs from the market, and a sampling of European opinion elicited a similar response.

At one time, such an overwhelming consensus of professional opinion would have been more than enough to deal with such a proposal, but today there is a strong commitment to the adversary procedure for settling such issues. If the question were to come up again, the case for the affirmative is likely to be thoroughly explored, and this case is surprisingly strong if we ask the simple question "Can we get along without OBPs?" Even the surveys that showed a 95 percent consensus against the proposal could be reinterpreted to show that the marked scattering of actual individual preferences means that the transition from OBPs to synthetics has already taken place, even if in piecemeal fashion, and that for every use of OBPs, one can find many physicians who prefer synthetics. The preferences are not only variable but they are contradictory.

Finally, it can be argued that there is a trend toward synthetics in actual volume of usage of certain natural compounds. For example, 435 kgm of morphine were used throughout the United States in 1971, but only 330 were projected for 1978. At this point, it becomes clear that different questions are being addressed when contradictory answers are given. Physicians generally were responding to the question "*Should* (not *can*) we get along without OBP; is it wise and what is to be gained or lost?" This brings up issues that have to do with (1) basic medical practices, (2) the need to use drugs with which the physician is familiar, and (3) the logic of making changes only when there is a clear advantage. Failure to deal with these factors leads to criticisms about "me too" drugs and to unpleasant surprises. Also, in the debate about complex issues, it is easy to forget the simple fact that codeine manufacture accounts for 95 percent of U.S. opium imports, and that codeine use has increased sharply despite rising prices: in 1967, the U.S. used 16,582 kgm (INCB, 1971), and the projection for 1978 is 46,700 kgm (INCB, 1977).

Thus, the final issue in this controversy, as is often the way with controversies, boils down to the issue "What is the question?" Also, one may ask, "Where does the burden of proof lie?"

References

AMA: Resolution of House of Delegates, 1973.

Brill, H.: Testimony before the House Select Committee on Crime. April 26, 1971.

Cochin, Joseph, and Harris, Louis: Synthetic substitutes for opiate alkaloids, a feasibility study. Washington, D.C., The Drug Abuse Council, 1975.

Eddy, Nathan B.: The National Research Council involvement in the opiate problem 1928–1971. Washington, D.C., National Academy of Sciences, 1973.

Eddy, N.B., Halbach, H., and Braenden, O.: Synthetic substances with morphine-like effect. Bull. WHO, 17:569–863, 1957.

Greentree, Leonard B. (editorial): No opium for pain—a threatening medical crisis. N. Engl. J. Med. 291:1411–1412, 1974.

IMS Research Group: The medical need for opium based products in the United States. A study of medical opinion and usage (Document commissioned by three domestic processors and several major formulators of products containing opium derivatives). Ambler, Pa., IMS, 1974.

International Narcotics Control Board: Statistics on narcotic drugs for 1971. New York, United Nations, 1972.

International Narcotics Control Board: Estimated world requirements of narcotic drugs and estimates of world production of opium in 1974 and 1978. New York, United Nations, 1973 and 1977.

Mallinckrodt Inc., Merck and Co., and S.B. Penick and Co.: Projected opium supply and demand in the United States 1974–78. Mimeograph report. September, 1974.

WHO (Report of a Scientific Group): Opiates and their alternates for pain and cough relief. Geneva, WHO Technical Report Series, No. 495, 1972.

The Medical Costs of Doing Without Opium Derivatives

William T. Beaver, M.D.
Georgetown University School of Medicine and Dentistry

The question of whether we can do without opium derivatives or, as it is more often phrased, whether opium derivatives (often referred to as *opiates*) are "indispensable" in the practice of medicine has been debated intermittently for about 30 years. As such, the issue presumably qualifies as a "controversy in therapeutics," although I have never encountered a clinician or researcher who argued that patients' interests would be better served if their physicians were denied the option of prescribing opium-derived medications. The issue has invariably arisen only in contexts extraneous to the choice of optimal therapy for particular patients requiring relief of pain, cough, or diarrhea or the use of a narcotic antagonist.

Historical Background

Initially, the question of the adequacy of totally synthetic drugs as substitutes for opium derivatives related to the public health implications of an interruption of the opium supply in the event of war. More recently, interest in substituting synthetics for opium derivatives was stimulated by concern over the rising tide of heroin abuse in the United States in the late 1960s. Cochin and Harris, in the preface to their feasibility study of *Synthetic Substitutes for Opiate Alkaloids* (1975), put the issue in this perspective:

> Heroin addiction in the United States had reached nearly epidemic proportions and the cost to the public, both individually and collectively, had become staggering. It is not surprising that in such an atmosphere, many diverse and radical proposals were put forth in an attempt to solve the problem. It was only natural for one of these proposals to be a worldwide ban on opium production. The rationale for this proposal was that since heroin comes from morphine and since morphine is extracted from the opium poppy, banning the growing of the opium poppy would result in the disappearance of heroin from our streets and in the successful solution of the narcotic abuse problem. This somewhat simplistic and naive proposal received serious attention from a number of government agencies and implementation of the policy was begun before the thorough study of its feasibility and implications was initiated.

In April, 1971, The Select Committee on Crime of the House of Representatives held hearings to establish the desirability of legislation that would ban the importation of opium for medical purposes into the United States as a first step in bringing about a total eradication of worldwide opium cultivation (Pepper, 1971). In June, 1971, President Nixon sent a message to Congress, which included the following policy statement:

> . . . it is clear that the only really effective way to end heroin production is to end opium production and the growing of poppies. I will propose that as an international goal. It is essential to recognize that opium is, at present, a legitimate source of income to many of those nations which produce it. Morphine and codeine both have legitimate medical applications.
>
> It is the production of morphine and codeine for medical purposes which justifies the maintenance of opium production, and it is this production which in turn contributes to the world's heroin supply.

The development of effective substitutes for these derivatives would eliminate any valid reason for opium production. While modern medicine has developed effective and broadly-used substitutes for morphine, it has yet to provide a fully acceptable substitute for codeine. Therefore, I am directing that Federal research efforts in the United States be intensified with the aim of developing at the earliest possible date synthetic substitutes for all opium derivatives. At the same time I am requesting the Director General of the World Health Organization to appoint a study panel of experts to make periodic technical assessments of any synthetics which might replace opiates with the aim of effecting substitutions as soon as possible (Nixon, 1971).

This policy and the associated Turkish Opium Pact of 1971, which brought about suspension of cultivation of the opium poppy in Turkey, coupled with the vagaries of economics and the weather, resulted in a shortage of opiates for legitimate medical and scientific use (Cochin, 1975; Greentree, 1974). The effect on the illicit heroin supply was, at best, transitory, with the rapid emergence of Mexico as the predominant source of street heroin (DuPont, 1975).

The Byzantine political motives and maneuvers surrounding the formulation and implementation of Nixon's policy, as well as its unfortunate direct and indirect consequences, were explored in a series of Senate hearings, the record of which is aptly entitled *Poppy Politics* (1975, 1977). The more amusing aspects of this saga, and the *dramatis personae* involved, have been chronicled by Epstein (1974) in his account of the Nixon Administration's "Incredible war against the poppies."

The goal of a worldwide ban on legal cultivation of the opium poppy and the forced substitution of synthetics in the practice of medicine was eventually abandoned by the Government as a potential solution to our heroin abuse problem (DuPont, 1975). This was presumably due to the realization that (1) street heroin was coming from illicit poppy fields and not from the diversion of opium from licit cultivation, (2) existing synthetics were not totally adequate substitutes for naturally-derived alkaloids, (3) neither physicians in the United States (Seitner, 1975) nor those abroad (Cochin and Harris, 1975) would cooperate with a forced change in prescribing practices that they felt was contrary to the best interests of their patients, and (4) international support for the goal could not be achieved because of the adverse economic impact both on opium-producing countries and on most of the other opium-consuming countries of the world, in none of which is heroin abuse considered a public health or social problem.

In 1974, Turkey unilaterally rescinded the Opium Pact and resumed cultivation of the poppy. However, the period of world opium shortage, which extended from 1972 to 1977, produced substantial increases in the cost to consumers of opium-derived drugs. This increase in price for raw materials has, in turn, encouraged various countries to commence or to increase cultivation of the opium poppy, which may, ironically, result in an oversupply of these materials and the possibility of an increased diversion to illicit channels.

Current Status of the Substitution Issue

For the moment, the "controversy" as to whether we can do without opium derivatives seems somewhat academic, because there appears to be no constituency currently advocating the desirability of making opiates unavailable for legitimate medical and scientific purposes. However, this chapter does provide an opportunity to review the significance of opiates in medical practice and biomedical research and to comment briefly on the circumstances in which synthetics do and do not constitute adequate substitutes.

Previous studies dealing with this question, including reports of various expert commissions and surveys of the opinions of practicing physicians, have come to apparently diametrically opposed conclusions as to whether total synthetics could adequately substitute for opiates. For example, a WHO Scientific Group (1972) concluded that ". . . the natural and semisynthetic opiates may be considered not indispensable in the practice of modern medicine." On the other hand, an AMA survey based on the reports of a stratified sample of over 5000 practicing physicians in the United States revealed that 51 percent rated codeine and 56 percent rated morphine as "indispensable" in their medical practice, and an additional 15 percent and 13 percent respectively rated these drugs indispensable in occasional situations (Seitner, 1975). In Western Europe, a sampling of the opinion of physicians who headed medical societies or who had public health responsibilities (Cochin and Harris, 1975) indicated that almost all felt that there was no adequate substitute for codeine, and some, particularly in Great Britain, felt that morphine was likewise "indispensable to good medical practice."

In 1960, in response to a query from the Division of Health Mobilization of the Public Health Service concerning the ability of synthetics to substitute for opiates "during a period of national emergency and mobilization," the National Academy of Sciences-National Research Council (NAS/NRC) Committee on Drug Addiction and Narcotics recorded the following resolution:

> . . . The Committee agreed unanimously that needs in medicine for pain relief and now also for cough relief so far as they are supplied by substances derived directly or indirectly from opium could be met fully by synthetic substances now available and that medical practice and the health of the nation would not suffer if codeine were not available.

However, the Committee, to preclude any possible misunderstanding of its position, subsequently added the following clarification:

> . . . The Committee did not say, nor did it mean to imply or recommend that synthetics replace substances of natural origin. It only said that under conditions of a national emergency such replacement would be possible, but many factors enter into the practicality of replacement under normal conditions (cited in Cochin and Harris, 1975).

It is apparent that, pertaining to the use of particular drugs in medical practice, the term *indispensability* means different things to different practitioners and clinical pharmacologists. The indispensability of almost any therapy depends on the context in which it is viewed. There is no doubt that we can "do without opium derivatives" in the event a national emergency cuts off their supply. Under those circumstances, medical practice could "make do" with synthetics, particularly if we had access to certain synthetics currently marketed in Europe but not in the United States. Synthetics may be freely substituted for opiates in many clinical situations, and they are drugs of choice in preference to opiates in certain of these situations. However, there are many situations in which opiates are drugs of choice in preference to existing synthetics. Furthermore, opiates are fundamental research tools. The appropriate question, then, is not "Can we do without opium derivatives?" but rather "What would be the cost in terms of optimal patient care and the furtherance of biomedical research of doing without opiates?"

General Importance of Opiates

No two analgesics have identical properties. Analgesics vary in potency, in the maximal analgesia obtainable by doses that have been proved safe, in speed of onset and duration of action, and in oral/parenteral potency ratio. Solubility considerations set practical limits on the parenteral dose of certain drugs, and tissue irritation may interfere with their chronic administration. Potent analgesics differ in their effect on mood, their tendency to produce sedation, their abuse liability, their side effect profiles, and the type of toxicity that occurs as the dose is elevated, Many of the newer synthetic agents have never been used to an extent adequate to establish their safety in special patient populations (e.g. children, women in early pregnancy, tolerant patients requiring very high doses of narcotics, or patients concurrently receiving potentially interacting medications).

Likewise, there are clinical situations in which only a single drug seems ever to have been given an adequate therapeutic trial. For example, morphine is so extensively and universally used to treat acute pulmonary edema that there is little evidence as to whether other narcotics would prove equally effective for this condition. Furthermore, patients exhibiting allergic or idiosyncratic reactions to one narcotic may tolerate another without difficulty. This fact alone justifies having a wide variety of alternative drugs available. Finally, although neither the natural nor the synthetic analgesics could be classified as expensive drugs, there are cost differentials that must be considered, particulary in the case of underdeveloped countries that must import synthetics.

Numerous totally synthetic analgesics and antitussives have been available for many years and have been heavily promoted by the pharmaceutical industry. Continued reliance on opiates by physicians cannot be adequately explained on the basis that physicians are ignorant of therapeutic alternatives. Analgesics such as aspirin, morphine, and codeine that have withstood the test of time have done so because both controlled clinical trials and vast clinical experience have shown them, in comparison with newer agents, to be drugs of choice.

The existence of a substantial body of clinical and experimental data on a drug greatly enhances its value in rational therapeutics. This information delineates the full spectrum of its therapeutic possibilities, defines precisely those situations in which the drug may be of particular value, and, by forewarning the physician, minimizes the likelihood of unexpected adverse effects. World literature on the opiates substantially exceeds that available for the synthetics. Were the opiates to become unavailable, the physician, and hence the patient, would lose the benefit of medicine's vast collective experience with these drugs. The therapeutic experience of the individual practitioner must also be considered. Many physicians routinely use opium-derived narcotics and antagonists as drugs of first choice in their practice, and they have become proficient in the use of these specific agents. The patient might therefore suffer from the unavailability of opiates not only by having a less thoroughly investigated and understood drug substituted for one whose therapeutic potential and adverse effects have been more clearly defined, but also because his physician has been deprived of the therapeutic tools with which he is most familiar.

In addition to its detrimental effect on patient care, doing without opiates would substantially impede both basic and applied research in developing superior analgesics, exploring the mechanism of action of narcotics and narcotic antagonists, understanding tolerance and psychic and physical dependence, and using antagonists for the prevention and treatment of narcotic addiction. Morphine, codeine, nalorphine, and naloxone are standards of comparison for agents in their respective classes. They have generally served as prototypes and tools in exploring the general pharmacology of narcotics and narcotic antagonists. The loss of these drugs would render obsolete a vast body of priceless experimental data in the world literature. It would be impossible to make any orderly progression along many lines of research without completely repeating masses of old experiments, substituting synthetic compounds for the opium derivatives originally used as standards.

Specific Opiates

Table 18–1 lists opium derivatives of medical interest that, with the exception of heroin, are currently marketed in the United States. Several promising but thus far unmarketed investigational agents have been omitted.

Although I regard only three of these drugs—morphine, codeine, and naloxone—as being of fundamental importance in medical practice and research, certain others are extensively prescribed and have particular properties that render them useful in special circumstances. For example, oxymorphone and hydromorphone are the only potent analgesics available as suppositories, a dosage form of particular value for children, the elderly, and patients with chronic pain (Beaver and Feise, 1977). Unlike most narcotic analgesics, the codeine congeners dihydrocodeine, hydrocodone, and oxycodone are characterized by excellent oral efficacy (Beaver et al., 1978). Throughout most of the world, paregoric and other crude opium prep-

Table 18–1. *Opium Derivatives of Medical Interest*

Opium	papaveretum (Pantopon, Omnopon), paregoric, etc.
Morphine and its Congeners	morphine heroin (diacetylmorphine, diamorphine) hydromorphone (dihydromorphinone, Dilaudid) oxymorphone (Numorphan)
	nalorphine (Nalline) naloxone (Narcan) } narcotic antagonists
	apomorphine – emetic
Codeine and its Congeners	codeine dihydrocodeine (Paracodin) hydrocodone (dihydrocodeinone, Hycodan, Dicodid) oxycodone (Percodan, Percocet, Tylox)
Thebaine	not used medically, but vital for synthesis of many drugs
Benzylisoquinolines	papaverine – commercial synthesis available noscapine (narcotine)

arations are the most widely used drugs for the treatment of diarrhea.

Morphine

Morphine was isolated from opium in 1803, and, in the intervening years, many semisynthetic derivatives and totally synthetic potent analgesics have appeared to challenge its therapeutic primacy. Although several of these have characteristics that indicate their use under certain circumstances, none is generally superior to parenteral morphine in the relief of severe pain. Morphine is the mainstay of therapy in severe pain associated with acute myocardial infarction and terminal cancer, and it is felt by many to be the general purpose potent analgesic of choice. Indeed, morphine is frequently used when other analgesics have been proven ineffective.

There are many clinical situations in which synthetic potent analgesics such as meperidine (Demerol), methadone (Dolophine), levorphanol (Levodromoran), and the antagonist-analgesic pentazocine (Talwin) may be substituted for morphine. The major problem in using these drugs as substitutes for morphine appears in patients with very severe pain or in tolerant patients who would require higher than ordinary doses of morphine for relief. In contradistinction to our knowledge concerning the effects of high doses of morphine, very little information is available concerning the effect of large parenteral doses of any of these synthetic agents. Large doses of meperidine may lead to convulsions, a complication not encountered with morphine. As the dose of injectable pentazocine is increased from 30 to 60 mg, the incidence of psychotomimetic side effects increases substantially (Hamilton et al., 1967; Wood et al., 1974). Again, this is an adverse effect rarely noted with morphine. None of the synthetics is available in a dosage form such as hypodermic tablets, which allow the injection of a large dose in a small volume, an important consideration for tolerant patients with poor muscle mass. Meperidine and, in particular, pentazocine are irritating to the tissues on repeated injection, and the latter drug can produce cellulitis and ulceration and hardening of the skin. Even less information is available concerning the effects of high doses of other morphine substitutes such as phenazocine and anileridine.

Lack of data or known contraindications also impose limitations on the use of synthetic morphine substitutes in special patient groups such as children, women in early pregnancy, and patients concurrently receiving other potent medications. For example, individuals being treated with monoamine oxidase inhibitors have died when given ordinary therapeutic doses of meperidine. Since this has not been observed when morphine is used, morphine is the recommended potent analgesic in such patients.

Meperidine is superior to morphine for use in labor and delivery because its rapid onset and short duration of action reduces the risk to the newborn infant. Meperidine and some of its congeners are also often used postoperatively, as adjuncts to anesthesia and as analgesics in brief, painful procedures. However, short duration of action constitutes a liability when the physician wishes to treat more prolonged pain. Physicians persistently overestimate both the potency and duration of action of meperidine, which frequently results in the undertreatment of pain with this drug and much needless suffering by patients (Marks and Sachar, 1973). Meperidine is obviously not an appropriate drug for the treatment of severe chronic pain associated with malignancy.

With the exception of pentazocine, all the potent synthetic narcotics have an abuse liability at least as great as that of morphine. Meperidine has been proven to cause much more of an abuse problem than morphine among doctors, dentists, nurses, and paramedical personnel, probably because of a lingering misconception that it is "safer" than morphine (Garb, 1969). Methadone currently constitutes our biggest single problem in terms of the diversion of medical narcotics to illicit use. A consideration of these two examples should dispel any notion that simply by virtue of being a synthetic, an analgesic has intrinsically less abuse liability than opium-derived narcotics.

As a research tool, morphine has been utilized as the standard of comparison in virtually all the modern controlled clinical trials of analgesic efficacy and adverse effect liability involving potent injectable analgesics. It has also been used at the Addiction Research Center in Lexington as the standard for evaluating the abuse liability of these agents. These comparative studies form the backbone of our knowledge of the relative therapeutic merits and liabilities of every potent analgesic currently available. The continued availability of morphine is essential if the quest for more effective and safer potent analgesics is to progress unhindered.

Morphine has also been used as the primary tool in the vast majority of studies of clinical and animal pharmacology aimed at elucidating the mechanism of action of narcotic analgesics and the interaction of these substances with narcotic antagonists.

Codeine

Codeine has properties that make it uniquely valuable among the narcotic analgesics. It has excellent oral efficacy (Beaver et al., 1978), substantially less abuse liability than other narcotics, and adjunctive antitussive and sedative effects. Along with aspirin, codeine has served as the preeminent standard of comparison for mild analgesics.

Propoxyphene (Darvon) is the only drug currently on the market with properties resembling those of codeine. Propoxyphene is definitely less potent than codeine (Beaver, 1966; Miller et al., 1970); the best available estimates indicate that 90 to 120 mg of propoxyphene must be administered to equal the effect of 60 mg of codeine. However, the maximum recommended dose of propoxyphene is 60 mg every 4 hours, whereas codeine is frequently used in doses of up to 120 mg every 3 to 4 hours. There is little documented clinical experience with repeated doses of propoxyphene above those recommended, but what experience does exist indicates that unpleasant cumulative toxic effects, including convulsions and toxic psychosis (Fraser and Isbell, 1960; Tennant, 1973), may appear when the total daily dose exceeds 600 to 800 mg. On the other hand, codeine may be administered over a wide dosage range to achieve successive increments of analgesia. The net effect of this discrepancy is that whereas propoxyphene, usually in combination with aspirin or other antipyretic analgesics, may be a useful substitute for codeine in the lower range of mild to moderate pain, it usually cannot substitute for codeine in the relief of moderate to moderately severe pain. Furthermore, propoxyphene has no useful antitussive activity.

Another consideration that makes propoxyphene a less than ideal substitute for codeine is the growing recognition that propoxyphene, alone and in combination with alcohol and other central nervous system (CNS) depressants, is responsible for an alarming number of drug overdose fatalities (Sturner and Garriott, 1973; Finkle et al., 1976; Hudson et al., 1977). It was this fact, as much as the long-recognized abuse liability of propoxyphene (Tennant, 1973; Maletzky, 1974), that led to the recent scheduling of propoxyphene products as Schedule IV controlled substances. For reasons that are unclear, propoxyphene seems to constitute a much greater hazard in terms of suicidal and accidental overdose death than does codeine, although the two drugs are currently prescribed to a comparable extent.

Oral pentazocine has been suggested as a potential substitute for codeine and has been shown to have the requisite analgesic potency and oral efficacy (Kantor et al., 1966; Beaver et al., 1968). However, oral pentazocine may produce alarming psychic reactions in certain patients (Kantor et al., 1966; Beaver et al., 1968; Wood et al., 1974). Although this is an acceptable risk in patients with chronic pain problems if the alternative is the use of potent narcotics, this risk is hard to justify if the pain could be equally well managed by codeine.

Codeine also has excellent antitussive activity and is generally regarded as the standard of comparison for other antitussives. The best nonnarcotic antitussive, dextromethorphan, is not generally regarded as fully equal to codeine in antitussive efficacy, particularly in more intractable cough problems.

Doing without codeine would necessitate the use of synthetics with substantially greater dependence liability, such as methadone, by some patients whose pain or cough are currently adequately managed by codeine, which is safer. Properly controlled analgesic studies exploring the interaction of synthetics such as methadone, levorphanol, or meperidine with aspirin or acetaminophen are, to my knowledge, nonexistent.

Naloxone

Naloxone, a derivative of thebaine, is unique in being a "pure" narcotic antagonist of exceptional potency without significant agonistic activity. As such, it has rendered both nalorphine and levallorphan obsolete in the treatment of narcotic poisoning. Nalorphine, the first narcotic antagonist introduced into medicine, is still of substantial theoretical and experimental interest as the prototype agonist-antagonist.

Naloxone is capable of swiftly and decisively reversing all the life-threatening aspects of acute narcotic overdose. It is also the only antagonist capable of reversing the respiratory depression and psychotomimetic effects produced by antagonist-analgesics such as pentazocine. However, when administered to an individual who has had no prior narcotics or to an individual with central nervous system or respiratory depression not produced by narcotics, naloxone produces no depressant effect of its own. It is this property that renders the use of naloxone safe as a diagnostic-therapeutic maneuver in patients with respiratory depression of uncertain etiology. There are no synthetics that are pure antagonists, and for those patients who need naloxone's unique properties, the availability of the drug could be a matter of life and death.

From the standpoint of biomedical research, it is difficult to overestimate the current and continuing importance of naloxone as an experimental tool in exploring the mechanism of action of narcotics and narcotic antagonists, the properties of the morphine receptor, and the biologic significance of the endorphins.

Impact on Directions of Current Research

A number of pharmaceutical firms, both in the United States and abroad, are engaged in research programs to develop new analgesics with reduced dependence liability and other advantages for the patient with severe pain. A few firms are also involved in the search for antagonists that would be useful in the treatment or prevention of narcotic addiction. Although many of the compounds under investigation are completely synthetic, several of the most promising are thebaine derivatives (e.g., nalbuphine, naltrexone, M-5050, buprenorphine), and any continued interest in these must presuppose the continued availability of thebaine.

Conclusion

Many patients with acute pain currently receive a great deal less than optimal pain relief from analgesic therapy, and the outlook is substantially worse for the patient with severe, chronic pain. These patients can ill afford to have their therapeutic options reduced by the loss of several of our most useful analgesics, nor are their interests served by the disruption of research vital to the improvement of analgesic therapy. It is apparent that the costs of doing without opium derivatives, both in terms of optimal patient care and medical research, would be substantial. I leave it to those who argue to the contrary to provide a convincing answer to the question "Why *should* we do without opium derivatives?"

References

Beaver, W.T.: Mild analgesics: a review of their clinical pharmacology (Part II). Am. J. Med. Sci. 251:576, 1966.

Beaver, W.T., and Feise, G.: A comparison of the analgesic effect of oxymorphone by rectal suppository and intramuscular injection in patients with postoperative pain. J. Clin. Pharmacol. 17:276, 1977.

Beaver, W.T., Wallenstein, S.L., Houde, R.W., and Rogers, A.: A clinical comparison of the effects of oral and intramuscular administration of analgesics: pentazocine and phenazocine. Clin. Pharmacol. Ther. 9:582, 1968.

Beaver, W.T., Wallenstein, S.L., Rogers, A., and Houde, R.W.: Analgesic studies of codeine and oxycodone in patients with cancer. I, Comparisons of oral with intramuscular codeine and of oral with intramuscular oxycodone. J. Pharmacol. Exp. Ther. 207:92, 1978.

Cochin, J.: The opium shortage; politics and health. N. Engl. J. Med. 293:990, 1975.

Cochin, J., and Harris, L.: *Synthetic Substitutes for Opiate Alkaloids.* Washington, D.C., The Drug Abuse Council, 1975.

DuPont, R.L. (Director, White House Special Action Office for Drug Abuse Prevention): Testimony before the Subcommittee to Investigate Juvenile Delinquency, March 5, 1975. *Poppy Politics; Cultivation, Use, Abuse and Control of Opium,* Vol I. Washington, D.C., U.S. Government Printing Office, 1975.

Epstein, E.J.: The incredible war against the poppies. Esquire, Dec., 1974. Reprinted in *Poppy Politics,* Vol I, 311, 1975.

Finkle, B.S., McCloskey, K.L., Kiplinger, G.F., and Bennett, I.F.: A national assessment of propoxyphene in postmortem medicolegal investigation, 1972–1975. J. Forensic Sci. 21:706, 1976.

Fraser, H.F., and Isbell, H.: Pharmacology and addiction liability of dl- and d-propoxyphene. Bull. Narc. 12:9, 1960.

Garb, S.: Drug addiction in physicians. Anesth. Analg. 48:129, 1969.

Greentree, L.B.: No opium for pain—a threatening medical crisis. N. Engl. J. Med. 291:1411, 1974.

Hamilton, R.C., Dundee, J.W., Clarke, R.S.J., Loan, W.B., and Morrison, J.D.: Studies of drugs given before anaesthesia. XIII, Pentazocine and other opiate antagonists. Br. J. Anaesth. 39:647, 1967.

Hudson, P., Barringer, M., and McBay, A.J.: Fatal poisoning with propoxyphene: report from 100 consecutive cases. South. Med. J. 70:938, 1977.

Kantor, T.G., Sunshine, A., Laska, E., Meisner, M., and Hopper, M.: Oral analgesic studies: pentazocine hydrochloride, codeine, aspirin, and placebo and their influence on response to placebo. Clin. Pharmacol. Ther. 7:447, 1966.

Maletzky, B.M.: Addiction to propoxyphene (Darvon): a second look. Int. J. Addict. 9:775, 1974.

Marks, R.M., and Sachar, E.J.: Undertreatment of medical inpatients with narcotic analgesics. Ann. Int. Med. 78:173, 1973.

Miller, R.R., Feingold, A., and Paxinos, J.: Propoxyphene hydrochloride: a critical review. JAMA 213:996, 1970.

Nixon, R.: Message from the President of the United States to the 92nd Congress. A draft of proposed legislation to establish a Special Action Office for Drug Abuse Prevention to concentrate the resources of the nation in a crusade against drug abuse. June 17, 1971. Reprinted in *Poppy Politics,* Vol. 2, 658, 1977.

Pepper, C.: *Narcotics Research, Rehabilitation and Treatment.* Hearings before the Select Committee on Crime, House of Representatives, 92nd Congress, 1st session. Vol. 1 (April 26, 27, 28, 1971), Washington, D.C., U.S. Government Printing Office, 1971.

Poppy Politics. Cultivation, Use, Abuse and Control of Opium. Hearings before the Subcommittee to Investigate Juvenile Delinquency of the Committee on the Judiciary, United States Senate, 94th Congress, 1st session. Vol. I (March 4 and 5, 1975), Washington, D.C., U.S. Government Printing Office, 1975; Vol. II (March 5 and 26, 1975), Washington, D.C., U.S. Government Printing Office, 1977.

Seitner, P.G.: *Survey of Analgesic Drug Prescribing Patterns.* American Medical Association, Center for Health Services Research and Development, Washington, D.C., The Drug Abuse Council, 1975.

Sturner, W.Q., and Garriott, J.C.: Deaths involving propoxyphene: a study of 41 cases over a two-year period. JAMA 223:1125, 1973.

Tennant, F.S., Jr.: Complications of propoxyphene abuse. Arch. Int. Med. 132:191, 1973.

WHO Scientific Group: *Opiates and Their Alternates for Pain and Cough Relief.* World Health Organization Technical Report Series No. 495, Geneva, 1972.

Wood, A.J.J., Moir, D.C., Campbell, C., Davidson, J.F., Gallon, S.C., Henney, E., and McAllion, S.: Medicines evaluation and monitoring group: central nervous system effects of pentazocine. Br. Med. J. 1:305, 1974.

19

How Useful Are Drugs in the Treatment of Hyperkinetic Children?

THE ROLE OF STIMULANT MEDICATION IN THE TREATMENT OF THE HYPERACTIVE CHILD

Paul H. Wender, M.D.

PROBLEMS IN THE USE OF STIMULANT DRUGS FOR HYPERKINESIS

Herbert E. Rie, Ph.D., and Ellen D. Rie, Ph.D.

But at three, four, five, and even six years the childish nature will require sports; now is the time to get rid of self-will in him, punishing him, but not so as to disgrace him.

Plato, *Laws*

A grievous burthen was thy birth to me;
Tetching and wayward was thy infancy.

Shakespeare, *Richard III*

The tired mothers found that spanking took less time than reasoning. . . . My mother spared the rod, because she preferred to use her hand.

Will Durant, *Transition*

Introduction

The "hyperactive child syndrome" means different things to different people. To some, it is a distressing behavioral abnormality, and those who suffer from it are a nuisance not only to their parents, siblings, and teachers but to themselves. To others, the syndrome is a pejorative authoritarian label used to justify the use of chemical straitjackets to inhibit perfectly normal young children who are protesting against a faulty social system or inept parents.

The truth seems to encompass these extreme positions as well as the ground in between. The grossly hyperkinetic child is a very real phenomenon indeed, and no parent, teacher, or doctor who has had to deal with such patients can doubt the reality of the problem. But almost certainly, stimulant (or other) medication has, at times, been sloppily doled out to children who hardly fit into the classic category.

As both Wender and the Ries point out, the study of hyperkinesis suffers from semantic confusion and inexactitude. Wender supplies his own criteria; the Ries seem to have such doubts about the syndrome (and its treatment) as to discredit the possibility of criteria.

Wender reminds us that imprecision in diagnostic criteria plagues much of medicine, not only psychiatry, and that empiric utility is not a bad thing if that is the best we have available. Not convinced of any serious danger from stimulant drugs, and convinced of their utility in at least some patients, he favors a short period of trial-and-error drug therapy. He is probably less worried by "overdiagnosis" than by "underdiagnosis," especially since the alternatives seem so unattractive and ineffectual. Nevertheless, he recommends that attention also be paid to nondrug approaches, either before drug treatment or in conjunction with it.

The Ries are much less sanguine. They question the existence of a true syndrome, or at least they doubt that it exists anywhere near as frequently as it is diagnosed. They also believe that the reputed benefits of stimulant drugs are trivial, temporary, and illusory, and that these drugs do not get to the heart of the matter. Finally, the Ries indict the physician for taking too readily to the "prescription pad" approach because it is easier, not because it works better.

LOUIS LASAGNA, M.D.

The Role of Stimulant Medication in the Treatment of the Hyperactive Child

Paul H. Wender, M.D.
University of Utah, Department of Psychiatry

Hyperactivity

The purpose of this paper is to support the proposition that stimulant medication plays an important and often an invaluable role in the treatment of hyperactive children. However, any discussion of treatment presupposes a general agreement as to the attributes and boundaries of the conditions treated. Such agreement does not exist with regard to hyperactivity. Some maintain that the syndrome has yet to be discovered, that it has only been invented and is the delusional product of inept observers (Schrag and Divoky, 1975). Some observe that a substantial fraction of children, particularly boys, are overly active—i.e., "hyperactive," and that to designate them as abnormal is to call a normal aspect of childhood a *disease*. Others acknowledge that hyperactivity exists but claim that it is extraordinarily rare (Rutter et al., 1970). Still others would contend that it is a pejorative term applied to normal children who fail to meet the expectations of parents, teachers, and child psychiatrists. Finally, some argue that it is a rare consequence of brain damage, and that most children diagnosed as hyperactive show no clinical signs or symptoms or laboratory evidence of brain damage and are, therefore, not hyperactive.

My assertion is that all these statements are, in varying degrees, incorrect. Their proponents have often been the unwitting victims of the names used to denote hyperactivity. Henceforth, I shall use the phrase *minimal brain dysfunction* (MBD) to refer to this disorder. I do so not because of personal devotion to this phrase but because it carries the least surplus meaning. Let me briefly discuss how semantics have led many astray.

Many MBD children are overactive. Some are not, but they manifest all the other signs and symptoms of the syndrome while being normally active or phlegmatic. Hyperactivity is not a pathognomonic feature of the syndrome. Many children—usually boys—are indeed very active (as many as half of all mothers will so characterize their sons). It has been argued by some that such a common symptom (to be accurate, a sign) cannot constitute a disease. This is correct. It is only one sign of many and is of significance *only* when it is seen as part of a behavioral cluster. The word *hyperactive* is thus apt to lead some to confuse one symptom with the entire syndrome. Based on the erroneous assumption that hyperactivity in isolation is often treated by the child psychiatrist (to the best of my knowledge this is not so), some authors assert that overactivity may only be a manifestation of the child's discomfort with a situation—e.g., school—and should not be treated. Inherent in this position is the belief that psychostimulant drugs are being forced down the throats of ebullient children to straightjacket them chemically or to anesthetize them into conforming to the demands of a repressive society.

Another phrase that has led people astray is *minimal brain damage.* Its abbreviation is unfortunately identical with the one I propose to use for *minimal brain dysfunction.* Based on the observation that some neurologically damaged children manifest the clinical picture of MBD, some clinicians have somehow reached the logically untenable position that all MBD children must (in order to have been diagnosed as such) manifest signs of brain damage. That is, if some brain-damaged children show signs of MBD, all MBD children must show signs of brain damage. The logical parallel would be that if some fish can fly, all flying animals are fish. Such clinicians, often neurologists, may evaluate a child, find normal EEGs and no neurologic signs, and conclude that the child in question does not have MBD. *Minimal brain dysfunction* itself is a phrase that has been taken to task. It is argued that (1) the syndrome need not be minimal, which is true; (2) it is trivial to assert that the brain is involved, since the brain is involved in all behavior, although the distinction is meant to emphasize a biologic rather than a psychologic dysfunction; and (3) the word *dysfunction* implies that we know something that we do not. Obviously, it would be best for all concerned if we could discover an obscure 17th century physician who had first described the syndrome. He might achieve eponymic distinction; we could refer to it as "Krankheit's syndrome," and all would be happy.

A second cause of concern to many is that it is impossible to specify exact symptomatic criteria that are necessary for the diagnosis of MBD. I would hasten to add that this is the rule rather than the exception in all of medicine, and it is true of many other psychiatric diagnostic categories. Confusion about this issue is often produced by an understandable lack of awareness of some general principles of nosology. Classification in biology—and this is relevant to all medical classification—may be either *monothetic* or *polythetic* (Sokal, 1974). In monothetic classification, membership in a class is defined by an individual having all of a set of specific characteristics. An example of a monothetic class would be that of mammals. A species is mammalian if it has hair and if it suckles its young. An example of a polythetic class would be rheumatic fever. For reasons that will be discussed presently, the Jones criteria specify that an individual can be so diagnosed if he has any two of five major criteria or one ot the major criteria and two of the minor criteria. It is obvious that two individuals may have rheumatic fever and yet have no symptoms in common. (For example, one might have carditis and Sydenham's chorea whereas another might have polyarthritis and erythema marginatum.) Unfortunately, there are no "Krankheit" criteria for MBD. Therefore, as is usually the case in the most primitive stages of an ailment, assessment is done by a clinician, whose diagnostic reliability is yet to be determined, for a perhaps heterogeneous classification of illness whose validity remains to be established.

If MBD is a polythetically defined illness, what are its attributes and what combinations of symptoms are necessary for diagnosis? Unfortunately, it is not possible to answer authoritatively. In the case of rheumatic fever, the clinician could appeal to the pathologist and the microbiologist. These scientists could inform him that a particular infection was associated with a variety of tissue reactions and that, accordingly, these tissue reactions might be clustered together meaningfully on the assumption that their appearance implied the previous existence of such an infection. This procedure cannot be employed in regard to MBD. The psychiatrist receives no aid from the pathologist. Unlike the internist, he cannot correlate signs and symptoms with ascertainable or definable tissue abnormalities. If we knew that MBD was associated with excessive deposits of cesium in the basal ganglia, we could correlate the signs and symptoms with tissue abnormalities and establish polythetic criteria. But we cannot. Accordingly, all that we can do is to state the major signs and symptoms that child psychiatrists *believe* cluster in MBD. These principal attributes seem to be as follows (Wender, 1971):

1. *Attentional deficits.* A short attention span that may be masked by perseverative interests. This may be a pathognomonic feature of the disorder.

2. *Motor abnormalities.* Hyperactivity, clumsiness, and soft neurologic signs.

3. *Deficits in impulse control.* Low frustration tolerance, impaired "stick-to-it-iveness," social impulsivity, and resistance to social demands—which varies as a function of increasing age with destructiveness, fire setting, stealing, lying, delinquency, and sexual "acting out."

4. *Altered interpersonal relations.* Increased independence (decreased separation anxiety); resistance to socialization by adults, manifested by refractoriness to reward and punish-

ment—i.e., obstinacy, negativism, stubbornness, imperviousness, impaired peer relations, obtuseness to the needs of others, bullying, domineering attitude, etc.

5. *Altered emotionality.* Increased affective lability (moody, easily depressed), overexcitability (lack of modulation), hot temper ("short fuse"), low self-esteem, anxiety.

6. *Perceptual and cognitive abnormalities.* Immature responses to perceptual tests and decreased performance in reading, writing, and arithmetic, despite the presence of normal intelligence. (Specific learning disabilities are apparently increased among children with other MBD characteristics, although such disabilities may occur in their absence. Whether such disabilities should be included as part of the MBD syndrome is not clear at present.)

7. *Congenital anatomic stigmata.*

These signs and symptoms constitute the raw material necessary to establish rational, polythetic, diagnostic criteria for MBD. Such criteria have yet to be established. Meanwhile, the fact that MBD must be regarded as a polythetically defined disorder does not make it, as some have asserted, either "unreal" or "mythical."

Is Minimal Brain Dysfunction (MBD) a Disease?

MBD appears to be a *syndrome.* Is it a *disease*? This is an important question, because to some, pharmacologic treatment appears warranted if and only if the syndrome has a biologic basis. To maintain this stance would be to demand certainty, which is not available for other psychiatric syndromes. Schizophrenias and depressive disorders are polythetically defined entities whose underlying biologic abnormalities are not yet determined. Nonetheless, identifying an individual as having schizophrenia or a primary affective disorder is of considerable utility in that such a classification reliably predicts therapeutic response to certain forms of medication. Parenthetically, we have strong circumstantial evidence that biologic factors do underlie these disorders. This evidence comes from family and adoption studies that indicate genetic transmission and therefore imply a mediating biologic mechanism. Similar family and adoption studies exist in regard to MBD, and they indicate the presence of a genetic factor in this syndrome. The facts that at least some forms of MBD are genetically transmitted and that some MBD children show congenital anatomic stigmata imply that at least some forms of MBD are biologically produced. This is, however, tangential. The issue at question is empirical: whether MBD children show a favorable therapeutic response to certain forms of medication.

Psychostimulant Treatment of MBD

Since Bradley's observation (Bradley, 1937) that children whom we would now designate as suffering from MBD benefit from stimulant medication, studies have repeatedly shown that psychostimulant medication (dextro-, levo-, and racemic amphetamines, methylphenidate, and pemoline) produces symptomatic relief in MBD children. These studies, which vary in efficacy of design, have documented that approximately 60 to 80 percent of MBD children derive symptomatic benefit from such treatment (Barkley, 1977).

What was present in Bradley's original study and what is missing from many of the later ones is clinical observation. Bradley saw his patients and talked to people who knew them. Many recent investigators have made contact with the patient only through rating scales. The latter approach may satisfy positivistic needs for precision, but it does so at the cost of diminished clinical observations. Precision may be inversely related to relevance. Many "precise" studies failed to observe that the response of many—but not all—MBD children to stimulant medication is qualitatively and quantitatively different from the response seen with other psychoactive drugs in other psychiatric syndromes. Antidepressants, when effective, may restore a depressed individual to his previous level of functioning. Neuroleptics relieve many of the symptoms of schizophrenia but often are only able to turn the process schizophrenic patient into a borderline schizophrenic. When psychostimulant drugs are efficacious in MBD children, they can have a profound effect. In that subgroup of MBD children who manifest an excellent response to such drugs, many aspects of behavior are affected.

Unlike other drugs used in psychiatry, which are at best able to restore the patient to the *status quo ante,* stimulant drugs may induce better functioning than had ever been seen before. In such instances, children not only become less restless (as do adults on stimulants) but they show decreased impulsivity, decreased affective lability, cooler tempers, and a markedly increased responsivity to social reinforcement. The last may be the most important effect. Children who were formerly refractory to reward and punishment and to blame and praise, and who seemed oblivious to the laws of classical and operant conditioning, may become very sensitive to social expectations. As a result, their behavior may be "improved" in relation to parents, teachers, and peers. These changes obviously are a relief to others. They may also (this is still questionable) benefit the child. With the help of medication, he may be able to practice and to learn more adaptive forms of behavior that will benefit him in the long run. But behavioral alterations—i.e., changes in signs—are not all we may expect. The child's symptoms may also change.

What are the subjective effects of psychostimulant medication in MBD children? This is difficult to ascertain. Most preadolescent children—and most treated MBD children are preadolescent—are not very good introspective reporters. What we see when treatment is begun is that some children appear sad. Some tell us so. Others report that they are calm. Some report changed feelings that appear secondary to the reactions their changed behavior produces. A typical example is that of a seven-year-old boy who stated that he liked the medicine because it made him a "good boy," so that other people liked him better, and that made him feel good.

Further insight may be obtained from observations of stimulant drug treatment of MBD in adults (Wood et al., 1976). These individuals frequently complain of lability of mood, with transient "highs" and "lows" that last from hours to days. They report that stimulant medication not only alleviates the lows but reduces the highs as well, producing a stability of mood that they find most relieving. Adult patients also report that medication helps them in doing what they normally would do and in avoiding what they normally would avoid. As a result, anxiety related to lack of self-control and guilt produced by transgression are reduced. If we can infer the subjective effects in children from those seen in adults, we may conclude that stimulant medications may relieve distressing symptoms in the younger age group as well as in the adults. If so, this is of considerable importance. The implication would be that we are providing these children with direct as well as indirect subjective benefit.

The Decision to Treat

In deciding to treat any patient, a physician must weigh four factors: (1) the consequences of nontreatment, (2) the benefits of treatment with a specific modality, (3) the risks of treatment with that modality, and (4) the availability of alternative forms of treatment. Let us examine the data concerning these factors in regard to minimal brain dysfunction.

Nontreatment. What are the consequences of nontreatment of MBD? There are both immediate and long-term implications. Right away, the nontreated MBD child is compromised in regard to his own behavior—the effects it has on him and on others—and he is burdened with the uncomfortable symptoms of the syndrome. The moderately to severely afflicted MBD child functions poorly with peers, teachers, parents, and siblings. His inability to function adequately frequently results in rejection by peers, criticism by teachers, and both punishment and criticism from parents. MBD children tell us that they do not like the negative feedback their behavior produces. And they also sometimes tell us that they are unhappy about their inability to control themselves. In addition to the indirect and direct consequences to themselves, they frequently generate turmoil and unhappiness in their families. They are provocateurs of family disruption. Friction with sibs, tension produced by them between their sibs and their parents, and conflict between the parents are frequent consequences of their behavior. Parents almost inevitably argue between themselves as to whose inept parenting has generated and/or perpetuated the problem. Another immediate consequence of nontreatment is the continuing subjective distress of the child.

What are the long-term consequences of nontreatment? The data necessary to answer this question fully are not available. Some noncontrolled follow-up studies, with and without treatment, indicate that MBD children, as a group, are at appreciably increased risk for school failure, juvenile delinquency, and institutionalization as delinquents or psychiatric patients (Menkes et al., 1967; Mendelsohn, 1971; Mendelson, 1972; Huessey and Cohen, 1976). Other studies do not indicate an increased risk (Hechtman et al., 1976). It may very well be that MBD children are simply lumped together inappropriately. It may also be that some subgroups (if they exist) are at no greater social or psychiatric risk than non-MBD children, whereas other subgroups are at appreciably greater risk. A reasonable clinical hunch is that the latter is true. It seems that the subgroup of MBD children who have "unsocialized aggressive conduct disorders" (children who manifest behavior such as physical aggression, hostility, defiance, destructiveness, lying, truancy, vandalism, and meanness) is the subgroup at greater risk—but it is uncertain. The ability to make the clinical distinction between those children at greater and lesser social and psychiatric risk would be of considerable practical importance, since in weighing the decision to treat we could consider the costs and benefits for each group separately.

Benefits of treatment. The available data concerning the long-term effects of treatment are difficult to interpret. Few studies exist, treatment assignment has not been random, control groups have not been employed, systematic ancillary treatments have not been used, and the duration of follow-up in general has been brief. Most unfortunate is that long-term double blind stimulant drug versus placebo trials have not been performed. Illustrative of the difficulties in interpreting the available data is a study conducted in Montreal (Weiss et al., 1975) in which children continuing to receive stimulant medication for approximately five years were found to be doing no better at follow-up than other children in the clinic for whom medication had been discontinued. The clarity of this finding was vitiated by the observation that the continuously treated children did worse when their medication was stopped than the children whose medication had been stopped earlier. The implication is that children in the first group had continued to receive psychostimulant medication because their problems had failed to abate.

A final difficulty in interpreting any drug studies is the recent finding that in some instances, MBD persists into adult life. In such cases, an interval of treatment might be expected to have no long-lasting effects. Like insulin in diabetes, phenytoin (Dilantin) in epilepsy, and chlorpromazine (Thorazine) in schizophrenia, psychostimulant medication is suppressive but not curative. Accordingly, in some instances one would anticipate the recurrence of symptoms when medication is discontinued.

Despite the absence of clinical evidence demonstrating the effectiveness of stimulant drug treatment in childhood on later psychologic adjustment, there are logical reasons for believing that it might be of benefit. An interesting possibility is that the use of psychostimulant medication early in the course of MBD might affect the child's ultimate adjustment by virtue of its effects on learning. Most MBD children have low self-esteem. Although this may be biologic in origin, it is also easy to see it as the indirect consequence of the child's presumably biologically produced behavior. Most psychiatrists believe that positive self-esteem develops as a consequence of positive feedback from the environment. The child who is liked by his peers and siblings, who does well in school, and who is positively regarded by his parents seems to incorporate these views and think well of himself. Conversely, the child who receives negative feedback thinks poorly of himself. If the MBD child's behavior can be altered so that he receives positive feedback, we might expect that this change would result in an increase of his self-esteem. In view of the fact that the degree of self-esteem acquired in childhood seems to persist into adult life, we would anticipate that the treated (as opposed to the nontreated) MBD child would have greater self-esteem in later life. The same comments apply to success in school. The child who performs well and receives praise for his performance and gratification from his accomplishments may be expected to develop a more positive attitude toward learning than the child for whom school performance is difficult, who experiences no sense of accomplishment, who is apt to be left back, and who is the frequent recipient of criticism. The foregoing is speculative but nevertheless plausible; psychiatric speculation is cheap and easy, and the absence of any data to support this position must be remembered.

Risks of treatment. What are the negative consequences of treatment with psychostimulant medication? Again, these may be divided into the immediate and the long-term. Immediate consequences are in virtually all instances trivial and readily controlled by adjustment of dosage. Idiosyncratic reactions to the amphetamines and methylphenidate are extraordinarily rare. (Such reactions appear to be more common with pemoline. In addition, this drug can produce abnormalities in liver function, which are apparently reversible when pemoline is discontinued. Fatal reactions have not been reported.) As a consequence, on a short-term basis, the physician need have little concern over conducting a therapeutic trial with amphetamines or methylphenidate. Immediate side effects of stimulant medication include excessive quieting; tearfulness and irritability; and a number of effects that appear sympathetic in origin, including headaches, stomachaches, and pallor. In almost all instances, these are the results of overmedication and can be eliminated by a decrease in dosage.

What of the negative long-term consequences of treatment with psychostimulant medication? A factor that has recently received much attention is that stimulant medication can decrease growth (Safer et al., 1972). The available data suggest that for the first year or two of treatment, there may indeed be a decrease in the expected rates of height and weight increase. Longer-term studies suggest that these effects are temporary and that despite the continuation of stimulant medication, growth patterns return to normal and the child eventually reaches his expected height and weight (Eisenberg, 1972; Gross and Wilson, 1974). The magnitude of the claimed decreases is relatively minor, but even if it were more appreciable, one would have to ask an important question. If stimulant medication does affect long-term psychologic outcome—and this needs to be determined—and if stimulant medication does reduce the child's eventual height—and this likewise remains to be determined—what would be more desirable? Would it be better to have an adult who was 5′9″ and psychologically well adjusted, or an adult who was 6′4″ and continued to suffer severe psychologic problems? The possibility of other detrimental long-term effects exists. Chronic use of sympathomimetic medication could, for example, produce changes in blood pressure. Such changes have *not* been reported (Gross and Wilson, 1974), but the possibility obviously dictates that blood pressure be monitored.

ALTERNATIVE TREATMENT. The last factor to be considered is the availability of alternative treatment modalities. These may be divided into the pharmacologic and the psychologic. Many drugs have been employed in the treatment of MBD. Aside from the psychostimulants, the most effective have been the antipsychotic drugs and the tricyclic antidepressants. Both classes of drugs have been found to be more effective than placebos but much less effective than the psychostimulants. Of equal importance is that both the antipsychotics and the antidepressants are capable of producing severe side effects. Long-term administration of antipsychotic drugs to adults has been associated with the development of an irreversible neurologic syndrome, *tardive dyskinesia*, and it has already been reported to occur in children receiving antipsychotic drugs as well. The tricyclic antidepressants produce a variety of toxic effects, and at least one death has been reported as a consequence of their therapeutic use in children. The last pharmacologic treatment, loosely speaking, that has been employed in the treatment of MBD is the "Feingold diet," which involves the removal of certain substances (initially salicylates and now food dyes) believed by Dr. Feingold to produce MBD and learning disabilities. A number of controlled trials have been conducted, and on balance, they seem to show that manipulation of diet affects a small fraction of MBD children and produces measurable but minimal benefit in this responsive subgroup (Wender, 1977).

What about psychologic therapies? A number of behavior modifiers have reported success in the treatment of MBD. With one exception, these studies have involved very small numbers of children and have focused mainly on one aspect of the MBD child's behavior; e.g., excessive motor activity. (The behavior modifiers seem to be unaware of many of the other signs of MBD or of the symptoms of the syndrome, and they make no claims that their intervention affects the child's subjective distress.) What is obviously necessary is a controlled study with a sample that is sufficiently large for statistical interpretation and that compares behavior modification techniques with pharmacologic intervention. One such study (Gittelman-Klein et al., 1976) compared the effects of behavior modification alone, medication alone, and a combination of behavior modification and medication. The results were clear: behavior modification was clearly more effective than no treatment, although the differences were not dramatic. Behavior modification alone was appreciably less effective than medication alone, and the combination of behavior modification and medication was no more effective than medication alone. Obviously, medication is the more effective treatment modality. But since behavior modification is not useless, it *might* be employed on an empirical basis with children whose signs and symptoms are comparatively minor.

That alternative techniques do not seem to be very effective when used alone does *not* mean that ancillary techniques will not be useful when combined with medication. Many MBD children have an academic performance below expectation, and the families of many MBD children are disrupted by the child's behavior. An effective treatment plan requires intervention in these areas. Even if medication reduces or eliminates any presumed biologic bases of the MBD child's impaired academic performance (such as attentional deficit or low frustration tolerance), medication can obviously not supply information that should have been but has not been acquired. In such instances, remedial education is mandatory. Nor can medication alone reduce family strife. Counseling, directed at enabling the parents to understand the origin of the child's problems and at helping them to manage the symptoms that medication does not eliminate, forms a necessary part of treatment.

Finally, the child, particularly when older, must be given an understanding of his own behavior. One useful consequence of this is that the child may be led to see that his receiving medication is neither a sign of his craziness nor a punishment for his misbehavior but a technique to help him to be more comfortable in his own life. This is particularly important as the MBD child approaches adolescence. Adolescents are notorious for their reluctance to take necessary medication; adolescent diabetics and epileptics often run into trouble because of their failure to do so. The uninformed MBD child is also likely to discontinue his medication. Working with the child and enlisting his cooperation often result in his willingness to continue to accept the most effective treatment modality available. There is an interesting analogy in adult psychiatry. Some drug advertisements—yielding to the widespread belief that psychotherapy is a universally effective treatment—state that antipsychotic drugs facilitate psychotherapy with schizophrenic patients. There is no evidence that psychotherapy has any effect on schizophrenic symptoms; medication seems to be the only effective treatment in this regard. It has been observed by one author that medication does not facilitate psychotherapy but that psychotherapy facilitates the patient's taking medication. I believe that this is true in MBD children and that this can be another benefit of psychotherapy for the MBD child.

Boundaries of the Syndrome: Consequences of Under- and Over-Diagnosis

In the absence of rational, widely accepted criteria for MBD, the clinician faces an insoluble diagnostic dilemma and is forced to adopt a strategic approach. He may decide, perhaps unwittingly, to diagnose MBD only when most of the listed attributes are present. By doing so he understands, or should understand, that he will decrease his number of false positives (instances in which MBD is diagnosed but does not exist) at the expense of increasing his number of false negatives (instances in which the disorder does exist but in which he fails to make the diagnosis). Conversely, he may decide to cast a broad diagnostic net. In this case, he will not require as many signs and symptoms to be present in order for him to make the diagnosis. By doing so, he decreases the number of false negatives at the expense of increasing his number of false positives. Deciding upon a strategy is not an empty academic—in the pejorative sense of the word—activity. Diagnosis is related to treatment. Accordingly, one must weigh the benefits and risks of treating those who do not require it and failing to treat those who would benefit from it.

What should a physician do for a child diagnosed as having MBD? First, he should intervene psychologically to eliminate as many stresses as possible in the school and the home. Next, if such intervention is ineffective—and this is the rule rather than the exception—I believe that he should cast the "broad diagnostic net" and offer a trial of psychostimulant medication. Whether medication is reported to be effective in 50 or 90 percent of MBD children is irrelevant. There is virtually no risk associated with a therapeutic trial, and the physician can determine within a week or two if medication affords the child appreciable benefit. It is presumed, parenthetically, that he is skillful in the use of such medication. Many psychostimulant treatment "failures" are the result of either inadequate dosage or the inadequate scheduling of doses. With regard to the former, the physician should gradually increase the dose until either therapeutic results become apparent or side effects indicate no further increase or a decrease in dosage. With regard to the latter, dosage must be spaced correctly throughout the day. Some physicians employ short-acting drugs such as methylphenidate on a morning only basis and infer on the basis of parental reports that the drug is useless. Since the parents are observing the child after school when the medication has worn off, this is to be expected. Another common cause of diminished success is failure to employ the aforementioned ancillary treatments. Medication can be very effective, but it does not teach children how to play the violin.

How long to employ medication is an important question. The possibility of long-term effects has not yet been determined. From a practical standpoint, the physician should periodically discontinue medication—which masks a child's symptoms—and see whether in the drug-free period, signs and symptoms have decreased. He may thus determine when further medication is necessary or if it may be discontinued.

Much criticism of the use of psychostimulant medication stems from its inadequate or exclusive usage. It is presumed, as with other psychiatric syndromes, that the physician will use all treatment modalities that afford the patient benefit. Confining therapy to the use of one modality in the treatment of MBD is inadequate. The unfortunate fact that some physicians use psychostimulant medication promiscuously and fail to monitor it, and neglect psychosocial factors in the etiology of the child's problems, is to be deplored. Such misuse is not a criticism of psychostimulant medication. It is a criticism of physicians who are indeed capable of misusing any effective drug. The doctor who treats uncomplicated colds with an antibiotic does not reflect unfavorably on the efficacy of antibiotics but on his own competency.

Conclusion

Finally, some are unhappy because the use of psychostimulant medication in the treatment of MBD is empirical. Physicians understandably feel more comfortable when treatment is rational. Increasing evidence, which cannot be summarized here, suggests that the psychostimulant treatment of MBD does indeed have a rational basis. Circumstantial evidence from a number of sources (Wender, 1978) suggests that many of the symptoms of MBD may be manifestations of underactivity of certain dopaminergic systems in the brain. If this is true, the use of psychostimulants would be a rational remedy, since the available agents all apparently act by amplifying the activity of dopaminergic systems. A rational basis for the treatment of MBD would be lovely.

As in the psychopharmacologic treatment of all psychiatric disorders, current treatment is empirical. At some time, we will know why psychostimulant medication is effective. In the interim, it appears that psychostimulant medication, not employed alone but together with psychologic and educational interventions, affords appreciable short-term benefit to MBD children and may afford long-term benefit as well.

References

Barkley, R.: A review of stimulant drug research with hyperactive children. J. Child Psychol. Psychiatry 18:137–165, 1977.

Bradley, C.: The behavior of children receiving benzedrine. Am. J. Psychiatry 94:577–585, 1937.

Eisenberg, L.: The hyperkinetic child and stimulant drugs. N. Engl. J. Med. 287:249–250, 1972.

Gittelman-Klein, R., Klein, D., et al.: Relative efficacy of methylphenidate and behavior modification in hyperkinetic children: an interim report. J. Abnorm. Child Psychol. 4:361–379, 1976.

Gross, M., and Wilson, W.: *Minimal Brain Dysfunction.* New York, Brunner/Mazel, Inc., 1974.

Hechtman, L., Weiss, G., et al.: Hyperactives as young adults: preliminary report. Can. Med. Assoc. J. 9:625–630, 1976.

Huessey, H., and Cohen, A.: Hyperkinetic behaviors and learning difficulties followed over seven years. Pediatrics 57:4–10, 1976.

Mendelson, N.: A 5-year followup study of 91 hyperactive school children. J. Am. Acad. Child Psychiatry 11:595–610, 1972.

Mendelsohn, W.: Hyperactive children as teenagers: a followup study. J. Nerv. Ment. Dis. 153:273–279, 1971.

Menkes, M., Rowe, J., et al.: A 25 year followup study on the hyperkinetic child with MBD. Pediatrics 39:393–399, 1967.

Rutter, M., Tizard, J., et al.: *Education, Health and Behavior.* Great Britain, Longman Group Ltd., 1970.

Safer, D., Allen, R., et al.: Depression of growth in hyperactive children on stimulant drugs. N. Engl. J. Med. 287:217–220, 1972.

Schrag, P., and Divoky, Deane: *The Myth of the Hyperactive Child.* New York, Pantheon Books, 1975.

Sokal, R.R.: Classification: purposes, principles, progress, prospects. Science 185:1115–1123, 1974.

Weiss, G., Kruger, E., et al: Effect of long-term treatment of hyperactive children with methyphenidate. Can. Med. Assoc J. 112:159–165, 1975.

Wender, E.: Food additives and hyperkinesis. Am. J. Dis. Child. In press, 1977.

Wender, P.: *Minimal Brain Dysfunction in Children.* New York, John Wiley & Sons, 1971.

Wender, Paul H.: Minimal brain dysfunction: an overview. In Lipton, M.A., DiMascio, A., and Killam, K.F., eds., *Psychopharmacology: A Generation of Progress,* New York, Raven Press, 1978.

Wood, D., Reimherr, F., et al: Diagnosis and treatment of minimal brain dysfunction in adults. Arch. Gen. Psychiatry 33:1453–1460, 1976.

Problems in the Use of Stimulant Drugs for Hyperkinesis*

Herbert E. Rie, Ph.D.
Ellen D. Rie, Ph.D.
Case Western Reserve University Department of Psychology

The past 15 to 20 years have witnessed not only a sudden and remarkable increase in the use of stimulant drugs for control of childhood behavior but a concomitant rise in the frequency with which disorders that are deemed treatable by these drugs are diagnosed. Certainly, the effects of stimulants on the behavior of children have been known for many years (Bradley, 1937). If their newfound popularity lacks adequate explanation, the increased number of diagnoses of stimulant-treated disorders is still more puzzling. In fact, it is uncertain whether there really is an increased prevalence of these disorders or whether their diagnosis has simply become increasingly convenient. To the advocates of stimulants, such issues may appear irrelevant, but they go to the heart of the question of who is treated and for what reason. Many new treatments are controversial initially and the decision for their use rests as heavily on the social climate, evolving professional mores, and personal predilection as it does on fact and reason. Stimulants used for behavior control are no exception.

A critical examination of the disorders for which stimulants have been prescribed, including minimal brain dysfunction, hyperkinesis, and learning disabilities, attests to the lack of precision, the controversy, and the reliance on unsubstantiated assumptions that have plagued both research and practice in this field (Rie, 1979; Satz and Fletcher, 1979).

Nature of the Treated Disorders

A disparity exists between generally accepted assumptions about the nature of the disorders being treated by stimulant drugs and the accruing facts about such disorders. To the extent that the assumptions underlie the decision for treatment and the choice of treatment, they are of concern.

It is frequently assumed that hyperactivity is (1) a syndrome that includes a variety of maladaptive behaviors, (2) either part of the ostensible syndrome of "minimal brain dysfunction" (MBD) or synonymous with it, (3) the result of central nervous system impairment ("dysfunction"), and (4) a medical problem by virtue of these assumptions. Hyperactivity is also thought to require medical treatment, and stimulants are the treatment of choice because of their relatively dramatic effect of reducing activity level, inattention, distractibility, and restlessness. Although the literature has contained many warnings against adopting these assumptions as facts, it is uncertain whether they

*Much of the research of the authors to which reference is made in this manuscript was supported by the Office of Program Evaluation and Research, Division of Mental Health, Ohio Department of Mental Health and Mental Retardation.

are heard or heeded in the real world of professional practice. In fact, the literature is replete with the often adamant restatement of these assumptions.

The idea of a *syndrome* of minimal brain dysfunction was codified with the publication of the report of the first phase of a three-phase project cosponsored by the Easter Seal Foundation and the National Institute of Neurological Diseases and Blindness (Clements, 1966). The widely adopted definition contained in the report refers to problems of "control of attention, impulse, or motor function." Hyperactivity appears first on the list of "ten characteristics most often cited by the various authors, in order of frequency." Furthermore, hyperactivity (or some closely related term) appeared prominently (9 times in 38 entries) among "terms used to describe or distinguish the conditions grouped as minimal brain dysfunction in the absence of findings severe enough to warrant inclusion in an established category . . ." (Clements, 1966). The link between hyperactivity and MBD has been stressed repeatedly, both implicitly and explicitly. A number of authors have written of treating minimal brain dysfunction with stimulants (Erenberg, 1972; Friedman et al., 1973; Garfinkel et al., 1975; Levitis, 1974; Levy, 1976). CIBA has advertised that "children with MBD can benefit from methylphenidate therapy" (1975), although it is obviously the elements of so-called *hyperkinesis* that are actually being treated. In a discussion of the effects of stimulants on "hyperactive children," Safer and Allen (1976) cite studies concerning children with MBD, behavior disorders, and learning disabilities.

Hyperactivity is said to be observed most often, if not exclusively, in the classroom, and only infrequently in the practitioner's office. As Denhoff et al. (1971) noted, ". . . generally, for school performance, it is the teacher who decides whether a child is hyperactive." If the "disorder" manifests itself in the classroom and not elsewhere, it is actually the teacher who makes the diagnosis.

More recent literature does not support the concept of a syndrome including the various elements that have been ascribed to it. In a number of studies of the relations among educational, psychologic, neurologic, medicohistorical, electroencephalographic, and other variables, it has been demonstrated consistently that no unitary syndrome of minimal brain dysfunction can be identified (Digman, 1965; Rodin, Lucas, and Simpson, 1964; Loney, Langhorne, and Paternite, 1978; Rie, Rie, Stewart, and Rettemnier, 1978; Routh and Roberts, 1972; Werry, 1968). It is therefore evident that equivalence among the designations "MBD," "hyperactivity," "learning disabilities," and variants thereof may not be assumed, and that justification does not exist for the treatment of one set of problems by methods deemed effective, by some criterion, in the treatment of another.

Effects of Treatment by Stimulants

Stimulants and Learning Disabilities

If one is inclined to dismiss the problem of conceptual confusion as hypothetical, improbable, or possible only in a limited number of cases of uninformed practice, one need only examine the literature. There are numerous references to the improved learning of children who are treated. Many studies have utilized the term *learning* to denote a variety of circumscribed functions such as paired-associate learning, continuous performance tasks, orienting response, and concept learning under different reinforcement conditions (Conners, 1971; Conners, Eisenberg, and Sharpe, 1964; Douglas, 1972; Sprague and Sleator, 1975). But children with learning problems have served as subjects in a number of studies on the effects of methylphenidate, and it has been reported that "these drugs have uniformly been shown to produce substantial academic and behavioral improvement . . ." (Conners, 1973). The frequently positive appraisals by teachers of the effects of stimulants on classroom performance, completion of work, and general quality of work, have tended to support these laboratory findings and have suggested that the effects on learning are as desirable as the effects on behavior.

Accruing data indicate that these findings have been inappropriately generalized and that the particular use of the term *learning* is critical. Teachers' observations are correct enough, so far as can be determined, since the moment-to-moment behavior of the treated children is more desirable from the perspective of classroom decorum. The children are more attentive, remain in their seats, and cause less disturbance than before treatment. They work more consistently and more neatly, and they tend to complete their assignments more often. Teachers tend to grant these students better grades, and classroom performance is enhanced.

However, studies utilizing more objective criteria of enduring scholastic achievement, and particularly of differential gains on medication for half a school year or longer, consistently fail to find any evidence of drug-enhanced scholastic achievement (Conrad et al., 1971; Rie et al., 1976a; 1976b; Sroufe, 1975). In fact, a recent survey of such research demonstrates convincingly that drug-enhanced improvement in scholastic achievement fails to occur in the overwhelming majority of cases (Barkley and Cunningham, 1977). Some of our own research (Rie and Rie, 1977) yielded the finding that children were better able to retain meaningful material for a short time (two hours) while taking methylphenidate than when not medicated, but that the differential retention did not persist for even two days. Such findings help to reconcile the seeming contradiction between teachers' reports of improved performance and the absence of improved scholastic achievement.

It is evident that stimulants are decidedly not the treatment of choice for "learning disabilities," and that it is essential that such problems be distinguished from hyperactive behavior and the more vague "minimal brain dysfunction". There is real danger that reliance on stimulants to treat learning disabilities will obscure the problem, reduce the amount of interaction between teacher and child, and result in the failure to offer appropriate help. After all, if the teacher misperceives the child's altered behavior as evidence of scholastic progress, there is no reason to seek further help to achieve such progress.

Problems of Measurement

Although problems in the measurement of hyperactivity could reasonably be subsumed under the discussion of definitional and conceptual problems affecting treatment, they are sufficiently distinct and important to merit separate comment.

It is evident that no generally accepted criteria of hyperactivity exist; "normal" variation in activity at different ages has not been established in any precise manner and measurement of the variables that constitute hyperactivity (by various definitions) is neither uniform nor reliable (Rie, 1975; Ross and Ross, 1976). Under these circumstances, hyperactivity is necessarily defined in part by the context in which the behavior occurs and in part by the observer who evaluates the behavior. Individual observers' levels of tolerance for high activity levels, the value they place upon them, and the extent to which their judgments are influenced by extraneous factors—i.e., the multiple sources of individual bias—form a confounding set of variables in the identification and appropriate selection of children for drug treatment. These factors grow in significance to the extent that the relevant behaviors of the child are not (as is often the case) independently observable in a different context (e.g., examining room). As Safer and Allen (1976) have pointed out, "The doctor's judgment of hyperactivity, based upon his observation of the child in his examining room, although more reliable than chance, offers little to the diagnosis . . ." Indeed, the value of a neurologic examination has been demonstrated to be of minimal value in the diagnosis of hyperactivity or minimal brain dysfunction (Kennedy and Ramirez, 1964; Clemmens and Kenny, 1972).

If one cannot identify hyperactive behavior reliably, except perhaps when it is extreme, one cannot select children reliably for treatment with stimulant drugs. The apparent increase in the frequency of the diagnosis of hyperactivity in the last decade strongly suggests that a variety of problems may be misdiagnosed or simply relabeled as *hyperactivity*, connoting all the implications of that designation. If drug treatment were confined to the identifiable, extreme cases of hyperactivity, we would not have witnessed this increase in the frequency of diagnosis. There is no doubt that hyperactivity is in vogue. As Kinsbourne (1973) has observed, ". . . we will soon be treating clumsiness with stimulant drugs."

The potential for measuring hyperactive behaviors should not be confused with the existing problems of measurement in practice. In fact, several rating scales have been developed. It is the variability of their application, the absence of norms, and the failure to utilize any explicit standard that constitute the principal problems of measurement in professional practice.

The Question of Benefit

The literature abounds with vague references to "effectiveness," "improvement," and "benefit" to imply satisfaction with the observed effects of stimulant drugs. Certainly many teachers and parents judge the affected behavior of the children to be desirable. The child behaves more acceptably in the classroom, is more tractable and compliant, often shows better classroom performance in certain respects, and gives the illusion of greater scholastic progress. There is not the slightest doubt that the child is less troublesome to caretaking adults, and the clamor for stimulant treatment by caretakers of children who have been difficult to manage has been well documented (Ross and Ross, 1976). Regardless of intent, much of the benefit accrues to the caretaking adult.

It has been noted (Wender, 1975) that parents are inclined to attribute the child's difficulties to their own failings or to the "malevolence" of the child, and the diagnosis of hyperactivity and prescription of stimulants may offer relief from such concerns.

The search for direct benefit to the child, in contrast to benefit to those in the child's immediate environment, is not reassuring. It is contended that drug-induced changes render the child generally more acceptable and elicit more supportive and constructive responses to him from which he therefore benefits (Safer and Allen, 1976). Several investigators have stressed improvement in the child's social relations, although the evidence is typically impressionistic. In our own studies (Rie et al., 1976a; 1976b), no differential effects of methylphenidate and placebo were found on classroom sociograms. Fish (1975) commented, "If a child has a problem in social interaction ... the drug could change only the excitability that made him act aggressively. But if he has already gotten into difficulties with other children, he will still feel badly about himself and other children." Although he is an emphatic proponent of the use of stimulants, Wender (1975) agrees that longstanding "psychological scars are often not relieved, even when medication is extremely effective. In these instances, limited psychotherapy ... may be of some benefit."

Data on the adaptation of children upon termination of long-term treatment with stimulants have not been supportive of the confident proclamations that psychologic growth occurs during treatment. Indeed, the limited data available suggest that socially and emotionally, the stimulant-treated child may be doing little more than marking time.

The follow-up studies at adolescence by the Montreal group (Weiss et al., 1971) revealed that the mothers' most frequent general complaint was the emotional immaturity of their children. Depressed moods were observed in many of the children and documented for a subgroup as lack of self-esteem. Riddle and Rapaport (1976) found that only 2 of 72 parents were free of serious concern about their children and that two thirds noted impulsive and immature behavior in their children on the two year follow-up. These investigators also found evidence of depressive tendencies. In a major survey of follow-up studies of children said to have minimal brain dysfunction, Helper (1979) reports that those who had been hyperactive "were still plagued by monumental difficulties in school performance and in self-management." Further, "depressive and self-critical reactions are noted ... prominently in follow-up of older MBD subjects." Mark A. Stewart is quoted as saying:

> They come off the drugs at fourteen or so, and suddenly they're big, strong people who've never had to spend any time building any controls in learning how to cope with their own daily stress. Then the parents, who have forgotten what the child's real personality was like without the mask of the drug, panic and say 'Help me, I don't know what to do with him. He's taller than I am and he has the self-discipline of a six year old. (Schrag and Divoky, 1975).

We have wondered, in the course of our own research, about the prospects of social and emotional development during the period of treatment. The consistently suppressed response to, or awareness of, emotionally charged phenomena has been impressive. This reduced responsivity, only rarely mentioned, could prove to be the side effect with the most serious implications. It is a difficult set of variables to measure reliably and objectively, particularly from moment to moment under conditions of varying stimulation and interaction, and this problem has received little attention thus far in the research literature.

It becomes logical to inquire, in light of the discovery that scholastic achievement is not enhanced in stimulant-treated children, why one would expect those children to learn more appropriate social adaptation and emotional modulation. The requisite tasks are, after all, far less structured, far less discrete, and far less repetitive than the tasks in the scholastic curriculum. In the context of reduced responsiveness to emotionally charged stimuli, the normal expected development of age-typical emotional controls, affect differentiation, and social skills may be impossible. In a subtle but real sense, the stimulant-treated child may actually be deprived of the opportunity to gain control of his behavior. Medication is a daily imposition of an external control and confirmation of the child's need for such control. Whereas formerly, the child was blamed for his unacceptable behavior, praiseworthy gains are now attributable to drugs. Far from reinforcing the child's increasing sense of control, the response he elicits reinforces continued reliance on medication.

Although the subjective responses of the treated children are not often of primary concern and may, in fact, be ignored, our subjects uniformly have been averse to the stimulants, have complained of strange and uncomfortable feelings, and have been delighted to terminate treatment.

Finally, the reduction of hyperactive behavior has been viewed generally as one of the most beneficial effects of the stimulants. But there is, after all, no unequivocal virtue in reducing a child's level of activity, nor should a high level of activity necessarily be met with opprobrium. For extremely hyperactive children who are literally intolerable in the classroom, this may be a most significant, temporary benefit, precluding their expulsion from school. But it has typically been assumed that the behavioral effects of the stimulants eliminate the presumed impediments to learning for all hyperactive children, most of whom are not threatened with expulsion, in our experience. It is now evident that even when these impediments to learning are eliminated by use of stimulants, the desired gains in achievement fail to occur for the majority of children. Is it not logical then, to inquire whether reduced activity is really beneficial to the learning process? To our knowledge, the question has not been raised in the recent research literature and, for now, one can only speculate.

In these speculations, one is struck by the differences between achieving and underachieving children with respect to enthusiasm, interest, curiosity, exploratory behavior, the search for relationships, the synthesis of data and experiences from a variety of sources, and the generally *active* rather than *passive* nature of the productive learning process. These are not recent or unique observations. So-called motivational factors have long been of concern, and active learning was at the heart of John Dewey's educational philosophy at the turn of the century. As activity level is reduced by medication, and even as attention becomes persistently focused on a delimited target, the potential impact of multiple cues is reduced, along with the potential for forming multiple associations. Further, the sensory modes through which information is gathered are necessarily reduced in number (e.g., a significant reduction in kinesthetic and proprioceptive stimulation), and with that reduction, there is necessarily a diminution of the potential for mutual reinforcement by two or more modes of input and response.

The search for a thorough understanding of the real benefits of stimulant drugs for hyperactive children is far from over. Indeed, in some respects it has hardly begun. The benefits derived by the child and those derived by others in his environment need to be more clearly distinguished. Immediate benefits (especially those that accrue primarily to the environment) must be more carefully weighed against possible impediments to the child's continuing development. And the seemingly obvious, presumed benefits need to be carefully reexamined.

"Responders"

The concept of stimulant drug "responders" has enjoyed some attention in the literature and has stimulated some research. It implies that differential responses to the stimulants occur that are contingent upon a variety of subject characteristics. "Responding" is a curious and almost superfluous concept in some respects. If stimulants are needed to alter hyperactive behaviors, and if, as contended, they are "unusually safe" and rapid in their effects (Wender, 1975), rendering a drug trial highly expedient, predicting response becomes rather an academic exercise.

Yet several predictors have been proposed if not validated. Safer and Allen (1976) cite six studies in support of the observation that "the more hyperactive the child, the better the clinical response." The conclusion is little more than a truism. The more hyperactive the child, the more *obvious* must the response be, since the nonhyperactive child has far less opportunity to respond dramatically with reduced activity level. This "predictor," furthermore, does not obviate the previously discussed problems of measurement, absent norms, and observers' biases. The predictor becomes totally irrelevant if the stimulants are prescribed for reasons other than hyperactivity (e.g., learning problems or simply minimal brain dysfunction without further elaboration).

It has also been contended that the more neurologically impaired the child, the more favorable his response to stimulants is likely to be (Barcai, 1971; Millichap, 1973; Safer and Allen, 1976). Noting that medication is the "most effective single treatment for MBD children," Wender (1975) observes that "responsiveness of many of the signs to the stimulant drugs is so prompt and marked as to have suggested their use as a diagnostic test."

In some instances, the rationale underlying this conclusion is circular. If the various hyperactive behaviors that respond to medication are taken as evidence of neurologic impairment, then so-called neurologically impaired children will respond more obviously to medication *by definition*. The conclusion is logical but meaningless. To render it meaningful, the neurologic impairment of hyperactive children would need to be independently established.

The assertion that neurologically impaired children respond more favorably to treatment than unimpaired children raises several questions that can be addressed empirically. Is there evidence that neurologic impairment assessed independently of hyperactive behaviors is predictive of drug response? Is there evidence that hyperactivity is the consequence of neurologic impairment? Is there evidence that children who are not neurologically impaired also respond to stimulants?

The ambiguity that pervades the concept of minimal brain dysfunction is evident once again. A recent review of biochemical research related to hyperactivity (Ritvo, 1975) concerned the work of only three investigative groups and did not bear directly on the current issues. In the same book (Cantwell, 1975), neurophysiologic studies with hyperactive children were surveyed by Satterfield, who summarized the work of his research group:

> (1) There is an identifiable subgroup of 'good responder' hyperactive children who are found to have low CNS arousal. (2) The pre-treatment CNS arousal level is negatively correlated with the severity of the child's behavioral disturbance; in other words, the lower the child's CNS arousal level, the greater his problem with motor control, attention span and impulsivity. (3) Stimulant medication in these low arousal hyperactive children functions like a stimulant—it increases the CNS arousal level. (4) Those hyperactive children with greatest increases in CNS arousal level resulting from stimulant medication obtained the best clinical response as measured by teacher rating scales.

Although these are the kinds of independent criteria of neurologic dysfunction that are needed, they have not been consistently confirmed, perhaps because of the problems of selecting comparable samples from study to study. Zahn et al. (1975) found no typical indicators of arousal to be "reliably different" between children diagnosed as having MBD and normal children. Prichep et al. (1971) contended that "hyperkinetic children" showed hypoarousal and that Ritalin "normalizes" the evoked potential in these children. However, the criterion of increased arousal on medication was met only under conditions of "uncertainty" (i.e., under conditions of increased demand for attention). In apparent contrast, Cohen, Douglas, and Morgenstern (1971), although observing drug-induced increments in skin conductance and heart rate, found that the orienting response ("readiness reaction") "was more pronounced" in response to placebo than to drug, with an increase in task demands.

Cantwell's (1975) summaries on this topic are perhaps of greatest relevance. With respect to electroencephalographic studies: "There are no EEG abnormalities specific to the syndrome"; with respect to neurophysiologic evaluations: "While it must be said that this appears to be a fruitful area for future research, these evaluations are currently not available to most practitioners and are generally only done in a research setting"; with respect to chromosome studies: "The only reported chromosome study of hyperactive children failed to find evidence of sex chromosome aneuploidy or other chromosome abnormality"; with respect to metabolic and biochemical studies: "Disorders of monoamine metabolism in hyperactive children have been proposed . . . but experimental evidence to support such abnormalities is sparse. Such investigations are only in the research realm at the present time"; and with respect to vitamin deficiencies, allergies to certain food additives, and disorders of glucose metabolism: "None of these claims has been substantiated as yet by proper studies."

In the search for evidence of neurologic impairment in minimal brain dysfunction and hyperactivity, some investigators have turned to the study of "minimal" or "soft" neurologic signs. Constituting a variety of criteria of ostensible neurologic integrity, including balance, fine and gross coordination, laterality, dexterity, tactile discrimination, and spatial orientation, the soft signs met with much opposition almost as quickly as they gained in popularity. Kinsbourne (1975) observed that developmental levels cannot be ignored, since "the child's age is the factor that determines whether the sign represents an abnormality." Schmitt (1975) argues more vehemently that "in general, soft neurological signs are not helpful findings. Most of them represent transient phenomena and disappear with age. At best they are evidence for neurological immaturity."

In a factor analysis of 22 neurologic soft signs and a variety of other variables (Rie et al., 1978), the soft signs did not factor together. Several factored with independent ratings of "neurocognitive dysfunction," and 11 (50 percent) factored with age. These appear to be indices of maturation rather than of neurologic impairment and, the analysis showed, the total number of soft signs was essentially irrelevant as a predictor of other characteristics.

Furthermore, a number of investigators report that various subgroups of hyperactive children with different etiologies can be identified. Ney (1974) distinguished among constitutional, conditioned, chemical, and chaotic hyperactivity that differed with respect to "sex ratio, family history, type of parenting, learning disability and response to treatment." Treatment with stimulants was explicitly recommended only for "chemical" hyperactivity, with environmental, parental, or school interventions proposed for the others in various combinations. Schmitt (1975) refers to "psychogenic hyperactivity", Fish (1975) notes that "the *symptom of hyperactivity* can occur in any one of the psychiatric disorders that occur in children," and Cantwell (1975) asserts that "the term *hyperactive child syndrome* should be used to denote a behavioral syndrome only, with no implications as to etiology."

The response of children without neurologic impairment has been evident virtually from the earliest days of experimentation with stimulants. Bender and Cottington (1942) used Benzedrine to treat children with a variety of disorders, including neurotic behavior disorders, psychoneuroses, and psychopathic personality, as well as organic brain disease. Among these, the majority had neurotic disorders, and they responded behaviorally. However, their therapeutic relationships were adversely affected, since they were deemed to be more resistant and evasive in contending with conflictual material. The organic and schizophrenic children failed to respond.

Similar observations were made by Sleator and Von Neumann (1974) in the responses of hyperkinetic children to methylphenidate. Only 10 of 46 children could have been diagnosed by office visit alone. "A most interesting finding was that the fraction of these obviously hyperkinetic children who were benefited by stimulant medication was smaller than in the group as a whole. Conversely, of the five children on whom the therapeutic effect of methylphenidate was profound, only one would have been deemed a classically hyperkinetic child..." (Sleator and Von Neumann, 1974).

In light of the popular, although essentially unsubstantiated, assumptions about the characteristics of "responders" to stimulants, the recently reported findings of Rapaport et al. (1978) are most telling:

> The behavioral, cognitive and electrophysiological effects of a single dose of dextroamphetamine (0.5 milligram per kilogram of body weight) or placebo was examined in 14 normal prepubertal boys (mean age, 10 years 11 months) in a double-blind study. When amphetamine was given, the group showed a marked decrease in motor activity and reaction time and improved performance on cognitive tests. The similarity of the response observed in normal children to that reported in children with 'hyperactivity' or minimal brain dysfunction casts doubt on pathophysiological models of minimal brain dysfunction which assume that children with this syndrome have a clinically specific or 'paradoxical' response to stimulants.

Analogous trends emerged in our studies on the effects of methylphenidate on underachieving children with behavior problems (Rie et al., 1976 a; 1976 b). Although active drug treatment was no more effective than placebo in enhancing achievement, the subgroup deemed to be free of neurocognitive dysfunction made somewhat greater gains in overall achievement during a 93-day period of drug treatment than did the subgroup with neurocognitive dysfunctions. The difference was greater when only gains in reading skills were compared.

There is little support for the contentions that hyperactivity is an "organic" disorder (except by definition), that children with neurological impairment are more responsive to stimulants than children without such impairment, and that response to stimulants is itself in some way diagnostic of the vaguely defined problems designated as *minimal brain dysfunction* and/or *hyperkinesis*. Some data are accumulating in contradiction to these assumptions. The net effect is that some of the professed guidelines for the prescription of stimulants offer little genuine justification for their use.

Context of Stimulant Drug Popularization

The foregoing material indicates that the popularity of stimulants is necessarily based on more than the available data and logic. The facts that data supportive of their use remain incomplete and that underlying assumptions are, in some instances, contradicted by more recent findings are not surprising or distressing. It is only surprising and distressing that underlying assumptions have been advanced with such certainty and that the value of the stimulants have been proclaimed with such confidence. This posture appears to be partly the product of the context in which it developed.

Prior to the conceptual development of a "syndrome" of minimal brain dysfunction and its variants, including hyperkinetic impulse disorder and the so-called educational counterpart of "learning disabilities," the dominant orientation toward maladaptation in this country was psychoanalytic or at least dynamic. The emphasis was clearly on functional disorders and psychogenesis, and enthusiasm for psychodynamic explanations of disorders and hence the inclination to propose psychodynamic psychotherapies pervaded the mental health fields. Disappointment with the results in many cases appears to have been the consequence of misapplication, and the impetus to seek alternatives. Although there is no dearth of antipsychoanalytic sentiment in the literature, the general context in which the stimulants were "discovered" is exemplified by Levy's observations (1976): "At the same time the impact of psychoanalytic theory exerted its influence, and soon reading and other school difficulties were explained on the basis of subconscious psychosexual disturbances and parent-child conflicts, a misconception still prevalent in some circles." Similarly, the generally accepted imprecise definition of minimal brain dysfunction (Clements, 1966) was formulated explicitly because it was believed that "although organicity is often recognized as a contributor to symptomatology, it is frequently ignored in the final diagnosis of the child, and in the treatment planning, unless it is grossly obvious." With a genuinely critical posture, one would not, of course, attempt to categorize or to explain any diverse group of childhood problems in the same way, nor should it be necessary in scientific affairs to swing with the pendulum from one extreme to another.

We live in a society in which the swing of the pendulum seems to be more the rule than the exception. We are subject to fads and momentary enthusiasms, and the belief in easy, immediate gratification of every sort is quite prevalent. Seductive advertisements in every medium encourage these wishful fantasies. The immediate and often dramatic behavioral response to stimulants is like the realization of such a fantasy, something approaching a panacea.

Finally, there are elements within the medical culture that similarly encourage reliance on stimulants. Demand for the services of primary care physicians virtually necessitates reliance on treatment that requires minimal commitments of time. Lengthy explorations that are necessary to comprehend the multiple determinants of childhood adaptive patterns, and the equally lengthy and repetitive efforts to coordinate multiple interventions and genuinely to monitor progress appear far too burdensome, if not impossible. Writing a prescription is, in contrast, quick and easy.

But if the time is lacking, so often is the inclination. Physicians who provide primary care tend to have limited interest in and commitment to "mental health problems." Such problems are of a different order from the biomedical problems that are of primary concern. Anyone who has taught in medical settings is aware of the effort required to stimulate interest in the "soft" data of child development and psychopathology, of the predominance of prescriptive approaches, and of the intolerance for the ambiguities of human adaptation, except of course in psychiatry. Additionally, the emphasis on treating and alleviating distress as quickly as possible, though laudable, can lead to uncritical and premature treatment. We believe that this occurs in the treatment of hyperactivity.

Conclusion

This is not the context in which to propose alternative modes of managing children with the various problems that have been designated as *minimal brain dysfunction* and *hyperkinesis*. Yet the adversely critical comments concerning stimulant drugs need to be placed in perspective, lest the proponents of their use dismiss these observations as extremist.

It is evident that stimulants are effective, and sometimes dramatically so, in altering behaviors of certain kinds during the period of drug administration in the majority of children, including nonhyperactive children. Such behavioral changes are essential, at least for short periods, in the relatively small number of cases in which the blatantly hyperactive behavior has grossly negative consequences for the child. But it is open to speculation, in the absence of research, whether reduction in activity levels is necessarily and invariably the blessing it is assumed to be. It is also evident that stimulants are ineffective in contending with a variety of other problems for the treatment of which they have been prescribed. Further, it is becoming increasingly clear that favorable outcomes may be the exception after long-term treatment, and that little is really known about long-term "side effects." Indeed, though the immediate side effects are familiar and, in many cases, apparently controllable by dose (and hence have not been addressed systematically in this chapter), it is not as clear as seems generally to be assumed that persistence of side effects is limited to a handful of children.

It is contrary to both fact and logic to proclaim MBD (in all of its ostensible manifestations) a medical or nonmedical problem *a priori*. Such diverse problems of adaptation will be neither understood nor properly treated by personnel who cannot, individually or in concert, bring to bear adequate sophistication in all relevant fields. One wonders how often it is lack of training and competence in a given realm rather than the attributes of the child that culminate in a given diagnosis or in failure to recognize a variety of related problems (Cummings and Finger, 1979).

Finally, multiple approaches are obviously required to contend with multiple problems. Just as it is naive to assume that stimulants are the treatment of choice for every child who exhibits hyperactive symptoms, it is equally naive to assume that stimulants are the sole necessary treatment for those who genuinely require it.

If social pressures, professional mores, limited data, and demands for service generated the familiar enthusiasm for stimulant drugs, it is time to shed unwarranted assumptions and to rely insistently on fact in diagnosing and treating children with maladaptive patterns. The result must inevitably be less reliance on stimulant drugs and more reliance on (or development of) alternative approaches that offer greater hope of fostering the child's development—socially, emotionally, and scholastically—not simply of suppressing behavior that is, or is deemed to be, undesirable.

References

Barcai, A.: Predicting the response of children with learning disabilities and behavior problems to dextroamphetamine sulfate. Pediatrics 47:73–79, 1971.

Barkley, R.A., and Cunningham, C.E.: Stimulant drugs and academic performance in hyperkinetic children: a review. In *Symposium on Hyperactivity in Children*, Annual Convention of the American Psychological Association, San Francisco, August 1977.

Bender, L., and Cottington, F.: The use of amphetamine sulfate (benzedrine) in child psychiatry. Am. J. Psychiatry 99:116–121, 1942.

Bradley, C.: The behavior of children receiving benzedrine. Am. J. Psychiatry 94:577–585, 1937.

Cantwell, D.P.: Diagnostic evaluation of the hyperactive child. In Cantwell, D.P., ed., *The Hyperactive Child*, New York, Spectrum Publications, 1975.

CIBA: MBD case history #1: (an advertisement for Ritalin). Clin. Pediatr. 14:836–838, 1975.

Clements, S.D.: *Minimal Brain Dysfunction in Children—Terminology and Identification.* Washington, D.C., Public Health Service Publication No. 1415, 1966.

Clemmens, R.L., and Kenny, T.J.: Clinical correlates of learning disabilities, minimal brain dysfunction and hyperactivity. Clin. Pediatr. 11:311–313, 1972.

Cohen, N.J., Douglas, V.I., and Morgenstern, G.: The effect of methylphenidate on attentive behavior and autonomic activity in hyperactive children. Psychopaharmacologia 22:282–294, 1971.

Conners, C.K.: Recent drug studies with hyperkinetic children. J. Learn. Disabil. 4:476–483, 1971.

Conners, C.K.: What parents need to know about stimulant drugs and special education. J. Learn. Disabil. 6:349–351, 1973.

Conners, C.K., Eisenberg, L., and Sharpe, L.: Effects of methylphenidate (Ritalin) on paired-associate learning and Porteus Maze performance in emotionally disturbed children. J. Consult. Psychol. 28:14–22, 1964.

Conrad, W.G., Dworkin, E.S., Shai, A., et al.: Effects of amphetamine therapy and prescriptive tutoring on the behavior and achievement of lower class hyperactive children. J. Learn. Disabil. 4:509–517, 1971.

Cummings, S.T., and Finger, D.C.: Emotional disorders. In Rie, H.E., and Rie, E.D., eds., *Handbook of Minimal Brain Dysfunctions: A Critical View*, New York, John Wiley and Sons, Inc., 1979.

Denhoff, E., Davids, A., and Hawkins, R.: Effects of dextroamphetamine on hyperkinetic children: a controlled double blind study. J. Learn. Disabil. 4:491–498, 1971.

Digman, J.M.: A test of a multiple-factor model of child personality. Progress Report NIMH MH 08659-01. Washingon, D.C., United States Public Health Service, March 1965.

Douglas, V.I.: Stop, look and listen: the problem of sustained attention and impulse control in hyperactive and normal children. Can. J. Behav. Sci. 4:259–282, 1972.

Erenberg, G.: Drug therapy in minimal brain dysfunction: a commentary. Ped. Pharmacol. Ther. 81:359–365, 1972.

Fish, B.: Stimulant drug treatment of hyperactive children. In Cantwell, D.P., ed., *The Hyperactive Child*, New York, Spectrum Publications, 1975.

Friedman, R., Dale, E.P., and Wagner, J.H.: A long-term comparison of two treatment regimens for minimal brain dysfunction. Drug therapy versus combined therapy. Clin. Pediatr. 12:666–671, 1973.

Garfinkel, B.S., Webster, C.D., and Sloman, L.: Methylphenidate and caffeine in the treatment of children with minimal brain dysfunction. Am. J. Psychiatry 132:723–728, 1975.

Helper, M.M.: Follow-up of children with minimal brain dysfunctions: outcomes and predictors. In Rie, H.E., and Rie, E.D., eds., *Handbook of Minimal Brain Dysfunctions: A Critical View*, New York, John Wiley and Sons, Inc., 1979.

Kennedy, C., and Ramirez, L.S.: Brain damage as a cause of behavior disturbance in children. In Birch, H.G., ed., *Brain Damage in Children*, Baltimore, Williams and Wilkins, 1964.

Kinsbourne, M.: School problems. Pediatrics 52:697–710, 1973.

Kinsbourne, M., editorial: MBD—a fuzzy concept misdirects therapeutic efforts. Postgrad. Med. 58:211–212, 1975.

Levitis, K.A.: Need for medication in minimal brain dysfunction (letter). Pediatrics 54:388, 1974.

Levy, H.B.: Minimal brain dysfunction/specific learning disability: a clinical approach for the primary physician. South. Med. J. 69:642–653, 1976.

Loney, J., Langhorne, J.E., and Paternite, C.E.: An empirical basis for subgrouping the hyperkinetic/MBD syndrome. J. Abnorm. Psychol. In Press, 1978.

Millichap, J.G.: Drugs in the management of minimal brain dysfunction. In DeLa Cruz, F.F., Fox, B.H., and Roberts, R.H., eds., *Minimal Brain Dysfunction*, New York, New York Academy of Sciences, 1973.

Ney, P.G.: Four types of hyperkinesis. Can. Psychiatr. Assoc. J. 19:543–550, 1974.

Prichep, L.S., Sutton, S., and Hakerem, G.: Evoked potentials in hyperkinetic and normal children under certainty and uncertainty: a placebo and methylphenidate study. Psychophysiology 31:291, 1971.

Rapoport, J.L., Buchsbaum, M.S., Zahn, T.P., Weingartner, H., Ludlow, C., and Mikkelsen, E.J.: Dextroamphetamine: cognitive and behavioral effects in normal prepubertal boys. Science 199:560–562, 1978.

Riddle, K.D., and Rapoport, J.L.: A 2-year follow-up of 72 hyperactive boys. J. Nerv. Ment. Dis. 162:126–134, 1976.

Rie, H.E.: Definitional problems. In: Rie, H.E., and Rie, E.D., eds., *Handbook of Minimal Brain Dysfunctions: A Critical View*, New York, John Wiley and Sons, Inc., 1979.

Rie, H.E.: Hyperactivity in children. Am. J. Dis. Child. 129:783–789, 1975.

Rie, E.D., and Rie, H.E.: Recall, retention and Ritalin. J. Consult. Clin. Psychol. 45:967–972, 1977.

Rie, E.D., Rie, H.E., Stewart, S., and Rettemnier, S.R.: An analysis of neurological soft signs in children with learning problems. Brain Lang. 6:32–46, 1978.

Rie, H.E., Rie, E.D., Stewart, S., and Ambuel, J.P.: Effects of methylphenidate on underachieving children. J. Consult. Clin. Psychol. 44:250–260, 1976a.

Rie, H.E., Rie, E.D., Stewart, S., and Ambuel, J.P.: Effects of Ritalin on underachieving children: a replication. Am. J. Orthopsychiatry 46:313–322, 1976b.

Ritvo, E.R.: Biochemical research with hyperactive children. In Cantwell, D.P., ed., *The Hyperactive Child*, New York, Spectrum Publications, 1975.

Rodin, E., Lucas, A., and Simpson, C.: A study of behaviour disorders in children by means of general purpose computers. In *Data Acquisition and Processing in Biology and Medicine*, 3, Proceedings of the 1963 Rochester Conference, New York, Pergamon Press Inc., 1964.

Ross, Dorothea M., and Ross, Sheila A.: *Hyperactivity: Research, theory, and action. Personality Processes.* New York, John Wiley and Sons, Inc. 1976.

Routh, D.K., and Roberts, R.D.: Minimal brain dysfunction in children: failure to find evidence of a behavioural syndrome. Psychol. Rep. 31:307–314, 1972.

Safer, D.J., and Allen, R.P.: *Hyperactive Children: Diagnosis and Management.* Baltimore, University Park Press, 1976.

Satterfield, J.H.: Neurophysiological studies with hyperactive children. In Cantwell, D.P., ed., *The Hyperactive Child*, New York, Spectrum Publications, 1975.

Satz, P., and Fletcher, J.M.: Minimal brain dysfunctions: an appraisal of research concepts and methods. In Rie, H.E., and Rie, E.D., eds., *Handbook of Minimal Brain Dysfunctions: A Critical View*, New York, John Wiley and Sons, Inc., 1979.

Schmitt, B.D.: The minimal brain dysfunction myth. Am. J. Dis. Child. 129:1313–1318, 1975.

Schrag, P., and Divoky, D.: *The Myth of the Hyperactive Child: And Other Means of Child Control.* New York, Random House Inc., 1975.

Sleator, E.K., and von Neumann, A.W.: Methylphenidate in the treatment of hyperkinetic children. Clin. Pediatr. 13:19–24, 1974.

Sprague, R.L., and Sleator, E.K.: Drugs and dosages: implications for learning disabilities. Paper presented at the NATO Conference on the Neuropsychology of Learning Disorders, Korsor, Denmark, June 1975.

Sroufe, L.A.: Drug treatment of children with behavior problems. In Horowitz, F., ed., *Review of Child Development Research*, 4, Chicago, University of Chicago Press, 1975.

Weiss, G., Minde, K., Werry, J.S., Douglas, V., and Nemeth, E.: Studies on the hyperactive child. VIII, Five-year follow-up. Arch. Gen. Psychiatry 24:409–414, 1971.

Wender, P.H.: The minimal brain dysfunction syndrome. Annu. Rev. Med. 26:45–62, 1975.

Werry, J.S.: Studies of the hyperactive child. IV, An empirical analysis of the minimal brain dysfunction syndrome. Arch. Gen. Psychiatry 19:9–16, 1968.

Zahn, T.P., Abate, F., Little, B.C., and Wender, P.H.: Minimal brain dysfunction, stimulant drugs, and autonomic nervous system activity. Arch. Gen. Psychiatry 32:318–387, 1975.

20

Is Hexachlorophene Too Dangerous to Use in Pediatric Nurseries?

THE ROUTINE USE OF HEXACHLOROPHENE (HCP) IN THE NEWBORN NURSERY SHOULD BE BANNED

Philip D. Walson, M.D., Rubin Bressler, M.D. and Vincent A. Fulginiti, M.D.

HEXACHLOROPHENE: A USEFUL AND LIFESAVING DRUG

Louis Gluck, M.D.

The skin calls for faculty of close observation and attention to detail.

Louis A. Duhring

The diseases of the young are in large part preventable diseases. Epidemics carry off in great proportion the healthy members of a community.

Sir William Withey Gull

Sickness is catching.

William Shakespeare,
A Midsummer Night's Dream

Introduction

Hexachlorophene (HCP), after years of widespread and apparently effective and safe use, has in recent years come under a cloud, and its former ubiquitousness in personal products is (at least for the moment) a thing of the past. Walson, Bressler, and Fulginiti argue that this is not only a good thing, but that (1) there is no "safe" level of human exposure to HCP, (2) better alternative measures are available, (3) epidemic staphylococcal disease in nurseries cannot be prevented by HCP, and (4) the routine use of HCP should be banned in all newborns.

Gluck takes a quite different position. Having personally seen the ravages of infectious outbreaks in newborn nurseries, and the decrease in such epidemics subsequent to the introduction of HCP, he is understandably reluctant to abandon its use in favor of procedures that seem unrealistic and that impede hospital care. Like Walson et al., Gluck acknowledges that HCP can cross the skin and reach tissues such as those in the brain, especially in certain kinds of patients, but he stresses that the avoidance of HCP in prematures and in children with widespread loss of skin integrity would render its use safe as well as effective. He believes also that the variations in epidemiologic statistics for nursery infection before and after the limitations on HCP represent cogent evidence in favor of the overall benefits of the antiseptic. He recommends its use whenever there is an outbreak of staphylococcal disease in a nursery and its application to all term babies, especially when there is a question of infection.

Has the pendulum swung too far—or not enough?

LOUIS LASAGNA, M.D.

The Routine Use of Hexachlorophene (HCP) in the Newborn Nursery Should Be Banned

Philip D. Walson, M.D.

Rubin Bressler, M.D.

Vincent A. Fulginiti, M.D.

Arizona Health Sciences Center, Tucson

Considerations in Hexachlorophene Use

The use of hexachlorophene (HCP) in neonatal practice has received much attention. Adversary positions that focus upon the benefits or risks of its use have been espoused. As with any therapeutic modality, the decision whether or not to use an agent can be made only after a careful analysis of both benefit and risk to the patient.

Cost-benefit analysis (Bressler et al., 1977) supports the contention that the widespread use of HCP in the newborn nursery is unjustified and at least potentially dangerous. Unfortunately, many supporters of the routine use of 3 percent HCP bathing of newborns ignore the following major considerations.

1. An infant residing in a newborn nursery may acquire staphylococcus organisms which can lead to clinical disease. Infection can occur while the infant is in the hospital nursery or after discharge. However, infections are usually mild and do not place the infant at substantial risk. This type of staphylococcal colonization and disease can be reduced by the use of 3 percent hexachlorophene bathing, especially if adequate attention is given to washing the umbilical cord stump.

2. Virulent ("hot") strains of staphylococcus that produce serious life-threatening disease do not appear to be prevented, contained, or aborted by hexachlorophene (Gehlbach et al., 1975; Sutherland, 1973). Such epidemics are cyclical in nature, have an unknown pathophysiologic basis, and may subside spontaneously.

3. Evidence suggests that as the staphylococcal colonization of the infant decreases with the use of hexachlorophene, the gram negative (pseudomonas, klebsiella) colonization rate rises. The increased gram negative flora may be associated with an increase in clinical infections due to these organisms.

4. There are alternatives to hexachlorophene bathing. HCP has no effect in a special nursery, where the environment is excellent and where personnel practice the highest level of asepsis 24 hours a day (Gezon, 1969). When the only alternative to this is to employ a potentially toxic product with as yet undetermined central

nervous system effects of long range implication, there really is no choice except to insist upon scrupulous technique.

The use of the cohort nursery concept with alternating use of rooms has been successfully employed in containing epidemics (Gehlbach et al., 1975; Shaffer et al., 1956). Although it requires more space than the usual nursery, it is an effective means of control.

Handwashing is crucial in preventing spread of infection in the nursery environment (Mortimer et al., 1962). More than any other single determinant, the transfer of bacteria—from infant to infant or from personnel to infant—on the hands (or equipment) of personnel accounts for nosocomial disease. Even without hexachlorophene "shielding" or some other protective method, strict attention to handwashing will keep infant contamination at a minimum if not eliminate it as a serious threat.

Bacterial interference (utilizing the staphylococcus strain 502A of Shinefield) has proven its usefulness in epidemic control (Shinefield et al., 1963). Substitution of the minimally invasive 502A for the bacterial flora of the newborn prevents colonization with virulent staphylococci. In epidemics, this method has been demonstrated to halt the spread of infection and terminate the episode.

Other alternatives, such as application of bacteriostatic dyes, use of antiseptics other than HCP, administration of antibiotics, and use of immunoprophylaxis with a variety of products are promising but have not been substantiated by appropriate controlled trials.

Background

HCP is a chlorinated biphenol that has been used extensively as a bacteriostat in soaps. To be effective, these soaps must deposit in the stratum corneum of the skin a residue of HCP sufficient to reduce the bacterial flora (Fahlberg et al., 1948; Philips and Warshowsky, 1958). The antibacterial activity of HCP is five to tenfold greater for gram positive than for gram negative organisms (Forfar et al., 1968).

Since its discovery in the 1940s, HCP has been used for the prophylaxis and therapy of cutaneous infections such as impetigo, carbuncles, furuncles, cradle cap, miliaria, diaper rash, mastitis, and other pyogenic skin infections.

HCP has been widely used in hospital nurseries since 1961, when Gluck and associates reported that daily bathing of newborn infants with a 3 percent suspension prevented colonization of the skin by coagulase-positive staphylococci (Simon et al., 1961; Gluck et al., 1961) and left a residue that reached a maximum after three baths.

In 1971, a series of studies in animals (rats and monkeys) showed that HCP could be absorbed from the intact skin and result in central nervous system damage (Kimbrough, 1973). A previous isolated report (Herter, 1959) had been largely ignored. As a result of these findings, HCP was limited to prescription use, and manufacturers were required to state on the label that 3 percent HPC is "not for routine prophylactic total body bathing" (Lockhart, 1973).

The current confusion concerning the safety and efficacy of HCP has its roots in the regulatory climate of the 1950s and early 1960s. Detailed efficacy and toxicity guidelines, which are now required prior to the clinical introduction of any drug, had not yet been established. During this decade, HCP attained widespread use in nurseries as a topical bacteriostatic agent deemed effective in control of Staphylococcus aureus colonization and disease, despite the absence of specific safety and efficacy studies. Clinical testing protocols for drug development were never applied to hexachlorophene, since they were not required at the time.

Potential hazards of HCP were brought to light by happenstance rather than through specific studies. HCP toxicity in humans has since been well documented (Herter, 1959; Kimbrough, 1973; Larsen, 1968). It is usually the result of accidental ingestion or application to large areas of burned or otherwise damaged skin. Systemic toxicity after such exposure is manifested in part by seizures and weakness of peripheral extremities. However, documented central nervous system lesions have also been reported in infants after routine use (Kimbrough, 1973; Schuman et al., 1974).

HCP can be absorbed through intact skin; this is the most significant pharmacologic fact to emerge from the human studies. Absorbed HCP is toxic to the central nervous system (CNS) and produces "spongy" degenerative vaculating lesions of the brain and spinal cord (Schuman et al., 1974). Maturity may play a role in skin permeability, detoxification by the liver, and the susceptibility of myelin to the drug's effects, since lesions associated with HCP bathing are much more common in premature than in mature infants.

Toxicity: Animal Studies

A large body of toxicologic information exists on the effects of HCP in animals, including monkeys (Kimbrough, 1973; Lockhart, 1973; Trout, 1973). Although it is difficult to extrapolate animal data directly to humans, there is no question that:

1. HCP can be absorbed from the gastrointestinal (GI) tract or skin of adult and newborn animals.
2. High doses produce neurologic signs such as leg weakness as well as identifiable morphologic lesions in the central nervous system.
3. Similar morphologic lesions (vacuolization of the white matter in the brain and spinal cord) can be produced with doses that produce neither death nor overt neurologic signs.
4. Morphologic brain alterations in rats and monkeys are found at plasma HCP levels of 2 to 3 μg/ml.

Animal studies have often used oral or parenteral rather than topical administration. Vehicles were used frequently to dissolve the HCP. These vehicles may have contributed to the absorption of the HCP or might even have had their own adverse effects. These methodologic problems and the well known differences in drug metabolism between various animal species make it difficult to extrapolate data to man. However, toxicity in humans has been clearly documented.

Toxicity: Human Studies

In light of the toxicity demonstrated in animals, concern arose about the use of HCP in human newborns.

Absorption through human skin was clearly documented to result in measurable blood levels. The higher blood levels were of the same order as those noted to produce vacuolar brain lesions in rats and monkeys. These studies are summarized in Table 20–1.

Table 20–1. *Percutaneous Absorption of HCP in Humans*

Study	Population	Exposure	Blood Levels Mean μg/ml (Range)
1	Newborn Infants (n = 53)	Baths with 5 cc of 3% HCP for 1–5 days with rinsing	0.345 (0.00–0.80)
2	Newborn Infants (n = 50)	"Routine" baths with 3% HCP for 1–11 days	0.109 (0.01–0.65)
3	Premature Infant (33 wks gestation) (n = 1)	24 daily baths with 3% HCP	1.10
4	Adult Volunteers	Hand washing with 5 ml of 3% HCP Q.I.D. for 28 days	0.07
5	Adult Volunteers	Hand and face washing with 3% HCP T.E.D.	0.196
6	Adult Volunteers	5 minutes of total body bathing with 3% HCP B.E.D. for 60 days	1.36° (0.50–2.16)
7	Adult Volunteers	10 minutes of bathing with 0.75% HCP for 21 days	0.52 males 0.28 females
8	Newborns (27–42 wks gestation) (n = 27)	3% HCP bath × 3 days; then 1.5% HCP bath × 9 days followed by rinsing	0.80 (0.15–2.78)
8	Newborns (25–40 wks gestation) (n = 27)	1.5% HCP × 6 days; then 3% HCP × 6 days followed by rinsing	0.97 (0.15–4.35)

° Summary of studies on the dermal absorption of HCP in man (Lockhart, 1972, plus data from Tyrala et al., 1977). Value with ° is serum rather than blood level. Blood levels are about one half serum levels.

There is no question that HCP is absorbed in significant amounts after repetitive use in newborns, infants, and adults. Although the reported cases of human toxicity from HCP have been due to inadvertent ingestion, there is no doubt that significant toxicity has occurred. In one report, a five-day old infant was bathed in a 3 percent HCP lotion by mistake (Gluck et al., 1961). After four days of liberal applications, excoriations appeared and the child experienced convulsions. The patient showed twitching, nystagmus, CNS irritability, and extensive excoriation on admission to the hospital. She improved following administration of fluids and was discharged from the hospital, apparently fully recovered. Six burned children also developed convulsions during the course of topical treatment with a 3 percent hexachlorophene compound (Larsen, 1968).

Two more recent events were of particular importance in causing the FDA to ban the routine use of HCP for bathing newborns. The first was the French report describing the deaths of hundreds of infants who were treated with a talcum powder that mistakenly contained 6 percent HCP (Lockhart, 1973). The powder was frequently applied, in an unspecified number of instances, to inflamed skin in the diaper region. These infants presented with a severe skin rash in the diaper region, gastroenteritis, lethargy, and pronounced hyperexcitability. Many infants demonstrated hypertonicity, hyperesthesia, clonic movements of the extremities, opisthotonus, and pyramidal tract signs. Some had papilledema. In severe cases, progression to decerebrate rigidity, respiratory arrest, and death were noted. Several children developed flaccid paraplegia. The use of a 6 percent HCP preparation under the equivalent of an occlusive dressing (a diaper) resulted in concentrated exposure. Examination of the CNS revealed spongy lesions in the brain consistent with HCP toxicity.

The second event was the report that examination of 248 brain stem sections from infants treated in two hospital nurseries revealed possible HCP toxicity (Schuman et al., 1974). In one hospital, 3 percent HCP was diluted 1:100 and applied only to limited skin areas such as the diaper region. At the other hospital, undiluted HCP was routinely used in daily whole body washes with rinsing. Of 248 brains studied, 21 showed vacuolization in the reticular formation and the various long tracts. All but one of the 21 infants were exposed to undiluted HCP, and the only exception had been exposed to HCP at another hospital prior to admission. All but two of the 21 infants had received three or more total body baths. None of the infants who were not exposed to HCP showed the lesions.

The data clearly indicate that HCP can be absorbed even through normal skin. Exposure to high (6 percent HCP) concentrations or repeated use can lead to toxic blood levels, and it may also be associated with characteristic, but nonspecific, lesions of the nervous system.

The potential toxicity of 3 percent HCP is made more likely by (1) the finding of definite human toxicity of a 6 percent product, (2) the demonstrated absorption through intact skin in infants, and (3) the association of neuropathologic changes and signs with certain blood levels.

Virtually any drug used in humans is toxic. In order to determine if a specific drug can be used clinically, the benefit-risk ratio must be determined. How efficacious is HCP as a bacteriostat? Are alternative agents of lower risk known? From toxicity studies, it appears that toxic levels of HCP are achieved with doses at or just in excess of those used clinically. To justify its continued use, HCP must be found to be singularly effective, and less toxic alternatives must not be available.

Efficacy of HCP

Prophylactic skin care with HCP was introduced to prevent virulent epidemic staphylococcal disease in hospitalized patients, including newborns. Epidemics of Staphylococcus aureus, of different specific phage types, reached a peak in 1958 in hospital nursery, maternity, and surgery units. The outbreaks were traced, at least in part, to the transfer of bacteria from infected to noninfected patients on the hands of hospital personnel (Mortimer et al., 1962). Newborns bathed with 3 percent HCP reportedly had a decrease in Staph. aureus colonization and infection (Gluck et al., 1961). Apparent confirmation was reported, establishing HCP as a highly effective bacteriostat (Gluck, 1973). However, dissenting reports have appeared (Plueckhahn, 1973; Kwong et al., 1973; Light and Sutherland, 1973) that question the effect of HCP use in a program of total skin and umbilical cord care.

Reservations concerning the effectiveness of HCP were voiced even prior to the emergence of information on its potential for toxicity (Gezon, 1969; Mortimer et al., 1962) and include the following:

The periodicity of staphylococcal disease. Staphylococcal disease (in both newborns and adults) follows an episodic history. Causes of the wave-like incidence and the changing virulence of the bacteria are not known. The epidemic incidence of serious staphylococcal disease in the late 1950s and early 1960s has not been sustained. Further, a longer view of the history of staphylococcal infection reveals an unpredictable periodicity of epidemics (Light et al., 1975). Certain phage types emerge, produce serious disease for a time, and then become less significant. There is no known reason for this. However, the combination of extensive antibiotic use plus abundant staphylococcal prevalence may encourage changes in the organism due to selection, lysogeny, and transduction (Jessen et al., 1969). A spontaneous decrease in incidence may be falsely attributed to the current modes of therapy. Thus, any decrease in incidence of staphylococcal infections may not be related to the use of HCP or to any other known factor. Partial evidence of the spontaneity of decreased infections is found in the observation that at least one major center observed this decline totally unassociated with HCP use (Light et al., 1975). The decline began prior to use of HCP in this institution, and incidence remained low after this product had not been used for four years. The most significant data came from the premature nursery, where colonization and infection declined and where HCP had never been used.

Failure of HCP in epidemics. Over the years of routine HCP use, this bacteriostat has failed to prevent or control staphylococcal epidemics, although it was used routinely in many nursery epidemics. In several cases, the addition of HCP failed to attenuate or to contain the epidemic (37 cases reviewed by Light and Sutherland, 1973). Thus, virulent ("hot") Staphylococcal aureus epidemics may not be amenable to hexachlorophene treatment.

Increase in other bacteria among the flora. Whereas the use of hexachlorophene has decreased the colonization and staphylococcal infection rate of Staphylococcus aureus, it has resulted in an increase in colonization and infection from gram negative bacilli (pseudomonas, klebsiella) (Light and Sutherland, 1973).

Reports of experience after discontinuing routine HCP bathing. Following the FDA recommendation limiting the routine use of 3 percent HCP bathing, a number of hospitals reported increases in the colonization rates of Staphylococcus aureus, sometimes associated with clinical infection (Campbell and Pitkewicz, 1972; Kaslow et al., 1973). Most of the reported infections were mild and superficial and occurred in the hospital; a number of instances of bullous impetigo of the diaper area occurred at home. One recent report noted bacteremia in seven human infants following cessation of routine hexachlorophene bathing (Hyams et al., 1975). Sixty-six hospitals reported their findings to the Center for Disease Control (CDC) following cessation of routine hexachlorophene bathing; 60 institutions reported increases in staphylococcal disease (Dixon et al., 1972). All the instances reported were of mild staphylococcal disease.

Many problems are raised in evaluation of these types of data. The reports were received following the FDA recommendation, which alerted the nursery units to expect an augmented infection rate. This might have resulted in increased awareness and greater surveillance. It is also possible that only hospitals with difficulties reported; what occurred in the vast number of hospital nurseries that did not report is not known. Thus, the data could have been weighted toward increased colonization and disease. Some hospitals have reported no increase (Dixon et al., 1972; Kaslow et al., 1973).

A retrospective study of 266 hospitals showed that there was, indeed, increased staphylococcal disease in most hospital nurseries following the discontinuation of routine use of hexachlorophene (Kaslow et al., 1973). In this survey, the incidence of staphylococcal disease rose sixfold with cessation of hexachlorophene, compared with nurseries that had never used HCP bathing, either before or after the 1971 FDA recommendations. These data suggest that staphylococcal disease in the first part of 1972 was increasing, and that the increase may have been spontaneous and not causally related to the change in HCP use (see Light et al., 1975 and Najem et al., 1975).

Summary

The question of the role of 3 percent hexachlorophene in prophylaxis is complicated by adversary positions on a complex problem. The major considerations have been touched on briefly.

In reviewing the HCP story, one is impressed

with the performance of the FDA. The regulatory agency not only was involved in the gathering and evaluation of pertinent information on the efficacy and toxicity of HCP but also was involved in the actual research (Kimbrough and Gaines, 1971; Lockhart et al., 1973). Moreover, the FDA remained in excellent communication with the medical community throughout the course of development of information. The recommendations made by the regulatory agency are consonant with the good practice posture of the pediatric community. In an overall consideration of benefit-risk potential, the FDA recommendations appear to be justified. Limitations on HCP use have certainly not left the physician "unarmed"; alternative therapies are available. Furthermore, the controversy has forced a close look at the HCP efficacy data and resulted in a modified view of its role in the neonatal nursery.

Studies are needed on the pharmacokinetics and biochemical pharmacology of HCP. Information is sparse concerning tissue storage; rate, extent, and type of metabolism; ability to permeate the skin; and effects of age or disease states on HCP toxicity or metabolism. Studies on the effect of gestational age and skin condition on HCP absorption and toxicity, such as those done by Tyrala et al. (1977), are to be encouraged, especially where HCP bathing is used to control staphylococcal epidemics.

Also, little is known of the significance of "silent" CNS lesions following hexachlorophene use. The fact that a child appears "normal" on a routine neurologic exam does not exclude pathologic changes or subtle abnormalities. Studies to determine the effects on school performance, IQ, or psychologic development long after hexachlorophene exposure are lacking.

Conclusion

Hexachlorophene bathing of newborn infants is unsafe in the light of known benefits and toxicity. There is evidence that HCP can decrease staphylococcal colonization and minor infections. However, HCP cannot prevent serious epidemic staphylococcal disease in the nursery. Further, HCP has no level of human exposure that is known to be safe. Finally, alternative preventive measures that are safe are available. HCP should be banned from routine use in newborn infants.

References

Bressler, R., Walson, P.D., and Fulginiti, V.A.: Hexachlorophene in the newborn nursery. Clin. Pediatr. 16:342, 1977.

Campbell, A.G.M., and Pitkewicz, J.S.: The incidence of infections in nurseries since the discontinuance of hexachlorophene. Pediatrics 51:361, 1972.

Dixon, R.E., Kaslow, R.A., and Mallison, G.F.: Staphylococcal disease outbreaks in hospital nurseries in the United States, December 1971 through March 1972. Pediatrics 51:413, 1972.

Fahlberg, W.J., Swan, T.C., and Seastone, C.V.: Studies on the retention of hexachlorophene (G-11) in human skin. J. Bacteriol. 56:323, 1948.

Forfar, J.O., Gould, J.C., and MacCabe, A.F.: Effect of hexachlorophene on incidence of staphylococcal and gram-negative infections in the newborns. Lancet 11:177, 1968.

Gehlbach, S.H., et al: Recurrence of skin disease in a nursery: ineffectuality of hexachlorophene bathing. Pediatrics 55:422, 1975.

Gezon, H.M.: Should nursery environmental control measures be reexamined? Pediatrics 44:636, 1969.

Gluck, L., Simon, H.J., Yaffe, S.J., and Wood, H.F.: Effective control of staphylococci in nurseries. Am. J. Dis. Child. 102:737, 1961.

Gluck, L., and Wood, H.F.: Effect of an antiseptic skin care regimen on reducing staphylococcal colonization in newborn infants. N. Engl. J. Med. 265:1177, 1961.

Gluck, L.: A perspective on hexachlorophene. Pediatrics 51:400, 1973.

Herter, W.B.: Hexachlorophene poisoning. Kaiser Foundation M. Bulletin 7:228, 1959.

Hyams, P.J., et al.: Staphylococcal bacteremia and hexachlorophene bathing: epidemic in a newborn nursery. Am. J. Dis. Child. 129:595, 1975.

Jessen, D., et al.: Changing staphylococci and staphylococcal infections, a ten year study of bacteria and cases of bacteremia. N. Engl. J. Med. 281:627, 1969.

Kaslow, R.A., et al.: Staphylococcal disease related to hospital nursery bathing practices—a nationwide epidemiologic investigation. Pediatrics 51:418, 1973.

Kimbrough, R.D., and Gaines, T.B.: Hexachlorophene effects on the rat brain. Arch. Environ. Health 23:114, 1971.

Kimbrough, R.D.: Review of the toxicity of hexachlorophene, including its neurotoxicity. J. Clin. Pharmacol. 13:439, 1973.

Kimbrough, R.D.: Review of recent evidence of the toxic effects of hexachlorophene. Pediatrics 51:391, 1973.

Kwong, M.S., Loew, A.D., Anthony, B.F., and Oh, W.: The effect of hexachlorophene on staphylococcal colonization rates in the newborn infant; a controlled study using a single bath method. J. Pediatr. 82:982, 1973.

Larsen, D.W.: Studies show hexachlorophene causes burn syndrome. Hospitals 42:63, 1968.

Light, I.J., and Sutherland, J.M.: What is the evidence that hexachlorophene is not effective? Pediatrics 51:345, 1973.

Light, I.J., Atherton, H.D., and Sutherland, J.M.: Decreased colonization of newborn infants with Staphylococcus aureus, 80/81: Cincinnati General Hospital 1960–1972. J. Infect. Dis. 131:281, 1975.

Lockhart, J.D., and Simmons, H.E.: Hexachlorophene decisions at the FDA. Pediatrics 51:431, 1973.

Lockhart, J.D.: How toxic is hexachlorophene? Pediatrics 50:229, 1973.

Lockhart, J.D.: Hexachlorophene and the FDA. J. Clin. Pharmacol. 13:445, 1973.

Mortimer, E.A., et al.: Transmission of staphylococci between newborns. Am. J. Dis. Child. 104:289, 1962.

Najem, G.R., et al.: Clinical and microbiologic surveillance of neonatal staphylococcal disease: relationship to hexachlorophene wholebody bathing. Am. J. Dis. Child. 129:297, 1975.

Philips, C.R., and Warshowsky, B.: Chemical disinfectants. Annu. Rev. Microbiol. 12:525, 1958.

Plueckhahn, V.D.: Hexachlorophene and the control of staphylococcal sepsis in a maternity unit in Gleelony, Australia. Pediatrics 51:368, 1973.

Schuman, R.M., Leech, R.W., and Alvord, E.C., Jr.: Neurotoxicity of hexachlorophene in the human. Clinicopathologic study of 248 children. Pediatrics 54:689, 1974.

Shaffer, T.E., Baldwin, J.N., Rheins, M.D., and Sylvester, R.F.: Staphylococcal infections in newborn infants. I, Study of an epidemic among infants and nursing mothers. Pediatrics 18:750, 1956.

Shinefield, H.R., et al.: Bacterial interference: its effect on nursery acquired infection with Staphylococcus aureus. V, An analysis and interpretation. Am. J. Dis. Child. 105:683, 1963.

Simon, H.J., Yaffe, S.J., and Gluck, L.: Effective control of staphylococci in a nursery. N. Engl. J. Med. 265:1171, 1961.

Sutherland, J.M.: Comment. Pediatrics 51(Suppl.):428, 1973.

Trout, M.E.; Hexachlorophene in perspective. J. Clin. Pharmacol. 13:451, 1973.

Tyrala, E.E., Hillman, L.S., Hillman, R.E., and Dodson, W.E.: Clinical pharmacology of HCP in newborn infants. J. Pediatr. 91:481, 1977.

Hexachlorophene: A Useful and Lifesaving Drug

Louis Gluck, M.D.
University of California, San Diego

Hexachlorophene (HCP) is truly a landmark drug. In its heyday in the late 1960s, HCP was ubiquitous; so widespread was its use that it was found not only in numerous personal products—including soaps, vaginal douches, antiperspirants, toothpaste, skin lotions, and shampoos—but in products such as furnace filters. It was even used as a fungicide on vegetables and citrus fruits. Nearly every home had a green squeeze bottle of pHisoHex with which almost every mother knew that her child's pustular rash or impetigo could be treated effectively. But HCP became controversial around 1969, after questions had been raised about its toxicity as an antiseptic compound and its widespread use in the bathing of newborn babies. This controversy is the focus of this discussion.

Background

What is HCP? Its chemical name is 2,2[1] methylenebis (3,4,5-trichlorophenol). It was first synthesized in 1939 from trichlorophenol and formaldehyde (Gump, 1941). HCP is a white powder that is insoluble in water, mineral oil, and glycerin, but is highly soluble in propylene glycol, ethyl alcohol, and acetone. Its most important use is as a highly effective antiseptic agent, especially against gram-positive organisms—staphylococci and streptococci in particular—and as a less effective drug against certain gram-negative organisms, including *Neisseria gonorrhoeae* and *Escherichia coli* (Gump and Walter, 1968). HCP has remarkable bacteriostatic properties, inhibiting the growth of *Staphylococcus aureus* in dilutions as great as 1:10,000,000 (Seastone, 1947). It is also bactericidal in higher concentrations. Of particular importance is the fact that there is almost no known resistance to HCP by *Staphylococcus aureus* or the *Streptococcus*, despite as many as 150 passages of *Staphylococcus* in HCP-containing agar broth (Meyer, 1956; Tanaka, 1957; Tanaka, 1958).

HCP is incorporated easily into a variety of compounds, but it is best known as the active antibacterial agent in 3 percent concentration in pHisoHex, used widely since 1949 as a skin antiseptic. In its most popular use—i.e., lathered on the skin—the HCP precipitates on contact with water. Ordinarily, two successive washings leave an antibacterial layer that persists up to 48 hours if it is not disturbed by washing with soap or with a lipid solvent (Gluck and Wood, 1961). Studies on animals showed it to be of extremely low toxicity as ordinarily used (Gump, 1969). Thus, HCP appeared to be the ideal compound for antibacterial surface use: it is highly effective against organisms that create clinical havoc, there is essentially no resistance to it by the usually susceptible organisms, and it can be readily layered on skin and persist there for a long time.

Of most interest and importance at the heart of the controversy is that HCP came into worldwide use for antiseptic skin and umbilical cord care in newborn nurseries. The first reports about the use of HCP-containing compounds on newborn skin concerned prophylaxis against infection with *Staphylococcus aureus* and were documented by Farquharson et al. (1952), Hardyment (1958), and Shaffer et al. (1958), all of whom noted reduction and elimination of pyoderma in newborn infants. Controlled studies by Simon et al. (1961), Gluck and Wood (1961, 1963), and Gezon et al. (1964) showed a very high degree of effectiveness of antiseptic skin and cord care regimens, using 3 percent HCP compounds, in reducing nasal and cord colonization by *Staphylococcus aureus*, and thereby essentially eliminating neonatal staphylococcal infections. Plueckhahn and Banks (1968) described 26,000 deliveries with outstanding success in controlling staphylococcal infection; Gluck et al. (1966) reported 25,000 consecutive deliveries without a single lesion due to *Staphylococcus aureus;* Williams and Oliver (1969) described a long experience with skin and cord care regimens utilizing 3 percent HCP compound with a very low incidence of colonization and disease, despite the elimination of restrictions such as caps, masks, and gowns and limitations on people entering nurseries. Similar experiences have been duplicated by many nurseries around the world.

These findings were (and are) of extraordinary significance, for with their series of controlled studies, Gluck and Wood (1961, 1963) and Simon et al. (1961) established that colonization and subsequent disease with staphylococcus is not the result of bacteria sailing through the air to infect babies, as had been the dogma regarding staphylococcal spread in nurseries, but that it results from cord and nose colonization of the babies, and that spread of organisms was a phenomenon of transfer by hands. This information and the ability to control staphylococcal colonization with pHisoHex made possible one of the most important advances in the 20th century, the *Newborn Intensive Care Unit.*

The Newborn Nursery

Bacterial infection with sepsis had been the scourge of newborn nurseries since its first description by Dunham in 1933. Streptococcus and Staphylococcus had early been identified as two of the murderous offenders. Care in newborn nurseries was given with difficulty, and it was a peculiar defensive care based upon the presumed necessity to hide from these organisms. Virtually everyone who practiced medicine in newborn and premature nurseries during the 1950s and early 1960s appreciated the near impossibility of giving adequate open care to babies in the face of stringent restrictive regulations emanating from health departments.

First of all, there were no newborn intensive care units. Premature nurseries existed, dating back many years to their founding by Dr. Julius Hess at Chicago's Michael Reese Hospital. These were able to provide the most important ingredients for survival (warmth and nutrition) for premature babies, but little else. Because of the fear of infections—there had been many epidemics of staphylococcal disease in newborn nurseries over the years—numerous regulations restricting the management of infants were implemented. Mostly these were in term nurseries, but they applied as well to premature nurseries. "Suspect" nurseries existed in both types, where babies who were suspected of being ill and especially of having sepsis were transferred for observation. Sick infants were transferred to pediatric wards, and therefore newborn and premature nurseries were largely areas in which custodial care for normal term babies and "normal prematures" was given.

The complexity of providing even the relatively primitive care of the era can be understood by considering that in the view of epidemiologists and infection control officers, the entire biologic environment—including attendant personnel and other infants plus the physical environment, including dust particles, equipment, walls, floors, blankets, laundry, and other fomites—somehow contributed to the pool of bacteria, (most notably Staphylococcus) in the air that in some way settled on the infants, infected their umbilical cords and skin areas and eventually got into their noses. Thereupon, infants became carriers and cross-infected each other, infected themselves, and infected their families. Frequently, within the first several weeks of discharge, infants were readmitted with pustules, sepsis, or meningitis or with the dreaded staphylococcal pneumonia. Among family members, pustules and boils were passed from one to another. Nasal carriage of the same organism by the infant, as established by Phage typing, could last as long as two to seven years, according to different studies.

Under the supposed threat from battalions of airborne organisms, a variety of recommendations, both reasonable and unreasonable, were made. In 1960, Wheeler asked "How can the conduct of our nurseries by improved?" The suggestions he listed were as follows:

1. One could eliminate nurseries altogether and send infants home after rooming-in with

the mother.

2. One could isolate each infant in his or her own air conditioned room.

3. The nurseries could rotate so that only those cohort babies born on a given day would stay together in the room and be discharged as a group, with no new admissions into the room until the cohort had been discharged. This was based on the mistaken notion that the babies somehow were protected against colonization if they stayed with other infants of the same age.

4. Common equipment in the hospital (such as bathing tables) should be eliminated.

5. Common equipment that could not be eliminated, such as bottle warmers, should be decontaminated, or disposable diapers, covers for scales, and towels should be used.

6. Ill personnel should be removed from contact with babies.

7. Nasal carriers of Staphylococcus should be treated with neomycin and bacitracin nasal jellies.

8. Personnel who harbor strains causing lesions should be removed from contact with babies. This could pose a severe problem, since as many as two thirds of the personnel in nurseries harbored offending organisms, most usually Staphylococcus.

9. Satisfactory diaper and linen disposal must be provided.

10. Laundry should be sterilized and kept separately for the unit.

11. Individual thermometers, soap, and oil should be used.

12. Vernix should be washed off because of its ability to harbor organisms.

13. Dust must be controlled by wet mops or sticky areas.

14. Ultraviolet light should be placed around the room to kill organisms in the air.

15. Mathematical principles of exchange transfusion should be applied to bacteria in the air, their numbers estimated, and then the number of air conditioning changes adjusted to keep the numbers of bacteria down.

16. If an outbreak does occur, susceptible infants should be converted to nonsusceptibles by appropriately treating all babies in the nursery with therapeutic doses of antibiotics.

The National Conference on Hospital-Acquired Staphylococcal Disease, the USPH-CDC, and the National Academy of Sciences-National Research Council (NAS-NRC) (1958) issued this recommendation: "It is possible to protect infants from colonization by administering an effective antibiotic in full therapeutic doses to all infants beginning immediately after birth and continuing until discharge. Antibiotic prophylaxis of this type effectively prevents colonization in the infant's nose and thus his skin." The incredible complexity of providing care was based on the fear of the Staphylococcus and specifically on the fear that the organisms would sail through the air and land on babies.

Not only was general care dictated by these fears, but so was the architectural design of nurseries. Recommendations for nursery design—for example, in an article by Eichenwald and Shinefield (1960)—were:

1. Few infants should share any common air supply; there should be no more than 4 to 6 per unit.

2. There should be wide separation of infants within the unit (30 sq.ft./infant/four-infant unit).

3. There should be a positive pressure ventilating system supplying from 12 to 15, draft free, clean air changes/hour.

4. A cohort rotation system on admission and discharge, plus an overflow nursery, are needed. Babies born the same day are discharged together and no new infants are admitted into their cohort until after discharge.

5. Careful exposure to attendants is essential. There should be contact with the least number of persons needed for adequate nursing care, the same nurses should care for the same infants during their hospital stay, frequent cultures of attendants should be done to detect carriers, and contact of infants with anyone with suspected staphylococcal disease or any respiratory infection must be rigidly avoided.

These concepts had little basis in fact, and were detrimental because they introduced impediments to care. It became clear, after the controlled studies on staphylococcal colonization, that organisms were not transferred primarily by the airborne route. Interesting studies done by the Sandia Corp. (Ballard, 1967; NASA, 1967) during development of laminar flow rooms (where smoke was introduced into conventional clean rooms even with potent air conditioning facilities) revealed remarkable turbulence, which was greatly enhanced by tables and other objects that increased turbulence to the point where particles were carried from floor level to table level. The implication here is that if airborne carriage of organisms was in fact so important, normal activity and equipment would enhance this to the point that the bulk of organisms would be concentrated about the height of the newborns' cribs. There was no evidence for this, however.

Other Studies on Colonization

Hardyment (1958), Farquharson et al. (1952), and Shaffer et al. (1958) had all used HCP compounds in an attempt to control staphylococcal colonization. In the report by Shaffer and his group (1958), infants were bathed at some time during their hospital stay with pHisoHex. This was done more or less haphazardly—i.e., at some time during the stay of the infant he or she was given an HCP bath. The rate of nasal colonization with this routine fluctuated between about 20 and 50 percent, and the rate of skin colonization ranged from 0 to 20 percent. When pHisoHex was stopped, colonization rates for both skin and nose shot up to over 80 percent, then dropped to previous levels with the reintroduction of occasional HCP baths. The findings were interpreted by the investigators as showing that somehow the wash with HCP prevented loose scales of skin from sailing through the air and infecting babies in distant parts of the nursery. Reports by Jellard (1957) showed that the longer babies stayed in hospitals (in England), the higher the incidence of nasal staphylococcal colonization of babies, remembering also that nasal colonization is important in the genesis of staphylococcal disease of newborns. Dr. Jellard found that when she painted the cords with triple dye (brilliant green, cresyl blue, gentian violet, and acriflavine), the incidence of colonization was retarded. In fact, many babies went home without nasal colonization, whereas those who were untreated had virtually 100 percent incidence of colonization.

We interpreted these studies, particularly those of Shaffer et al. (1958) and Jellard (1957), to mean that skin and cord colonization was paramount to the nasal acquisition of Staphylococcus and that this was preventable by adequate antiseptic skin and cord care. Thereupon, a controlled study was undertaken at the Yale-New Haven Hospital (Gluck and Wood, 1961, 1963). First of all, babies were cultured to establish the normal incidence of nose and cord colonization, which was about 51 percent of the 500 babies sampled. The infants then were put on an antiseptic skin and cord care regimen; right after birth each infant was lathered with full strength (3 percent) pHisoHex. This was rinsed off and the baby was dried thoroughly. Special attention was paid to the cord to make sure that it was cleansed. On admission to the nursery, a second pHisoHex bath was given, again with particular attention to the cord. Every day, a total body bath was given with special care to the cord.

On this regimen, colonization of nose and cord of the next approximately 1000 babies fell from 51 percent to 3 percent. Because it was not certain that we had not simply reduced the numbers of flakes of infected skin sailing through the air, we mixed the babies at random so that approximately one of every three was given antiseptic skin and cord care and put among other infants who were only rinsed with water. Before we did this, all washing with pHisoHex was stopped. The incidence of colonization of skin (and cord) and nose crept back up to about 36 percent. At this point, it was difficult to go back to former "neglect" and not wash these babies with pHisoHex, since nurses had become accustomed to clean infants without pustules or other lesions. The random study washing only one baby and leaving two unwashed continued for the next approximately 400 infants and showed about a sixfold difference (34 percent as compared with 6 percent) between the infants who were not washed and those who had antiseptic skin and cord care.

This established without question the value of antiseptic skin and cord care, and suggested that a pool of staphylococci exists—from many sources including colonized attendant personnel, colonized infants, laundry, blankets, equipment, dust, walls, airborne particles, floors, and the delivery room itself—and that these organisms could be carried to the infants' skin and cord areas and from there to their noses by the infants' own random movements, by nurses, and by clothing, which then contribute further to the pools of staphylococci and cause the infants' problems with colonization. By simply cutting the link between the pool of staphylococci and the infants' skins colonization, incidence took a great plunge.

On the strength of these studies, the world's first Newborn Special Care Unit (Newborn Intensive Care Unit) was founded in 1960 at the Yale-New Haven Hospital. Careful records and bacteriologic surveillance kept both in the normal nurseries and in the special care unit showed that some 25,000 consecutive deliveries occurred without any lesions, and in the Newborn Intensive Care Unit, overall incidence of sepsis decreased from about 2 per thousand live births to 1.7, nearly all of which occurred in the first 48 hours of life, suggesting that they were maternally associated. This is compared with the majority of infections occurring after 48 hours, prior to the introduction of HCP, suggesting that these had been nosocomial (nursery-incurred) infections (Gluck, Wood, and Fousek, 1966).

Further studies with staphylococcal prevention continued, including an important community study. Allegations had been made that stopping normal nasal colonization or disrupting the normal ecology of the nose and skin would result in particularly susceptible infants in the community who would go home uncolonized with Staphylococcus and succumb to an infection once in the community. To this end, 180 families were enrolled in a study in the New Haven area with a total of about 1000 people—babies, their siblings, and their families (Payne et al., 1966). Three groups of infants were followed: (1) those who had been given pHisoHex baths daily and were not colonized at the time of discharge, (2) those who had no pHisoHex and who were colonized at discharge, and (3) those who had no pHisoHex and had not been colonized at discharge. Cultures were taken from these infants weekly; any infections were followed up with cultures taken from the entire family. When bacteria were isolated, the staphylococci were phage-typed. Over 15,000 cultures were taken.

The group of infants who had gone home without staphylococcal colonization and who had been washed with pHisoHex had not a single clinical lesion in either the index infant or his family for the first 12 weeks; during the remainder of the year, there were only five family members with lesions. Only after nine months had passed did the first baby show up with a lesion; by year's end there were only two of these. Contrary to this, among the infants who were colonized on discharge, within the first 12 weeks, 13 family members and six babies had significant clinical lesions. During the course of the year, nine more of these family members and four more infants were affected. Among those who had not used pHisoHex and were not colonized at discharge, during the first 12 weeks, one baby and four family members had clinically significant lesions. During the rest of the year, there were 15 more family members and two more babies with lesions. There was 11 times more chance of disease with Staphylococcus among family members and babies in those not washed with pHisoHex during the hospital stay than in those who were. This was highly significant statistically.

Newborn Intensive Care Units and HCP

The important spinoff of this study was the development of Newborn Intensive Care Units, once one could show that infants required relatively little to prevent cross infection. These units housed infants of various sizes and ages who had different medical, surgical, and infectious problems so that they could receive optimal observation and care. The United States had had perinatal death rates (newborn deaths and stillborns) well in excess of 25/1000 live births. In the 1950s and early 1960s, in many areas this had been as high as 40/1000 live births. Today, with the advent of neonatal intensive care units, which began with the unit we founded at the Yale-New Haven Hospital in 1960, the neonatal mortality rate has dropped into the range of 4 to 5/1000, with a total perinatal mortality rate of only 7 to 8/1000 live births. This figure begins to approach an irreducible minimum. Newborn intensive care units will continue to be inestimable contributions to human lives and their productivity for the future. These units are not without drawbacks, especially in posing many ethical problems, but the general impact has been stupendous, with many babies now alive and doing well that just a short time previously would not have survived and would not have been expected to survive.

However, around 1969, ominous rumblings began to be heard and frightening questions began to be raised. Studies by Kimbrough and Gaines (1971), Curley et al. (1971), and others began to question the safety of HCP. In particular, the studies suggested that absorption of HCP from the skin occurred in newborns. Some of these studies measured blood levels of HCP. These reports elicited emotional responses from clinicians, especially following terrifying studies by Kimbrough and Gaines (1971) showing lesions in the brains of rats that had been fed or injected with HCP. After the initial period of terror, a number of studies followed in various species of animals, all of which showed that with rather high doses of hexachlorophene, cystic lesions appeared in the cerebral cortex. Monkey studies (Winthrop Labs., 1971) showed that HCP tended to affect nervous tissue inside the spinal cord, with lesser lesions in ganglia and peripheral nerves. HCP also attacked the optic nerve in monkeys. In 1973 (Powell et al.), we reported the first lesions witnessed in human infants. These tended to be in infants under 1400 gm who had been washed frequently and all of whom were gravely ill.

The lesions appeared to be accumulations of water with formation of cystic areas (Powell and Lampert, 1977). When a mouse brain was examined after 14 days on HCP, the water content had risen from 76 to 82 percent. This persisted slightly above normal until about six weeks off HCP (Powell and Lampert, 1977). There were no changes in lipid composition or content; merely a water change. In electron micrographs, fluid was seen within the myelin sheaths, splitting them. When HCP was stopped, slight vacuolization persisted as well as proliferative astrocytosis, and the myelin collapsed. After two weeks off HCP, some degeneration still was found, so that stopping HCP still left some lesions—although admittedly few. It is believed that the lesions are generally reversible once HCP is stopped.

It is important to add that once the frequency of washing was cut down, in our experience, even in infants under 1400 gm, the lesions virtually disappeared. Even in the very sickest babies lesions were no longer seen, so that factors other than simple toxicity of HCP apparently were involved. Furthermore, *at no time has any term baby ever been found to have had a lesion.* Lesions have occurred only in infants under 1400 gm.

The HCP Mechanism

Following the initial reports of the absorption and toxicity of HCP, many questions were asked, especially concerning the facts that HCP (1) can cross the placenta, (2) is absorbed from the skin, and (3) may be toxic. How were these missed following its use for so many years? This is not a unique situation. Many drugs in use today have never been evaluated adequately by current standards. A sort of "grandfather clause" exists by which drugs that have been in widespread usage for a long time without any noticable toxicity are assumed to be safe. With the popular acceptance of HCP as an antiseptic agent, and no obvious toxicity in ordinary use, the action of HCP was assumed to be known and understood. Furthermore, the great insolubility of HCP also may have been important in quieting fears about potential toxicity. Possibly the most important single reason for the failure to detect problems with HCP much sooner is the fact that no valid analytic technique that was capable of detecting the parts per million or even per billion of HCP in blood was available until the end of the 1960s (Browning et al., 1968). Perhaps it should have been suspected that HCP was capable of absorption, since in its most widespread use it is suspended in an emulsion containing surface tension lowering agents, which could facilitate absorption through the keratin of the skin and thereby allow HCP to penetrate into hair follicles, sebaceous glands, and pores. Since HCP is soluble in fats and fat solvents, it would have seemed plausible for HCP to be absorbed into the blood, especially through thin skins such as those of newborns.

HCP Toxicity

The cases of human poisoning that had been reported after HCP came into wide use were almost always caused by ingestion of HCP. Only one case had been reported of toxicity from its use on skin. This was in a five-day-old infant whose mother misunderstood the use of 3 percent HCP compound as a wash and used it instead as a lotion (Herter, 1959). The baby was lathered liberally for four days until excoriations appeared and the baby began having seizures. She was admitted to the hospital with twitching, nystagmus, CNS irritability, and extensive excoriations. She was treated with fluids, showed marked improvement, and was discharged from the hospital after 16 days, fully recovered.

In 1968, Larson reported on six children from the Shriners' Burn Hospital in Galveston who developed convulsions during the course of extensive topical treatment with 3 percent HCP compound for burns. Blood levels of HCP were measured and were shown to be elevated. The methods for the analysis of HCP came under question: the levels reported were extremely high and the methods were considered unreliable. (They have since been surpassed by highly accurate techniques.) This was true also for a study reported on experimental burns produced in rats, in which the absorption of HCP from this abnormal skin was measured. Blood levels of HCP in these rats were extraordinarily high, which were later also shown to be due to erroneous analytic techniques.

In December 1968, Browning et al. described a new, highly sensitive and valid analytic technique to measure HCP. Early in 1970, we measured blood levels in 50 infants who had been washed daily with 3 percent HCP compound. These levels were reported to the FDA and subsequently became part of a report by Lockhart (1972).

Reports prior to those on absorption of HCP from babies' skins and on the toxicity of HCP included a note of alarm regarding the alleged increased colonization and infections with gram-negative organisms in nurseries (Forfar et al., 1968; Williams and Oliver, 1969). Presumably, by reducing gram-positive organisms, infections with gram-negative organisms increased. This actually was a relative issue; the total number of infections with the use of HCP *decreased.* The relative proportions of organisms not susceptible to HCP, namely the gram-negative organisms, did increase; but the total number of infections was down (Gluck et al., 1966).

Other toxicities reported included irritation of scrotal skin (McDonald and Woodruff, 1961) and gastrointestinal and CNS toxicity from accidental ingestion (Wear et al., 1962) or from treatment for liver flukes (including diarrhea, vomiting, anorexia, coma, convulsions, weakness of lower extremities, twitching of extremities, and ocular abnormalities). These invariably disappeared after stopping HCP. Photosensitivity and melanosis were also seen.

Blood Levels of HCP

However, the important aspects of HCP's real and potential toxicity came out initially in the report by Kimbrough and Gaines (1971), who studied rats fed a diet containing 500 ppm of HCP. An intermyelinic edema of the white matter in the central nervous system was seen, which was reversible on stopping HCP. If HCP continued to be fed, the rats developed paralysis and died. Curley et al. (1971) then compared blood levels in rats poisoned by being fed HCP with blood levels of infants who were washed with HCP by total body bathing. It was found that blood levels in infants ranged up to as much as 50 percent of those in rats. A study by Feldmann and Maibach (1970) showed that HCP penetrates intact skins in both animals and man. According to their study, 3.1 percent of a topical dose of radioactive labeled HCP passed through intact skin in five days.

Studies generally have suggested that the concentration of HCP in blood is related to the concentration of HCP in the product applied to the skin surface. In part this is correct, but HCP does not accumulate in blood, apparently, with continued use. Additionally, blood levels would scarcely be an adequate reflection of tissue absorption, tissue binding, and tissue toxicity. As with other compounds, blood levels by themselves, unless accompanied by data on blood-tissue equilibria, may be misleading, as appears to be the case with HCP. However, it is fair to say that the highest blood levels of HCP with commercial 3 percent HCP cleanser in infants was about 0.38 mcg/ml, which is about 33 percent of the level producing brain damage in rats by long-term feeding, as reported in 1971 by Curley et al. (see also Cunningham and Tsoulos, 1972; Lockhart, 1972). Total body washing with 3 percent HCP produces blood levels that appear to be less than 10 percent of the toxic levels observed in rats.

In addition to the studies from our institution reported by Powell et al. (1973), other studies (Shuman et al., 1974) reported a large number of very small, ill infants (weighing under 1400 gm) who had undergone total body washing with HCP to show vacuolization of the white matter in the brain. It is important again to emphasize that there is no evidence that any full term baby with normal skin, even with the total body washed in the usual manner, has ever shown untoward effects. Cunningham and Tsoulos (1972) reported a follow-up study of 80 infants washed with 3 percent HCP compound for periods of from 3 to 82 days who showed no apparent ill effects in regard to neurologic status or developmental patterns.

HCP has a half-life of 19 hours and is largely excreted within 24 hours following absorption, being completely eliminated after four to seven days. Almost 85 percent is excreted unconjugated in feces and urine within 96 hours following a single dose local application (Gluck, 1973). Evidence of absorption through the skin of premature infants was shown in a report (Cunningham and Tsoulos, 1972) of a concentration of 1.59 mcg/ml in an infant of 822 gm following daily washing. In another report, a single washing per day with 5 ml of 3 percent HCP produced levels in the blood of between 0.75 and 1.20 mcg/ml, two to four days following application (Gluck, cited in Lockhart, 1972).

Most recently, Plueckhahn and Collins (1976) reviewed 81,756 live births and 858 infant deaths in Victoria, Australia. Autopsy records and histologic sections of brain were available in 245 of the children, and 63 cases of vacuolization of the CNS were found. All were in infants weighing less than 2000 gm at birth. An association of vacuolization was also found with elevated serum bilirubin in low birth weight babies. The assertion was made in this study that vacuolization of the brain has little effect on babies, since those who survived the premature period were mentally and physically normal.

HCP Regulations

The Food and Drug Administration (FDA), in 1972, taking into account these various reports of toxicity and, additionally, a report from France stating that infants who were accidentally exposed to high concentrations of hexachlorophene (6 percent) in talcum powder suffered brain damage, moved to ban all nonprescription uses of HCP. The agency restricted HCP to prescription use only as a surgical scrub and a handwash product for health care personnel. Prior to this, on December 8, 1971, the FDA warned against prophylactic total body bathing of infants with HCP. This was the signal in hospitals in the United States to cease prophylactic bathing of newborns with HCP. Outbreaks of neonatal staphylococcal disease followed, confirmed by the Center for Disease Control (CDC) (1972). Subsequently, there were discussions among the FDA, the CDC, and the Committee on the Fetus and Newborn of the American Academy of Pediatrics about these outbreaks. Accurate assessment of their significance was difficult because staphylococcal disease is not routinely reportable. It also was difficult to determine how severe the illnesses were and whether the handwashing practices of nursery personnel during these outbreaks had changed. It was concluded from these meetings that good nursery practice (aseptic technique) should be emphasized as a preventive measure and that a prophylactic bathing of infants with 3 percent HCP once daily followed by rinsing should be considered when a nursery infection is present.

Soon after the recommended cessation of prophylactic total body bathing, reports of outbreaks of staphylococcal disease were received by the CDC. The CDC actively encouraged state health authorities, hospitals, and manufacturers to report outbreaks in nursery staphylococcal disease for a four-week period beginning January 16, 1972. These reports continued to be received. Between December 31, 1971, and March 25, 1972, 60 epidemiologically investigated nurseries experienced confirmed outbreaks, involving 467 infants in whom there had been discontinuation of HCP bathing.

In order to eliminate any biases due to voluntary reporting of outbreaks, about 300 hospitals in the United States were selected randomly in February 1972. These were polled by telephone by the CDC about their use of HCP for handwashing by personnel and for bathing of infants. More than 95 percent of the hospitals polled had continued to use HCP (or even iodophors) for handwashing of nursery personnel; 243 of these hospitals were chosen by epidemiologists from the CDC or the State Health Department to obtain more information on nursery staphylococcal disease. A number of hospitals were excluded, and finally, 208 hospitals were surveyed.

Hospital Studies of HCP

In 102 hospitals that had discontinued bathing with HCP and used dry skin care or washed with nonmedicated soap and tap water or with tap water alone, there was an increase of staphylococcal disease to 6 cases per 1000 live births. In 58 hospitals in which bathing with HCP emulsion alone had been continued, no increase in disease rates occurred. The difference between the two groups of hospitals was statistically significant at the 5 percent level. In 26 hospitals in which HCP-emulsion bathing had been replaced by bathing with other antimicrobial agents, including antibacterial bar soaps and iodophors, increases in infection rates comparable to those seen in hospitals that had used only dry skin care or nonmedicated soaps or plain tap water were seen. In 22 hospitals in which no antibacterial bathing agent was used at any time during the study, staphylococcal disease rates in newborns increased over a two-month period as compared with the previous six-month period. The difference in rates during the two periods was not significant at the 5 percent level, however.

It is important to recognize that increased awareness did not appear to be an important factor in staphylococcal disease among newborns in nurseries in which HCP bathing routines were discontinued. Serious staphylococcal disease, including bullous impetigo, bacteremia, enterocolitis, and osteomyelitis, increased at about the same rate as did milder staphylococcal disease, and it accounted for about 20 percent of all infections during both time periods.

The National Nosocomial Infections Study of the CDC corroborated this, prospectively polling some 77 hospitals to submit data on surveillance to the CDC from January 1971 through March 1972. Thirty-two hospitals that had nurseries and bathing practices comparable to those chosen for analysis in a random survey reported results consistently. There was, among these 32 hospitals, a rise in staphylococcal disease comparable to that observed in the randomly selected hospitals. A sharp increase had occurred in December 1971 in the rate of staphylococcal disease among hospitals discontinuing HCP emulsions for infant bathing. Monthly rates subsequently remained above those for hospitals using HCP emulsions. A slight increase, furthermore, in the total incidence of staphylococcal disease among all hospitalized patients was noted in the combined group of 77 reporting hospitals. This was attributable to a substantial increase in skin disease with Staphylococcus, primarily in newborns, although no increase was observed for infections at other sites.

The CDC, on the basis of their studies, recommended that total body bathing of neonates with HCP not be done when there is absolutely no evidence of infection. However, it was recommended that nurseries experiencing staphylococcal infection should consider HCP bathing, as had been recommended previously. It was further recommended that this should be limited generally to short-term, in-hospital use and that infants with denuded skin surfaces not be bathed with HCP. Furthermore, careful rinsing must follow the bathing, and any bathing of infants after discharge from the hospital should be under the direction of a physician. The CDC also suggested other infection control practices reminiscent of the aforementioned recommendations made by Wheeler, with strict guidelines on adequate handwashing. Additional suggestions included isolating the infected neonate promptly, having adequate personnel, avoiding crowding of facilities, and developing the practice of cohorting infants routinely.

Effects of HCP on Pregnancy

Recently, new concerns have arisen about the safety of hexachlorophene, again causing the FDA to sound a note of alarm. A study in Sweden of pregnant hospital personnel exposed to hexachlorophene through handwashing was done by Halling (1977). At a New York Academy of Sciences meeting on June 27, 1978, Halling presented a paper entitled "Suspected Link Between Exposure to Hexachlorophene and Malformed Infants." She presented evidence that medical personnel produced a high number of malformed babies in association with HCP handwashing during the first trimester. Unfortunately, this is a poor study and has been criticized in Sweden by the NBHW, the Swedish equivalent of the FDA. Halling investigated the hospital staffs at six Swedish hospitals, all of whom had been exposed several times a day to handwashing with HCP emulsion. She studied 460 mothers, 25 of whom gave birth to severely malformed children. Forty-six other children were born with minor malformations. A control group of 233 offspring showed no major malformations but did show 8 minor ones.

This report created a sensation. Criticism included that by Professor Bengt Kallen, of the NBHW reference group on malformations and developmental disturbances, who felt that there is no evidence at all that HCP may produce fetal damage (1978). The problem is that Halling did not include a random assortment of hospitals. There are many hospitals in which HCP is used and the number of malformed children born to hospital personnel is even below average, according to Professor Kallen. Further, he questioned the fact that no severe fetal damage had been found in the control group of 233 offspring. He considered this a mathematical impossibility, since the statistical average should be between 2 and 3 percent.

On the basis of Halling's report, the FDA has issued a warning. The FDA Drug Bulletin of August/September 1978 stated:

> As an interim precaution until the issue of whether or not hexachlorophene is associated with increased risk of birth defects is resolved, FDA considers it prudent for surgeons, nurses, and other health care personnel who are or may become pregnant to avoid hexachlorophene antibacterial scrubs. They should substitute other safe and effective products.

The FDA acknowledged the reservations about the study because of its technical deficiencies, and it has been in touch with the Swedish academy. But the FDA also felt that it must act, and that published research fails to provide insurance that HCP is safe for use in women who are or could become pregnant. The transfer of HCP across the placenta had previously been reported in studies on cord bloods by Curley et al. (1971). Thus, this must remain an open issue, pending the results of further studies now under way in the United States and Sweden.

Decreased HCP Usage

One of the most impressive changes that has occurred concurrently with the diminution in widespread use of HCP in personal products has been a profound change in the types of organisms that now affect newborns. Whereas the incidence of gram-positive and gram-negative organisms was approximately equal (or there was perhaps a slight preponderance of gram-negative organisms) prior to HCP, with HCP usage, a reduction was seen both in gram-positive organisms and in total infections, with a relative rise in gram-negative organisms. But now there is a reversion to preponderance with gram-positive organisms and a particularly potent lethal organism, group B Streptococcus (GBS). This organism has now become the number one killer and main cause of sepsis in newborns. Because it exists in two clinical forms, infection with GBS can overwhelm an infant shortly after birth or it can occur late in the first week of life, when the primary infection usually is meningitis and seems to be far less lethal. GBS has been identified in the female vagina and in the male urethra and it is a true venereal disease. The high incidence of this disease occurring simultaneously with the decreased use of HCP may not be a coincidence. Many previously available douches and other products that contained HCP would have killed this organism, which is exquisitely sensitive to HCP. Furthermore, standard preparation of the vagina prior to delivery included a scrub containing HCP in most institutions. Thus, the organism may have been eliminated inadvertently and not have infected the baby during birth, as seems to be the major problem today. Therefore, the current rise in GBS disease may well be associated with the general decline in use of HCP in personal products. It would be important to examine the possibility that this has occurred.

Conclusion

It is difficult to place HCP and its use in nurseries in true perspective because of the relative paucity of useful data about many minor points. However, some major factors seem quite clear. In the case of documented infection, including outbreaks, the use of HCP can be lifesaving. It is highly effective as a control measure against staphylococcal as well as streptococcal disease in nurseries.

HCP should therefore never be withheld in nursery outbreaks of staphylococcal disease. Its routine use, with at least a washing after delivery, is encouraged in all term babies, particularly when there is any question whatever about the presence of infection. Overall, its value far exceeds its drawbacks, although we understand the many problems that have been seen, particularly when it has not been used properly—such as on raw skin or in excessive concentrations. Whether the drug is to be totally banned in the future or revived and used in more widespread fashion, one truth is inescapable—hexachlorophene appeared at a time in clinical history when the need for it was essential, and it has resulted in the saving of countless thousands of infants in intensive care units around the world. It is more than a landmark drug; it was an essential drug at a crossroad in medical history.

References

Ballard, D.W.: Contamination control at Sandia Laboratories. Sandia Laboratories Bulletin SC-M-67-423, Jan. 1967.

Browning, R.S., Jr., Grego, J., and Warrington, H.P., Jr.: Gas chromatographic determination of hexachlorophene in blood and urine. J. Pharm. Sci. 57:2165, 1968.

Center for Disease Control (USPHS) and National Academy of Sciences-National Research Council: Recommendations of the National Conference on Hospital-Acquired Staphylococcal Disease. Atlanta, Ga., Sept. 1958.

Center for Disease Control (USDHEW, PHS): Investigation of hospital use of hexachlorophene and nursery staphylococcal infections. Morbidity and Mortality Weekly Report for week ending Feb. 5, 1972. Atlanta, Ga., Feb. 11, 1972.

Center for Disease Control (USDHEW, PHS): Follow-up on nursery staphylococcal disease and its relationship to the use of hexachlorophene. Morbidity and Mortality Weekly Report for week ending July 29, 1972. Atlanta, Ga., Aug. 4, 1972.

Contamination control principles (SP-5045), Washington, D.C., National Aeronautics and Space Administration, 1967.

Cunningham, M.D., and Tsoulos, N.G.: The growth and development of newborns with known hexachlorophene (HCP) levels, abstract. Pediatr. Res. 6:431, 1972.

Curley, A., Kimbrough, R.D., Hawk, R.E., Nathenson, G., and Finberg, L.: Dermal absorption of hexachlorophene in infants. Lancet 1:296. 1971.

Dunham, E.C.: Septicemia in the newborn. Am. J. Dis. Child. 45:229, 1933.

Eichenwald, H.F., and Shinefield, H.R.: The problem of staphylococcal infection in newborn infants. J. Pediatr. 56:665, 1960.

Farquharson, J.H., Penny, S.F., Edwards, H.E., and Barr, E.: Control of staphylococcal skin infections in nursery. Can. Med. Assoc. J. 67:247, 1952.

FDA Drug Bulletin (USDHEW, PHS): Hexachlorophene and newborns. Rockville, Md., Dec. 1971.

Feldmann, R.J., and Maibach, H.I.: Absorption of some organic compounds through the skin in man. J. Invest. Dermatol. 54:399, 1970.

Forfar, J.O., Gould, J.C., and MacCabe, A.F.: Effect of hexachlorophene on incidence of staphylococcal and gram negative infection in the newborn. Lancet 2:177, 1968.

Gezon, H.M., Thompson, D.J., Rogers, K.D., Hatch, T.F., and Taylor, P.M.: Hexachlorophene bathing in early infancy: effect on staphylococcal disease and infection. N. Eng. J. Med. 270:379, 1964.

Gluck, L., Wood, H.F., and Fousek, M.D.: Septicemia of the newborn. Pediatr. Clin. North Am. 13:1131, 1966.

Gluck, L.: A perspective on hexachlorophene. Pediatrics 51(Suppl. II):400, 1973.

Gluck, L., and Wood, H.F.: Effect of an antiseptic skin care regimen on reducing staphylococcal colonization in newborn infants. N. Eng. J. Med. 265:1171, 1961.

Gluck, L., and Wood, H.F.: Staphylococcal colonization in newborn infants with and without antiseptic skin care. N. Eng. J. Med. 266:1265, 1963.

Gump, W.S.: Dihydroxyhexachlorodiphenylmethane and method of producing same. U.S. Patent 2,250,480, July 29, 1941.

Gump, W.S.: Toxicological properties of hexachlorophene. J. Soc. Cosmetic Chemists 20:173, 1969.

Gump, W.S., and Walter, G.R.: The bisphenols. In Lawrence, C.A., and Block, S.S., eds., *Disinfection, Sterilization and Preservation*, Philadelphia, Lea and Febiger, 1968.

Halling, H.: Suspected link between exposure to hexachlorophene and birth of malformed infants. Läkartidningen 74:542, 1977.

Hardyment, A.F.: Control of infections of newborn infants. Pediatr. Clin. North Am. 5:287, 1958.

Herter, W.B.: Hexachlorophene poisoning. Kaiser F. Med. Bull. 7:228, 1959.

Jellard, J.: Umbilical cord as a reservoir of infection in a maternity hospital. Br. Med. J. 1:925, 1957.

Kallen, B.: Quoted in Chemical Week, July 12, 1978.

Kimbrough, R.D., and Gaines, T.B.: Hexachlorophene effects on the rat brain. Arch. Environ. Health 23:114, 1971.

Larson, D.L.: Studies show hexachlorophene causes burn syndrome. Hospitals. J. Am. Hosp. Assoc. 42:63, 1968.

Lockhart, J.: How toxic is hexachlorophene? Pediatrics 50:229, 1972.

McDonald, H.P., Jr., and Woodruff, M.W.: Scrotal reaction to pHisoHex. J. Urol. 86:226, 1961.

Meyer, G.: Studies on the question of increased resistance of bacteria to hexachlorophene. Z. Hautkr. 20:320, 1956.

Payne, M.C., Wood, J.F., Korakawa, W., and Gluck, L.: A prospective study of staphylococcal colonization and infections in newborns and their families. Am. J. Epidemiol. 82:305, 1966.

Plueckhahn, V.D., and Banks, J.: Antiseptic skin care of newborn infants with hexachlorophene. Med. J. Aust. 1:247, 1968.

Plueckhahn, V.D., and Collins, R.B.: Hexachlorophene emulsions and antiseptic skin care of newborn infants. Med. J. Aust. 1:815, 1976.

Powell, H.C., and Lampert, P.W.: Hexachlorophene neurotoxicity. In Roisin, L., Shiraki, H., and Greevic, N., eds., *Neurotoxicity*, N.Y., Raven Press, 1977.

Powell, H.C., Swarner, O., Gluck, L., and Lampert, P.W.: Hexachlorophene myelinopathy in premature infants. J. Pediatr. 82:976, 1973.

Seastone, C.V.: Observations on the use of G-11 in the surgical scrub. Surg. Gynecol. Obstet. 84:335, 1947.

Shaffer, T.E., Baldwin, J.N., and Wheeler, E.E.: Staphylococcal infections in nurseries. In *Advances in Pediatrics*, vol. 10, Chicago, Year Book Publishers, Inc., 1958.

Shuman, R., Leech, P., and Alvard, E.: Neurotoxicity of hexachlorophene in the human. I, Clinicopathologic study of 248 children. Pediatrics 54:689, 1974.

Simon, H.J., Yaffe, S.J., and Gluck, L.: Effective control of staphylococci in a nursery. N. Eng. J. Med. 265:1171, 1961.

Tanaka, J.: Acquired resistance of bacteria to diphenyl methane derivatives. I, Variation in biological functions of the resistant strains. Nippon Saikingaku Zasshi 12:327, 1957.

Tanaka, J.: Acquired resistance of bacteria to diphenyl methane derivatives. II, The sulfhydryl content nutritional requirements of the G-11 and phenol-resistant strains. Nippon Saikingaku Zasshi 13:329, 1958.

Wear, J.B., Jr., Shanahan, R., and Ratliff, R.K.: Toxicity of ingested hexachlorophene. JAMA 181:587, 1962.

Wheeler, W.E.: Infections and nursery problems. Am. J. Dis. Child. 99:722, 1960.

Williams, C.P.S., and Oliver, T.K., Jr.: Nursery routines and staphylococcal colonization of the newborn. Pediatrics 44:640, 1969.

Winthrop Laboratories: Unpublished data submitted to the FDA by Winthrop Laboratories, 1971 (monkey studies of toxicity).

21

Should Estrogens Be Used in Postmenopausal Women?

A STATEMENT IN FAVOR OF ESTROGEN REPLACEMENT THERAPY
Nathan Kase, M.D.

THE NEGATIVE SIDE OF LONG-TERM POSTMENOPAUSAL ESTROGEN THERAPY
Harry K. Ziel, M.D.

If you want to be a dear old lady at seventy, you should start early, say about seventeen.

Maude Royden

No one who is not female can be in a position to make accurate statements about women.

Otto Weininger, *Sex and Character*

Thy bones are hollow.

Shakespeare, *Measure for Measure*

A woman does not take the gout, unless her menses be stopped.

Hippocrates, *Aphorisms*

Introduction

Not all postmenopausal women have symptoms related to estrogen deficiency, but many do. There are, in addition, a variety of organic changes that are either definitely attributable to hormonal changes or are suspected to be.

As these two essays indicate, considerable disagreement exists as to both the efficacy and safety of estrogen replacement therapy. Kase reminds us that women differ enormously in their physiologic and psychologic response to menopause. There is probably least argument about the ability of estrogens to control the "hot flash" syndrome; when such therapy is both low-dose and short-term, there would seem to be little cause for concern. Much more argument prevails about long-term therapy for prevention of osteoporosis, a regimen that Kase believes to make more sense than treatment after the osteoporosis is moderately advanced. Prevention of atherosclerosis no longer appears to be a legitimate indication for estrogen therapy during menopause.

Kase and Ziel both seem to accept endometrial cancer as a risk of estrogen therapy, although they differ on its magnitude and implications. (For the record, there are some who remain unconvinced about the etiologic relationship.)

Ziel is also concerned about a possible increase in breast cancer, hepatomas, cholelithiasis, hypertension, diabetes, and thromboembolic disease. He concludes that at best, one should treat only women who appear to be at risk according to the Singh index, and he prefers to withhold estrogen until all other therapeutic modalities have failed. If estrogen is to be used, he urges the addition of a potent 19 nor-progestin. Kase, although much less apprehensive about estrogen therapy during menopause, also recommends the addition of progestin.

Louis Lasagna, M.D.

A Statement in Favor of Estrogen Replacement Therapy

Nathan Kase, M.D.
Yale University School of Medicine

The thesis of this presentation is that estrogen replacement therapy can be administered to hypoestrogenic women safely and effectively, provided that standard elements of prudent medical practice—careful patient selection, judicious dosage, and meticulous followup—are observed.

In support of this argument, (1) menopause, the most common phase of prolonged hypoestrogenicity, will be defined endocrinologically, and the clinical symptoms will be listed; (2) the advantages of estrogen replacement therapy in spontaneous and induced menopause will be reviewed and evaluated; (3) the disadvantages and dangers of estrogen replacement therapy will also be considered; and (4) a scheme for clinical management of the menopause will be proposed, which includes the circumstances and methods whereby the benefits of estrogen therapy outweigh the risks.

Although this analysis of benefit and risk is directed toward a professional readership, it can form the basis for physician input in the dialogue leading to the informed patient's consent. There are few instances in medicine comparable to estrogen therapy in which patient self-assessment and guided self-determination are as crucial to the effectiveness and safety of the evolving pattern of therapy.

The Female Climacteric

Clinical implications of the female climacteric result from the impact of three factors.

Amount and Rate of Estrogen Depletion

Although most attention focuses on the menopause, ovarian function begins to wane years before the last menstrual period. Women in their late 30s experience decreasing frequency of ovulation, which is accompanied by relative infertility and variable menstrual cycles. Serum follicle stimulating hormone (FSH) levels begin to rise, and some women may even display vasomotor flushes during this premenopausal decline in estrogen. At some point in her early 50s, a woman's estrogen production becomes inadequate for endometrial proliferation to cause menstrual flow. The cessation of menses is call the *menopause.* In the postmenopausal period, despite amenorrhea, estrogen continues to be produced in lesser amounts, which are sufficient to sustain secondary sexual characteristics for many years. Vaginal and vulvar atrophy may not occur until the seventh or eighth decade (Fig. 21–1).

The ovary is not the source of the estrogen produced after the menopause (Fig. 21–2). The adrenal cortex is the origin of the prehormone Δ^4-androstenedione, which is converted to estrone at peripheral nonendocrine metabolic sites, the most important of which is fat. This estrone production is not under the control of the usual factors modifying pituitary-ovarian interactions that ordinarily maintain physiologically appropriate quantities of estradiol during the reproductive years (Siiteri and MacDonald, 1973).

In the absence of this feedback mechanism,

Figure 21-1. From Clinical Gynecological Endocrinology and Infertility, By Leon Speroff, Robert Glass, and Nathan Kase, Williams and Wilkins.

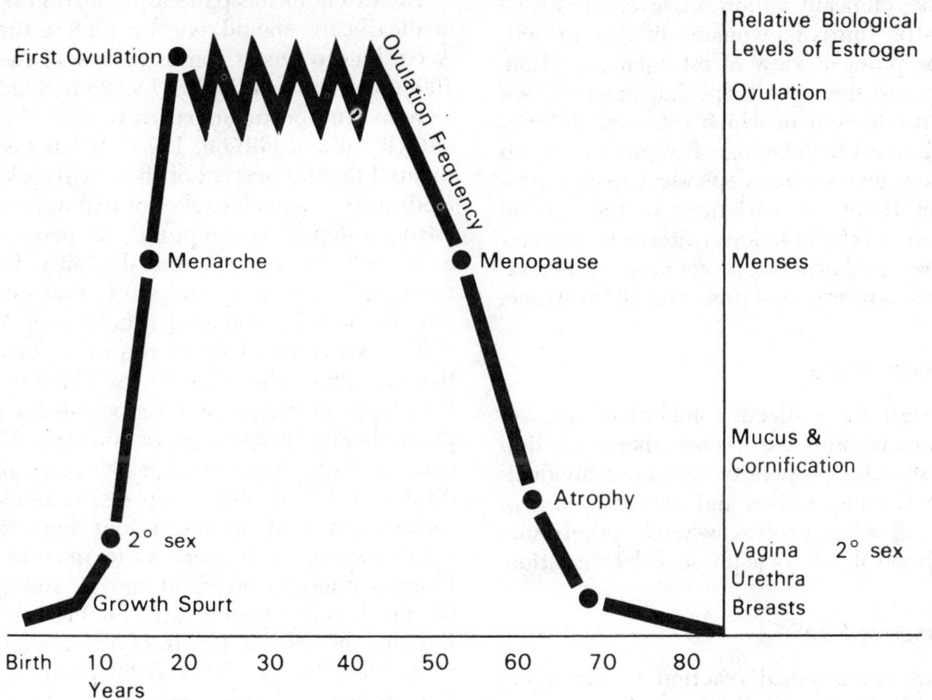

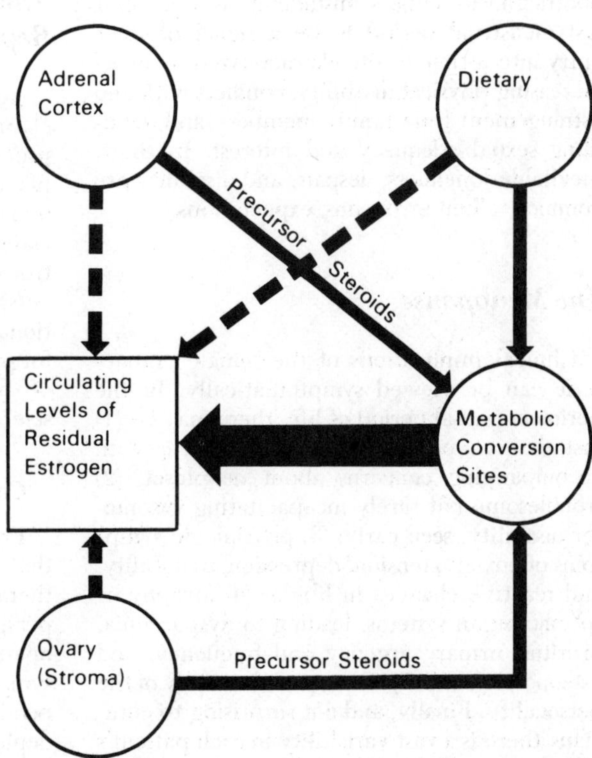

Figure 21-2. From Clinical Gynecological Endocrinology and Infertility, By Leon Speroff, Robert Glass, and Nathan Kase, Williams and Wilkins.

aging, stress, and obesity become important elements that lead to production of variable, sometimes clinically important, levels of estrone in the latter third of a woman's life. As a result, from the point of view of estrogen depletion, not only are there early and late stages of estrogen production in which estrogen declines from relatively high biologically effective levels to the low levels when dependent tissues atrophy, but there are variations in the *rate* of decline in which depletion is altered by increasing either prehormone production or the efficiency of conversion of prehormone to estrone.

Tendency to Age

Although the collective inherited and acquired mechanisms are obscure, there is a clinically observable propensity for some individuals to resist the impositions and manifestations of the overall aging process, whereas others succumb all too obviously to physical deterioration.

"Change of Life"

Just as the physical reaction to the aging process is variable, so is the psychologic impact of the implications of menopause. In some women, accommodation to the psychosocial and physical implications of aging is simple and nontraumatic. Others mistakenly assume their last menstrual period to be a signal of their entry into a time of life characterized by ever-increasing physical disability, conflicts with and estrangement from family members, and dwindling sexual adequacy and interest. In short, inevitable loneliness, despair, and disability are common, albeit erroneous, expectations.

The Menopause

Clinical implications of the female climacteric can be viewed symptomatically. In the perimenopausal period of life, there may be (1) disturbances of the menstrual pattern, with accompanying concerns about neoplasia; (2) troublesome but rarely incapacitating vasomotor disability, seen early; (3) physiologic symptoms of anxiety, tension, depression, irritability, and reactive changes in libido; (4) atrophy of specific organ systems, leading to dyspareunia, pruritus, urinary urgency and frequency, and osteoporosis; and (5) self-imposed atrophy of the personality. Finally, and not surprising to clinicians, there is a vast variability in each patient's presentation and personal perception of her situation.

The extent of this patient population seeking medical care should not be underestimated. According to recent census figures, of the over 100 million women in the U.S., 25 to 30 million were in their postmenopausal years (>50 years old) (Ryan and Gibson, 1973). It has been estimated that 60 percent of these will seek some medical assistance for relief of real or imagined estrogen depletion symptoms; 25 percent will have such severe vasomotor disability, leading to disruption of sleep and work, that estrogen therapy will be required (Stadel and Weiss, 1975). Atrophic changes requiring estrogen therapy afflict the majority of older women. Finally, postmenopausal osteoporosis is a major public health problem. Approximately 25 percent of white women over 60 years of age display vertebral body compression, and symptomatic spinal osteoporosis is four times as common in women as in men. An increase in distal forearm fractures begins at age 45, and by age 60, the female-to-male ratio for these is 10:1. Finally, the risk of hip fracture in women is 20 percent by age 90, and 80 percent of all hip fractures display preexisting osteoporosis (Heaney, 1971).

Advantages of Estrogen Replacement Therapy

Advocates of estrogen replacement therapy claim that estrogen loss, coupled with the aging process (even if it does not accelerate aging) places an unnecessary additional burden on females. Accordingly, several advantages are claimed for estrogen replacement therapy: control of vasomotor reactions, prevention or reversal of atrophic conditions, reduction of emotional reactions to the climacteric, opportunities for preventive medicine, prevention and control of osteoporosis, and prevention of atherosclerosis.

Control of Vasomotor Reactions

From clinical experience, there is no question that one clear gain of estrogen replacement therapy is control of the episodic flush and perspiration ("hot flash") of the early postmenopausal period. The extent to which vasomotor symptoms appear and become troublesome depends upon the rapidity with which estrogen depletion occurs. Perhaps 20 percent of women experience sufficient difficulty as a result of this symptom to seek therapeutic relief. This can be achieved easily and completely by intermittent, low-dose, short-term estrogen replacement therapy.

Reversal of Atrophy in Estrogen-Dependent Tissues

Whereas vasomotor instability is a feature of the early postmenopause, atrophic changes and resulting dysfunction in vaginal, urethral, bladder, and gum mucous membranes occur only after prolonged estrogen loss. The major difficulties pertain to the vagina, where atrophic vaginitis and vulvitis often yield dyspareunia, vaginismus, pruritus, bleeding, and malodorous discharge. Urethral and bladder neck anatomic alterations and inflammatory reactions are associated with urge and stress urinary incontinence and recurrent cystourethritis. Low-dose estrogen therapy reverses the atrophic processes and relieves the associated symptoms in all but those rare situations complicated by nonestrogen-oriented processes.

Reduction of Emotional Reactions to the Climacteric

Although there is little biophysical evidence to support the contention that depletion of estrogen alters brain function and thus causes psychologic disturbances, empiric observations suggest that estrogen replacement therapy may be associated with alleviation of these difficulties. Whether the benefits of this therapy are direct—i.e., biologic in the replacement phenomenon—or indirect—i.e., psychologic in that the patient gains by "having something done" for her symptoms—they should be acknowledged but not overemphasized.

In a double-blind study conducted in a home for the aged in Texas, psychometric evaluation was performed every three months for a three-year period on women aged 60 to 90 (the majority were over 75 years of age). The women were placed into estrogen- and placebo-recipient groups. The tests evaluated communication, interpersonal relationships, care of self, social responsibilities, work activities, and recreation. In the placebo group, the scores fell gradually over time. In the estrogen group, there was a one-year improvement followed by a decline—but in this group, scores remained higher than those for the placebo group (Kantor et al., 1973).

Opportunities for Preventive Care

All too frequently, the postmenopausal patient attributes a variety of symptoms to a mystical "change in life" mechanism. As a result, major disease entities can be ignored until serious consequences or irreversible changes have occurred. Advocates of estrogen replacement contend that the surveillance this therapy requires enables the primary physician to examine the patient periodically, evaluate symptoms, and take preventive measures. Semiannual examinations are helpful in disclosing vascular or colonic disease as well as the pulmonary problems common in this age group.

Prevention and Control of Osteoporosis (Heany, 1971, 1976)

Age-related bone loss is seen more frequently in white females than in males. In humans, bone mass reaches a peak at age 35, plateaus for several years, and decreases within the sixth or seventh decade. The reduction in mass and density occurs in both cortical and cancellous bone. Reduction in overall density results in bone fragility and subsequent disabilities, manifested by the higher frequency of spinal compression and fractures of the hip and distal part of the forearm in females than in males.

Unquestionably, various exercise programs and dietary plans have a beneficial effect on osteoporosis, but the fact that osteoporosis is age-related and pronounced in white females raises the following questions. Is it related to estrogen depletion? Can estrogen replenishment be beneficial? The loss of density in long bones is at least temporally related to estrogen loss. There is evidence that estrogen replacement therapy can retard the loss of density in specific bones, such as the phalanges, as well as the symptomatic manifestations and x-ray appearance of postmenopausal osteoporosis (Nachtigall et al., 1976). There is also an elevation of the plasma calcium and phosphate levels in the menopause, and this can be reversed by estrogen. There is a decrease in renal tubular reabsorption of phosphate and an increased absorption of calcium from the bowel when estrogen replacement therapy is given to postmenopausal women. As a result, a positive calcium balance can usually be noted during therapy. Finally, as measured by calcium-tracer techniques, estrogens appear to suppress bone resorption to an extent sufficient to enhance further the positive calcium balance. This can be noted even in such osteoporotic disease states as poliomyelitis. It appears that estrogen administration is beneficial in osteoporosis in that bone density is preserved via an effect on calcium balance and bone resorption. However, the relationship of bone density to fracture incidence remains to be determined by continued prospective double-blind studies.

Although estrogen therapy has a retarding effect on the reduction in bone density in these women, unfortunately there is also an associated decrease in bone formation within three to nine months of initiation of estrogen replacement therapy that results in a stabilized, lower rate of bone turnover. The clinical implication of this is that if estrogen therapy is to be most beneficial in preventing osteoporosis, it must be instituted early, before serious loss of bone density has occurred. Estrogen replacement therapy does not result in important quantities of new bone formation.

Prevention of Atherosclerosis

Traditionally, three types of evidence have been cited to support estrogen replacement therapy for retardation of atherogenesis in the aging woman (Wuest et al., 1953): (1) retrospective autopsy data indicated that women receiving estrogen replacement therapy had less atherosclerotic change in large vessels than did control groups; (2) there was evidence that the pattern of serum lipoprotein constituents was converted beneficially by estrogen replacement therapy to imitate that of younger women; and (3) evidence that the risk of death from coronary vascular disease was significantly higher in men than in women was attributed to the fact that women were protected in some way by estrogen.

Current information and controlled studies no longer substantiate the contention that estrogen replacement therapy has a beneficial influence on atherosclerosis. Only in low-dose replacement of long-standing estrogen-deficient castrates (loss of ovaries prior to age 30) has estrogen appeared beneficial in reducing cardiovascular deaths in recipients (Johansson et al., 1975).

Disadvantages of Estrogen Replacement Therapy

The disadvantages of estrogen therapy are related to the undesirable metabolic and cardiovascular effects and to the development of cancer in estrogen-dependent tissues such as those of the endometrium and the breast.

The once hoped for benefit of estrogens in the prevention of atherosclerosis has been dashed by a series of negative findings (Furman, 1971; Coronary Drug Project, 1973; Ryan and Gibson, 1973; Report of the VA Cooperative Study, 1966; Stadel and Weiss, 1975; Bailar and Byar, 1970). The evidence is strong that high-dose estrogen replacement therapy can contribute to the risk of thromboembolic disease, cerebrovascular accident (CVA), and coronary artery disease. The effects are dose related, and the risk increases with age.

Other metabolic effects of estrogen can also be considered detrimental to the aging woman. The increased incidence of hypertension as a result of progestin-estrogen therapy, the peripheral decrease in insulin activity with the subsequent stress on insulin reserves, and the increase in gallbladder disease are seen as distinct disadvantages to administration of high-dose estrogens to aging females. Bloating and edema are additional burdens of estrogen treatment.

Cancer. The risk of cancer must be considered the major disadvantage of estrogen replacement therapy, if it can be proven that there is a causal rather than casual relationship between the therapy and the incidence of breast and endometrial carcinoma.

An increase in frequency of breast carcinoma is seen in men given estrogen therapy for prostatic carcinoma, in the treatment of men undergoing transsexual conversion, and in Bantu men with gynecomastia. Although there is a continual rise in the incidence of breast carcinoma in women after the menopause, the increase is known to begin before the menopause. Two major studies have yielded conflicting results (Burch et al., 1974; Hoover et al., 1976). At the moment, there is no evidence to support a cause-and-effect relationship. Prospective studies of the effect of birth control pills on the incidence of benign and malignant breast disease have thus far failed to show a definitive relationship.

Although there is no demonstrated causal relationship between estrogen therapy and breast carcinoma, there is a relationship between elevated levels of endogenous estrogen and estrogen therapy and the incidence of endometrial hyperplasia and carcinoma (Sartwell, 1976; Smith et al., 1975; Ziel and Finkle, 1975). In general, certain constitutional stigmata are present in patients with a high incidence of atypical adenomatous hyperplasia, and endometrial cancer appears with progressive aging and obesity. These stigmata occur with an inappropriately early incidence in patients with polycystic ovary disease and functioning ovarian tumors, but they are rarely seen, however, in individuals with senile vaginitis or those complaining of vasomotor symptoms. Thus a relationship between the presence of endogenous estrogen and evolving endometrial hyperplasia and early cancer has been observed clinically.

Increased production of endogenous estrogen can be manifested by two mechanisms in postmenopausal individuals (Siiteri et al., 1974; Hemsell et al., 1976). Factors that increase the production of the prehormone androstenedione or that increase the conversion of androstenedione to estrone would lead to increases of estrone, which would affect the endometrium. Both have been noted in individuals who developed postmenopausal bleeding, adenomatous hyperplasia, and endometrial carcinoma. In the case of excess androstenedione production, one can observe, as possible causative factors, stress, various tumors, liver disease, congestive heart failure, and, less frequently, obesity. Among the factors increasing the conversion of androstenedione to estrone, obesity has appeared to be dominant, and progressive aging has played a role in specific cases. The contention is that the constitutional stigmata lead to increased production of endogenous estrone, which results in endometrial hyperplasia and carcinoma. A claimed disadvantage of estrogen therapy is that it mimics the constitutional endogenous estrogen situation, resulting in endometrial stimulation and endometrial neoplasia. Statistical support for this view has recently been presented in studies noting an increased incidence of endometrial carcinoma in association with estrogen replacement therapy (Mack et al., 1976; Sartwell, 1976; Ziel and Finkle, 1975). The increase in incidence is suggested to be four to ten times that in control patients, with an increased risk with higher dose and longer duration of therapy.

Although the relationship displayed by these retrospective studies is valid, there is reason to believe that the reported odds ratio is falsely excessive. This is due to the fact that endometrial carcinoma may exist in an occult asymptomatic state for years (approximately 20 percent of all cases) and may come to diagnosis because of bleeding induced by exogenous estrogen therapy. The apparent association between estrogen and endometrial cancer may in large measure represent increased rates of disease detection in women with uterine bleeding and estrogen exposure. Further, there is a diagnostic surveillance bias applied to estrogen recipients leading to early biopsy. This is reflected in lower stage and grade tumors seen in estrogen recipients than in control patients. Finally, tumor formation can be prevented by addition of periodic progestin to the estrogen therapy (Nachtigall et al., 1976) and can be reversed by progestin therapy (Editorial, 1977) or by simple elimination of the hormone therapy (Silverberg and Makowski, 1975).

In summary, if estrogen is given continually or in injudicious doses to recipients who have increased endogenous estrogen, estrogen therapy can exaggerate or possibly uncover a constitutional predisposition to endometrial neoplasia. However, low-dose therapy covered by periodic progestin controls the problem (Mack et al., 1976).

Principles of Estrogen Replacement Therapy

1. In the early menopause, in obese women over the age of 50 who have amenorrhea but display significant cervical mucous or vaginal cornification, progestin alone should be administered. If progestin-induced withdrawal bleeding does not occur, the decline of endogenous estrogen can be determined by simple observation of symptoms, vaginal cornification, and cervical mucus.

2. In nonobese individuals in the early menopause with little or no biologic evidence of estrogen, or in castrates, estrogen therapy—conjugated equine urinary estrogens 0.3 to 0.6 mg per day for courses of three weeks, or ethinyl estradiol 0.01 to 0.02 mg per day for courses of three weeks, with a one-week rest period between courses—can be utilized.

Because of the increased concern over endometrial hyperplasia as a result of this therapy, it is advisable to add a progestin daily during the last week of estrogen administration as an antimitogenic agent and also as a determinant of withdrawal bleeding. If endometrial bleeding should occur under these circumstances, office aspiration or biopsy must be performed. If endometrial bleeding does not occur, progestin may be administered on an every-third-cycle basis and biopsy should be performed annually.

3. In the late menopause, when atrophy is clearly evident, 0.625 mg of estrogen, or perhaps 1.25 mg at most, can be administered cyclically. Again, inclusion of progestin is advised.

4. I cannot conceive of many circumstances in which it would be necessary to administer these estrogens parenterally, but when there are medical complications or restriction of oral intake, Depo-Provera may be useful. Vaginal placement of estrogen may be a useful therapeutic technique in certain individuals, although systemic absorption can occur when estrogens are given by that route.

5. The usefulness of androgen is often considered. In some patients, the addition of methyltestosterone (5 to 10 mg) provides a sense of well-being that some physicians have found effective in patient management.

6. There must be full physician-patient dialogue to achieve understanding of the therapeutic limits of estrogen replacement therapy and its advantages and disadvantages.

Conclusion

1. Hot flashes and genital atrophy are unique features of the menopause and are responsive to low-dose estrogen replacement.

2. Estrone can be produced after the menopause. It can alter the clinical course of the climacteric and have an influence on dosage and effectiveness of therapy.

3. Although estrogen deprivation does not appear to be the sole factor in osteoporosis, the higher occurrence of osteoporosis in females than in males, and its increase in the postmenopausal period, are noted. Estrogen replacement therapy probably retards the rate of osteoporotic change but cannot reverse it.

4. There is a higher incidence of myocardial infarction in males than in females that is not understood. In prophylactic and therapeutic trials, the results with higher doses of conjugated estrogens included increases in the incidence of a variety of thromboembolic disorders, cerebrovascular accidents, and myocardial infarction. Furthermore, there is evidence that the larger the dose of estrogen, the more likely the risk of thromboembolic disease, cerebrovascular accident, and, possibly, coronary disease.

5. The suggestion that breast disease may be related either to continuous production of endogenous estrogen or to administration of estrogen is not supported by available data. On the other hand, estrogen replacement therapy has been shown to be associated with progression of endometrial stimulation to hyperplasia and even carcinoma. Although avoidable and correctable, this possibility must be considered in the cost-benefit analysis of estrogen replacement therapy in a particular patient.

In my opinion, at present it is not reasonable to deny relief of menopausal symptoms to patients by withholding moderate- to low-dose cyclic estrogen therapy, nor is it acceptable to extol estrogen as a solution for aging, degenerative disease or psychic disturbances after the menopause. Estrogen obviously should not be used indiscriminately in the hope of correcting nonspecific ailments or complaints.

References

Bailar, J.C., and Byar, D.P.: Estrogen treatment for cancer of the prostate. Cancer 26:257, 1970.

Burch, J.C., Byrd, B.J., Jr., and Vaughn, W.K.: The effects of the long-term estrogen on hysterectomized women. Am. J. Obstet. Gynecol. 118:778, 1974.

Coronary Drug Project Research Group. JAMA 226:652, 1973.

Editorial: Hormonal replacement therapy and endometrial cancer. Lancet 1:577, 1977.

Furman, R.H.: Coronary heart disease and the menopause. In Ryan, K.J., and Gibson, D.C., eds., Menopause and Aging, DHEW Publication No. (NIH) 73–319, Washington, D.C., U.S. Government Printing Office, 1971.

Heaney, R.P.: Estrogens and postmenopausal osteoporosis. Clin. Obstet. Gynecol. 19:765–825, 1976.

Heaney, R.P.: Menopausal effects on calcium homeostasis and skeletal metabolism. In Ryan, K.J., and Gibson, D.C., eds., Menopause and Aging, DHEW Publication No. (NIH)) 73–319, Washington, D.C., U.S. Government Printing Office, 1971.

Hemsell, D.L., Grodin, J.M., Brenner, P.F., Siiteri, P.K., and MacDonald, P.C.: Plasma precursors of estrogen. II. Correlation of the extent of conversion of plasma androstenedione to estrone with age. J. Clin. Endocrinol. Metab. 38:466, 1976.

Hoover, R., Gray, L.A., and Cole, P.: Menopausal estrogen and breast cancer. N. Engl. J. Med. 295:401, 1976.

Johansson, B.W., Kaij, L., Kullander, S., Lenner, H.C., Svanberg, L., and Astedt, B.: On some late effects of bilateral oophorectomy in the age range 15-30 years. Acta Obstet. Gynecol. Scand. 54:449, 1975.

Kantor, H.I., Michael, C.M., and Shore, H.: Estrogen for older women. Am. J. Obstet. Gynecol. 116:115, 1973.

Lindsay, R., Hart, D.M., Aitken, J.N., MacDonald, E.B., Anderson, J.B., and Clarke, A.C.: Long term prevention of osteoporosis by estrogen. Lancet. 1:1038, 1976.

Mack, T.M., Pike, M.C., Henderson, B.E., Pfeffer, R.I., Gerkins, V.R., Arthur, M., and Brown, S.E.: Estrogens and endometrial cancer in a retirement community. N. Engl. J. Med. 294:1262, 1976.

Meema, S., Bunker, M.L., and Meema, H.E.: Arch. Intern. Med. 135:1436, 1975.

Nachtigall, L.E., Nachtigall, R.H., Nachtigall, R.B., and Beckman, E.M.: Letter to the editor. N. Engl. J. Med., 294:848, 1976.

Report of the VA Cooperative Study of Atherosclerosis, Neurology Section: An evaluation of estrogenic substances in the treatment of CV disease. Circulation 33(SII):3, 1966.

Ryan, K.J., and Gibson, D.C., eds.: Menopause and Aging, DHEW Publication No. NIH 73–319. Washington, D.C., U.S. Printing Office, 1973.

Sartwell, P.E.: Estrogen replacement therapy and endometrial carcinoma: epidemiologic evidence. Clin. Obstet. Gynecol. 19:765–825, 1976.

Siiteri, P.K., and MacDonald, P.C.: Role of extraglandular estrogen in human endocrinology. In Geiger, S.R., Astwood, E.B., and Greep, R.O., eds., Handbook of Physiology, Section 7, Endocrinology, Washington, D.C., American Physiology Society, 1973.

Siiteri, P.K., Schwarz, B.E., and MacDonald, P.D.: Estrogen receptors and the estrone hypothesis in relation to endometrial and breast cancer. Gynecol. Oncol. 2:228, 1974.

Silverberg, S.G., and Makowski, E.L.: Endometrial carcinoma in young women taking oral contraceptive agents. Obstet. Gynecol. 46:503, 1975.

Smith, C.C., Prentice, R., Thompson, D.J., and Herrman, W.L.: Association of exogenous estrogen and endometrial carcinoma. N. Engl. J. Med. 293:1164, 1975.

Stadel, B.V., and Weiss, N.: Characteristics of menopausal women: a survey of King and Pierce counties in Washington, 1973–1974. Am. J. Epidemiol. 102:209, 1975.

Wuest, J., Dry, T.J., and Edwards, J.E.: The degree of coronary sclerosis in bilaterally oophorectomized women. Circulation 7:801, 1953.

Ziel, H.,K., and Finkle, W.D.: Increased risk of endometrial carcinoma among users of conjugated estrogens. N. Engl. J. Med. 293:1167, 1975.

The Negative Side of Long-Term Postmenopausal Estrogen Therapy

Harry K. Ziel, M.D.
Southern California Permanente Medical Group

The only potentially valid long-term use of estrogen is for combating the development of osteoporosis. Only one report, in abstract form, has appeared that claims that long-term estrogen therapy prevents fractures (Hutchinson et al., 1978a). Unfortunately, no one has to date shown that fracture prophylaxis might not be accomplished by exercise or protein, calcium, fluoride, or vitamin D supplements—without estrogen.

Pharmaceutical companies currently promote estrogen therapy with the goal of osteoporosis prevention in mind. A huge financial bonanza would accrue to estrogen manufacturers were it deemed that postmenopausal women should take estrogens.

Recker et al. (1977) have shown that as little as four 10-grain calcium carbonate tablets daily stabilize bone density nearly as well as 0.625 mg of conjugated estrogen and 5 mg of methyltestosterone taken daily. Perhaps, with the addition of an exercise regimen or with protein, fluoride, or vitamin D supplementation, bone density would equal or even exceed the density achieved with estrogen. To its detriment, estrogen actually stops osteoblastic activity and, accordingly, any new bone growth.

Risks of Estrogen Therapy

Eleven retrospective case control studies (Smith et al., 1975; Ziel et al., 1975; Mack et al., 1976; Ziel et al., 1976; McDonald et al., 1977; Gray et al., 1977; Hoogerland et al., 1978; Horwitz et al., 1978 as interpreted by Hutchinson et al. 1978b; Jick et al., 1979; Antunes et al., 1979; Hammond et al., 1979) have associated estrogen use with the development of endometrial cancer. The cases in one of the reports (Gordon et al., 1977) were histologically reviewed by three international experts in endometrial pathology. In 99 percent of the cases, at least one expert concurred in the original diagnosis of cancer. When the risk ratio was recalculated using cases in which there was unanimous concurrence in the diagnosis of cancer by all three experts, the risk estimate increased from 7.6 to 8.1.

These studies have been attacked on every conceivable basis, but they have withstood the criticisms and the test of time. The association of endometrial cancer with estrogen exposure is nearly as strong as the association of lung cancer with cigarette smoking. In fact, the association is so well established that no further research grants are offered to study it.

The retrospective case control studies showed that both the daily dosage of estrogen and the duration of estrogen use correlate directly with cancer incidence. The risk of endometrial cancer is dramatically enhanced when estrogen is given over many years, the same long-term use proposed by the advocates of estrogen for prevention of osteoporosis.

Hoover et al. (1976) have reported an association of long-term estrogen use with the development of breast cancer. Because breast cancer is far more common and far more lethal than endometrial cancer, long-term estrogen therapy may portend greater harm than benefit on the breast neoplasm issue alone. In addition, the postmenopausal breast exposed to estrogen has greater turgor than one not exposed to estrogen and it resists tactile detection of early malignancies. Further, the denser estrogen-stimulated breast requires more irradiation to obtain xeromammograms.

Other documented concerns are associated with estrogen use. The incidence of hepatomas correlates strongly with estrogen use. Cholelithiasis, diabetes, hypertension, and hyperlipidemia are associated with estrogen therapy. Induction of hypercoagulable states as witnessed by pulmonary embolus, coronary occlusion, and cerebral infarction add no small measure of concern to estrogen treatment.

Conclusion

How should we proceed? First, not every woman is at risk of developing significant osteoporosis. Only thin-boned caucasians are predisposed to vertebral, wrist, and femoral fractures. Women who are uniquely at risk must be identified for therapy. It is inappropriate to treat all women indiscriminately. The simplest test to detect women at risk is the grading of the femoral head and neck trabecular pattern as obtained by an anterior-posterior x-ray view of the hip rotated 15 degrees internally (Singh index).

Next, the least risky therapy should be employed. Simple calcium carbonate dietary supplementation may prove adequate to stabilize bony integrity. Addition of a graded exercise program (Aloia et al., 1978) that stresses the bones will not only benefit the skeleton but in addition will benefit the cardiovascular and neuromuscular systems. Added protein, fluoride, and vitamin D supplements are integral components of low-risk therapy.

If these modalities of treatment should fail to halt loss of bony substance, estrogen should be added as a last resort. Before and during estrogen therapy, the endometrium, breasts, blood pressure, blood sugar, blood lipids, and liver should be monitored.

The monthly addition of a progestin to a course of estrogen did not prevent all endometrial cancers in young women taking sequential oral contraceptives (Silverberg, 1975). Postmenopausal women, who are certainly at greater risk for endometrial neoplasia, would have even less protection from endometrial cancer than younger women taking a sequential formulation of estrogen and progestin.

I believe that a potent 19 norprogestin should be combined with each estrogen tablet. The progestin would serve to reduce the number of estrogen receptors in the endometrial cytoplasm. The addition of a progestin would accordingly protect the endometrial DNA from excessive estrogenic stimulation.

References

Aloia, J.F., et al.: Prevention of involutional bone loss by exercise. Ann. Intern. Med. 89:356–358, 1978.

Antunes, C.M.F., et al.: Endometrial cancer and estrogen use. N. Engl. J. Med. 300:9–13, 1979.

Gordon, J., et al.: Estrogen and endometrial carcinoma: an independent pathology review supporting original risk estimate. N. Engl. J. Med. 297:570–571, 1977.

Gray, L.A., et al.: Estrogens and endometrial carcinoma. Obstet. Gynecol. 49:385–392, 1977.

Hammond, C.B., et al.: Effects of long-term estrogen replacement therapy II, Neoplasia. Am. J. Obstet. Gynecol. 133:537–547, 1979.

Hoogerland, D.L., et al.: Estrogen use—risk of endometrial carcinoma. Gynecol. Oncol. 6:451–458, 1978.

Hoover, R., et al.: Menopausal estrogens and breast cancer. N. Engl. J. Med. 295:401–405, 1976.

Horwitz, R.I., et al.: Alternative analytic methods for case-control studies of estrogens and endometrial cancer. N. Engl. J. Med 299:1089–1094, 1978.

Hutchinson, G.B., et al.: Editorial: Correcting a bias. N. Engl. J. Med. 299:1129–1130, 1978b.

Hutchinson, T., et al.: A new application of case-control research, demonstrating that postmenopausal estrogens protect against hip and radial fractures. Clin. Res. 26:486A, 1978a.

Jick, H., et al.: Replacement estrogens and endometrial cancer. N. Engl. J. Med. 300:218–222, 1979.

Mack, T.M., et al.: Estrogens and endometrial cancer in a retirement community. N. Engl. J. Med. 294:1262–1267, 1976.

McDonald, T.W., et al.: exogenous estrogen and endometrial carcinoma: case control and incidence study. Am. J. Obstet. Gynecol. 127:572–580, 1977.

Recker, R.R., et al.: Effects of estrogen and calcium carbonate on bone loss in postmenopausal women. Ann. Intern. Med. 87:649–655, 1977.

Silverberg, S.G.: Endometrial carcinoma in young women taking oral contraceptive agents. Obstet. Gynecol. 46:503–506, 1975.

Singh, M., et al.: Change in trabecular pattern of the upper end of the femur as an index of osteoporosis. J. Bone Joint Surg. 52–A:457–467, 1970.

Singh, M., et al.: Femoral trabecular pattern index for evaluation of spinal osteoporosis. Ann. Intern. Med. 77:63–67, 1972.

Singh, M., et al.: Femoral trabecular pattern index for evaluation of spinal osteoporosis. Mayo Clin. Proc. 48:184–189, 1973.

Smith, D.C., et al.: Association of exogenous estrogen and endometrial carcinoma. N. Engl. J. Med. 293:1164–1167, 1975.

Ziel, H.K., et al.: Increased risk of endometrial carcinoma among users of conjugated estrogens. N. Engl. J. Med. 293:1167–1170, 1975.

Ziel, H.K., et al.: Association of estrone with the development of endometrial carcinoma. Am. J. Obstet. Gynecol. 124:735–740, 1976.

SECTION III

Sociolegal Issues

22

Should New Drugs Be Evaluated in Children Before Marketing?

Children are not simply micro-adults, but have their own specific problems.

Béla Schick

If we had paid no more attention to plants than we have to our children, we would now be living in a jungle of weeds.

Luther Burbank

The days of childhood are but days of woe.

Robert Southey

Introduction

In the years since the Nuremberg Trials, certain ethicists, scientists, and "patient advocates" have been preoccupied with the alleged abuse of "captive" populations as research subjects; e.g., prisoners, the mentally ill, the retarded, and children. These essays focus on this last group and on the problems that arise for sick children if research studies are not performed on them.

Some have argued that children should *never* be the subjects of experimentation, but this posture ignores an irrefutable fact of life: the application of new drugs, or new operations, or new medical devices for the first time to a patient population that has not been previously studied does in fact constitute an experiment, whether or not we call it that. The alternative is to make children "therapeutic orphans" and simply to deny them any new advances in medicine.

Clearly the latter philosophy will not work, so the question becomes how and when to do the pediatric research, not *whether* to do it.

Finkel reminds us that for many of the drugs in the Physician's Desk Reference (PDR), there are restrictions on their use in children, although the Elixir Sulfanilamide and thalidomide tragedies that resulted in the 1938 and 1962 Drug Acts in fact occurred in children. We also know that children differ from adults in ways that can be expected at least occasionally to alter to a significant degree their reaction to drugs.

She further argues that the number of studies she envisions as necessary in children will not exhaust the available scientific resources for performing them, and that drug companies have more than adequate incentive for performing these studies. Finkel sees no great ethical constraints on pediatric research of this sort.

When should this research be done? Finkel favors mandatory premarketing studies for drugs that seem to be major therapeutic advances and for "novel" drugs that are likely to be widely used in children. However, she expresses a willingness to allow postmarketing studies to be done if withholding the drug from adults will deprive them of important therapy.

Finkel would like postmarketing studies for drugs that represent some advantage over already available drugs and are likely to be used on children to a significant extent. (One wonders whether any drugs are submitted for approval these days whose manufacturers would *not* deem them to represent "some" advantage.) Premarketing studies should generally be short-term; for some drugs, postmarketing chronic studies would have to be done.

Christensen seems to agree with Finkel on the problem of drugs "with a reasonably large potential for use in children." Where they may well disagree is on the definition of which drugs might be predicted to have a pediatric use that "is small relative to the total use of the drug."

He points out that some studies are going to be difficult to perform if the disease entity is uncommon in children, such as juvenile rheumatoid arthritis. Also worth considering are the methodologic problems in children, which range from blood sampling to the inability to elicit subjective responses in patients below a certain age. The element of time (which also means money) becomes vital if one has to do studies sequentially in adults, adolescents, and younger and younger children.

Christensen mentions that drugs expected to have substantive use in children are already being studied prior to marketing. (Finkel's data at the end of her paper tend to support Christensen on this point, at least partially.) As one reads both essays, it does not seem that the two experts are all that far apart *in theory* in regard to the timing or the nature of the studies. I suspect, however, that between theory and reality there may be considerable slippage.

Finally, Christensen raises a valid but troubling point. If pediatric studies are to be required, why not also require studies on the elderly, on diabetics, etc.? It would certainly be helpful to the practitioner to know all these facts when a drug is first sold, but to perform all the studies would be to keep drugs off the market even longer than is the case now. The realistic compromise, which would allow the manufacturer to start earning back some of the funds invested in the drug, would seem to be a postmarketing accumulation of data by the manufacturer. Such data have, to be sure, been collected in the past, but perhaps a more systematic voluntary commitment by the drug industry to this issue might obviate unreasonable regulatory demands.

LOUIS LASAGNA, M.D.

Certain New Drugs Should Be Evaluated in Children Before Marketing

Marion J. Finkel, M.D.
Bureau of Drugs, Food and Drug Administration

For the purposes of this discussion, the term *children* will be confined to those in the postnatal period. Although it is of importance to determine the effects of a drug administered to a pregnant woman on the developing child, few would argue that such studies should be completed prior to marketing of the drug, except in the case of drugs used to treat disorders of pregnancy.

The Necessity of Drug Studies in Children

Since Dr. Harry Shirkey introduced the term *therapeutic orphans* in 1963, few papers decrying the paucity of drug studies in children are considered complete without reference to it. As used by Shirkey, the term refers to the deprivation, actual or potential, of sick children of drugs that might be useful to them, owing to statements in package inserts that such drugs have not been adequately studied in children and therefore are not recommended for use in children (Shirkey, 1968). Many package inserts are, in addition, silent with respect to use of the drugs in children, providing neither dosage nor any other information pertinent to usage. Whereas in the latter case, practicing physicians might be more sanguine from a medicolegal standpoint in prescribing such drugs than in prescribing those with a package insert statement warning or cautioning against use in children, neither situation is desirable for children and prescribers; often, it is not desirable for the drug manufacturers, either.

Wilson, in a review of 2000 drugs listed in the 1973 edition of the Physicians' Desk Reference (PDR), found that for 78 percent of them, there was some restriction regarding their use in children—either a statement not recommending their use, certain pediatric age limitations because of lack of information, or no reference at all to children (1975). He did not undertake the laborious endeavor of judging for which drugs such negative information truly resulted in a therapeutic loss and for which it merely represented an inconvenience or even a superfluity; nor did he undertake the still more laborious task of determining for how many drugs adequate information on their safe and effective use in children actually exists in the published medical literature.

The irony of package insert warnings regarding the use of drugs in children has been pointed out by Done (1974) and Shirkey (1970), who noted that the two most recent changes in the Food, Drug and Cosmetic Act—the amendments of 1938, which declared that new drugs must be shown to be safe prior to marketing, and those of 1962, which declared that new drugs must also be shown to be effective prior to marketing and that study of investigational drugs must be monitored by the Food and Drug Administration (FDA)—were precipitated by therapeutic tragedies in which children died (Elixir Sulfanilamide) or were maimed (thalidomide).

Of what actual importance is the lack of adequate pediatric drug studies? Beyond the age of infancy, the utilization of scaled down adult doses has usually met with no discernible untoward effects beyond those that are encountered in some adults. Even in infancy, the relatively wide margin of safety of many drugs may compensate, for example, for undetected differences in rate of metabolism between infants and older children or adults. There are many instances, however, in which failure to conduct adequate studies in children has led to serious toxic effects or, in some cases, to lack of adequate therapeutic effects. Among the most frequently cited are sulfisoxazole-promoted kernicterus due to drug displacement of bilirubin from albumin binding sites; chloramphenicol-produced cardiovascular collapse ("grey syndrome") in neonates due to immaturity of metabolic pathways and consequent elevated levels of serum chloramphenicol; neurotoxicity in hexachlorophene-bathed premature infants due to enhanced percutaneous absorption; and subtherapeutic effect of digitoxin in infants because of deficiency in enzymatic biotransformation of digitoxin, the activity of which depends upon such transformation.

Infants and even older children may differ from adults in rate of drug metabolism, rapidity of gastrointestinal transport, size and permeability of absorptive surface, volume of drug distribution, storage and uptake of lipid-soluble drugs, and rate of renal excretion. In addition, certain drugs given for prolonged periods may affect growth and development—e.g., the masculinizing and epiphyseal maturation effects of androgens and the impairment of longitudinal growth by corticosteroids. A field little explored is the effect of chronically administered drugs on learning and behavior.

Reasons for the Paucity of Drug Studies in Children

The "therapeutic orphans" situation has been ascribed to many factors: (1) lack of sufficient pediatric clinical pharmacology centers and pediatric clinical pharmacologists, (2) inaction by drug manufacturers, (3) inaction by the federal government, and (4) societal concerns for the risks of drug studies in general and for the ethicality of drug studies in children in particular. To these might be added the relatively slow development of pediatric clinical pharmacology into the sophisticated discipline that exists today.

Insufficient Facilities and Inaction by Pharmaceutical Manufacturers

Regarding the lack of sufficient resources and trained individuals, I would agree that such is the case for the field of pediatric clinical pharmacology as a whole but would disagree that this is of consequence for the study of those few new drugs that emerge each year that are potentially valuable for pediatric therapy. Should pediatric studies be required as a condition for marketing approval of such drugs, they would have to compete with other interests of pediatric clinical pharmacologists. Nevertheless, when drugs appear that are of potential therapeutic advantage for adults over those already available, pharmaceutical manufacturers encounter little difficulty in obtaining outstanding clinical investigators to study those drugs. Consequently, one would expect that pediatric clinical pharmacologists could be found to perform the necessary studies of drugs that would appear to be advantageous to children. For drugs with no demonstrable advantage in adults over other available drugs but that nevertheless would be expected to be used widely in children, the acquisition of investigators to perform studies in children may be more difficult. Drug manufacturers, however, when spurred by the economic incentives of potential widespread use of a new drug in a pediatric population—e.g., an antibiotic, a bronchodilator, or a burn preparation—have encountered little difficulty in persuading well-trained pediatric clinical pharmacologists and experienced pediatricians to study these drugs, and such studies are completed prior to submission of a new drug application (NDA) to the FDA for permission to market the drug. When a drug, even if it is a therapeutic advance, is expected to have relatively little use in children—e.g., an antihypertensive or a drug for the treatment of peptic ulcer—there is no incentive to perform studies in children before marketing and little inclination to perform such studies in the postmarketing stage. Even in the case of marketed drugs that have attained widespread use in children because of an unanticipated need or a serendipitous discovery, firms rarely initiate controlled studies to provide adequate information on safe and effective use for the labeling of the drug for pediatric indications. Or, in the event that controlled studies have been performed independent of the firms, the firms rarely even gather the published data for submission to the FDA, despite the fact that they are profiting from such widespread use. To be sure, once a drug has gained widespread use and appears to be both safe and effective, it is difficult to persuade well trained and experienced investigators to perform controlled clinical trials.

Federal Government Inaction and Societal Concerns

In 1965, the American Medical Association (AMA) Board of Trustees, acting on the recommendation of the AMA Council on Drugs, urged the members of the Pharmaceutical Manufacturers Association to include, when appropriate, data for use of drugs in children when submitting a new drug application to the FDA, and, when data are inadequate, to state on the labeling that "information on the use of this drug in children is not available" (Editorial, 1965). Such labeling was considered preferable, from the medicolegal standpoint, to an actual labeling proscription on use of a drug in children, since the drug might have to be used in a child despite the inadequacy of formal studies in children. The AMA noted that, in general, the industry was favorably inclined to this labeling recommendation, and that various drug companies did attempt to obtain data on new drugs in children but were encountering difficulty in finding sufficient investigators and facilities. Thus, the AMA and individual pediatricians are on record as urging amelioration of the "therapeutic orphan" situation.

The federal government, on the other hand, has been attacked for its inaction. Criticism of the government has involved three areas: financial support, new drug regulations, and FDA inaction relative to "therapeutic orphans" labeling. The federal government has been criticized for not recognizing the need to provide training for a greater number of pediatric clinical pharmacologists and support for additional pediatric research centers. I do not venture an opinion on the merits of this criticism and on the priorities placed upon various types of research by those who allocate federal research dollars. I think, however, that this criticism is not relevant to, and therefore is unfairly applied to, the issue of adequate study of drugs in children. As noted earlier, such studies, if limited to important new drugs or those of widespread utility in children, would require a small fraction of the resources of pediatric pharmacology centers.

The new drug regulations attendant upon the 1962 amendments to the Food, Drug and Cosmetic Act have been cited as inhibiting research in children because of the requirement of informed consent and the presumed reluctance on the part of investigators to ask for, and of parents to give, consent for research in children. Forces outside the regulations, however, have been instrumental in a growing reluctance of society to participate in research. Snider (1967) summarized the many reasons for the unfavorable climate surrounding new drug evaluation, including Nazi atrocities; the thalidomide tragedy; the Supreme Court decision on civil rights; the financing by the federal government of medical care for the indigent, making them no longer dependent on research for their medical care; the criticism of physicians for excessive incomes and, in some cases, unethical practices; the increase in malpractice suits; and many articles on unethical research.

The usual new drug research in children is of a type, however, that arouses little controversy: extensive studies in adults have preceded introduction of a drug to the pediatric population (except in rare instances in which children are the only appropriate subjects); older children receive the new drug before the younger ones; and the drugs are administered with the intent to benefit a sick child who (1) often has responded inadequately to other therapy, (2) is expected to have a greater therapeutic benefit or lesser risk from the new agent than from available agents, or (3) is at least expected not to be exposed to a greater risk from the new drug. Again, I mention the relative ease with which pharmaceutical firms accumulate data in children treated with drugs for common illnesses. Where the research involves no greater intervention than would occur in good medical practice consonant with the condition of the patient, obstacles are few. Additional intervention, such as drawing of blood samples for monitoring of serum levels of drugs, are clearly justified when there is particular benefit to be gained from the new drug. The recent recommendations of the National Commission for the Protection of Human Subjects of Biomedical and Behavioral Research with respect to studies in children will go a long way toward easing the fears of those investigators reluctant to perform research in children, and in assuring parents that due care has been taken to insure proper safeguards for their children involved in studies of new drugs.

The FDA has been cognizant of the "therapeutic orphans" situation for some time. In 1967, it sponsored a Conference on Pediatric Pharmacology, the main purpose of which was "to develop a comprehensive statement identifying, if possible, and within the scope of current knowledge, a program for drug evaluation which may serve to assist the Commissioner to promulgate regulations leading to maximum benefit for infants and children." It was apparent that the disenfranchisement of a large segment of the population from the benefit of adequate drug studies and of adequate directions for use of drugs in the labeling for these products was undesirable and should be eliminated. In addition, several FDA officials publicly stated that steps would be taken to assure that appropriate studies are performed in children. For example, in 1972, former FDA Commissioner Edwards stated:

> It is not a question of whether drugs should be studied in children, but rather, when, how, in whom, and under what circumstances . . . . I am committed to this effort and to the goal of advancing the (new drug application) process toward the ideal where any new drug with a potential for use in children is tested for that purpose and approved for that purpose at the same time that the drug is approved for adults.

Because of the public concern about drug testing at that time, particularly in groups deemed to be disadvantaged, it was felt desirable to delay formal implementation of this policy, or some modification thereof, until there was a resolution at the national level of the legal and ethical issues of research in children. In 1975, former Secretary of Health, Education and Welfare Weinberger stated: "There is no way to abide by the [1962 amendments to the Food, Drug and Cosmetic Act] as it applies to drugs for children without first having a clear mandate on the ethical issues of testing drugs on children as subjects".

In 1974, Congress established the National Commission for the Protection of Human Subjects of Biomedical and Behavioral Research to develop guidelines for the ethical conduct of research in various segments of the population. The Report and Recommendations of the Commission on Research involving children was issued in September 1977. It concerned research in both children who did and who did not stand to derive immediate benefit therefrom. The Commission stated that research is necessary in both groups, and it recommended that such research may be conducted if "an institutional review board has determined that (a) the research is scientifically sound and significant; (b) where appropriate, studies have been conducted first on animals and adult humans, then on older children, prior to involving infants; (c) risks are minimized by using the safest procedures consistent with sound research design and by using procedures performed for diagnostic or treatment purposes whenever feasible." In addition, the Commission recommended that provisions be made for protection of privacy of children and parents and for maintenance of confidentiality of data, and that subjects be selected in an equitable manner so that no stratum of society is involved disproportionately. The Commission further recommended that for cases in which an intervention that may be of direct benefit to a child or is required for his wellbeing carries the potential for more than minimal risk, it may be instituted—provided that a review board has determined that the risk is justified by the anticipated benefit and that the benefit-risk ratio is at least as favorable as that provided by available alternative procedures. Examples of this situation are when (1) alternative therapies in cases of serious illness have failed and (2) alternative approaches for less serious illnesses have achieved only partial success. However, in the latter case the new therapy must offer at least an equally favorable benefit-risk ratio.

In research involving more than minimal risk, when no direct immediate benefit is to accrue to the child, the Commission recommended that it be conducted only if an institutional review board has determined that the increased risk is minor, the procedures are reasonably commensurate with those that the subjects or others with the disorder under study would ordinarily experience, and the research is expected to yield information that would be of benefit to those with the disorder under study, including possibly the subjects themselves.

Finally, the Commission recommended that research be conducted only with the permission of parents or guardians and the assent of children seven years of age and older, unless such children are incapacitated and cannot be consulted. The objection of a child of any age should be binding except in cases where the intervention has the potential for direct benefit. Under certain circumstances, mostly those involving adolescents, parental permission can be waived.

The Commission's recommendations, if adopted, will be converted into proposed regulations for research conducted under the support of the Department of Health, Education and Welfare. These regulations will also be adopted by the Food and Drug Administration for drug research that it monitors.

When Should Drug Studies Be Conducted in Children?

Now that ethical principles for conduct of research in children have been published by the National Commission, the FDA is in the process of developing regulations defining the conditions under which new drugs should be studied in children either in the premarketing or postmarketing stage. The FDA's final regulations will be influenced by comments from interested parties in medical, pharmaceutical, sociologic, and other circles. The FDA has not been idle, however, while awaiting the outcome of the National Commission's deliberations. In the past few years, it has contracted with the American Academy of Pediatrics for its Committee on Drugs to develop guidelines for studies of drugs in children. The Committee has produced general guidelines and seven guidelines for studies of specific drug classes. Several of the FDA's own advisory committees have drafted guidelines for study of various drug classes in children. In addition, the FDA has requested manufacturers of certain drugs that would appear to have advantages in children, or that would be expected to be used because of their appeal as an interesting new molecule, to perform studies in children in the postmarketing phase. Such requests have been made as a condition for marketing approval of these drugs. There has also been a growing tendency upon the part of manufacturers to recognize their responsibilities toward the pediatric population and to perform studies voluntarily for drugs that were not traditionally studied in a controlled manner in children. However, not all new drugs that could be used in children should be studied in children. Of those that are chosen for this research, some should be studied before marketing and others afterwards.

Premarketing pediatric drug studies should be completed for (1) drugs representing *major* therapeutic advances and thus likely to be used in children and (2) drugs not representing major advances but likely to be used widely in children because of their novelty (e.g., the first new antiinflammatory agent in 10 years) or because of their applicability in the treatment of diseases that occur commonly or characteristically in children (e.g., acute leukemia). Application of these criteria should be flexible in order not to delay the availability of significant new drugs for use in adults. For example, marketing approval of a major drug for the treatment of hypertensive emergencies should not be withheld until the required studies are completed in children, in view of the limited availability of an adequate pediatric population with severe hypertension. In such cases, postmarketing studies in children should be performed. Postmarketing pediatric drug studies should also be performed for drugs that represent *some* advantage over other available drugs and are likely to be used in children to a significant extent, but not as widely as in (2), above.

Because of limited pediatric pharmacology facilities, pediatric studies should not be required for drugs that appear to offer no advantage over those already available. Instead, these drugs should be required to contain the usual label disclaimers. A manufacturer could, if he wishes, voluntarily perform studies in children with such drugs in order to provide label information on the use of those drugs in children.

It is safe to assume that the proposed regulations would not call for studies in normal children, because investigational drug studies can be considered to involve more than minimal risk. This policy would be consistent with the National Commission's recommendations. It would also be consistent with the clinical guidelines developed by the American Academy of Pediatrics and the FDA's advisory committees, which recommend that studies of investigational drugs be conducted in children with the condition of interest and only after adequate study in adults (with the exception of rare toxic drugs, such as anticancer drugs, intended only for use in children). Studies in children, therefore, would ordinarily be performed with drugs for which chronic toxicity studies in animals have been performed, and for which there are pharmacokinetic data and evidence of effectiveness and defined risk in adults. The studies would be performed in ill children in whom the drug would be expected to have a reasonable chance for providing benefit.

What Types of Drug Studies Should Be Conducted in Children?

The types of studies to be performed in children in order to gain approval to label a drug for pediatric use should generally be short-term and aimed at obtaining safe and effective dosages. Depending upon the nature of the drug and its indications, long-term studies might be required in the postmarketing phase to determine possible drug-related effects on growth and development and other physiologic or pathologic parameters of particular interest.

Whereas this scheme, if adopted, would provide for pediatric coverage of new drugs, it would have no impact on already marketed drugs that have either pediatric disclaimers or no pediatric information, except insofar as it might cause physicians to switch, in some cases, to drugs that are adequately labeled. The FDA has not determined whether it will attempt to obtain a review of available data in the published literature or ask manufacturers to do this, so that those drugs for which data exist that are considered adequate for labeling purposes can be labeled for pediatric use. It has asked interested individuals and drug manufacturers to consider voluntary efforts in this regard, and one of the FDA's advisory committees has undertaken to perform such a review for drugs in its area that are used commonly in children. The FDA has also not reached a conclusion on whether it will request manufacturers of marketed drugs that are widely used in children but unlabeled for such use, and for which adequate data do not exist in the literature, to undertake controlled clinical trials.

It should be noted that requests by the FDA for clinical studies once a drug is marketed have met with little success. The only sanction the FDA has in the case of a noncomplying firm is the implied threat of withdrawal of approval for marketing of the drug. Since requests for new clinical trials are generally made on the basis that the drug appears to be of importance in the treatment of a disease, such an implied threat is an idle one because patients would stand to lose more from the unavailability of the drug than from its continued availability in its inadequately studied state. New drug legislation pending before Congress would require that studies be conducted on marketed drugs when the FDA so requests. Passage of such a provision will not, of course, guarantee that the studies will be conducted, but a law does serve the purpose of emphasizing the importance of the issue.

Impact on Pediatric Pharmacology Units

The impact of requirements for studies of new drugs on pediatric pharmacology units will be minor. The following figures support such a conclusion. A retrospective analysis utilizing the aforementioned criteria for drugs to be studied in children was carried out on the new chemical entities or drugs with significant new dosage forms or new uses that were approved for marketing between 1972 and 1977. Of a total of 95 drugs in these categories, 53 would require no pediatric studies, 15 would require postmarketing studies, and 27 would require premarketing studies. Of the 27 requiring premarketing studies, 13 were subjected voluntarily to adequate premarketing studies by the pharmaceutical company sponsors, and another two were the subject of voluntarily initiated postmarketing studies. Of the remaining 12, 7 are involved in ongoing postmarketing studies at the request of the FDA. Among the 15 drugs for which postmarketing studies would be required, one was subjected to adequate studies in children prior to marketing, one is involved in postmarketing studies on the initiative of the pharmaceutical firm, and three are the subject of postmarketing studies at the request of the FDA.

Thus, of the 27 drugs that would require completion of studies in children prior to marketing, 13 were in fact subjected to such studies. Therefore, over the six-year period, an average of only two additional drugs per year would be added to the premarketing pediatric study "burden." Of the 15 drugs that would require postmarketing studies in children, two were voluntarily subjected to such studies. Thus, an average of two additional drugs per year would be added to the postmarketing "load."

Conclusion

Not only would children benefit from the performance of adequate studies in their age group before drugs are widely used in this group, but physicians would be provided with greater confidence in their initial use of new drugs in children, thus resulting in safer use and unimpeded selection of the best drug for the particular situation. When so much is to be gained, it is well worth the extra effort required to achieve it.

References

Done, A.K.: Pediatric drug problems. Presented at the Gordon Research Conference on Drug Metabolism, Plymouth, N.H., July 25, 1974.

Editorial: A therapeutic gap. JAMA 193:536, 1965.

Edwards, C.C.: Keynote address at the annual meeting of the American Academy of Pediatrics, Oct. 16, 1972.

Shirkey, H.C.: Conference of Professional and Scientific Societies, Chicago, June 27–28, 1963 (Sponsored by Commission on Drug Safety, Chicago, Ill.).

Shirkey, H.: Therapeutic orphans (editorial). J. Pediatr. 72:119, 1968.

Shirkey, H.C.: Therapeutic orphans: who speaks for children?, South. Med. J. 63:1361, 1970.

Snider, A.J.: The role of the communication industry in creating a climate of public opinion which will make drug testing in minors an acceptable procedure. Proceedings Conference on Pediatric Pharmacology, Feb. 19–21, 1967, Washington, D.C., U.S. Department of Health, Education and Welfare.

Weinberger, C.W.: Keynote address at National Academy of Sciences' Forum: Experiments and Research with Humans: Values in Conflict, Feb. 19, 1975.

Wilson, J.T.: Pragmatic assessment of medicines available for young children and pregnant or breast-feeding women. In Morselli, P.L., Garattini, S., and Sereni, F., eds., *Basic and Therapeutic Aspects of Perinatal Pharmacology*, New York, Raven Press, 1975.

Should Trials of Drugs in Children Be Required Before Market Approval for Use in Adults Is Granted?

C. N. Christensen, M.D.
Eli Lilly and Company

The suggestion that pediatric trials should be required before drugs are approved for marketing arises from the fact that the package inserts for many drugs on the market today include a statement similar to one of the following: "Adequate data for use in children under twelve years of age are not available"; "There have been no studies in children; therefore the safety and effectiveness of this drug in children are unknown"; "This drug is not recommended for use in children because documented clinical experience has been insufficient to establish safety and a suitable dosage regimen in the pediatric age group."

Despite the lack of adequate data, many of the drugs that carry these warnings have a legitimate place in pediatric practice. It has been the concern of many physicians that children are being deprived of optimal treatment because adequate studies to support use are not available and FDA approval has not been granted. Harry Shirkey took note of this phenomenon in 1968 and coined the phrase *therapeutic orphans* to apply to the deprived children. Much has been written about the subject since then.

Pediatric Drug Trials

Some new drugs are studied in children, and their labeling carries directions for use in pediatrics. There is generally no problem in arranging adequate pediatric studies for drugs that have a reasonably large potential for use in children. The problem lies primarily with those drugs for which the anticipated use in pediatrics is small relative to the total use of the drug.

From 1974 to 1976, 43 single chemical entities were approved for marketing in the United States. The labeling for 20 of them states that data are inadequate to support their use in children. In nine of them, mostly topical preparations, no mention is made in the labeling about use in children. Fourteen carry dosage recommendations for use in children; in some cases with limitations—e.g., there may be a caution about use in neonates or very young children. Nevertheless, these particular compounds had at least some evaluation in children.

A review of the compounds by therapeutic class is revealing. Of the eight antiinfective compounds, six had directions for use in children and one should probably not be used in children because of toxicologic findings in immature animals. Thus, in this class of compounds, which could be expected to have wide use in children, only one of eight had not been studied in children.

Compounds with less potential for use in children were less frequently studied. There were six compounds in the neuropsychopharmacologic class and five in the cardiovascular class. Two of these eleven drugs have directions for use in children. Among the drugs were four nonsteroidal antiinflammatory drugs (NSAIDs); none are currently recommended for use in children. This class of drugs is now being used extensively in adults with rheumatoid arthritis and osteoarthritis. The incidence of rheumatoid arthritis in children is much lower than it is in adults, and anticipated use of the drugs in children will be proportionately much less than it will be in adults. Yet therapy for juvenile rheumatoid arthritis is far from ideal, and it would seem important that the potential utility of these drugs be established in children.

Deterrents to Drug Studies in Children

The case of NSAIDs illustrates some of the reasons why drugs are not studied in children, at least initially. A relatively small patient population is available in which the drugs can be tested. As noted earlier, the incidence of juvenile rheumatoid arthritis is low. Another reason it is difficult to study such drugs in children is the limited number of investigators available to do the studies. This occurs because only a few have adequate patient populations in which to conduct the trials. Another reason for lack of investigators is the neglect accorded to the training of pediatricians in the discipline of clinical pharmacology. Although perhaps desirous, it is not necessary or imperative that drugs be studied by people trained in clinical pharmacology—but in pediatrics, there has been little emphasis on even modest training programs. Hence, few pediatricians deem themselves qualified to undertake drug studies.

Why have pediatricians not embraced the field of clinical pharmacology to the same extent as their colleagues who care for adults? There is an element of "Catch-22" in the answer to this question. Those who have tried to establish formal training programs in pediatric clinical pharmacology have had difficulty in obtaining federal funds for this purpose. The granting agencies, it seems, require some evidence that a program will be effective before funding is granted. Without funds, originators of the projected programs are unable to develop evidence that an effective program can be established (Done, 1968). It has not been easy to break into this cycle, as attested by the few centers available in the U.S. for the study of pediatric clinical pharmacology.

Another deterrent to obtaining adequate studies in children is the lack of suitable methods for many types of studies. The study of pharmacokinetics in children is impeded by such simple considerations as the volume of blood required to determine the level of drug in repeat serum samples. Newer methods for detection of small amounts of drug in small samples are being developed, but often the pediatric clinical pharmacologist must settle for a research design that would be considered inadequate by those who study adults.

The understanding and comprehension of pediatric patients apparently has also been a factor in the ability to carry out certain drug studies. Thus, studies of drugs whose effects are largely subjective present very real problems in pediatrics. Although they are useful in pediatrics, oral analgesics have rarely been evaluated for effectiveness in children; the methods used in adults have not been found adequate to obtain a reliable measure of analgesic potency in children.

Some investigators have noted that the problem of obtaining consent has been an impediment to drug trials in children. The National Commission for the Protection of Human Subjects of Biomedical and Behavioral Research (1977) has studied the moral and ethical considerations presented by the use of children as research subjects. The Commission has recently affirmed that children must not be denied the benefits that can be obtained from research utilizing them as subjects. However, the Commission stresses that the vulnerability of children because of their dependence and immaturity raises questions about the ethical validity of involving them in research. Nevertheless, the Commission recognizes that research involving children is important for their health and well-being. To conduct such research, proper safeguards must be established to provide maximal protection and minimal risk. The Commission has made a series of recommendations that it feels should be observed when research is conducted in children. Among these is the provision that, whenever possible, research involving risk—and all drug research involves some risk—should be conducted first in animals, then in adults, and subsequently in younger and younger patients. Except under very specific conditions, the Commission recommends that the pediatric research subject should stand to obtain some direct benefit from the research; this for all practical purposes eliminates the use of "normal childhood volunteers" as the subjects of drug research. The evaluation of vaccines may be an exception, but in this instance, children stand to benefit individually and as a group. Although this raises problems and further limits the available patient population, the problems are surmountable given adequate time.

Despite these problems, should drug studies be done in children? The answer, I think, is yes. Children deserve to benefit from drug therapy as much as adults.

Drug Research Sponsors

Who should sponsor these studies? It would seem appropriate for the drug manufacturer to take the responsibility of sponsorship. It has been suggested in the past that pediatric studies have not been supported by drug manufacturers because of the limited market for these drugs. There is undoubtedly some truth in this accusation; however, the many factors noted previously have also played a significant role. In recent years, these has been more awareness in industry of the importance of doing drug studies in children when one can anticipate that a drug will be used in children.

Premarketing and Postmarketing Studies

To encourage manufacturers to perform pediatric studies, should the drugs be withheld from the market until pediatric studies are completed? My answer is no—at least, this concept should not be made into a policy.

The need or desirability of doing studies in children should be determined for each drug on an individual basis. If a drug has no potential use in children, it is obvious that studies should not be attempted in children. At the other extreme are drugs that one can anticipate will have substantial use in children. In this instance, a policy or requirement for drug studies in children prior to approval is not needed; such studies are being done now.

In between is the large gray area—drugs that will be used primarily in adults but almost certainly will have some place in pediatric practice. The projected limited use in children will reflect the size of the pediatric patient population available for testing. Because this population is relatively small, it can be anticipated that pediatric data will be accumulated slowly. Because of the delay in completing studies in children, these drugs should be allowed on the market when safety and efficacy have been established in adults, but before studies in children are complete.

It would not be in the interest of the public health to deprive adults of the benefits of these medications while data are being collected in children!

Whether drugs are evaluated in children before general approval or after general approval, it is customary, and in keeping with the recommendation of the National Commission for the Protection of Human Subjects of Biomedical and Behavioral Research, to obtain data in adults before proceeding to children. Furthermore, the usual sequence in testing drugs in children is to begin in teenagers and later to gain experience in successively younger age groups. The reason for this sequential approach relates to toxicity. Each age group of children may have toxicities that are different from those observed in adult populations; therefore, each age group must be studied to evaluate this potential. Differences in metabolism, maturity of enzyme systems, maturity of excretory processes, and the influence of compounds on growth and development are only a few of the reasons why toxicity may differ in different age groups. Experimental models, as yet, are not adequate to predict all adverse experiences that may be encountered in young patients. Much of what we have learned in the past has come from sad experience—e.g., the kernicterus associated with the use of certain sulfonamides and the "gray" syndrome associated with chloramphenicol. These experiences have taught us, however, to approach the evaluation of drugs in children with great caution.

Studying a drug in successively younger age groups in tandem takes longer than proceeding immediately to all age groups. However, it is believed that by this process, risks may be minimized to the greatest extent possible and the investigator can have greater confidence as he proceeds to the younger population.

Because of the obstacles that have confronted pediatric studies, great care must be exercised in planning such studies, and overly extensive trials should not be expected. As noted, a prime consideration in research in children is the evaluation of toxicity, and it is appropriate that this be a prime goal of pediatric studies. Similarly, the pharmacokinetics of a drug may be much different in children than in adults, and studies to elucidate these differences are needed. In addition, the pharmacokinetic studies will help to establish proper dosage regimens for children, an essential to proper drug usage. Extensive controlled comparative studies for efficacy, however, should probably not be required for most drugs. The basic effectiveness of the drug should be established in adults and it should then be sufficient to show that children respond similarly to adults. The limited study population and the available investigators should be used as efficiently as possible.

Another reason why drugs should be allowed on the market before studies are completed in children relates to economic considerations. A sizable investment is required to support the development of every new chemical entity. This investment is bringing no return to the company during periods of delay. The monetary return should be available so that it can be applied to the discovery and development of other new chemical entities that might be useful both in adult medicine and in pediatrics. It has been estimated reliably that the cost of delay exceeds $5 million per year, a sum that would support a considerable amount of research.

It would be particularly inappropriate at this point to change the current policy of allowing drugs on the market before completion of pediatric studies. The report of the National Commission for the Protection of Human Subjects of Biomedical and Behavioral Research has only recently become available, and its impact on drug studies in children needs to be assessed before changing the approval process. The Commission recommends that not only should parental permission be obtained in order for a child to participate in an investigation, but, in addition, children older than six should give their assent to such participation. The Commission points out that as children mature, they are more able to act in their own best interest. Thus, although parents may override the objections of school-aged children to participation in research, that decision becomes more burdensome with the increasing maturity of the child. Further, the Commission suggests that only children who have good relationships with their parents or guardians and their physician are suitable candidates as research subjects. These recommendations could significantly increase the time required to carry out pediatric studies, and their full effect should be determined before there is a change in the policy of new drug approval.

Finally, requiring that pediatric studies be completed before approval is granted ignores the many other population groups to which the same principle might be applied. Studies in the elderly might as reasonably be required. Studies in subpopulations of individuals with various diseases in addition to the target illness could be mandated—e.g., the response to antibiotics of diabetic patients with infections. Studies in various racial groups or in patients with specific enzyme alterations—e.g., G6PD deficiency—could as logically be required.

It should be recognized that no drug can ever be completely evaluated before it becomes available for general distribution. Approval for marketing is only a license to allow a drug to be widely used and to allow its eventual value in the practice of medicine to be assessed from the experience of critical physicians over a period of years.

Conclusion

In summary, some drugs have no use in children and, obviously, need not be evaluated in children. Other drugs have a wide potential for use in children, and it can be anticipated that, as in the past, data available at the time of submission of a new drug application will be sufficient to approve the drug for use in both adults and children. A large number of drugs will have limited use in children. They should be studied in children, but the relative scarcity of qualified investigators, the limited patient population available for study, and ethical considerations dictate that the studies will not be completed until long after studies are completed in adults. These drugs should be allowed on the market before pediatric studies are finalized, but there should be a commitment by the sponsor to complete the studies so that all drugs to be used in children will have adequate directions for that use.

References

Done, A.K.: Problems of Drug Evaluation in Infants and Children. Report of the 58th Ross Conference on Pediatric Research, Ross Laboratories, 1968.

National Commission for the Protection of Human Subjects of Biomedical and Behavioral Research: Report and Recommendations, Research Involving Children, DHEW Publications No. (OS)77-0004, Superintendent of Documents, Washington, D.C., U.S. Government Printing Office, 20402, 1977.

Shirkey, H.: Therapeutic orphans, (editorial). J. Pediatr., 72:119, 1968.

23

Should All Venereal Disease Contacts Be Treated?

But do not hope to see the end of the scourge that is afflicting you. This disease shall be eternal . . . . Apollo has sworn it by the Styx and by immutable Destiny.

Fracastorius, *Syphilis*

Pox'd by her love.

Alexander Pope, *Satires and Epistles Imitated*

Two minutes with Venus, two years with Mercury.

J. Earle Moore

Introduction

In many countries, venereal disease (VD) is a major problem, made even more serious by the failure of many physicians to consider the possibility that it may be responsible for the patient's presenting complaints. Medical school curricula now neglect to teach students adequately about the diagnosis and treatment of VD, let alone the epidemiologic aspects of sexually transmitted illness.

Lively controversy exists about the so-called "epidemiologic treatment" of VD; i.e., the routine treatment of contacts of identified cases. King takes the position that such contacts should not be treated without examination or investigation because it creates needless anxieties in noninfected individuals and may provide inadequate treatment if the contact suffers from diseases other than the one suspected. He has little patience with lack of skills and facilities as an excuse for epidemiologic treatment. King also points out that antibiotic treatment itself is not without risk, and that the list of individuals who are at high risk for syphilis may be very lengthy indeed. He grudgingly grants that there are a few rare situations where "diagnosis before treatment" is not possible.

Willcox is more willing to engage in the treatment of contacts, but has a catechism for helping to decide when epidemiologic treatment is justified. These include the preventability of disease, good history of exposure, multiplicity of sexual exposures without precautions, consultations within the incubation period, quality and availability of diagnostic facilities, likelihood of default, and number of other individuals at risk.

Although Willcox and King see eye-to-eye on a few issues, their respective philosophies suggest a radically different clinical stance. A Willcox-oriented physician will treat a good many more asymptomatic contacts than would a doctor who espouses the King point of view. The reader will have to decide for himself which approach will, on average, do more good than harm.

LOUIS LASAGNA, M.D.

All Venereal Disease Contacts Need Not Be Treated

A. J. King, M.B.B.S., F.R.C.S.
The London Hospital, London

Problems of Epidemiologic Treatment

Everyone accepts the need to trace venereal disease (VD) contacts and to treat them if they are found to be infected. But the question considered here raises broader issues. Should contacts who show no evidence of infection be treated? Is it legitimate to treat contacts without submitting them to examination and tests? These are the problems of what is often called *epidemiologic treatment.*

To the conscientious clinician, treatment without examination and investigation is highly objectionable. It is the concept of the chair-borne epidemiologist who is not in touch with the problems and anxieties of patients and is, in fact, prepared to regard them as subhuman, like sheep who are immersed in sheep dip and sent on their way. Epidemiologists should be profoundly dissatisfied with such a procedure because it gives no opportunities for further contact tracing and may lead to ineffective treatment. If the patient is suffering from venereal disease, he may have more than one infection, and the remedy used may not render him noninfectious. In any case, there is no possibility of establishing the fact of cure. It is sometimes argued that treatment of this kind, although far from ideal, becomes necessary in certain parts of the world in which skills and facilities are not available and the incidence of VD is very high. The answer to this is that it is time someone supplied these areas with skilled personnel and facilities and the necessary organization to make them effective. Very large sums of money are spent by the World Health Organization (WHO) on less worthy causes.

What of the patient who is believed to be at risk but in whose case no evidence of disease has been found? One of the most important aphorisms in medicine is *diagnosis before treatment.* It embodies a very sound principle, and any physician who departs from it regularly is practising unsound medicine. Nevertheless, departures from it are regularly recommended by some eminent people, and the matter has to be argued in detail. To give an example, the following paragraph is included in recommendations for the treatment of syphilis by the Venereal Disease Control Advisory Committee to the VD Control Division of the Bureau of State Services of the United States (1976):

> Patients who have been exposed to infectious syphilis within the preceding 3 months and other patients who on epidemiologic grounds are at high risk for syphilis should be treated as for early syphilis. Every effort should be made to establish a diagnosis in these cases.

The final sentence has some saving grace, but I submit that the recommendation is faulty in principle. Leaving out the unreliability of the histories obtained from some patients, there is good evidence that patients exposed to infectious syphilis quite often escape infection. The reported results of what we may call *suppressive treatment* indicate only that such treatment diminishes the proportion of those patients who, exposed to infection, develop the early signs of the disease. Patients treated in this way have not been observed long enough and in sufficient numbers to indicate whether the infection is truly eliminated or merely suppressed in the early stages. Patients who have received such treatment should be observed and tested as though they had truly suffered from syphilis, but they seldom are. If observed and tested in this way, anxiety that with adequate observation and tests (but no treatment) might have been limited to 3 months is prolonged for one or perhaps two years, depending on the methods of the clinician. The introspective patient may spend the rest of his life worrying about a serious disease he has never had. The patient may well have had other contacts; are they to be rounded up and treated? If he had syphilis, this would be important, but there could hardly be medical or legal justification for dealing with them in this way when the data are so unclear.

The quoted paragraph includes the statement that epidemiologic treatment should be applied to "other patients who on epidemiologic grounds are at high risk for syphilis." Does this mean that we are to treat all prostitutes, all practising homosexuals, all seamen, and all promiscuous people? The list can be prolonged almost indefinitely; the further we go, the more extraordinary the recommendation seems. How often are we to treat them and are we to bear in mind that even penicillin is not without its dangers?

There are circumstances in which such treatment may be justified, as, for instance, when a woman late in pregnancy has been exposed to a serious risk, or a seaman is about to embark on a long voyage or a traveller on a long journey. Occasionally, too, there is a patient who will not submit to investigation but is willing to have an injection. These exceptions are few, and it behooves the clinician to consider them carefully and to use his best judgment. If he departs from principle, he should do so unwillingly, with the realization that it is an unsatisfactory compromise dictated by circumstances. Compromises of this kind are welcomed and freely used by careless and indifferent physicians, of which our profession, sad to say, has some.

Objections to this kind of procedure are also valid in cases of gonorrhea and other venereal diseases, although because of the nature of the diseases, the objections are less weighty than in cases of syphilis. It is sometimes difficult to establish the diagnosis of gonorrhea, especially in females, and delay may result in pelvic complications. Some of these patients, too, will not submit to the delays and inconveniences involved in a series of tests. Again, the clinician has to use his judgment, but he should still regard *diagnosis before treatment* as a fundamental principle, any departure from which should be regarded as an undesirable expedient. The physician is justified in making, and acting upon, a clinical diagnosis in the exceptional conditions where time and circumstance do not permit confirmation from the laboratory, but the omission of detailed and careful investigation is bad for the patient because it leads to anxiety and uncertainty. It is also bad for the clinician, because, if practised extensively, it leads to careless work and deterioration of standards.

Should Venereal Disease Contacts Be Treated? A Qualified Yes.

R. R. Willcox, M.D., F.R.C.P.
St. Mary's Hospital, London, England

In many countries, the legally definable venereal diseases are syphilis, gonorrhea, soft sore, lymphogranuloma venereum, and granuloma inguinale. However, the question really relates to the broader field of sexually transmitted disease, which includes also nonspecific genital infection, trichomoniasis, candidiasis (at least in the male), pediculosis pubis, scabies (in adults), venereal warts, molluscum contagiosum, and genital herpes—figures for which are collected for statistical purposes in some countries (e.g., the United Kingdom). Numerous other organisms—e.g., mycoplasmas and the virus of hepatitis B—are also spread sexually.

Considerations that determine whether contacts should be treated are listed in Table 23-1.

Table 23-1. *Criteria for the Treatment of VD Contacts*

Positive Criteria	Negative Criteria
Disease preventable	Disease not preventable
Good evidence of exposure to preventable disease	Precise diagnosis indefinite
Several exposures with no precautions	Single or doubtful exposure with precautions
Contact seen within incubation period	Contact seen outside incubation period
Poor diagnostic facilities	Good diagnostic facilities
Likelihood of default	Little likelihood of default
Others at risk	No others at risk

Prevention

Preventive, so-called epidemiologic treatment of contacts, if properly applied, can be effective against infectious syphilis and gonorrhea and is widely used for these conditions at least on a selective basis, and it is often given for nonspecific urethritis and lymphogranuloma venereum. Epidemiologic treatment is used also for trichomoniasis, pediculosis pubis, and, sometimes, for scabies. The effective agents are not yet available for the prevention of viral infections such as venereal warts, molluscum contagiosum, and genital herpes (or viral hepatitis B).

Exposure to Preventable Disease

Good Evidence

As there is no single drug that will abort the development of all the preventable sexually transmitted diseases, it is therefore very important that the physician know exactly what condition is involved so that the most appropriate treatment can be applied.

For example, an injection of repository penicillin (benzathine penicillin—2.4 mega units) is necessary to prevent syphilis but would be poor protection against gonorrhea, for which double the amount of the shorter-acting procaine penicillin (or oral ampicillin plus added probenecid by mouth) may be required. The penicillins will not, however, prevent nonspecific urethritis, for which a more prolonged course of tetracyclines or erythromycin is necessary, whereas a nitroimidazole derivative is obligatory for trichomoniasis and antiparasitic lotions and powders are necessary to prevent scabies or pediculosis pubis.

Indefinite Evidence

Although the true diagnosis of the condition can frequently be obtained from discreet inquiries between hospitals and clinics, this is not always possible, particularly when the information has been by hearsay or the infected person has left town.

In these circumstances, the decision has to be made whether to treat or to observe the patient. Sometimes treatment will be given for syphilis if the source patient has a sore (which may be herpes) and for gonorrhea to a female patient if the man had a discharge, although the latter therapy would not be effective if the condition was nongonococcal urethritis (NGU). If the source contact was a female complaining of a discharge, the male would require treatment for trichomoniasis, although gonorrhea might also be present. Sometimes, a history shows that the source patient had been treated without having undergone laboratory tests.

In general, unless the evidence is concrete, it is best to withhold treatment and to make repeated tests, but since humans are fickle, default rates are high, and in some groups (e.g., those in mobile occupations), treatment may be justified if the opportunities for follow-up are reduced.

Widespread antibiotic treatment after exposure to people in whom there was no evidence of disease is not approved. Postexposure antibiotic treatment can be given, which will certainly prevent gonorrhea and probably syphilis and other preventable venereal diseases, but in promiscuous people (amongst whom prevention is most important), frequently administered antibiotics may encourage microbial resistance. What is good for the commissars is not good for the troops! Nevertheless, treatment is occasionally given when other indications are strong.

Number and Nature of Exposures

Also important is the number of exposures with the infected person. Syphilis infection is more likely to require multiple exposures than gonorrhea, but who knows for venereal warts and some other conditions? Without using local precautions, the heterosexual male is one third or one quarter less likely to acquire gonorrhea from a single exposure than the female in whom infection from a single exposure is virtually certain, but very little, if anything, is known regarding the other previously mentioned conditions.

Although only one exposure to a defined disease may be sufficient justification for treatment, inquiries should be made as to the nature of the exposure. A hand-genital contact, for example, would not be sufficient to contract gonorrhea. Also, risks are very largely reduced if the male used a properly applied condom.

Relationship With Incubation Period

The decision to treat VD contacts is bound to the incubation period of the disease. Treatment is no longer necessary, providing proper tests are taken, when the incubation period for the disease in question has been exceeded.

For example, if contacts of patients with syphilis are seen three months or more after exposure and their VDRL and TPHA serum tests for syphilis are negative, no treatment is required. Experience has shown that of those admitting to contact with infectious syphilis within 30 days, one in every four or five will develop the disease unless given prophylactic treatment. If exposure was more than 30 days before and the contact is sero-negative without clinical signs of the disease, relatively few will subsequently develop infection. The latter group is best untreated and simply observed until three months have elapsed.

In the male, if no clinical or microscopic signs of gonorrhea are seen after two weeks following exposure, no treatment is necessary. The same applies to the female contact, although here two sets of microscopic tests and bacterial cultures are desirable.

Insufficient data are available concerning chlamydial infections such as nonspecific urethritis.

Facilities for Diagnosis

The importance of adequate diagnostic facilities is particularly applicable to gonorrhea. If there is a readily available service providing bacterial cultures, the necessity for treatment of contacts without overt signs of disease is less pressing, and treatment will be implemented on a more selective basis. On the other hand, when facilities for diagnosis are less reliable or nonexistent, treatment of contacts becomes mandatory because it is then a principal weapon of control (e.g., in many developing countries in which facilities for culture tests are lacking, Gram smears are performed on males with discharges and treatment is given to female contacts whether the smear is positive or negative). The same applies in countries in which it is extremely difficult to persuade women to be examined. Unfortunately, such treatment may have to be given even without examination.

Likelihood of Default

Even when diagnostic facilities are good, selected contacts will be treated appropriate to the disease, owing to the likelihood of default. Defaulters include those unlikely to visit the doctor or clinic for reason of occupation and those with a previous tendency toward noncompliance. When facilities for diagnosis and treatment are poor, all patients may be considered likely defaulters and treatment of contacts becomes the rule.

Others at Risk

If the suspect disease is unknown, diagnostic facilities are good, there is little likelihood of default, and no others are likely to be at risk (e.g., the contact being a single and usually nonpromiscuous individual), there may be no need for epidemiologic treatment.

If, on the other hand, the suspect disease is known to be preventable, regardless of the diagnostic facilities or the likelihood of default, epidemiologic treatment will be justified if others are at risk. A man exposed to syphilis or gonorrhea who has not yet had sexual relations with his wife or regular partner will desire such preventive treatment. This is especially so for syphilis, due to its long incubation period (9 to 90 days but usually 21 to 28 days). Likewise, if the regular partner of someone with a known case of syphilis, gonorrhea, or another preventable condition has already been exposed, treatment of that partner is desirable not only to prevent infection in that person but also to prevent so-called "ping-pong" reinfection of the original patient.

Contacts who are known to be promiscuous either from their past record of venereal infections or from their admitted number of sexual exposures should likewise be treated as if they were in fact incubating the disease, since even if the patient underwent tests—which is unlikely to be the case—others would probably be exposed if the disease were allowed to develop.

Finally, risk to the fetus or baby at birth has to be taken into account when the contact is pregnant.

Conclusion

Should VD contacts be treated? Yes, depending on circumstances.

Factors that favor the use of epidemiologic treatment of VD contacts include (1) firm evidence of exposure to a preventable disease, especially multiple encounters with no precautions; (2) if the contact is seen within the incubation period of the disease in question; (3) availability of only poor diagnostic facilities; (4) the likelihood that the patient may not return for follow-ups; and (5) if other people are likely to be at risk if the contact is not treated.

Not advocated is the indiscriminate treatment of suspected contacts or contacts without examination. All those treated should have a clinical examination, with the best available laboratory backing.

If used with discrimination and judgment, epidemiologic treatment of VD contacts is a valuable method of control.

References

Willcox, R.R.: Treatment before diagnosis in venereology. Br. J. Vener. Dis. 30:7–12, 1954.

Willcox, R.R.: 'Epidemiological' treatment in non-venereal and in treponemal diseases. Br. J. Vener. Dis. 49:107–115, 1973.

Willcox, R.R.: 'Epidemiological' treatment in venereal diseases other than syphilis. Br. J. Vener. Dis. 49:116–125, 1973.

24

Should the Public Have the Legal Right to Use Unproven Remedies like Laetrile and DMSO?

Quacks are the greatest liars in the world except their patients.

Benjamin Franklin

By quack I mean impostor, not in opposition to but in common with physicians.

Horace Walpole

It is better to have recourse to a quack, if he can cure our disorder, although he cannot explain it, than to a physician, if he can explain our disease, but cannot cure it.

Charles C. Colton, *Lacon*

Don't cry out against the quack; find out wherein his success lies—and be a better quack.

Martin H. Fischer

For diverse ills are remedies diverse.

Euripides, *Fragments*

Introduction

The question of public rights in regard to the use of "unproven" remedies goes to the heart of some fundamental assumptions about our society and is, therefore, a matter of basic importance.

Weiner tackles the problem head-on. Can public servants impose their own will and judgment on others? Does the public need to be protected against itself? He suggests that informed patients, aided by qualified physicians, should have the right to decide for themselves about remedies whose status is controversial. Weiner points out that some people have gotten so fed up with governmental intervention as to suggest doing away with the Food and Drug Administration (FDA), but he does not go that far. Instead, he suggests a return toward the less constrained atmosphere that prevailed prior to 1962, and he proposes that Laetrile, anticoagulants, beta blockers, and drugs of possible benefit against rare diseases all need a less heavy regulatory hand. Weiner's essay ends with some specific plans for handling "special status" drugs.

Hutt, a former general counsel for the FDA, reviews the history behind our current dilemma and spells out the legal requirements for approving a new drug. The reader will note that the law and the regulations promulgated to implement the statute allow for considerable latitude with respect to such matters as "controls." How to speed up new drug approval is a tricky question, as Hutt points out, especially since one has to deal with what he calls the "siege mentality" of FDA bureaucrats.

The practicing physician is likely to be concerned about the proposals to alter present governmental controls over drug distribution and prescribing. One can only hope that we adopt any proposed changes only after full and thoughtful discussion of their implications.

Hutt also suggests that an inflexible regulatory approach to such alleged remedies as Laetrile may force us as a society into radical counterefforts, which will be harmful in the long run.

The last two essays discuss two of the most fascinating new drugs of the last decade—Laetrile and dimethyl sulfoxide (DMSO). Their acceptance as legitimate therapies has suffered at least in part from the unorthodoxy of the approaches they typify. The unfamiliar always has to battle the prejudice felt in many quarters of the medical establishment. Such bias is not necessarily a bad thing—most ideas that sound strange turn out to *be* strange. But not all.

Moss presents the case for Laetrile with skill and thoroughness. He argues that the data in favor of Laetrile are not inconsequential, and that the ready dismissal of the drug has perhaps been both unfair and unscientific. In the long run, the final decision on the utility of Laetrile in cancer patients will have to come from careful clinical investigation, which thus far has lagged behind the animal research.

For most scientists, Laetrile seems to be the krebiozen of the 1970s. Krebiozen was under a cloud from its inception. Its mysterious nature and the questionable tactics and ability of its producers turned many against it before any valid examination of its true merit could be carried out. As with Laetrile, some cancer patients had improved on krebiozen in the absence of other, conventional therapy, but cancer remissions have been recorded in the absence of any therapy. Few now lament the passing of krebiozen, and most doctors probably see equally little promise in Laetrile.

The DMSO story is more comforting. Although it is also an unconventional therapy, DMSO has never been under the same cloud as Laetrile. Its fascinating properties have long been apparent, although its full therapeutic potential is still not known. Human studies were stopped for a considerable period on the basis of animal toxicity tests that were probably irrelevant, and now there are significant bureaucratic obstacles to full investigation of the drug's clinical utility. Unlike Laetrile, DMSO has been approved for marketing, although for fewer indications than many who have worked with it would like to see. The DMSO affair is thus only a partial success story, but an illuminating one nevertheless.

LOUIS LASAGNA, M.D.

Should The Public Have the Legal Right to Use Unproven Remedies? Yes.*

Murray Weiner, M.D.
Merrell Research Center, Cincinnati

Defining the Issues

Let us agree from the start that no society can long exist if it does not recognize that the rights of individuals must at times be subservient to the requirements of the common good. However, a key index differentiating a society that respects human rights—such as we aspire to be—from one with little real concern for human rights is the manner and frequency with which the will and opinion of one group, no matter how large or prestigious, is imposed upon all. The controversy about the use of unproven drugs is in some respects a microcosm of this broader societal issue. Where and when is governmental control a legitimate requirement in the public interest rather than a counterproductive bureaucratic invasion of individual prerogative? Several distinctions need to be considered in making these judgments.

Regard for the public welfare can legitimately justify the imposition of the judgment of health authorities on everyone if the noncompliance of some would create a threat to the welfare of others, or if the solution of a serious public health problem required limitations on individual choice. But if the issue involves individualized treatment of specific patients who alone will be hurt or helped by a given remedy, it takes a strange morality and considerable conceit on the part of public servants to demand that they have the right to impose their judgment on all. The will of the individual who consciously desires to pursue his own judgment should not be lightly overruled.

"But," says the opposition, "this poor individual doesn't understand what he is doing, and we must protect him from being misled into harming himself." This attitude rings a familiar note, historically characteristic of the despot who defends his assumption of power over others as a necessity to "protect" the public against its own ignorance. Protection against thieves, charlatans, and fakers is one thing; but prohibiting reputable, learned professionals from acting in accordance with their own judgment and conscience is something else. When an authority seeks and gets blanket power to prevent well informed physicians from following their own judgments as to what is best for their individual patients, the action must stand condemned as interfering with basic human rights. The *de facto* blocking of availability of medications, as is now practiced, is an example of such interference.

When an agent is shown beyond reasonable doubt to have significant toxicity without any redeeming features, there is a legitimate basis for restricting its availability to very special circumstances. But when a new medication has received an evaluation that suggests significant

*The opinions expressed are those of the author, and do not necessarily represent those of any of the organizations with which he is affiliated.

utility in the judgment of some qualified experts, it is difficult to understand why the use of the agent by such qualified people must be forbidden until some agency has officially ruled that it may be used. Many medications acknowledged to be valuable today were prohibited to doctors who may have wanted to use the drug months or years ago to benefit their patients but were prevented by law from following their judgment. It is one thing to prohibit drugs shown to be dangerous or inactive. It is something else to impede the availability of promising new agents until a cumbersome bureaucratic system catches up with all the "documentation" and professional fault-finding in a legalistic framework.

A public responsibility exists to block attempts to mislead the ignorant and gullible with unproven remedies. But when a competent, informed physician and his patient agree that for *this* patient—with the current state of knowledge, imperfect as it may be—the benefit-risk assessment for the use of the "unproven" remedy is in favor of its use, it is neither morally nor scientifically proper for a governmental agency to preclude that option.

Today, a "sponsor" may be given permission to make individual shipments of unproven drugs to practitioners who request them for patients with a distinct need for them. To stay within the law, the procedure requires a deceptive statement to the effect that each doctor recipient is an "investigator" studying an "investigational new drug." A practicing physician who is not an "investigator" has to sign documents saying that he is, in order to treat a patient according to his considered judgment. Why is such a charade tolerated? This complex process by which our FDA gets around its own excessive legal restraints when they become morally intolerable causes thousands of practitioners to go against their better judgment, and let the patient do without. The situation is particularly sad when the FDA has already acknowledged, in principle, that a drug is safe and effective, but many months go by while some fine print on the labeling goes through serial "final" approval processes across the desks of innumerable lawyers and administrators, with intermediate stops at the typing pool. Meanwhile, the physician and his patient stand by and suffer the consequences.

In short, when I argue for the *legal right* of the *public* to use *unproven drugs,* I am referring to the treatment of informed individuals by their qualified physicians with the status of the drugs truthfully described. This right is nonexistent today, despite public pronouncements to the contrary. If a medication is not available on prescription in a hospital pharmacy, and it can be obtained only after petitioning as an "investigator" for the review and official approval of third parties, *de facto,* the medication is not available.

Present Status and Goals

Even the strongest defenders of individual rights acknowledge the public need for protection against the unconscionable con man as well as the sincere but misguided fanatic who might persuade the gullible to buy and use potentially harmful, untested remedies. On the other hand, even the most ardent proponents of strict new drug regulations disclaim any desire to have regulations replace the practicing physician or to deny the role of qualified practitioners in prescribing potent medications. Everybody agrees that the search for better drugs should be encouraged, and that promising new agents should be tested efficiently so as to determine their true relevant properties; that useful new drugs should be made available with appropriate labeling to guide their optimal use as soon as possible; and that few things are 100 percent safe and effective, so that one must try to achieve a proper benefit-risk balance. Nor is there any opposition to the concept that sick people should be encouraged to seek the advice of competent physicians and to follow that advice.

It is the practitioner who must balance the risks of a variety of possible therapeutic approaches, including the risk of doing nothing, in deciding on the management of each patient. The issue under discussion can therefore be described in terms of the options open to him. Current United States regulations blindly forbid use of any agent that has not yet cleared the bureaucracy, and bitter experience demonstrates that the bureaucracy can hold up clearance because of concern over a thousand different trivia, even after all the significant scientific questions have been answered satisfactorily.

What ought to be done about patients who may need a drug during the very considerable interval between the first evidence of a promising effect and the final ruling, many years later, that the agent is "safe and effective as labeled"? Paradoxically, as scientific methods become increasingly sophisticated, the time necessary to come to a decision as to if, when, and how a drug should be used becomes longer rather than shorter. Since new skills, not available years ago, can now generate information that might possibly help evaluate a drug, a system has evolved that demands that massive amounts of new types of information be generated, analyzed, documented, and submitted before an approval judgment will be undertaken. All too often, there is little serious thought as to whether the new information, which requires considerable time and research to generate, makes a significant contribution to the evaluation of the efficacy and safety of the new drug. These poorly reasoned demands contribute to the ever increasing time interval between discovery and approval for marketing.

The practical objective of drug study is to determine how a drug might be used to accomplish the most benefit and the least harm. The learning process is continuous, and the vast majority of drugs fall by the wayside. Those that continue to be pursued past the first phases of clinical study fit into a pattern of ongoing experience, which leads to progressively sounder judgments about their utility. Under the current regulatory system, a politically dominated bureau is given the awesome power to say how much of what kind of test results is *adequate* (an indefinable term) before qualified practitioners are offered the option of deciding that a new drug may be of value to one of their patients. The bureau is a massive and frequently clumsy machine that tends to be more sensitive to political pressure than to scientific reality. It is the centralized locus of this ever increasing power in regard to the use of unproven drugs that is really at issue.

Is it in the public interest that the development, supply, and use of drugs are so powerfully and centrally controlled? Is such control an unfortunate but unavoidable facet of the government's responsibility to see that all drugs are properly tested before they are marketed? I think not.

Historically, control of the availability of drugs to the American public started with frontier-type freedom, with the occasional tar and feathering of a medicine showman if the people caught up with him after they recognized his expensive nostrums as fakes. Protection of the public took a series of legal steps now universally recognized as proper:

1. The label on a bottle should properly represent its contents and use (Pure Food & Drug Act of 1906).
2. New drugs should be prepared and tested by appropriate experts, and they should be made available for use in humans only to physicians competent to handle them (Food, Drug and Cosmetic Act of 1938).
3. Standard drugs recognized as dangerously potent should be available only by the prescription of a licensed physician (Durham-Humphrey Act of 1951).

In 1962, the thalidomide tragedy resulted in the passage of amendments to the existing laws. An objective historical review of circumstances just prior to this event must conclude that the problem that precipitated passage of these amendments was primarily a reflection of inadequate scientific knowledge, not of inadequate regulation.

It is not these amendments but the advance of science in response to a demonstrated need that has led to the laudable development of teratology and many other subspecialties that contribute to the improved drug testing procedures available today. In fact, much time now spent by teratologists on conducting legally mandated studies would be better spent in the public interest if these experts were freer to adapt their tests to the problem at hand rather than to the regulatory requirement.

Alternative Approaches

In considering possible ways of protecting the public without compromising the availability of new drugs, it would be helpful to review the options, old and new. Too often, one sees such strong habituation to the existing mode that other points of view are dismissed blindly.

Implement Stronger Controls

Some of the most counterproductive actions have resulted from hasty decisions to "do something" in response to a problem. Tightening control has become the easiest thing to do when faced with a problem, and too often this is pursued without thinking through the critical question: control of what by whom? The potential for harm is enormous, even with the best of intentions. The fact that former problems were reasonably attacked by instituting regulations does not mean that current problems can best be handled in the same way.

Seekers of stronger new drug controls still delight in citing the ancient use of blood-letting and cathartics as proof that the practicing physician is a pompous fool who must be ordered to treat patients in accordance with some superior wisdom that is now available from on high—i.e., the governmental bureau. Were there a government bureau in the 19th century with the power to impose the teaching of the times on all therapists, as we have today, we might still be treating patients with blood-letting and strong catharsis. More than anything else, it was the right of free and intelligent clinical observers to differ with the leading authorities that made it possible to show the truth of new ideas and the error of some old ones. I have little doubt that 50 years from now, people looking back at us from their vantage point will see some of our currently popular treatment as we now see blood-letting, and they will wonder how our society could have been so shortsighted as to demand conformity under penalty of law.

In fairness to our blood-letting ancestors, we should remember that they practiced without the benefit of an effective diuretic or antiarrhythmic, and with only crudely standardized and poorly understood digitalis preparations. Since so many illnesses terminated in congestive heart failure, blood-letting and catharsis were probably the only treatments, albeit very poor by modern standards, to delay congestive deaths.

Do away with the FDA. If we now look with historic perspective at the 1962 amendments, and particularly at the brazen expansion of those amendments by ever broader regulatory and administrative interpretations, it becomes apparent that the amendments probably cost, and continue to cost, more lives (and perpetuation of misery among the sick) than they have saved. Some scholars have actually reached the serious conclusion that, on balance, it would be in the public interest to do away with the FDA (Friedman, 1973). I do not propose elimination of the FDA as a desirable option, but let it be recorded that matters have gone so far that it has been proposed as the most straightforward way out of our current quagmire.

Return to Former Control Standards

Perhaps a more reasonable option, voiced at the risk of being labeled Neanderthal and a bucker of the inevitable tide, is to return to the regulatory concepts as they existed prior to 1962, adapted to the current, more advanced state of medical science. Government would not approve or disapprove drugs. Government would not mandate indications and dosages to create a basis for malpractice suits of the type that have sacrificed the best interests of the patient to the need to practice defensive medicine and that have contributed to the soaring cost of medical care. Government would not take responsibility for, nor edit, every word of the scientific report that a sponsor is obliged to prepare over his own signature. Investigators and practitioners would not be obliged to wait hat-in-hand for a new agent while a small army of desk-bound scientists, statisticians, and lawyers study other people's data to determine who shall and who shall not be allowed what treatment.

Revise Licensing Procedures

Another option discussed from time to time is an *extension* of the licensing procedure. Practicing medicine, driving a truck, teaching in public schools, and practicing law are all regulated by the government on the basis of appropriate examinations to assure that the practitioners possess the background, training, experience, and morality necessary to make the judgments required of their profession. The truck driver doesn't have to file in advance and defend his plan to take a new route to his destination, and then await government permission to proceed. A teacher with an innovative lesson plan does not await clearance by the federal government. Why not license new drug developers, investigators, and other specialists on the basis of competence, and let them "do their thing" without item-by-item approval of every project and every patient regimen by bureaucrats?

This licensure option does not address itself directly to the issue of the clinical availability of unproven drugs, though it would tend to expedite their study and therefore hasten availability. To attack more directly the issue at hand, prestigious medical centers, and possibly individuals, may be licensed as competent to prescribe unproven drugs. Through these centers, general practitioners and patients could have access to promising though unproven remedies on a more direct, immediate, and practical basis.

Maintain Current Practices

The final option is to retain the current practice, which has a built-in tendency to attack every problem by more and more controls and limitations on new drug availability. Contributing to this inertia is the experience of the staff of the bureaucracy, which teaches that their careers are advanced by finding fault and developing excuses to put off affirmative decisions. It takes only a handful of professional faultfinders to discourage thousands of conscientious bureaucratic employees from making practical, straightforward, scientific judgments.

The political influence on what should be scientific judgment is exemplified by the page one headline reporting of the complaints of a handful of FDA employees at a congressional hearing on August 14, 1974. The presiding senator's news release contained the widely reported charge of this small group that "their recommendations to approve new drugs have never been questioned, but their recommendations to disapprove drugs were almost always questioned."

Unfortunately, there was no example cited of a recommendation to approve a new drug by members of this group, and the forum was hardly a good one to argue the scientific merits of their frequent disapprovals. They won their point largely in the press. The lesson taught by this and other similar events cannot escape the attention of many reasonable, knowledgeable, dedicated career scientists in the FDA who are compelled to learn to avoid or delay decisions or to regard negative decisions as the easiest way to survive.

Sooner or later, this situation must lead to revolt by the public to reestablish its rights in its own interest, or to the sad specter of ever tighter controls eventuating in abject hopelessness and lethargic acceptance. Given enough time, the public may no longer realize the awful loss it is suffering in the name of the public welfare. Centralized unbridled control of unproven drugs can become the accepted norm, with its inevitable adverse effect on the quality of medical care. This is the least satisfactory of all the options reviewed, and it is the direction in which we are now heading.

Forbidden Drugs

Unproven drugs that are now forbidden to the public may be categorized into several types. The following are scenarios of what can be expected to happen, or has happened, under current regulations, in contrast to what might be expected if there were more reasonable public access to these agents.

Type 1: The Unproven "Faddist" Medication

This imprecise terminology is meant to cover agents that generally arise outside the mainstream of pharmaceutical research and tend to be associated with emotional, zealous adherents. The drugs are usually common substances, often of natural origin with little apparent toxicity. The alleged utility is likely to have been discovered by incidental rather than organized or planned clinical observations. Recent examples of agents in this class include Laetrile for cancer and megavitamins (particularly ascorbic acid) for many purposes.

I shall make my arguments under the assumption that these treatments are in fact worthless, and I shall review the scenarios that develop under the current FDA attitude—i.e., the FDA has the obligation and power to ban their public availability—in comparison with the attitude that qualified practitioners and their informed patients should have the right to proper supplies of such agents for use in accordance with their own judgment. The Laetrile situation will serve this purpose well.

Despite scientific advances, there is still a large patient population, particularly among cancer victims, who are admittedly beyond cure. There is a growing concern among these patients and their doctors for the quality of life and the dignity of death that makes some of them reject radical surgery and disabling forms of radiation or chemotherapy, even though the statistics might show a few months longer mean survival with such treatment. Although there has recently been a most laudable series of advances in the control and even cure of a variety of previously hopeless malignancies, the practitioner must still often engage in the art of human counsel when his science fails to meet the challenge adequately. To be honest and frank, he must tell some patients he has little or nothing to offer. What then?

If one man says "I offer no hope" and another says "I offer a slight chance," where would one expect a cancer patient to go? No one denies the power of placebo to relieve. Is it fair to deny the desperate patient the benefit of this power? Is it honest to say that we *know* Laetrile (or anything else) is ineffective, when what we really mean is that we have not yet seen any impressive evidence of efficacy, and have no reason to believe that it works?

Today, the desperate patient is driven away from his own doctor, with a good chance of winding up in the hands of a Laetrile fan who might ignore other useful measures that the original doctor might have planned. He may be treated with material from uncertain sources. Science loses control and the issue becomes politicized. State legislatures get into the act and confusion reigns.

The scenario might be different if every cancer clinic that so desired could stock and use Laetrile as they saw fit. Note that I speak of use, not "clinical investigation," with all its filings, forms, and approvals. Were I the physician in such a clinic, I would regularly tell my inquiring patients that I saw no value in the drug. Yet, every now and then, I'm sure I would find a patient whose condition and attitude were such that I might decide that the use of the drug in this instance was worthwhile. The patient would remain under good general medical care and would continue to have other appropriate measures available. Nobody would be obliged or tempted to leave my clinic because I did not have the option of treating with Laetrile. If, in fact, Laetrile is ineffective, I have no doubt it would lose its popularity much sooner under these circumstances.

The regulatory argument against proposals to make a Laetrile-like drug available tends to take several forms. Since the drug is ineffective, they say, anyone who uses it is unscientific or fraudulent or both, and he must therefore be stopped. Thus, the proof of your error lies in the fact that you disagree with the agency decision. But the agency has been wrong in some of its past judgments as to what is reasonable and scientifically correct, and I see no evidence of infallibility in their present scientific conclusions. Equally important, their understandable preoccupation with statistics and numbers has reinforced a disinterest in and limited comprehension of the totality of individual patient care, in contrast to the average (or group) response "documented" under the rigid and frequently artificial conditions of controlled studies in a population with characteristics that may or may not be applicable to the total problem in a specific case. Individual situations and experiences are annoyances brushed aside by the FDA as useless "testimonials," unless, of course, the testimonial can be interpreted as a side effect, in which case it deserves prompt and wide communication to all, and serves as another weapon to justify centralized, rigid control of availability. I think the FDA is right in taking seriously the possibility that a "testimonial" side effect report might be the first reflection of an important reality. By the same token, however, "testimonial" experiences of efficacy shouldn't be ignored when balancing the risks of using versus not using an unproven drug. The practitioner and his patient have the right not to ignore this information, with all its limitations, and the right to have supplies if they decide they wish to risk using the drug.

Type 2: Drugs Involving Difficult Value Judgments of Therapeutic Benefit-risk

Many of the most important pharmaceutical contributions to therapy go through long periods of evaluation, with varying degrees of agreement as to the proper indications, dosage, and degree of risk. At any point, denying the availability of a drug is tantamount to forcing practitioners to act as if the drug didn't exist or had been proven too dangerous or ineffective to use; that is, the practitioner becomes legally bound to behave contrary to the facts. So often, it is not realized that "not to act, is to act" (Eisenberg, 1977).

With this type drug, the issue is not just a matter of the ultimate statistical judgment of benefit-risk, which is never final, but the right of individual physicians to make that determination for each individual patient. The coumarin anticoagulants and the beta blockers can be used as examples.

At the time of the National Academy of Sciences/National Research Council (NAS/NRC) review of marketed drugs in the late 1960s, the coumarin anticoagulants were given a "possibly effective" rating. They had already been marketed for over 20 years and were the subject of thousands of publications, but there was no unanimity among experts about their place in therapy. In the legal interpretation of this scientific classification, more data were necessary to prove the drugs "effective" or they would have to come off the market. Experts who had followed these anticoagulants from their start knew that it was highly unlikely that any data generated in the next couple of years would answer the outstanding questions definitively. To this day, after 30 years of study, the experts still differ on the proper role of these anticoagulants.

The FDA finally ruled the anticoagulants "effective" on the basis of much the same body of knowledge (and differences of opinion) that existed at the time of the NAS/NRC review that rated them "less than effective." Thus, with the anticoagulants, as with other older drugs, the FDA recognized that availability to the practitioner cannot be restrained because major questions have not or cannot be resolved in the current state of the art. Logic prevailed, and physicians use these drugs as they see fit.

The betablocker situation was different in two respects. First, there was only one representative of the group on the U.S. market (propranolol) and second, this drug has a remarkable history of strictly limited approved indications. It was originally made available for the treatment of tachyarrhythmias in 1969, and it took about five years more before it was approved for angina. It was longer still before it could be used in hypertension without risking the consequences of daring to prescribe without governmental blessing. Since the drug was available, it was occasionally prescribed for hypertension, despite FDA efforts to dissuade doctors from making individual judgments outside of "labeling."

But what about other agents with new drug applications pending for years, which are not yet marketed for any purpose? By denying their availability during prolonged periods of continuing clinical evaluation—decades in some instances—the FDA is once again not merely withholding judgment but imposing the full consequences of a negative decision when, by its own admission (i.e., the existence of an active IND application), the drug has promising characteristics at least deserving of further study.

In the view of many experts, propranolol has several serious limitations not shared equally with some of the "second generation" betablockers that have been available abroad for years. Unfortunately, American physicians who would prefer to put their confidence in the experience of prestigious clinicians at home and abroad are obliged to use the more dangerous older drugs until the FDA finishes evaluating the new agents. With the betablockers, U.S. investigations were delayed for years because of a highly controversial presumption of carcinogenicity based on an unusual strain of mice. This fear has since been cleared away for several of the agents.

The misconceptions concerning the availability of unproven drugs are reflected in the following exchange between a senator and a witness at the 1974 hearings on the U.S. "drug lag":

> *Senator*: . . . But they also established a policy that makes oxprenolol available to any patient who gets adverse reactions from the available drug which is now in the marketplace. What is wrong with that procedure . . .?
>
> *Witness*: . . . From the public health point of view, that borders on the useless. The number of people who might well have benefited from oxprenolol over propranolol is much larger than the number that would actually be in a position to go through the procedure . . . special requests and so forth.
>
> *Senator*: The FDA did not specify any particular procedure, except that it was available to be prescribed by a physician in those cases where the patient does not tolerate the drug that is available in this country. What is wrong with those procedures?
>
> *Witness*: I doubt if it is available in any pharmacy . . . in the United States.

Of course, the drug was not available from a pharmacy with a prescription, but only to doctors who agreed to follow the "investigator" procedure.

Type 3: Empirically Unproven but Rational Medication

The progress of modern therapeutics is largely dependent on understanding the mechanism of disease and finding a drug that attacks the mechanism. Frequently, the therapeutic endpoint is very difficult to prove, whereas the attack on the mechanism of action may be easily demonstrated.

The effects of anticoagulants on blood clotting are obvious in a day, but after decades of research, there are still questions about the influence of these drugs on some types of thrombosis. Of course, empirical proof of efficacy is the most useful goal of clinical research. But who should say what ought to be done with a patient for whom a rational drug exists, but empirical proof of efficacy is not yet at hand? Should a mandatory judgment be made by a central authority and imposed indiscriminately on all? Would not the public be better served if each patient's situation were individually evaluated by the physician most familiar with his particular problem?

The use of thiazides for hypertension is a case in point. Several compounds in this class were approved for the treatment of severe hypertension in the early 1960s. For a number of years, the manufacturers were obliged not to discuss mild to moderate hypertension in anything considered "labeling" because the FDA had not yet gotten around to the official opinion that the data supported use in such patients. Since the drugs were, in fact, on the market, many physicians did prescribe them for mild to moderate hypertensives, but many others were dissuaded by FDA statements that such use was "outside the label," making the prescribing physician subject to malpractice suits and possibly to other legal action.*

Years later, mild to moderate hypertension became an approved indication, based on slowly developed empirical mortality and morbidity data. "Well controlled studies" (VA Cooperative Study, 1970) eventually showed that medical control of mild to moderate hypertension did indeed reduce mortality. A placebo-treated group, whose death rate was quite similar to that noted in the standard statistics of hypertensive populations in general, had about twice the mortality of the treated group.

There are over 20 million hypertensives in the U.S. who have a distinctly higher cardiovascular morbidity and mortality than their nonhypertensive counterparts. Since about one quarter of the almost one million cardiovascular deaths per year in the U.S. are related to hypertension, medical control of hypertension is now recognized to be a personal and public health matter of urgent importance. This year, millions of dollars are being spent by the government and heart associations to find and to treat mild and moderate hypertensives. And only a few short years ago, physicians already impressed with the value of antihypertensive therapy had to ignore the existing FDA rulings in order to treat such patients!

Let us now review what the situation might have been if the regulatory powers did not take the attitude that all "unproven" drug use is forbidden until they get around to declaring otherwise. The agents that can control mild and moderate hypertension might well have been employed several years earlier, and thousands now dead might still be alive. Was the toxic potential of these drugs in uncomplicated mild and moderate hypertension really so great as to justify FDA insistence that patients ought to risk the well recognized incidence of fatal and crippling strokes and heart attacks associated with uncontrolled hypertension rather than the hypothetical dangers of using the unproven drugs? In fact, the nature and frequency of thiazide side effects in uncomplicated hypertensives is so low as to have no discernible mortality or significant morbidity. The tragedy might have been much greater if the drugs in question had not previously achieved marketability as diuretics. How many people would have died if the use of penicillin for syphilis had been forbidden until statistical data concerning mortality due to tertiary syphilis was generated, instead of giving weight to extrapolations from the observed conversion of positive serology tests? If polio vaccine were to be developed in today's regulatory atmosphere, is there any doubt that its development and approval would be years slower than was the case in the 1950s?

Type 4: The Unusual Drug for the Rare Disease

There is universal concern about the low priority likely to be assigned to drugs of this type as opposed to drugs with potentially broader utility. However, there is more interest in such drugs at the research level, both industrial and academic, than is generally acknowledged. Responsible management is often willing to follow scientific advisors when the scientists say that the medical importance of a promising new agent makes its pursuit a moral obligation despite low commercial potential. The major problem arises when the regulators exhibit their usual disinterest in the scientific requirements as opposed to the regulatory ones and in the limits of time, facilities, and funds available to the research community.

For example, a simple analog of the chelating agent EDTA was found to be the most effective agent known to reduce the plutonium body burden if given intravenously promptly after acute plutonium poisoning. Responsible health officers in the few laboratories with a low (but real) potential for a plutonium accident wanted to stock a reasonably labeled supply of the agent in injectable form in case of emergency. The

* Such veiled threats to physicians are a common ploy by which the FDA influences the practice of medicine even beyond the considerable power granted it by law. The FDA has no legal power to prevent a physician from using a marketed drug differently from the label recommendations. Nevertheless, there have been discussions of ways to discourage authors of medical texts from suggesting the use of drugs in doses or for indications that have not been approved. Such limitations are imposed on material considered to be advertising.

company scientists persuaded the management that they had a moral obligation to make the material available—which is not an insignificant commitment, considering modern production and quality control requirements. They also foresaw an additional limited utility for the chelator in detecting subclinical lead intoxication or iron overload by urine analysis after a single modest dose of the agent. The FDA reviewed the data and made a series of demands, including long-term toxicity evaluations of three doses in each of two species if the drug were to be approved, even though the use would be limited to single-dose or short-term emergency treatment. The toxicity of large daily intravenous doses for a month had already been studied, and no remarkable effects had been found.

With this demand, the product had to become a full-fledged project that would consume time and facilities for studies of questionable scientific need. The project took its place in the priority list, in competition with projects for which chronic toxicity studies were truly important. The management response to the FDA demands was first to wonder whether their own scientists had exaggerated the need to make the product available. Instead of some modest recognition of their willingness to do a public service, they had to defend themselves against thinly veiled accusations of trying to "cut corners." In the end, managers took the attitude that they were willing to lose money to fill a human need, but they did not feel obliged to fight for the privilege. The project was dropped.

Pharmaceutical innovators go along with regulators' demands, whether rational or not, when dealing with products of economic importance, because they have no choice. But when the regulators insist on going "by the book" instead of by logic in special cases, the pharmaceutical people feel relieved of any moral responsibility to make the agents available, and real opportunities are doomed to oblivion. This sad situation with important but limited-use drugs would be markedly alleviated if there were an effective mechanism that allowed for the availability of unproven drugs to qualified physicians.

With all four classes of unproven drugs described, there are major problems that exist only as a consequence of the current rigid, centralized control. They could be largely resolved if all concerned had a little more respect for the wisdom and morality of our licensed physicians and a little more skepticism about those same qualities in the politically dominated bureaucracies.

It has become popular in recent years to evaluate physicians who practice and do medical research by the documents they produce, rather than by the logic and reality of the conclusions they reach. In any effort as complex and judgmental as the development and use of unproven drugs, accompanied by the collection of masses of data, there are bound to be technical and recording imperfections, the vast majority of which are inconsequential. There are also bound to be rare instances of significant misjudgment and even malfeasance. In order to keep proper perspective in regard to the seriousness of the problem and the justification of the dislocations caused by attempts at regulatory solutions, it is critically important not to confuse the incidence of minor errors found in retrospective reviews of thousands of bits of recorded data with the rare significant abuse of professional trust. In recent years, there has been an unconscionable practice of citing in detail an isolated, deplorable event and then pointing to some survey alleging a high frequency of "deficiencies" in the conduct of practice or research. The "deficiencies" cited are mostly inconsequential and innocent, and often based on inspection of old records with after-the-fact criteria. They are rarely a legitimate basis for disqualifying sound scientific conclusions. This type of unfair attack is not really new. It was well described by the following comment in a review of medical ethics over a century ago:

> The errors of good men and the crimes of knaves are never discriminated by the vulgar, who have a keen relish for detecting blemishes in all who are by position and knowledge superior to themselves (Review of Medical Ethics, 1852).

Conclusion

There is an urgent need to change our current system so that unproven drugs will be made available to qualified practitioners in the interest of their patients. Adequate precedents exist for arrangements by which potential misuse of valuable drugs is controlled without the obstruction of their proper use. The special category of prescription drugs, as contrasted to over-the-counter drugs, was voluntarily introduced by the medical and pharmacy professions over a century ago and has since become legally formalized at the federal level (Durham-Humphrey Act of 1951).

To correct the current anomaly, in which the practice of medicine has been limited by law in regard to unproven drugs, I propose the creation of a new special category for such agents, defining practical and reasonable precautions under which these "special status" drugs can be distributed for prescription or direct use by qualified physicians. Again, I emphasize therapeutic use; this need not be "investigational," and it is intended first and foremost for the benefit of specific patients. No filings with the federal government are to be required. There is to be no time limit as to how long a drug may remain in the "special status" category. There are to be no monitoring requirements beyond those normally practiced by physicians and reports a doctor may voluntarily agree to send, if requested. "Special status" drugs will, however, carry some special requirements that distinguish them from "approved" prescription drugs:

1. The prescription or order form signed by the physician shall confirm that he is familiar with the drug and its special status.

2. Physician records shall include a statement signed by the patient or responsible guardian indicating that he is aware that a "special status" drug is being prescribed.

3. Advertising shall be limited to statements as to the availability of the drug, its intended use, and a presentation of, or an invitation to the physician to write for, a complete listing of the relevant literature.

4. At its option, the FDA may require inclusion of its own statement of whatever opinion or concerns it may wish to express as part of the literature packet available to physicians. These statements, however, shall be introduced with a phrase indicating that they have no official or legal status beyond that of any other review that the practitioner may evaluate in deciding on a course of therapy.

The law bringing the "special status" category into being will call upon the FDA to create a licensure system to assure proper facilities and the professional talent, ethics, and experience of practitioners and organizations licensed to use "special status" compounds made available to them by similarly licensed manufacturers. The FDA shall have the authority to inspect facilities and records and to review the license of any "special status" user or manufacturer for cause. A summary of available information as furnished to the profession shall be filed with the FDA to aid in their review of licenses, but copies of data, full reports, etc., available for on-site inspection or spot checks, will not be duplicated for filing at the FDA. The FDA will *not* have the responsibility of making scientific evaluations of the safety and efficacy of each compound or of determining whether a compound may or may not be made available under this category. Licensed producers will be expected to take responsibility for the proper manufacture and proposed use of individual products, and they will take the initiative in limiting distribution to appropriate certified specialists or major clinics.

In considering the above suggestion, the legal mind will, no doubt, raise the question of abuse by the few unscrupulous or irrational individuals to be found in any large professional group. I believe that the licensing power will take care of this problem. It is the intent of this approach that the agency not involve itself with value judgments, which can be better done by on-the-spot licensed experts who are directly involved with the product. The agency will be in a position to investigate and to suspend or refuse license to the incompetent or dishonest, but not to make individual product-by-product scientific judgments.

No manufacturer is likely to get rich on an unadvertised, "special status" drug. The current status of unproven drugs as prime subjects of protracted, adversary-type debate between sponsors and the FDA will largely be replaced by more dispassionate examinations, by and on the initiative of those in the scientific community who have particular interest and knowledge concerning each agent. Clinical scientists who now shy away from the formalities and handicaps imposed by the current IND system will regain the opportunity to contribute to clinical drug evaluation and to take advantage of unique opportunities for study as they arise. Drugs that deserve to become generally used "approved" drugs will reach that status sooner and more smoothly to the benefit of all concerned. Some drugs will remain available for the relatively few patients who need them, and others will fall into disuse and disappear. A small army of scientists and other government employees will be able to turn their attention to more fruitful activities and will be in a better position to encourage rather than interfere with research. A new respect for the ethics and motives of both investigators and regulators will be generated, and this will foster an increasing sense of responsibility to live up to that respect. Most important, more people will be better treated by physicians with full therapeutic options, and a renewed sense of judgmental responsibility and opportunity in the interest of the patient will tend to replace defensive medicine.

There is indeed a great deal at stake in reestablishing the availability of unproven drugs. The pendulum has swung altogether too far in the direction of centralized dominance over individual judgment, and it is high time it started swinging the other way.

In the final analysis, it is not regulatory requirements but the state of science and the enlightened self-interest of research-oriented, ethical (in the literal sense) pharmaceutical manufacturers that make for the safe development and availability of new drugs. Moral responsibility, for which there is no substitute in medical science, is certainly not the exclusive domain of government bureaucrats, and it cannot be legislated. We sorely need to reestablish the principle that the physician is in the best position to determine what is proper therapy for each patient, and the availability of "unproven" drugs needs to be restored to him and his patient. The government's mission should once again be surveillance against the criminal, the immoral, and the incompetent, without the suppression of scientific diversity, which is the key to progress and the public welfare.

References

Eisenberg, L.: The social imperatives of medical research. Science 198:1105, 1977.
Friedman, M.: Frustrating drug advancement. Newsweek, Jan. 8, 1973.
Friedman, M.: Barking cats. Newsweek, Feb. 19, 1973.
Joint Hearings, Subcommittee on Health on S.3441 and S.966, Aug. 16, 1974, p. 2933.
Review of medical ethics. Am. Med. J. 23:149, 1852.
Smith, R.D.: The Laetrile papers. Science 18:10–13, 1978.
V.A. Cooperative Study Group on Antihypertensive Agents: Effects of treatment on morbidity in hypertension. JAMA 213:1143–1152, 1970.

The Legal Requirement that Drugs Be Proved Safe and Effective Before Their Use

Peter Barton Hutt, Esq.
Covington & Burling, Washington, D.C.

The complexity of the controversy surrounding the federal statutory requirement that drugs be proved safe and effective before they may be marketed lawfully is illustrated by the fact that the very physicians and scientists who supported this requirement most strongly in testimony before Congress in 1962 are now among those who criticize the Food and Drug Administration (FDA) implementation of the requirement most vehemently today. Current provisions of the law and their implementation by the FDA are attacked from one side as being too weak and ineffective to protect the public against dangerous drugs and incompetent prescribing by physicians, and from the other side as being too broad and stringent to permit the rapid marketing of lifesaving drugs that would greatly benefit the public. There is general agreement, on all sides, that the drug provisions of the Federal Food, Drug, and Cosmetic Act should be revised and modernized. But there is massive disagreement about the form that any new law should take, and thus the prospects for rapid enactment of a new statute are uncertain (Ballin, 1979).

It is essential, at the outset, to understand at least the broad outline of the current law and the regulations under which the FDA controls the marketing and the use of drugs in this country. Once the current law and regulations are understood, it is possible to isolate major policy issues that must be resolved in fashioning future regulatory control of the marketing and use of drugs under the current law or in enacting new statutory provisions.

Current Law and Regulations

The Federal Food, Drug, and Cosmetic Act, as enacted in 1938 (P.L. 75-717, 52 Stat. 1040, 21 U.S.C. 321 et seq.), defined a "new drug" as *any drug (whether available over-the-counter or only on prescription) not "generally recognized as safe" (GRAS) by qualified experts for its intended uses.* The law considered that a new drug would first be subject to limited clinical testing by appropriately qualified scientists as an "investigational drug." When safety was proved through this clinical investigation, the manufacturer would submit a new drug application (NDA) containing all the safety data. Within 60 days (postponable by the FDA to a maximum of 180 days) after submission of the NDA, the FDA was required either to permit the NDA to become effective or to deny the NDA on the ground that it failed to show adequately the safety of the drug. If the FDA did nothing within the prescribed time period, the NDA automatically became effective. The sole authority of the Food and Drug Administration in reviewing an NDA related to safety, not effectiveness.

The new drug provisions of the law remained unchanged from 1938 to 1962. During this time, NDAs became effective for a few hundred nonprescription drugs and about seven thousand prescription drugs.

In 1962, as a result of the public attention focused on new drugs because of the thalidomide tragedy, Congress amended the new drug provisions of the law in several important respects (P.L. 87–781, 76 Stat. 780). The investigational new drug provisions of the law were tightened to require the submission to the FDA of reports justifying proposed clinical testing of an investigational drug (now called an *investigational new drug application* or *IND*) and informed consent of all subjects involved in this testing. The law was also changed to add (1) a requirement that the FDA affirmatively approve a new drug application (rather than just allow it to become effective by inaction), (2) a requirement that a new drug be proved effective as well as safe, (3) a requirement that effectiveness be shown by adequate and well controlled clinical studies, and (4) a number of other new provisions governing the manufacturing, labeling, and advertising of drug products. The effect of the 1962 Drug Amendments on the availability of drugs in the United States has been the subject of major controversy for the past 10 years.

Major Current Issues

For most consumer products, there are only two approaches by which government regulation can be accomplished: labeling and banning. Under the labeling approach, the product may be marketed as long as its relevant characteristics are accurately and truthfully conveyed by informative labeling. It is then left to the individual consumer to decide whether, in light of that information, he wishes to use it. The sole function of the government under this approach is to assure that all the information relevant to an informed decision is provided to the consumer and that the information is in fact accurate.

Under the banning approach, the government makes the decision for the consumer by determining that the product inherently is too deceptive or too unsafe to be marketed at all, even with fully informative labeling. The consumer therefore has no opportunity to make his own decision in the matter, except indirectly by participation in the administrative and legislative processes by which the government decision is made.

Drug products, however, are unique, because society has established a third category of regulation.* A drug product can be placed in *prescription* status, which means that it is made available to consumers only if or when prescribed by a physician. This form of limited distribution, which applies uniquely to drugs and medical devices, uses the physician as an independent control mechanism on the hypothesis that consumers, by themselves, do not have sufficient technical information to insure the safe and effective use of the product.

There is, of course, a wide variety of specific enforcement mechanisms by which these basic regulatory approaches are implemented. As might be expected, it is these specific mechanisms, embodied in the Federal Food, Drug, and Cosmetic Act, that are at the heart of the controversy about current drug regulatory policy.

Most of the current FDA drug regulatory policy is the result of administrative decisions rather than specific statutory mandates. The Federal Food, Drug, and Cosmetic Act, like virtually all regulatory statutes, for the most part expresses its mandate in relatively general terms. It is then left to the FDA to implement the statutory objectives. In pursuing this, the FDA has wide latitude, as long as it does not contravene any specific provision of the law and can justify the specific requirements it imposes as a reasonable exercise of its administrative discretion under the statute.

Several major issues that have provoked controversy over the past few years are discussed here. This is not an exhaustive list, but the issues raise the problems on which public attention has focused most frequently. For each, there is no "right" or "wrong" answer. Resolution involves as much one's own personal philosophy about the roles of the government and the individual in a free society as it does an understanding of the medical or legal issues involved. It is therefore not surprising that feelings on all sides of these issues run very strong, and they are guided as much by emotion as by reason.

Proof of Effectiveness

As already noted, the requirement that a new drug be proved effective before it can be approved for marketing by the FDA was first included in the law as part of the Drug Amendments of 1962. Moreover, in enacting this provision, Congress did not leave it to the FDA

*Under the Federal Insecticide, Fungicide, and Rodenticide Act, as amended by the Federal Environmental Pesticide Control Act of 1972, (P.L. 92–516, 86 Stat. 973), a pesticide may similarly be registered for "restricted use" only by or under the direct supervision of a certified applicator, 7 U.S.C. 136a(d).

to determine what would constitute adequate proof of "effectiveness"— Congress specifically defined it in 21 U.S.C. 355 (d) to mean:

> . . . evidence consisting of adequate and well-controlled investigations, including clinical investigations, by experts qualified by scientific training and experience to evaluate the effectiveness of the drug involved, on the basis of which it could fairly and responsibly be concluded by such experts that the drug will have the effect it purports or is represented to have under the conditions of use prescribed, recommended, or suggested in the labeling or proposed labeling thereof.

This definition was included in the law at the request of prominent pharmacologists, who felt that the opinion of experts or the uncontrolled experience of practicing physicians is inadequate to demonstrate the effectiveness of a drug, and that double blind clinical studies are the only reliable basis for determining drug effectiveness.

The statute contains no exception whatever to the requirement for controlled clinical studies. If the law were interpreted and applied literally, such studies would be required even when they would be unethical or impossible. Recognizing that Congress could not have intended this, the FDA issued regulations providing for exemptions from the requirement of controlled studies when good reasons can be proved [21 C.F.R. §314.111(a)(5)(ii)(*a*)].

Faced with the regulatory need to particularize the broad statutory requirement that all new drugs be proved effective by controlled clinical studies, the FDA promulgated regulations defining the required elements of such studies. Those regulations, which have not been changed since they were set forth in 1970, are set forth in 21 C.F.R. §314.111(a)(5)(ii) as follows:

> (i) The following principles have been developed over a period of years and are recognized by the scientific community as the essentials of adequate and well-controlled clinical investigations. They provide the basis for the determination whether there is 'substantial evidence' to support the claims of effectiveness for 'new drugs' and antibiotic drugs.
>
> (a) The plan or protocol for the study and the report of the results of the effectiveness study must include the following:
>
> (1) A clear statement of the objectives of the study.
>
> (2) A method of selection of the subjects that (i) Provides adequate assurance that they are suitable for the purposes of the study, diagnostic criteria of the condition to be treated or diagnosed, confirmatory laboratory tests where appropriate, and, in the case of prophylactic agents, evidence of susceptibility and exposure to the condition against which prophylaxis is desired;
>
> (ii) Assigns the subjects to test groups in such a way as to minimize bias;
>
> (iii) Assures comparability in test and control groups of pertinent variables, such as age, sex, severity, or duration of disease, and use of drugs other than the test drug.
>
> (3) Explains the methods of observation and recording of results, including the variables measured, quantitation, assessment of any subject's response, and steps taken to minimize bias on the part of the subject and observer.
>
> (4) Provides a comparison of the results of treatment or diagnosis with a control in such a fashion as to permit quantitative evaluation. The precise nature of the control must be stated and an explanation given of the methods used to minimize bias on the part of the observers and the analysts of the data. Level and methods of 'blinding,' if used, are to be documented. Generally, four types of comparison are recognized:
>
> (i) No treatment: Where objective measurements of effectiveness are available and placebo effect is negligible, comparison of the objective results in comparable groups of treated and untreated patients.
>
> (ii) Placebo control: Comparison of the results of use of the new drug entity with an inactive preparation designed to resemble the test drug as far as possible.
>
> (iii) Active treatment control: An effective regimen of therapy may be used for comparison, e.g., where the condition treated is such that no treatment or administration of a placebo would be contrary to the interest of the patient.
>
> (iv) Historical control: In certain circumstances, such as those involving diseases with high and predictable mortality (acute leukemia of childhood), with signs and symptoms of predictable duration or severity (fever in certain infections), or in case of prophylaxis, where morbidity is predictable, the results of use of a new drug entity may be compared quantitatively with prior experience historically derived from the adequately documented natural history of the disease or condition in comparable patients or populations with no treatment or with a regimen (therapeutic, diagnostic, prophylactic) the effectiveness of which is established.
>
> (5) A summary of the methods of analysis and an evaluation of data derived from the study, including any appropriate statistical methods.

PROVIDED, HOWEVER, That any of the above criteria may be waived in whole or in part, either prior to the investigation or in the evaluation of a completed study, by the Director of the Bureau of Drugs with respect to a specific clinical investigation; a petition for such a waiver may be filed by any person who would be adversely affected by the application of the criteria to a particular clinical investigation; the petition should show that some or all of the criteria are not reasonably applicable to the investigation and that alternative procedures can be, or have been, followed, the results of which will or have yielded data that can and should be accepted as substantial evidence of the drug's effectiveness. A petition for a waiver shall set forth clearly and concisely the specific provision or provisions in the criteria from which waiver is sought, why the criteria are not reasonably applicable to the particular clinical investigation, what alternative procedures, if any, are to be, or have been, employed, what results have been obtained, and the basis on which it can be, or has been, concluded that clinical investigation will or has yielded substantial evidence of effectiveness, notwithstanding non-conformance with the criteria for which waiver is requested.

(b) For such an investigation to be considered adequate for approval of a new drug, it is required that the test drug be standardized as to identity, strength, quality, purity, and dosage form to give significance to the results of the investigation.

(c) Uncontrolled studies or partially controlled studies are not acceptable as the sole basis for the approval of claims of effectiveness. Such studies, carefully conducted and documented, may provide corroborative support of well-controlled studies regarding efficacy and may yield valuable data regarding safety of the test drug. Such studies will be considered on their merits in the light of the principles listed here, with the exception of the requirement for the comparison of the treated subjects with controls. Isolated case reports, random experience, and reports lacking the details which permit scientific evaluation will not be considered.

These criteria were based on the views of leading clinical pharmacologists as expressed in the medical literature at that time. In 1973, the United States Supreme Court upheld those regulations and their implementation by the FDA in four decisions that broadly supported the FDA's enforcement of the Drug Amendments of 1962 (Weinberger v. Hynson, Wescott and Dunning, Inc., 412 U.S. 609 (1973); Ciba Corp. v. Weinberger, 412 U.S. 640 (1973); Weinberger v. Bentex Pharmaceuticals, Inc., 412 U.S. 645 (1973); USV Pharmaceutical Corp. v. Weinberger, 412 U.S. 655 (1973)).

Most of the early controversy about the effectiveness requirement of the law focused on specific studies conducted with respect to particular drugs. It is not the function of this paper to debate the merits of any particular decision with respect to the studies conducted on any specific drug.

More recently, however, the controversy has taken on broader ramifications. First, it has been contended that because of the effectiveness requirements of the 1962 Amendments, there is both a reduction in new drug development and a delay in marketing new drugs in the United States, as contrasted with those in many European countries, with a resulting harm to the health of American citizens (Peltzman, 1974). This is the so-called "drug lag" issue. Second, the advocates of such unproven drugs as Laetrile have built upon the drug lag issue to contend that citizens are inappropriately being denied their constitutional right to use whatever remedy they wish (see 42 Fed. Reg. 39768, August 5, 1977). This is the "freedom of choice" issue.

Drug Lag

With respect to the drug lag issue, it should be apparent to anyone that the requirement of proof of effectiveness prior to marketing a new drug will, in fact, delay the marketing of that drug. If no regulatory controls existed of any kind, there would be no marketing lag of any kind. Thus, the issue is not whether there is indeed a drug lag, but rather whether that lag results in a decrease in public health protection for the United States or in other detriments to the public that should lead to a change in policy.

There does not appear, at this time, to be agreement on the question whether the drug lag caused by the Drug Amendments of 1962 has resulted in an increase or decrease in public health in this country. Since the issue ultimately is subjective (because the importance of new drugs that are marketed at a later time here cannot be measured in objective terms), it is not feasible to offer a definitive resolution of this issue.

It is not necessary to resolve the issue, however, in order to conclude that some modification of the drug approval process, more specifically the task of reviewing proof of effectiveness, is warranted. The FDA has never contended that the current process cannot be improved. Several study groups, both inside and outside the agency, have recommended specific changes for improving it (Final Report, 1977). Without question, changes that will reduce the drug lag can be made.

Freedom of Choice

The freedom of choice issue, in contrast to the drug lag issue, involves far more basic and philosophic questions. The drug lag issue revolves largely around the question of how the process of proving safety and effectiveness of new drugs, and of governmental approval for marketing, can be expedited. The freedom of choice issue, on the other hand, is based on the hypothesis that the government should have no say in this process whatever. Those who advocate absolute freedom of consumer choice contend that the Federal Food, Drug, and Cosmetic Act should be repealed, the FDA should be abolished, and the fate of drugs should be left solely to the workings of the marketplace in a free enterprise system.

Under this arrangement, any person would be free to market any drug, and any consumer would be free to obtain any drug of his choice. If the drug were unsafe or ineffective, people would no longer use it, and if anyone were harmed as a result, he would have access to the courts for redress under traditional tort law. Although they do not always explicitly state it, advocates of this approach presumably depend heavily upon the provision of information to consumers on the basis of which they can then make a truly informed choice.

This concept does, of course, have enormous attractiveness in a society that is fundamentally based on the free enterprise system and the belief that individual choice should be maximized. In the context of governmental regulation of food, I have argued strongly for reducing the number of situations in which the government bans a product (thus taking away from consumers their right to free choice), and for increasing the number of situations in which products are allowed to remain on the market with fully informative labeling (thus leaving to consumers a full choice on the matter, in light of complete and accurate information) (Hutt, 1977, 1978). It must be recognized, however, that foods and drugs are quite different types of products, and that totally different factors are involved in a consumer's decision to purchase or to use them. A direct analogy between the two is impossible.

Even the potentially most "dangerous" food product has an infinitely greater margin of safety than most drugs of the same category. Food is chosen primarily for recreation and pleasure. Although we must all eat in order to live, a person's decisions with respect to which of an enormous variety of nutritious foods to consume are dictated more by personal preference and enjoyment than by any specific nutritional reason.

Drugs, in contrast, are purchased and used (except in unusual circumstances) for specific medical purposes. The choice of a drug is dictated solely by the consumer's desire to achieve a particular result, not by any broad desire to consume drugs in general.

Moreover, the specific information needed to determine the appropriateness of a prescription drug—both to achieve effectiveness and to minimize risk—is not only not available to consumers generally, but even if made available through informative labeling would largely be beyond the knowledge or comprehension of most consumers. The circumstances under which many prescription drugs are taken—when the consumer is ill and is searching for something that promises to cure or alleviate the disease—further detract from the possibility that he can make a well reasoned choice among competing alternatives.

This is not to say that consumers should have no choice whatever, under any circumstances, in determining their medication. I believe that consumers should indeed (1) be permitted freedom of choice whenever feasible, (2) be brought into the decisional process when free choice is not feasible, and (3) under very limited conditions, be permitted access to unproven remedies. As a rule, however, it is difficult to believe that many consumers could make a fully informed and free choice for most prescription drugs. The doctrine of free choice, which contends that all governmental control of drugs should be abandoned, is inappropriate.

Perhaps the most important impact of the recent debate on Laetrile has been that it has required many physicians and scientists who have been critical of the drug effectiveness requirements to reevaluate their position. Fewer are stridently calling for an end to all governmental regulation of drug effectiveness. There is a growing consensus that proof of effectiveness for new drugs is indeed wise, but that the implementation of this requirement needs further improvement. Some of the specific issues discussed here address proposals that have been made for improving the system.

Rapid Approval for Marketing

Proposals to speed up the approval of new drugs by the Food and Drug Administration have focused on a wide variety of remedies, virtually all of which have been used at one time or another.

Relax Effectiveness Requirements

As already noted, many physicians and scientists who have supported a legal requirement that a new drug be proved effective prior to marketing have nonetheless criticized the FDA for implementing this requirement too rigidly and thus imposing unnecessary barriers to the early marketing of new drugs in this country. Several changes have been proposed, ranging from amendment of the new drug provisions to changing the "attitude" of those who approve new drugs in the FDA.

It is doubtful that statutory changes will have any significant impact on this mattter. Although it would be wise to amend the Federal Food, Drug, and Cosmetic Act explicitly to state that the FDA need not require adequate and well controlled clinical studies where they are not necessary, it must be recognized that this will merely codify existing agency practice. It is evident that the degree to which the FDA enforces the present requirement for proof of effectiveness for a particular new drug depends upon a wide variety of factors, including the medical importance of the drug, prevailing medical opinion, and other nonstatutory considerations. Although these other considerations cannot be discussed publicly by representatives of the agency (and, indeed, must be explicitly denied by them), any realistic understanding of FDA actions must take them into account.

Thus, it is largely in the area of "attitude" that any relaxation of the requirements for proof of effectiveness must come. And it is clear that the precise wording of the statute has little or nothing to do with the attitude of those who enforce it.

To the extent that a rigid attitude about proof of effectiveness currently exists in the FDA, it is in large part the product of the atmosphere in which the agency has been working for the past few years (Hutt, 1977). The FDA has repeatedly been attacked by leading members of Congress, consumer advocates, and the media for the perceived failure to protect the public adequately from unsafe and ineffective drugs. Under these conditions, it is not surprising that some agency employees have developed a "siege mentality," preferring to deny approval or simply to make no decision in order to avoid potential public controversy and criticism that has often resulted from approval of a new drug for which the benefit-risk ratio may be small. It is only through a change in this atmosphere, rather than a change in the statute, that this "siege mentality" will gradually subside. As long as FDA employees are threatened with public disgrace for approval of new drugs, and promised public accolade for disapproval or inaction, any substantial change in the current rate of approval of new drugs will be unlikely, regardless of changes in the governing act.

Make Withdrawal of Drugs from the Market Easier

The FDA has argued that one reason for the current reluctance of the agency to approve any new drug is that, once approved, requirements for withdrawing the drug from the market are extremely cumbersome, difficult, and lengthy. Accordingly, the FDA contends that as long as it is difficult to remove an unsafe or ineffective drug from the market once it is approved, it must make absolutely certain that the drug is in fact safe and effective before initial approval is given. The agency has suggested that if drug withdrawal provisions were made easier and more flexible, it would have no serious objection to making the drug approval process correspondingly easier and more flexible.

The current provisions of the Federal Food, Drug, and Cosmetic Act require that the Secretary of Health, Education and Welfare (HEW) find that a new drug represents an "imminent hazard" (a determination that is nondelegable) before the FDA may order its immediate removal from the market without first going through all the administrative proceedings. In 1977, this provision was invoked for the first time in order to remove phenformin from the market (Forsham v. Califano, 442 F. Supp. 203 D.D.C. 1977). If in fact this signals an increased willingness by the FDA to pursue immediate removal from the market of drugs concluded to be unsafe or ineffective, the agency may be more willing in the future to permit more rapid approval of new drugs even without changes in the Federal Food, Drug, and Cosmetic Act.

Grant Conditional Approval of New Drugs (Phase IV)

The FDA has for several years approved some new drugs for which there was persuasive evidence of safety and effectiveness, but for which additional confirmatory animal or clinical data were thought to be desirable (see 21 C.F.R. §310.303). Probably the best known was levodopa, which was approved on the condition that long-term animal and clinical studies be completed in order to assure the drug's long-term safety and effectiveness. Other drugs have received similar conditional approvals.

The FDA has made the related point that more rapid approval of new drugs is difficult in this country because of the lack of an adequate postmarketing surveillance system. In response, the pharmaceutical industry has established a Joint Commission on Prescription Drug Use, composed of representatives of government, industry, and the public, with the approval of Senator Edward Kennedy, to determine the feasibility of adequate postmarketing drug surveillance. The work of this commission is still in progress, and it is premature to predict the outcome.

Use Expert Advisory Committees

In the late 1960s, the FDA began to establish advisory committees consisting of independent experts with specialized knowledge and background in particular fields of medical practice relevant to prescription drug categories—e.g., dental, cardiovascular and renal, gastrointestinal, and ophthalmic drugs. These advisory committees have been used by the agency to provide advice with respect to the approval of new drug applications and to other issues relating to drugs within those categories (see 21 C.F.R. §14.160 et seq.).

This is the most effective procedure that has been tried for avoiding unnecessary caution and delay in the approval of new prescription drugs. Advisory committees cannot and should not be permitted to substitute for thorough review of a new drug application by FDA personnel. But it must also be recognized that the agency can never hire as full-time employees the best experts in the country in all these medical categories. Accordingly, it is essential that their expertise be available through an advisory committee if the agency is to make the best medical and scientific judgments on pending applications in the shortest time possible.

At present, these advisory committees are established by administrative order, and they are not required by statute. When Congress enacted the Medical Device Amendments of 1976 (P.L. 94–295, 90 Stat. 539), it included a virtually identical mechanism for new medical devices (21 U.S.C. 360e(c)(2)). An amendment that would formally incorporate the outside advisory committee process into the new drug approval process would be an important step forward, and would preclude the possibility that the FDA would use advisory committees only when it wished to do so and not in all instances in which their advice would be useful.

Governmental Control Over Drug Distribution and Prescribing

There are two ways in which the FDA can control the use of drugs. First, it can require that a drug be available on prescription only. Second, it can require informative labeling and advertising for a prescription drug. At present, the FDA does not have legal authority to control the distribution and prescribing of prescription drugs (see *APLA v. Matthews,* 530 F.2d 1054(D.C. Cir. 1976), affirming 377 F.Supp. 824(D.D.C. 1974), and 37 Fed. Reg. 16503, August 15, 1972), but numerous legislative proposals have been made to change the law to permit additional controls of this nature.

Nonprescription or Prescription Status

Under the Federal Food, Drug, and Cosmetic Act, all drugs must be marketed on a nonprescription basis unless they meet the legal criteria for a prescription drug or are limited to prescription status in an approved NDA. The law defines a prescription drug as *any drug which, because of its toxicity or other potential for harmful effect, or the method of its use, or the collateral measures necessary to its use, is not safe for use except under the supervision of a physician.*

In practice, the decision of the FDA with respect to the prescription status of a drug has, with very rare exception, met with virtually universal agreement (see Parke, Davis and Co. v. Califano, 564 F.2d 1200 (6th Cir. 1977); United States v. An Article of Drug . . . Decholin, 264 F. Supp. 473, E.D. Mich. 1967). Accordingly, the agency is able to control, through this long-accepted and recognized procedure, those drugs that will be available directly to consumers through their own purchasing choices, and those that will be available only through the independent judgment of a physician. There has been very little controversy about this system and no suggestions that it be changed.

Prescription Drug Labeling and Advertising

Under the Federal Food, Drug, and Cosmetic Act, the FDA has broad authority to prevent false or misleading labeling or advertising of a prescription drug. Through the new drug control mechanism, it has the legal authority to require the preparation of a package insert, which states in detail the indications, warnings, contraindications, and other prescribing information for the drug.

No one complains about the basic concept of this form of governmental regulation. The use of this authority by the FDA has, however, been subject to substantial criticism. Some contend that the current package inserts are far too detailed, lengthy, and comprehensive to be of any assistance to busy physicians. They also argue that much of the information is trivial and is included solely to avoid responsibility by the pharmaceutical industry or the FDA for failure to warn about even the most remote possibility of a reaction. Others contend that the package inserts should give even stronger and more pointed warnings to physicians and should be more detailed and comprehensive. These people argue that neither the FDA nor the pharmaceutical industry is adequately warning the physician about the dangers of prescription drug use.

These controversies can, of course, be resolved only on an individual drug basis. Suffice it to say that issues of drug safety will undoubtedly remain judgmental for many years to come, and that these specific controversies will continue to rage, without resolution, into the indefinite future.

Other Proposed Control Mechanisms

Those who contend that giving a drug prescription status and requiring the provision of adequate prescribing information to the physician is insufficient to insure adequate protection of the public have, in the past 15 years, advocated a wide variety of changes in the law and in government policy in order to reduce wrongful prescribing. It is not feasible to list all the suggestions they have made. The following are those that have been most prominently suggested.

IMPROVEMENTS IN THE PACKAGE INSERT. These improvements would include greater emphasis on warnings and contraindications, use of standardized warnings for common problems such as the lack of detailed data about safety for use in infants or pregnant women, and a requirement that the labeling specify the relative frequency of adverse reactions (see 21 C.F.R. 201.56; 40 Fed. Reg. 15392, April 7, 1975).

PATIENT PACKAGE INSERTS (PPIs). It has been proposed that some or all prescription drugs be accompanied by a special patient package insert that is given directly to the patient (see 21 C.F.R. §§310.502 and 310.515; PMA v. FDA, CCH Food Drug Cosmetic Law Reports paragraph 38,130, D. Del. 1977). The PPI explains both how to take the drug and all the important warnings, contraindications, and adverse reactions. Many physicians have opposed this concept on the ground that it will interfere with the traditional physician-patient relationship. Others have contended that it is the only method of bringing the patient into the decisional process and have pointed out that every individual has the fundamental right to understand any risk to which he subjects himself. Perhaps the most difficult issue to resolve with respect to this matter is the degree to which warnings, contraindications, and adverse reactions will be included in any patient labeling. To the extent that some of this information is included, it could scare the patient away from needed medication, but to the extent that some of it is excluded, it could mislead the consumer into believing that the product is safer than it is.

INFORMED PATIENT CONSENT. It has been suggested that for some or all prescription drugs, the patient should be given all the information relating to possible hazards—either orally or in writing—and should then be required to give informed consent—either orally or in writing—before it is prescribed (see 21 C.F.R. §310.501a, stayed in 39 Fed. Reg. 38226, October 30, 1974). There are serious practical obstacles to implementation of any such approach.

PUNISHING PHYSICIANS FOR IMPROPER PRESCRIBING. At least one bill introduced in Congress would have imposed criminal penalties (including a jail sentence) on any physician who prescribed a drug under any condition for which it was not approved by the FDA as shown in the approved package insert (S. 2697, 1975). At present, the FDA has taken the position that it is not a violation of federal law for a physician to prescribe an approved new drug for an unproven use, and it is unlikely that Congress will change the law in this respect (see 37 Fed. Reg. 16503, August 15, 1972).

Limited licensing of doctors to prescribe drugs. Particularly in view of the increasing toxic potential of highly specialized drugs like the new anticancer agents, it has been suggested that only those physicians specifically licensed to prescribe certain types of drugs, or only those doctors with specific qualifications (e.g., specialty board certification), would be permitted to prescribe them (see 21 C.F.R. §310.505 (methadone)).

Limiting the distribution channels of drugs. As an alternative, or in addition to limited licensing of physicians to prescribe drugs, it has been suggested that the distribution channels of some drugs also be limited in order to preclude widespread prescribing. For example, the distribution of some drugs might be limited solely to hospitals, meaning such drugs would not be generally available in all pharmacies. Supposedly, this would encourage prescription of these drugs only by physicians with specialized knowledge in their use, rather than by the general family practitioner.

Special educational programs about drug prescribing for physicians. It has been argued that many doctors receive relatively little information about drugs once they leave medical school, and in any event, that most of the educational material they do receive about drugs after medical school comes from the pharmaceutical industry. Accordingly, some have suggested that special educational programs on drug prescribing be required for all physicians in order for them to retain their authority to prescribe drugs.

Increasing malpractice liability. The common law concept that a physician is subject to monetary liability for damages caused by misprescribing of drugs has been cited many times as the principal mechanism controlling that problem today. Although some have argued that the malpractice liability of physicians is already too high and should be decreased, others have contended that the malpractice liability for wrongful prescription of a drug should be increased in order to force physicians into learning more about proper drug prescribing and taking more care in their decisions about prescription drugs.

More strict enforcement of licensure laws. In theory, a physician who consistently misprescribes a drug is subject to disciplinary action, including loss of his license to practice medicine. In practice, such disciplinary action occurs only rarely. Another means of greater public control over drug prescribing would be greater self-scrutiny of drug prescribing by the medical profession, accompanied by more strict enforcement of the licensure laws to prevent persistent misprescribing.

Elimination of refillable prescriptions. For most drugs (amphetamines would be one exception) that have been classified in Category II, III, or IV under the Controlled Substances Act (Title II of P.L. 91–513, 84 Stat. 1236), a physician may lawfully authorize any prescription to be refilled continuously without limitation. Some have felt that eliminating the use of refillable prescriptions, for some or even all drugs, would require physicians to make better decisions about the use of the prescription drugs (Cf. 21 U.S.C. 829).

The length and breadth of these suggested changes in the handling of drug prescribing are staggering. They illustrate the seriousness with which the issue of drug prescribing is viewed by many people. Although it is unlikely that any of the more drastic suggestions will be adopted, it is clear that this will remain an important area of concern and will be the subject of continuing proposals into the foreseeable future.

Orphan Drugs

One of the more perplexing problems in the past has been how to handle drugs for which there is only a very small market and for which there is thus no economic incentive to conduct the testing necessary to show safety and effectiveness or to handle the expensive administrative process for submitting and obtaining approval of a new drug application. For years, these so-called "orphan drugs" have survived in the twilight zone in which they have been made available to the medical profession by pharmaceutical firms. This is a permanent investigational new drug plan, without any pretense of performing an actual clinical investigation or of having an intent eventually to pursue approval of a new drug application.

The current status of these drugs quite properly leaves the FDA, the pharmaceutical industry, the medical profession, and the public very uneasy. It is apparent that sooner or later a better mechanism must be found to assure that these drugs meet proper standards of safety and effectiveness, and that the investigational new drug mechanism not be misused in order to hide the inadequacies of the current drug approval system.

One proposal has been for the federal government, and in particular the National Institutes of Health (NIH), to sponsor appropriate safety and effectiveness studies for any drug that is of medical significance but for which there is an inadequate market to justify development by the pharmaceutical industry. The NIH has, of course, undertaken such studies for a number of anticancer and other new drugs. NIH officials are quick to point out, however, that their entire budget could be consumed by expensive studies of this type. They quite properly argue that if Congress intends that they undertake this additional function, additional funds must be added to their budget.

Drugs Used in Terminal or Incurable Illness

Finally, there is no subject more filled with emotion today than the issue of whether a terminal or incurable patient has a constitutional right to choose any remedy he desires, regardless of whether there is a scientific basis for suggesting that it is any more effective than a placebo. A closely related issue involves the use of nontherapeutic drugs solely for palliative purposes in such circumstances.

Until now, Congress and the FDA have declined to make any distinction between drugs used in terminal or incurable illness and those used at any other time. Faced with emotional pleas from terminal cancer patients who properly point out that there is no known effective cure for their disease, however, some courts have recently prohibited the FDA from interfering with the right of these individuals to use the controversial drug Laetrile (see Rutherford v. U.S., 399 F.Supp. 1208 (W.D. Okla. 1976), aff'd, 542 F.2d 1137 (10th Cir. 1976), on remand, 424 F.Supp. 105 (W.D. Okla. 1977), 429 F.Supp. 506 (W.D. Okla. 1977), aff'd, 582 F.2d 1234 (10th Cir. 1978), reversed and remanded for further consideration of the constitutional issues (U.S. Sup. Ct., 1979)). The courts have concluded that even if there is no evidence whatever that Laetrile is effective, and since there is no other effective remedy, a terminal patient should be allowed to exercise his right of free choice in this matter. It is certainly not difficult to understand why a court is willing, under these circumstances, to grant to a dying man what is, in effect, his last wish, particularly because it cannot possibly hurt anyone else.

It is clear that Congress and the FDA must now face up to the very difficult issues posed by this problem. Although it is reprehensible to allow anyone to market an untested drug, it is equally reprehensible for the government to deny a terminal or incurable patient a drug that may at least put his mind at ease. By fighting against some form of compromise solution to this problem, the FDA may unwittingly be providing the strongest arguments for those who contend that all requirements for proof of effectiveness should be eliminated from the current law.

Admittedly, the use of Laetrile or the so-called "heroin cocktail" must be rigidly circumscribed to prevent abuse. This will inevitably raise close questions of judgment with respect to the circumstances under which use will be permitted. Those judgments are no more difficult, however, than those made every day by physicians and relatives about other forms of therapy, including the ultimate judgment to withdraw life support systems. A reasonable statutory and administrative framework must therefore be developed before the courts thrust their own system upon the FDA.

Conclusion

One is always left, after any review of current controversies in the regulation of prescription drugs, with the feeling that the issues are basically insoluble. In many respects, the questions facing the Food and Drug Administration today are the same as those that have faced it for the past 20 years. It is unlikely that the next 20 years will see any definitive resolution of these issues. Improvement will come at the margin, in slow and painstaking steps. Those who seek easy or quick solutions or believe that new legislation will make a major difference simply fail to appreciate the complexity of the issues.

I have long believed that if the FDA did not exist, it would have to be invented. Society cannot tolerate the wholly unregulated marketing of drugs. We are left, then, with doing our best to improve a system that we all know is imperfect and that, in the nature of things, can never become perfect. An opportunity now exists, in new legislation, to confront these issues and to make some improvements in the process. Only with good will and understanding on all sides is even this modest goal likely to be achieved.

References

Ballin, J.C.: Legislation, regulation, drug lag, and new drugs. JAMA 241:1405, 1979.

Final Report of the Review Panel on New Drug Regulation, HEW, 1977.

Hutt, P.B.: The basis and purpose of government regulation of adulteration and misbranding of food. 33 Food Drug Cosmetic Law Journal 505 (October 1978).

Hutt, P.B.: Balanced government regulation of consumer products. Food Technol. Jan. 1977.

Hutt, P.B.: Public policy issues in regulating carcinogens in food. 33 Food Drug Cosmetic Law Journal 541 (October 1978).

Peltzman, S.: Regulation of pharmaceutical innovation: the 1962 amendments. American Enterprise Institute, 1974.

In Defense of Laetrile

Ralph W. Moss, Ph.D.
Second Opinion, Bronx, New York

The Problem

Few controversies in therapeutics have been as fierce or prolonged as that over the proposed anticancer agent, Laetrile.

According to the Food and Drug Administration (FDA), "Laetrile has been sold for treating cancer for around 25 years, yet there is still no sound, scientific evidence that it is either effective or safe. It is therefore classified as a 'new drug'" (FDA Consumer Memo, 1975). In simpler terms, Laetrile is "goddamned quackery."

According to its proponents, Laetrile is neither "new" nor really a "drug." And far from being quackery, when used correctly as part of an overall nutritional program, it is one of the most promising and effective treatments for cancer.

The widespread fear of cancer and the growing bitterness over "orthodox" medicine's failure to find a cure, despite billions of dollars spent, has fueled the Laetrile controversy. According to Dr. Charles Moertel of the Mayo Clinic, Laetrile is "a dominant unresolved problem for American medicine today" (Moertel, 1978).

To understand why this is so, it is necessary to look more closely at the substance itself and the long history of its use.

Laetrile and Folk Medicine

Although the term *Laetrile* is of relatively recent coinage, the chemical most often sold as Laetrile has been used as a folk remedy for cancer and related diseases for many centuries. *Laetrile* is a trade name for amygdalin, a glycoside that occurs frequently in living organisms, especially in plants and their derivatives. All glycosides have one thing in common: in reactions with water, they can be split into a sugar (or sugars) and a noncarbohydrate substance(s). Usually, an enzyme must be present to facilitate this cleavage.

There are different kinds of glycosides in nature. The kind we are concerned with releases cyanide (HCN) when broken down. It is therefore called a *cyanogenic* (or *cyanogenetic*) *glycoside.* Included in this category are plant chemicals such as prunasin, found most commonly in wild cherry bark; dhurrin, found in sorghum; lotusin, from the Lotus arabicus plant; and, of course, amygdalin.

Amygdalin, or, as it is popularly called, Laetrile, is found all over the globe, occurring naturally in about 1200 different plants. One could compare it, in its ubiquity, to glucose. Like sugar, Laetrile does not normally occur in a purified, pristine form, but it can be extracted readily from its sources.

We have all ingested amygdalin, or "taken Laetrile," at one time or another, and some of us take it every day without knowing that we are engaging in medical controversy. Chickpeas and lentils, lima beans and Chinese sprouts, cashews and alfalfa, barley, brown rice and millet—all these foods, and many more, contain Laetrile. For commercial purposes, Laetrile is derived from the kernels of apricots, peaches, and bitter almonds, after which amygdalin is named (Greek: amygdale = almond).

Laetrile-rich foods, including fruit kernels, were eaten by our ancestors, including, according to some experts, Peking Man (Brothwell and Brothwell, 1969). Laetrile's use in medicine dates from at least the time of the Great Herbal of China, credited to the legendary Emperor Shen-Nung (2838–2698 B.C.), which lists kernel preparations as useful against tumors. Ancient Egyptian, Greek, Roman, and Arabic physicians were all familiar with the biologic properties of "bitter almond water" *(aqua amygdalarum amarum)*. Celsus, Scribonius Largus, Galen, Pliny the Elder, Marcellus Empiricus, and Avicenna all used preparations containing Laetrile to treat tumors. The same is true of the medieval pharmacoepia (Halstead, 1977; Summa, 1972).

Such ancient use does not, of course, constitute proof that Laetrile is effective. For those familiar with the course of medical history, however, it does remove Laetrile from the realm of simple quackery and make it a prime candidate for serious scientific testing. Other natural products have already demonstrated their usefulness in the treatment of cancer. Antibiotics such as bleomycin, dactinomycin, doxorubicin, mithramycin, and mitomycin C, plant alkaloids such as vincristine and vinblastine, and biologicals such as mixed bacterial vaccine (Coley's toxins), BCG, and C. Parvum have all proved their usefulness, sometimes after initial resistance from medical "orthodoxy."

Folk remedies in particular are a promising field of cancer research. The National Cancer Institute (NCI) is currently conducting tests of maytansine, a drug derived from an East African shrub. This drug was discovered after investigators found that a mixture containing maytansine had been used for many years by Africans in the treatment of cancer.

In addition, the Penobscot Indians used mayapple as a treatment for tumors, and this fact was even published in a medical book in 1849. An extract of mayapple, VM-26, has now been found by NCI investigators to be effective against some cases of brain cancer (Cancer News, 1975).

Because of the antiquity of its use and its natural origin, Laetrile would be a likely candidate for scientific investigation, even if the current controversy had not developed.

Holistic Medicine

"There is no proven case of a person with bona fide cancer who has received no other treatment than Laetrile being cured of his disease," Dr. Howard Goldstein, an anti-Laetrilist, said recently (Journal-News, December 21, 1977).

Even if this statement were true—and there are qualified physicians who would dispute it—it misses the point of this entire debate. Laetrile involves much more than the use of a single drug for the treatment of cancer. Laetrile and the movement that has grown up around it pose a major challenge to the current methods of treating cancer as they are practiced at most medical centers. This challenge has not only medical but philosophic and socioeconomic aspects as well.

Laetrilists are advocating the marketing of not just a single substance but a new kind of treatment for the patient's body and mind. There is an apparently irreconcilable difference between Laetrilists and anti-Laetrilists in how they understand cancer.

Orthodox oncologists, since the time of John Hunter (1728–1793), have tended to see cancer as a localized disease that, as Hunter said, "only produces local effects" (Shimkin, 1977). Such a disease should therefore be curable through localized means; e.g., removing the growth through surgery or other techniques.

Hunter's views led to an enormous increase and improvement in surgical techniques. Nevertheless, experiments in our century and especially in the last two decades have proved that the body has natural immune mechanisms against cancer, analogous to those that function in microbial infections. The logical corollary of this view is that cancer can be controlled by enhancing the body's normal immune functions.

Laetrilists are not alone in adopting this view, but they propose some novel methods of influencing the body's natural curative powers. First of these is with the cyanogenic glycosides, consumed either through the ingestion of Laetrile-rich foods or introduced as medicine in a concentrated form. Since Laetrilists regard this class of substances not as drugs but as "vitamin B-17," they advocate its daily ingestion for the maintenance of a cancer-free state, as well as its use in concentrated form when cancer has already developed.

In addition, they utilize "megadoses" of recognized vitamins such as (emulsified) vitamin A and vitamin C, as well as other vitamins and minerals (e.g., selenium) believed to have anticancer properties.

Enzymes are usually added to this regimen,

following the theory of Krebs (1970) and Beard (1911) that the pancreatic enzymes—trypsin and chymotrypsin—are intrinsic antineoplastic factors. To free these enzymes to kill cancer cells, Laetrilists advise their patients to eat only small amounts of animal protein. They advise their patients to eat large amounts of fresh fruits and vegetables, in part to make up for the loss of animal protein and in part for the other enzymes and nutrients that these foods contain. Enzymes are often given in the form of "Wobe Mugos," which contain enzymes from pancreas, calf thymus, pisum sativum, lens esculenta, and papaya (Wolf and Ransberger, 1977).

The "Laetrile diet" also forbids such items as alcohol, coffee, soft drinks, white bread, ice cream, butter, canned foods, etc., and it encourages the use of "health foods" such as whole grains, herb teas, and honey.

In addition, Laetrilists sometimes employ other relatively nontoxic and "unorthodox" therapies such as Staphage Lysate, hydrazine sulfate, or the Livingston-Jackson cancer vaccine (Gold, 1975; Livingston, 1972).

Finally, Laetrile-using physicians usually attempt to treat the whole person; i.e., body, mind, and spirit—hence the designation *holistic medicine*. Although there is no single method of psychotherapy employed, there has been a great deal of interest in the work of Dr. O. Carl Simonton, who attempts to use biofeedback techniques to concentrate a patient's conscious and subconscious mind on the destruction of his tumor and the restitution of his health.

All this adds up to a new and radically different approach to cancer, one that many patients report to be a positive experience. This is in sharp contrast to the methods currently employed in "orthodox" medicine that, whatever their medical value, are extremely trying for the patient's mind, body, and bank account.

Opponents of the Laetrile movement sometimes make the mistake of regarding the idea of holistic medicine as a clever ruse being used to fool a gullible public that simply doesn't want to take some very bitter medicine. Such an attitude is contradicted by the observations of two sociologists, neither of whom is connected to this movement, who view holistic medicine as a radical challenge to orthodoxy:

> In these revolutionary periods, nothing less than the very definition of the discipline is at stake. After a new paradigm emerges, all previous research in an area may be defined as irrelevant, if not false.
>
> Laetrile research is clearly an attempt at paradigm creation or revolutionary science (Markle and Petersen, 1977).

The fact that Laetrile therapy threatens to change the methods of treating a major disease with its new philosophic concepts and practices accounts in part for the vehemence with which it has been opposed by the medical "establishment."

Is Laetrile a Vitamin?

Laetrilists contend that purified amygdalin is not a drug, new or old, but a food factor—specifically that it is "vitamin B-17" (Krebs, 1970 and 1977; Burk, 1975). This concept has been attacked by Greenberg in an article entitled "The Vitamin Fraud in Cancer Quackery" (1975), in which he proposes several properties that distinguish a bona fide vitamin:

1. It is a nutritional component of organic composition required in small amounts for the complete health and well-being of the organism.
2. Vitamins are not utilized primarily to supply energy or as a source of structural tissue components of the body.
3. A vitamin functions to promote a physiologic process or processes vital to the continued existence of the organism.
4. A vitamin cannot be synthesized by the cells or the organism and must be supplied *de novo*.
5. In man and in other mammals, deficiency of a specific vitamin is the cause of certain rather well defined diseases.

Vitamin B-17 certainly conforms to requirements two and four. Whether it conforms to the others hinges on a single, central issue: does it help to prevent cancer? If it does, it would certainly seem to be a vitamin, even by Greenberg's criteria.

Greenberg states that "no evidence has been adduced that laetriles are essential nutritional components"; "laetriles have never been shown to promote any physiological process;" and "no specific disease has been associated with a lack of laetrile in any animal." Yet no studies of the effect of Laetrile on cancer are cited by this author, although such studies do exist.

There are three main arguments in favor of Laetrile's vitamin status. None of these is ironclad, but each suggests that this theory deserves a serious reception.

First, as Krebs points out, cancer is a chronic, metabolic disease, and such diseases have almost always been solved by factors normal to human metabolism (Krebs, 1970). For a long time, rickets was treated by surgically breaking and resetting bones, and pellagra was widely believed to be caused by an unknown infectious agent. Both these diseases were proved—against great opposition from conservative "experts"—to be caused by the lack of a naturally occurring food factor. Why should we rule out the possibility that cancer, or at least some forms of it, could be prevented or controlled by naturally occurring factors?

Second, there are epidemiologic data to suggest that populations that have relatively large amounts of Laetrile in their diets are also relatively free of cancer. The Hunzakuts have often been reported to be virtually free of cancer, and it is an established fact that apricots and apricot kernels form a staple in their diet to a degree unparalleled in the rest of the world (Leaf, 1976).

Third, experiments performed to test Laetrile's preventive value at New York's Sloan-Kettering Institute for Cancer Research did show a prophylactic effect, according to veteran researcher Kanematsu Sugiura. In a 30-month experiment with a strain of mouse bred to develop breast cancer (CD_8F_1), 72 percent of the saline-treated control mice developed lung metastases, whereas only 17 percent of the Laetrile-treated mice developed such metastases (Stock et al., 1978; see also Second Opinion, 1977). Sugiura also noted positive effects in experiments with AKR leukemic mice, including a dramatic reduction in the size of internal organs in treated mice.

The idea of Laetrile as vitamin B-17 is therefore not simply a ruse or cancer quackery but a scientific hypothesis that deserves serious attention.

Biochemistry of Laetrile

In the late 1940s, biochemist Ernst T. Krebs, Jr., purified a crude apricot kernel preparation and proposed a biochemical rationale for the use of cyanogenic glycosides and their derivatives in the treatment of cancer.

On the basis of extensive work reported in the scientific literature, Krebs proposed a "cyanide theory" to explain Laetrile's effect on cancer. Bruce W. Halstead, a toxicologist, recently summarized the long debate over Laetrile's mode of action (Halstead, 1977).

Two separate pathways have been suggested for Laetrile's activity in the body (Figure 24–1), the first of which is not controversial. The second, the one proposed by Krebs, has been sharply questioned by a number of critics (Greenberg, 1975; Ross, 1975).

According to this second pathway, the glucuronide form of amygdalin is synthesized in the liver of individuals ingesting natural amygdalin. This glucuronide is then degraded at the tumor site to release cyanide, which selectively attacks the cancer cells, but spares normal cells.

Some scientists have in fact found glucuronide formation in the liver, and to a lesser extent, in the intestine and kidneys (references in Halstead, 1977).

In order for this glucuronide to be broken down it requires the enzyme β-glucuronidase. In some studies, this enzyme has been found in cancerous tissues of the breast, uterus, stomach, mesentery, abdominal wall, and esophagus, in amounts about 100 to 3600 times more than is present in noncancerous tissues (references in Halstead, 1977). More recently, Sloan-Kettering Institute researchers have found that "in many cases β-glycosidase and glucuronidase activities were higher in cancerous than homologous normal tissues . . ." (SKI Annual Report, 1974).

The breakdown of Laetrile by β-glucuronidase at the site of the tumor would cause general cyanide poisoning in normal cells were it not for the presence of another enzyme, rhodanese, which is capable of detoxifying HCN.

Rhodanese was discovered by Lang in 1933, and a number of scientific reports have shown that normal cells contain a relatively high concentration of rhodanese and low levels of β-glucuronidase (references in Halstead, 1977). Sloan-Kettering researchers found variable levels of rhodanese.

If the glucuronide is in fact formed in the liver, as Krebs postulated, and if this glucuronide then reaches the tumor site, where it is broken down by the high level of β-glucuronidase, the resulting HCN could conceivably poison cancer cells deficient in rhodanese, while sparing those normal cells that have high levels of this enzyme, since HCN depresses enzyme functions in cells. At the same time, benzaldehyde, a known pain-killer, would also be released, accounting perhaps for the analgesic properties often associated with Laetrile.

Recent reports from Japan indicate that benzaldehyde itself may be efficacious in the treatment of human lung cancer (Science News, 1979).

Figure 24-1. Biochemical Pathways of Amygdalin (From Halstead, Bruce: Amygdalin Therapy. Los Altos, Ca.: The Committee for Freedom of Choice in Cancer Therapy, Inc., 1977.)

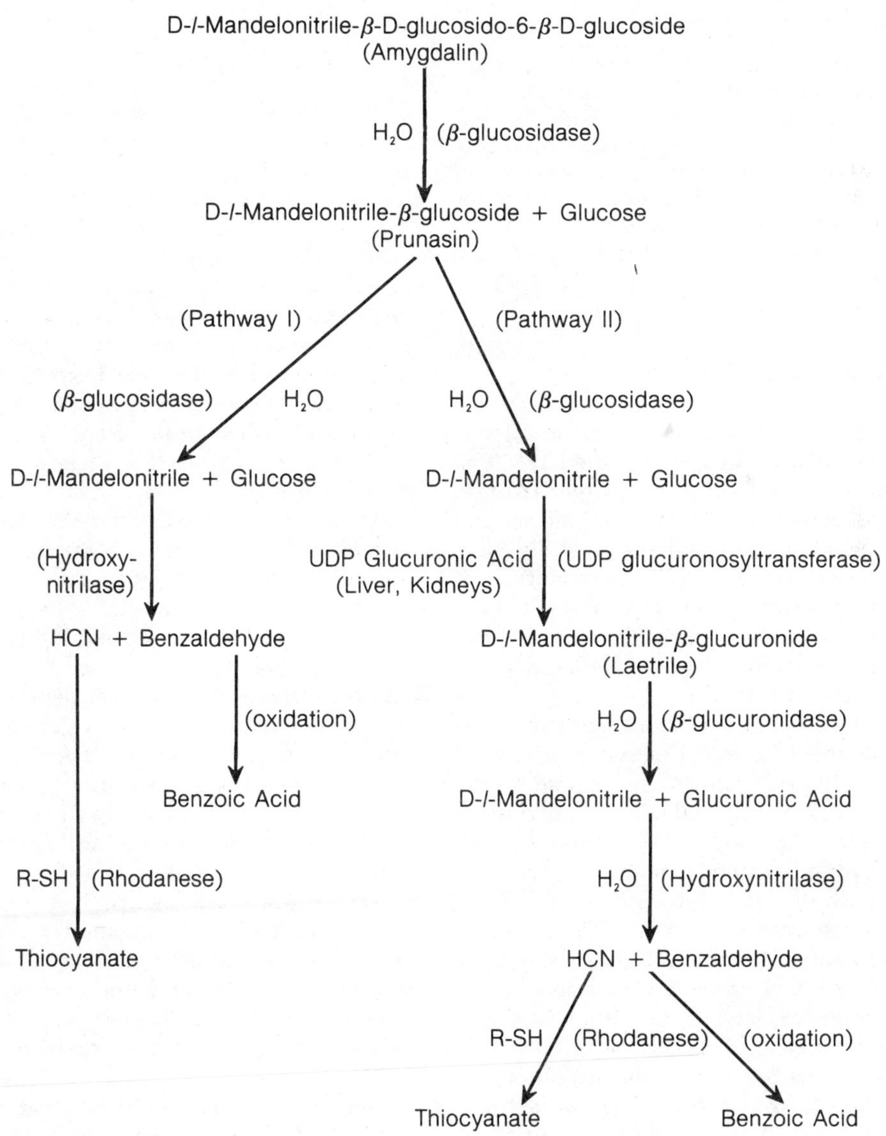

A number of other possible mechanisms of Laetrile activity have also been proposed, including those of Passwater (1977), McCarty (1975), and Brekhman and Dardymov (1969) (the "adaptogen" concept). Krebs's explanation is still widely respected among Laetrilists and in some ways is the most appealing, since it comes close to the long sought "magic bullet" for cancer, which could kill cancer cells while leaving normal cells unharmed. Halstead has summarized the current state of the controversy over Laetrile's mode of action:

> Despite Krebs' critics and a number of unanswered questions about the "cyanide theory," it continues to remain the most biochemically rational explanation of some very complex chemical events revolving around the use of amygdalin (Laetrile) in cancer metabolic therapy. This theory is now under critical review by a number of investigators and only time and further research will determine its ultimate reality (Halstead, 1977).

The Question of Toxicity

A great deal has been made of the alleged toxicity of Laetrile. In 1977-78, the FDA took the extraordinary step of posting large "Laetrile Warning" posters in 10,000 post offices and sending an FDA drug bulletin on the subject (November-December, 1977) to hundreds of thousands of health workers. As a result, Laetrile, once known as a remarkably nontoxic form of therapy, is today widely considered to be a dangerous and toxic drug.

The FDA bulletin contained numerous misstatements about Laetrile. For example, it stated that "this glycoside [amygdalin] contains cyanide." Of course, amygdalin does not contain cyanide, but it can be hydrolyzed into benzaldehyde, hydrogen cyanide and two sugars given the presence of beta-D-glucosidase and beta-oxynitrilase (Greenberg, 1975). This is more than a semantic difference. Unless the proper conditions are met, cyanide is as firmly bound in the amygdalin molecule as a brick in a solid brick wall. One might as well state that table salt is poisonous because it contains chlorine!

According to the poster, 37 poisonings and 17 deaths have been caused by "ingestion of Laetrile ingredients (apricot and similar fruit pits)." Apricot pits are not ingredients of Laetrile. If anything, Laetrile is an ingredient of apricot pits (kernels), which also contain other substances, such as enzymes, not found in purified amygdalin. (The whole kernel contains only 2 to 4 percent Laetrile). The 37 poisonings, culled from the entire world over many years, refer to circumstances quite different from those encountered by cancer patients ingesting Laetrile as medicine.

In the United States, one death has definitely been attributed by the government to Laetrile—that of an 11-month old girl in Attica, New York, in June 1977. According to the FDA bulletin, "she accidentally ingested up to 5 tablets (500 mg/tab) of Laetrile." This contention is firmly rejected by the child's mother, who holds that the child was free of danger until hospital personnel administered an anti-cyanide medicine. The child subsequently slipped into a coma and died (personal communication, January, 1978).

The FDA Bulletin contains other "warnings" that appear to be designed to frighten cancer patients away from an alternative form of cancer therapy. For example: "Indeed, some deaths ascribed to cancer, particularly in debilitated patients, may have been either due to or accelerated by cyanide from the drug." A frightening prospect—but what is the evidence for this? "Further studies should be undertaken to determine whether this is true or not" (FDA Bulletin, 1977).

At present, it is estimated that between 50 and 100,000 cancer patients are ingesting over one million grams of Laetrile a month (Moertel, 1978). So far, one or possibly two deaths have been reported from accidental ingestion of this substance. Two cases of minimal toxicity have also been reported. Based on these facts, Laetrile does not seem to be a "dangerous" or "toxic" substance when it is taken correctly.

Recently, anti-Laetrile researchers killed dogs by infusing massive doses of prehydrolyzed amygdalin into their stomachs (Ross, 1978). This "finding"—that Laetrile, when allowed to break down by enzymatic action, will poison those who ingest it—made headlines, but is not really news. The potentially poisonous nature of a slurry of bitter almond kernels has been known since the time of the Pharaoh, when it was used as a means of executing prisoners (Summa, 1972).

Since 1837, it has been known that amygdalin can be hydrolyzed to release hydrogen cyanide under the proper chemical conditions. The fact is, however, that this does not normally happen to a dangerous extent in the human gut, and certainly not when purified amygdalin (without enzymes) is administered parenterally.

As an FDA spokesman once said, "Laetrile

is not a significantly toxic substance. I don't know of any deaths or serious injuries of persons injecting Laetrile" (personal communication, 1977).

This observation is borne out by Sloan-Kettering's five-year study of Laetrile. In one case, Laetrile was administered intraperitoneally to mice in doses as high as eight grams/Kg/day, with no sign of acute or chronic toxicity. This is equivalent to giving a human being a pound a day of this "toxic" substance! In another test, mice were given 2 grams/Kg/day for 30 months. Sugiura reported that the treated mice in his experiments exhibited better health and well-being than the controls, which did not receive Laetrile (Stock et al., 1978).

When advocates of orthodox chemotherapy accuse Laetrile of being toxic, it is a case of the pot calling the kettle black. Most standard chemotherapeutic agents are truly toxic in the extreme. Methotrexate, for example, produces anemia, leukopenia, thrombocytopenia, liver atrophy, necrosis, cirrhosis, fatty changes, fetal death, congenital abnormalities, diarrhea, and ulcerative stomatitis—and, occasionally, death from intestinal perforation (Physician's Desk Reference, 1972).

In comparison with such agents, Laetrile is indeed nontoxic, although one could certainly imagine situations in which it *could* be toxic or even fatal (the same is true of water or air). Paracelsus (1493–1541), sometimes called the "Father of Chemotherapy," could have been commenting on this controversy when he wrote, "All substances are poisons; there is none which is not a poison. The right dose differentiates a poison and a remedy."

Testing of Laetrile in Animals

Although spokesmen for orthodox medicine continue to deny that there have been any animal data in favor of Laetrile, this is contradicted by a number of studies.

For example, the SCIND Laboratories in California conducted several experiments in preparation for an Investigative New Drug (IND) application filed by the McNaughton Foundation in 1970. (The application was approved and then suddenly rescinded.)

In the second study on Walker 256 carcinosarcoma of rats, with amygdalin in dosages of 500/mg/Kg injected intraperitoneally on days one, three, and six after tumor take, the following results were found:

Days of Survival

Controls: 19, 19, 19, 20, 20, 22, 22, 22, 24, 24, 24, 25, 25, 26, 26, 26, 26

Treated: 27, 28, 28, 28, 29, 29, 29, 30, 30, 30, 30, 30, 31, 32, 32, 32, 60, 60, 60, 60

The median survival time of the controls was thus 24 days, whereas for the amygdalin-treated group it was 30 days. Note that the survival time of *every* amygdalin treated animal was greater than that of *every* control animal.

As Dr. Carl Baker, then Director of the National Cancer Institute, wrote in a letter to Congressman Edward Edwards, "The data provided by the McNaughton Foundation certainly indicates some activity in animal tumor systems" (McCarty, 1975). In Europe as well, a number of experiments were performed that appear to show anticancer activity in animal systems. For example, in a test by Dr. Paul Reitnauer, a chief biochemist of the Institute Manfred von Ardenne in Dresden, 20 of 40 H-strain mice were given bitter almonds, in addition to their standard chow. Bitter almonds contain relatively high levels of Laetrile.

Fifteen days after initiation of this regimen, all 40 mice were inoculated with one million Ehrlich ascites cells. The 20 control mice lived an average of 21.9 days following this injection. The 20 mice receiving the bitter almond supplement lived an average of 25.8 days ($p < .05$ by t-test) (Reitnauer, 1973).

Dr. T. Metianu, director of research in pharmacology-toxicology of the Pasteur Institute, Paris, using an adenocarcinoma adapted for mice, showed that 10 mice treated subcutaneously two to three times per week for 20 to 25 days with 500 mg/Kg amygdalin lived an average of 58 days past the time of tumor take, whereas a group of 10 control mice averaged 21 days survival time. A repetition of this experiment showed 47 days survival for the Laetrile-treated mice and 27 for the controls. Less striking results were observed at higher dosages, and no effect was seen at 100 mg/Kg in this system (cited in Burk, 1975).

The Sloan-Kettering Controversy

The most extensive animal experiments with Laetrile were performed at the Sloan-Kettering Institute (SKI) for Cancer Research, New York, between 1972 and 1977. Results were consistently negative in transplantable tumor systems. However, when Kanematsu Sugiura (member emeritus of SKI) switched to spontaneous tumor systems, he got dramatically positive results.

In a series of six experiments with CD_8F_1 mice, which spontaneously develop mammary tumors, Sugiura found:

1. A reduction in the incidence of lung metastases, from 80 to 90 percent in the control animals to 20 percent in the Laetrile-treated mice.
2. Temporary stoppage in the growth of small tumors (1 cm in diameter or less), with no effect on larger tumors.
3. Increased health and well-being in the Laetrile-treated animals.

Laetrile used alone did not appreciably diminish the size of the primary tumors, nor did it significantly extend the lifespan. However, the effect on metastases was considered to have clinical relevance, since metastasis is often the actual cause of death in cancer.

Sugiura saw virtually identical effects in a prevention experiment with CD_8F_1 mice, the Swiss albino mouse system, and in 12 treatment and prevention experiments with AKR leukemic mice. In the latter system, he consistently saw a marked diminution in the size of the internal organs, such as the thymus, the inguinal lymph nodes, and, to a lesser extent, the spleen.

In other work at Sloan-Kettering in 1973-74, Lloyd Schloen, working under SKI vice president Lloyd Old and along with technician S. Jacobs, saw virtually identical results in the Swiss albino mouse system: those animals receiving the highest dosage of Laetrile were healthier, lived longer, and showed retarded tumor growth and a lower rate of metastases. This work remained unpublicized until 1977, however (Second Opinion, 1977).

Sugiura's key finding was the marked inhibition of metastases. A great deal of confusion and disappointment ensued when other investigators were apparently unable to reproduce Sugiura's positive results.

Part of the problem may have been that these investigators departed from many of Sugiura's protocols in their own experiments. Thus, while Sugiura used a combination of macrovisual and histologic examinations of the lungs to detect metastases, Dr. E. Stockert employed only macrovisual observation. Dr. F. Schmid, also of SKI, employed only macrovisual observations in his first two experiments, and in the second of these he utilized only one fiftieth of Sugiura's dosage level (40/mg/Kg/day instead of 2000/mg/Kg/day).

It may be significant, therefore, that when Schmid followed Sugiura's protocols closely in his third experiment and utilized the microscope, he *was* able to confirm Sugiura's work and see a statistically significant difference between the treated and the untreated mice with respect to metastases (Stock et al., 1978).

Thus, three different experimenters (Sugiura, Schloen, and Schmid) did see positive results with Laetrile between 1972 and 1975.

Another researcher who collaborated in these studies, Dr. Daniel S. Martin of the Catholic Medical Center in Queens, New York, was unable to duplicate the results. He also made a number of departures from Sugiura's protocols, which may have influenced his findings. Instead of using histologic examination of the animals' lungs, he switched to a relatively novel type of "bioassay" and shunned microscopic examination. In the bioassay system, he claimed to see no difference between treated and control animals.

A "blind" test at Sloan-Kettering, in which Sugiura participated, also failed to reveal any significant difference between the two groups. It is possible, however, that this test may have been flawed. Forty percent of the mice in the control group showed initial tumor stoppages, whereas only 27 percent of the treated group showed such stoppages. Initial tumor stoppage in small growths was characteristic of Laetrile injections in Sugiura's earlier experiments. Since the treated and control animals were housed in the same cages in order to make the test completely blind, Sugiura felt that the treated mice may have accidentally received saline solution and the control mice may have received Laetrile at times. He therefore has rejected the validity of this experiment and holds to his belief that Laetrile stops the spread of cancer and has palliative effects (personal communication, 1979).

In standing by his often-repeated results, Sugiura is certainly in good company. Nobel laureate Sir Peter Medawar has written about a similar challenge he himself once faced with controversial results:

> Several people tried to repeat our work and failed. There were, however, always good reasons why they did so; either they had introduced into our techniques little 'improvements' of their own, or they were too clumsy or something. These failures did not disturb us in the very least; we knew we were right—and we were—so we did our best to tell those

who were struggling with our techniques how best to carry them out (Medawar, 1976).

After 60 years in the field of cancer chemotherapy research, Sugiura certainly has a right to believe in the validity of his own work and techniques, and reasonable people have a right to agree with him without being labeled quacks.

The Sloan-Kettering results were released to the press in 1977 and published in a scientific journal in 1978 (Stock et al., 1978). Although these papers provide much valuable information, the reader should be aware that the conclusions of the report have been the subject of sharp criticism. The gist of this criticism is that Sloan-Kettering presented the data in such a way as to discredit Sugiura's positive work. The most extensive criticism was "Second Opinion Special Report: Laetrile at Sloan-Kettering," written by a number of employees of Memorial Sloan-Kettering Cancer Center, including the author (Second Opinion, 1977; summarized in Science, 1977).

Sugiura has publicly associated himself with this criticism, writing to one of its authors, "Your critical review of my positive results and negative results of three investigators at Sloan-Kettering Institute is very well done and accurate. Please accept my sincere congratulations."

Combination Therapy

Recent experiments have focused on the use of Laetrile in combination with other nontoxic agents.

Harold Manner, chairman of the Biology Department of Loyola University in Chicago, has reported 89.3 percent complete regressions in mice with spontaneous mammary tumors (C3H/HeJ) and partial regression in the other 10.7 percent when he used a combination of Laetrile, emulsified vitamin A, and "Wobe Mugos" enzymes intratumorally (Manner, DiSanti, and Michaelsen, 1978).

Manner's results are highly unusual, if not unprecedented, for spontaneous animal tumors, which are notoriously difficult to cure by any means. Manner's initial experiment did not separate the contribution of each of the three agents, and specifically did not determine if Laetrile in and of itself is an anticancer agent. Tests currently underway are intended to do so.

Manner's experiments were preceded by an unpublished work of Schloen at Sloan-Kettering, which came to light during the controversy over Sugiura's work. Schloen achieved 100 percent complete regressions in mice with transplantable tumors when he used a combination of Laetrile and the enzyme bromelain (Second Opinion, 1977).

Clinical Studies

In modern times, Laetrile was one of the first purified chemicals to be tried for cancer treatment in a hospital setting. The substance was used by a Russian physician, Fedor J. Inosemtzeff, in 1844; after several months, "the patient was declared cured, and he left the hospital. He had received about one and a half ounces of pure amygdalin without showing any signs of toxicity" (Gazette Medicale de Paris, 1945).

Laetrile was employed in the treatment of cancer in the early 1950s by Ernst T. Krebs, Sr., a San Francisco physician, and a Los Angeles doctor, Arthur Harris. In a 1962 paper, Harris claimed that of the 82 cancer patients treated with Laetrile between 1951 and 1953, three were alive and free of disease almost ten years later, 24 were alive with their cancers under control, and 55 had received only temporary, palliative results (Beard, 1962).

These and other early clinical reports were challenged in a retrospective study of 44 cancer patients treated with Laetrile in an article by the California Cancer Commission (CCC). The Commission claimed that Laetrile was "completely ineffective" in man, in laboratory animals or *in vitro* (California Medicine, 1953).

For many years, this report stood as the definitive anti-Laetrile study, but it has come under sharp attack in recent years. For example, all the doctors questioned by the CCC reported important subjective benefits from Laetrile, and the laboratory studies showed anti-cancer "toxic cellular changes" that were omitted from the official 1953 report. In addition, the patients had all received either very few injections or dosages considered to be minute by today's standards.

Since that time, Laetrile has been used by an extraordinary number of cancer victims and physicians. Although the aura of illegality that has surrounded Laetrile in this country has undoubtedly discouraged scientific publication, there are a number of clinical papers that report positive results with regard to both safety and efficacy.

In 1962, for example, John A. Morrone, an attending surgeon at the Jersey City Medical

Center, reported "a dramatic relief of pain" in ten cancer patients treated with Laetrile, as well as other effects that "suggest regression of the malignant lesion."

Ettore Guidetti of the University of Turin and his colleagues reported positive effects of Laetrile on cancer patients at both the sixth and the ninth International Cancer Congresses, sponsored by the International Union Against Cancer (Guidetti, 1955; Rossi, 1966).

One of the most prolific authors in the field has been a Philippine physician, Manuel D. Navarro. He has written almost 20 articles on his experiences with Laetrile therapy since 1954 (bibliography in McNaughton Foundation, The Laetriles, 1967). Navarro has called Laetrile "the ideal drug for the treatment of cancer."

Dr. Hans A. Nieper is a well known West German oncologist who uses Laetrile and synthetic analogs of Laetrile in his medical practice. He is the author of several papers on Laetrile, including "Amygdalin therapy (60 patients)" (Z. Blut Geschwulstkrank., 1971).

In 1977, Dr. John A. Richardson published detailed case histories of cancer patients treated by him at his Albany, California clinic, selected from about 4000 patients whom he claims to have treated with some success: "Almost all of them have shown a positive response to their initial course of therapy before returning home."

In addition, there have been numerous journalistic accounts of the Clinica del Mar of Dr. Ernesto Contreras in Tijuana, Mexico, where cancer patients have been treated with Laetrile since the early 1960s. According to these accounts, Contreras claims that 35 percent of his patients (most of whom were terminally ill at the inception of treatment) experienced no response at all; 65 percent received some benefit from Laetrile, but almost half had recurrences of the disease after its temporary arrest. In about 30 percent of the cases, there were "more definite responses," ranging from slight improvement to the dramatic disappearance of all symptoms. Contreras estimates that perhaps 5 percent of the terminal patients he has seen have been actually "saved." These are modest claims, which belie the picture often painted of the Tijuana clinic as the haunt of crackpots and thieves.

There has been no lack of clinical studies attesting to Laetrile's effectiveness, especially as a palliative. What has been lacking is the randomized, double blind study that is a standard part of new drug testing in the United States. Responsibility for the lack of such double blind tests rests with the federal government and especially the FDA, which has opposed such a test, even when it has been proposed by established cancer scientists.

Instead, the National Cancer Institute undertook a retrospective study of cancer victims treated with Laetrile. This study came under criticism from the Laetrile movement because it placed its main emphasis on tumor shrinkage as an index of anticancer effect, and it omitted reduction in pain or other palliative aspects of Laetrile's action.

Of the 22 cases deemed "evaluable" by NCI, two showed complete responses, i.e., total elimination of their tumors; four showed partial responses, i.e., greater than 50 percent reduction in tumor size; nine cases had "stabilized disease"; and "three additional patients showed increased disease-free intervals." Thus 18/22, or 82 percent, appear to have had a beneficial response to Laetrile therapy (Ellison et al., 1978).

Although NCI officials adduced other possible reasons for these results, shortly afterwards the director of NCI called for a double blind clinical study with Laetrile.

Conclusion

In part because of the federal government's intransigence on the question of testing, Laetrilists have taken to the courts and the legislatures. Laetrile has been legalized in 17 states and action is pending in a number of others. In New York, pro-Laetrile bills were passed by wide margins in the state legislature, only to be vetoed by an anti-Laetrile governor.

Currently, despite FDA obstruction, cancer patients can receive Laetrile legally from their physicians under an affadavit system set up by federal judge Luther Bohanon. If Bohanon's landmark decision of December 5, 1977 is upheld (it is currently under appeal by the FDA), Laetrile will be officially "grandfathered" (i.e., not subject to "new drug" regulations) and will be freely available in the United States.

In a review of the entire controversy, Bohanon wrote:

> Unquestionably, the administrative record in this case reveals a substantial and well-developed controversy among medical professionals and other scientists as to the efficacy of Laetrile.

Advocates of Laetrile's use in cancer treatment include many highly educated and prominent doctors and scientists whose familiarity and practical experience with the substance vastly exceeds that of their detractors. To deem such advocacy "quackery" distorts the serious issues posed by Laetrile's prominence and requires disregarding considerable expertise mustered on the drug's behalf.

While the record reveals an impressive consensus among the nation's large medical and cancer-fighting institutions as to Laetrile's ineffectualness, a disconcerting dearth of actual experience with the substance by such detractors is revealed . . . .

The current debate is fierce. The issue appears largely unresolved as to Laetrile's true effectiveness, in large part because FDA has prevented adequate testing on humans . . . .

It is only when the substance is openly used, and its results carefully observed and fully reported that this controversy will be resolved.

It is urgent that Laetrile and other promising, unorthodox therapies be made freely available to physicians, for it is from clinical practice that the truth is most likely to emerge.

References

American Cancer Society: Plants that cure and cause cancer. Cancer News, Vol. 29, no. 2, 1975.

Beard, Howard H.: A New Approach to the Conquest of Cancer, Rheumatic and Heart Diseases. New York, 1962.

Beard, John: The Enzyme Treatment of Cancer and its Scientific Basis. London, Chatto & Windus, 1911.

Bohanon, Luther [Hon.]: "Opinion" case of Glen L. Rutherford v. United States of America, Joseph A. Califano, Secretary of Health, Education and Welfare; Donald Kennedy, Commissioner of the Food and Drug Administration, et al., December 5, 1977 in the United States District Court for the Western District of Oklahoma.

Brekhman I.I., and Dardymov, I.D.: New substances of plant origin which increase nonspecific resistance. Ann. Rev. Pharm. 9:419–430, 1969.

Brothwell, Don, and Brothwell, Patricia: *Food in Antiquity*. New York, Frederick A. Praeger, 1969.

Burk, Dean: *A Brief on Foods and Vitamins*. Sausalito, California, The McNaughton Foundation, 1975.

California Cancer Commsssion: The treatment of cancer with 'Laetriles'. Calif. Med. 78, no. 4 (April, 1953).

Ellison, N.M., Byar, D.P., and Newell, G.R.: Special Report on Laetrile: The NCI Laetrile Review, New Eng. J. Med., 299:549, 1978.

Food and Drug Administration: Laetrile. DHEW Publication, Consumer Memo, 1975.

Gold, Joseph: Use of Hydrazine Sulfate In Terminal and Pre-terminal Cancer Patients. Oncology 32:1–10, 1975.

Greenberg, David M.: The vitamin fraud in cancer quackery. West. J. Med. 122:345–348, 1975.

Guidetti, Ettore: Observations preliminaires sur quelques cas de cancer traites par un glycuronoside cyanogenetique. Acta Unio Internationalis Contra Cancrum 11:156–158, 1955.

Halstead, Bruce W.: Amygdalin (Laetrile) therapy. Los Altos, California, The Committee for Freedom of Choice in Cancer Therapy, Inc., 1977.

Krebs, Ernst T.: The nitrilosides (vitamin B-17)—their nature, occurrence and metabolic significance. J. App. Nutrition, Vol. 22, 1970.

Leaf, Alexander: *Youth in Old Age*. New York, McGraw-Hill, 1976.

Livingston, Virginia: *Cancer: A New Breakthrough?* Los Angeles, Nash Publishing, 1972.

Manner, H.W., DiSanti, S.J., and Michaelsen, T.L.: *The Death of Cancer*, Advanced Century, Chicago, 1968.

Markle, Gerald E., and Petersen, James C.: Laetrile and cancer: the limits of science. Paper prepared for presentation at the 1977 annual meeting of the Midwest Sociological Society.

McCarty, Mark: Burying Caesar: an analysis of the laetrile problem. Triton Times, University of California at San Diego, Nov. 29, 1975.

McNaughton Foundation: The Laetriles-Nitrilosides—in the prevention and control of cancer. Sausalito, California, 1967.

Medawar, Sir Peter: *The Strange Case of the Spotted Mice*. The New York Review of Books, April 15, 1976.

Moertel, Charles: A trial of laetrile now (editorial). N. Engl. J. Med. 298:219, 1978.

Passwater, Richard: In defense of Laetrile. Let's Live, June, 1977.

Reitnauer, P.G.: Prolonged survival of tumor bearing mice following feeding bitter almonds. Arch. Geschwulstforsch. 42:135, 1973.

Ross, Joseph F.: Laetriles—Not a vitamin and not a treatment. West. J. Med. (editorial). April, 1975.

Rossi, B., Guidetti, E., and Deckers, C.: Clinical trial of chemotherapeutic treatment of advanced cancers with L-mandelonitrile-beta-diglucoside. In The Laetriles-Nitrilosides—in the Prevention and Control of Cancer, Montreal, McNaughton Foundation, 1967.

Schmidt, E.S., Newton, G.W., Sanders, S.M., Lewis, J.P., and Conn, E.E.: Laetrile toxicity studies in rats. JAMA 239:943–947, 1978.

Laetrile's "secret" cancer weapon, Science News 115:71, 1979.

Second Opinion Special Report: Laetrile at Sloan-Kettering. P.O. Box 548, Bronx, New York, 1978.

Shimkin, Michael B.: Contrary to nature. Washington, D.C., U.S. Department of Health, Education and Welfare, DHEW Publication, 76–720, 1977.

Sloan-Kettering Institute for Cancer Research: Annual Report, New York, 1974.

Stock, C. Chester, et al.: Antitumor tests of amygdalin in spontaneous animal tumor systems. J. Surg. Oncol. 10:89–123, 1978.

Summa, Herbert M.: Amygdalin, a physiologically active therapeutic agent in malignancies. Krebsgeschehen 4 (1972) (West Germany).

Wolf, Max, and Ransberger, Karl: *Enzyme Therapy*. Los Angeles, Regent House, 1977.

The Case of Dimethyl Sulfoxide

Robert Herschler, B.S.
Stanley W. Jacob, M.D.
University of Oregon Department of Surgery

History

There is a span of roughly eight decades from the first recorded synthesis of dimethyl sulfoxide (DMSO) to the investigation of its diverse parameters of biologic usefulness.

Various factors in the early 1950s reawakened general scientific interest in DMSO. Principally, there was a technologic need for a superior polymer solvent. Also, a worldwide research effort was initiated to utilize forest-derived waste chemicals such as lignin, one of many potential sources of the methyl radical needed to prepare precursor dimethyl sulfide (DMS).

Commercial development was first undertaken circa 1953. In this pioneering effort, DMSO was promoted with emphasis on its superior solvent properties. An attempt was made to substitute DMSO for ethylene glycol as an antifreeze additive to coolant waters. Lovelock and Bishop utilized this property of DMSO to protect cells against freezing damage. Their publication (1959) is the first record of experimentation with DMSO in a biologic system.

Research defining the primary pharmacology of DMSO (Herschler and Jacob, 1963 to 1975) began in 1959, with studies following the movement of marker molecules across membranes when dissolved in DMSO. These experiments employed both animals and plants. Initially, four aprotic solvents were investigated, but dimethyl formamide (DMF), dimethyl acetamide (DMAC), and acetone were later dropped due to toxicities seen with diverse biologic models.

The pharmacologic effects recognized by Herschler and Jacob that stimulated initial clinical evaluations were:

1. Membrane penetration with DMSO alone and when DMSO functions as a solute "carrier"
2. Antiinflammation
3. Analgesia
4. Bacteriostasis
5. Diuresis
6. Reduction of abdominal adhesions in the rat
7. Antibiotic potentiation
8. Relief of swelling induced by trauma
9. Muscle relaxation
10. Vasodilation
11. Collagen modification

Some of these clinical applications are discussed later in this paper.

Preparation

"Cracking" lignin to free methyl radicals for dimethyl sulfide synthesis is not a convenient method of laboratory preparation of DMSO. The sole advantage to the use of the by-product lignin is cost. The actual process is credited to the Swedish inventors Hägglund and Enkvist (1955).

Several oxidants readily convert DMS to DMSO. Catalyzed hydrogen peroxide is clean and convenient, but expensive. The more economic and hence principal commercial process employs a catalyst of nitrogen oxides plus oxygen or oxygen-bearing gases. One drawback to nitrogen tetroxide-catalyzed systems for DMSO production is the potential of side reactions with feedstock impurities, which could yield toxicants of an insidious nature. Only well purified chemicals should be used for industrial applications, and only highly purified DMSO should be used for any drug purpose.

Purification

Several methods are available whereby DMSO of medical grade purity is prepared. The production of drug grade DMSO for clinical studies in the United States utilizes a process in which commercial purity DMSO is first placed in contact with strong base, metal oxide, and activated charcoal—and then distilled carefully in a vacuum (Lackey, Jacob, and Herschler, 1965).

Physical and Chemical Properties

Dimethyl sulfoxide is the lowest and most stable member of the aliphatic sulfoxides. When pure, the highly polar chemical is essentially odorless, infinitely miscible with water, and very hygroscopic. DMSO's attraction for water is phenomenal, as shown by its ability to remove water from such common "drying" chemicals as potassium hydroxide, calcium chloride, and silica gel.

The clinician should realize that DMSO is a truly unique chemical, as demonstrated by both its physical and chemical properties. As a solvent, it will dissolve most unsaturated and aromatic hydrocarbons, other organosulfur compounds, organic nitrogen compounds, and a number of inorganic salts, particularly those with halide or nitrate as the anion. It is an excellent solvent for several synthetic polymers utilized in clothing fiber manufacture, such as rayons, acrylics, urethanes, and vinyls. Patients using DMSO are best clothed in cotton, wool, polyester, or nylon, as DMSO generally is not a solvent for these materials at room temperature.

Clinical Ban and Related Toxicity

The Food and Drug Administration (FDA) on November 11, 1965, terminated clinical studies with DMSO. Though rescinded, in part, at a later date, this decision was made on the basis of toxicity findings in lower animals, which were seen as changes in the lens of the eye. It is suggested, considering the technicalities of the toxicity findings, the procedures used with the ban, and the resultant side-effect pattern in many ongoing research studies, that the FDA may have overreacted.

The lens change, seen first with dogs, was noted during a Merck-supported study. It is a credit to the pharmaceutical industry that its evaluation detected even the subtle and different expression of toxicity seen with DMSO. Follow-up studies demonstrated that DMSO can alter the nucleus of the lens of the eye in lower animals when given at sufficiently high dose for sufficient time. Interestingly, there were no lens changes in rhesus monkeys receiving DMSO at a dosage of 5 grams/kg/day for 100 days (Rubin and Mattis, 1966).

The FDA further relaxed restrictions on clinical studies following completion of a controlled study in man. The FDA assisted in the design of this study, which involved human volunteers (Brobyn, 1975). The findings were summarized as follows:

> A very extensive toxicology study of DMSO was conducted at 3 to 30 times the usual treatment dose in humans, for three months. DMSO appears to be a very safe drug for human administration, and in particular, the lens changes that occur in certain mammalian species do not occur in man under this very high prolonged treatment regimen.

Since DMSO possesses such a wide variety of drug activities, particularly when therapeutic benefit is seen in otherwise intractable disorders, supportive studies have continued to this date. Much research emphasis has centered on the question of toxicity. At the time of this writing (1979), all available findings suggest that DMSO is generally safe when given at any reasonable dose, by any route, to any animal model.

The FDA, in recent years, has been especially cooperative and helpful. Without the assistance of Drs. Merle L. Gibson and K.C. Pani, and members of their division, there would not be a single prescriptive approval in the U.S.

This writing is not intended to serve as a general review of DMSO toxicology. The National Academy of Sciences (NAS) conducted an extensive review of this matter (1974) and reported:

> Compared to most drugs or commonly recognized toxic agents, DMSO is relatively impotent on a weight or molar dosage basis. The compound is not innocuous, however, especially when administered at high concentrations (greater than 50%) and can give rise to serious, acute, toxic reactions. For

instance, if such concentrations are given intravenously, hemolysis will result leading to hemoglobinuria, anemia, pulmonary obstruction and edema, hemorrhage, hypotension, etc. Large doses of high concentrations of DMSO orally produce gastroenteritis and bowel hemorrhage or when given by other routes produce analogous, toxic effects appropriate to the avenue of administration.

The Ban in Retrospect and Comparative Considerations

It should be noted that at the time of the ban, no participating body or individual, public or private, had seen and reported a single case of serious toxicity in man attributable to DMSO. Clinical termination of the drug therefore came as a great surprise and a grave disappointment to many physicians familiar with DMSO.

The clinical findings of the prior two years (1964 to 1965) indicated that the overwhelming majority of investigators recognized dual benefit for their patients: clinical improvement coupled with apparent freedom from concern of serious drug-related side effects. During this time, each drug being used for musculoskeletal disorders presented a recognized danger—even an occasional serious, irreversible toxic reaction.

A comparison of DMSO with approved substances serving dually as drugs and drug vehicles may be helpful in illustrating the concern of those who believe that DMSO was treated unfairly in 1965.

Ethanol serves as both a drug and a vehicle. It can be administered to lower animals and to man by the same routes as DMSO. Ethanol is reported to have a lethal dose (LD) 50 (oral) in the rat of 13.7 gm/kg. DMSO is variously reported to have an LD 50 (oral) in the rat of 19.7 to 28.3 gm/kg (Brown et al., 1963; Sommer and Tauberger, 1964; Willson et al., 1965). Toxicologists have suggested that if ethanol had been substituted for DMSO in certain of the toxicity studies of concern, many of the involved laboratory animals would have expired before a change in the nucleus of the lens was seen.

An unresolved issue is the effect that maximum tolerated doses of ethanol would have on the lens of the eye of lower animals. Ethyl alcohol, and other agents at hyperosmotic strengths, appear to influence the electrical activity of the lens by decreasing the activity of the sodium pump (Yorio and Bentley, 1976).

One can also make a logical comparison of coal tar and DMSO. In so doing, there is no intent to tamper with traditional medicine. DMSO is a single, pure chemical—a lignin derivative. Coal tar is a heterogenous composition derived from the destructive distillation of ligneous substrates (as is pine or juniper tar). Both DMSO and tars have a common, though distant, ancestry. With coal tar, various phenols such as cresols and guaiacol are present as active ingredients while serving dually as solvent and vehicle. Additionally, naphthalene, anthracene, and a mixture of other polycyclics are present. The more common chemical compounds of the mixture, such as the phenols, are significantly more toxic than DMSO by any route of administration.

By direct comparison, there seem to be advantages to the preferred use of DMSO as a drug vehicle, based on the drugs' characteristics. DMSO is:

1. A single, water-white chemical, suggesting the probability of better clinical reproducibility of action.
2. A superior drug solvent.
3. Strikingly lower in dermal and systemic toxicity.

Fate and Metabolism

Absorption. DMSO in aqueous solution is absorbed through the skin barrier at a rate dependent on the concentration. Increasing absorption is seen to approximately 90 percent w/v strength. Since DMSO is optimally absorbed through the skin in the concentration range of 70 to 90 percent, most clinical experience has been with this range.

Lower concentrations are employed when the solution is applied to other membranes. Excellent penetration of the bladder is seen with 15 percent aqueous DMSO (Jacob et al., 1964).

Kolb et al. (1967) studied the rapidity of DMSO's appearance in the blood of the rat, beagle dog, and man using sulfur-35 and tritium-labeled DMSO applied to the skin. Label was detected in the blood of man with the first drawn sample taken at five minutes. With samples taken over several days, both DMSO and $DMSO_2$ were isolated and identified.

Distribution. Kolb and associates carried out distribution studies one hour after topical application to laboratory animals and found distribution of label throughout the body.

Denko et al. (1967) determined the distribution of radioactive DMSO when administered dermally to the rat. These investigators found that radioactivity rapidly accumulated in both soft and hard tissues and was thereafter relatively rapidly excreted.

Biotransformation. The recognized metabolites of DMSO are dimethyl sulfide (DMS) and dimethyl sulfone ($DMSO_2$). Both metabolites are found as normal constituents of many food substances eaten by man.

Excretion. Unchanged DMSO was shown to be rapidly cleared from the body in studies by Gerhards and Gibian (1967).

Properties of Major Metabolites —DMS and $DMSO_2$

Dimethyl sulfide (DMS), CH_3SCH_3, the simplest aliphatic thioether, is a stable liquid. Although it is immiscible with water, solutions form with many organic solvents.

DMS is referenced in many clinical reports as the causative agent for the sulfurous, garlic, onion-like, or oysterish malodor of the breath of patients receiving DMSO. It is only a part of the odor. Dimethyl sulfide, when ultrapure, possesses a not unpleasant, penetrating ether-like odor. It serves in industry as an odor enhancer and is critical to the fresh odor of seafoods, vegetables, milk, coffee, and tea.

Dimethyl sulfone ($DMSO_2$), $CH_3SO_2CH_3$, the simplest aliphatic sulfone, is an odorless compound. Although it is very soluble in warm water, it is but slightly soluble in cold water. The exceptional chemical stability of $DMSO_2$ possibly accounts for the long-term residence of this metabolite in the blood of animals after a single DMSO challenge.

Basic Biologic Considerations

The imposed ban on DMSO clinical studies, although temporary, also effectively terminated many valuable basic studies designed to elucidate the pharmacology of DMSO. The effect was not temporary. Almost overnight, it was difficult for investigators to obtain new or renewed funding for DMSO research. The flow of basic pharmacologic reports with DMSO continues, but many studies now stem from research supportive of clinical work in other countries. New findings in the literature, both basic and clinical, are numerous and diverse. It is beyond the scope of this writing to discuss or even reference the majority of these.

Jacob, Rosenbaum, and Wood (1971) have provided a summary text that serves as a status review of the scientific knowledge prior to November 1965 up to about 1970. The reports of two symposia sponsored by the New York Academy of Sciences on DMSO, published as separate annals (1967 and 1975), contain data supportive of various clinical studies with DMSO. Since these pertinent references are less widely available, selected findings are abstracted.

Görög and Kovac (1975) employed topical 90 percent DMSO compared with 90 percent DMSO containing 2 percent hydrocortisone. The model was fully developed adjuvant-caused arthritis induced by killed Mycobacteria injected into the rat. DMSO alone, and in combination, was an effective antiarthritic when evaluated according to (1) antiedema effect, (2) radiographic study, and (3) the "plasma inflammation unit." These investigations suggested a tenfold enhancement of hydrocortisone effectiveness when this steroid was used with DMSO.

The concentration of steroids used to stabilize lysosomes could be reduced from 10- to 1000-fold when the steroids were predissolved in DMSO (Weissman et al., 1967).

Ward et al. (1967) prevented or suppressed the local Schwartzman phenomenon in the rabbit with DMSO applied topically to the preparatory site at intravenous challenge time.

Ashwood-Smith (1967) reviewed the antiradiation usefulness of DMSO in studies with protein, microorganisms, mammalian cells, and entire organisms.

DMSO is an effective carrier of solutes across membrane barriers, even the skin. Franz and Van Bruggen (1967) demonstrated that DMSO can produce a marked change in frog skin influx-efflux ratios. Finney et al., (1967) demonstrated the use of DMSO associated with oxygen (as H_2O_2) as a pericardial perfusate for experimental anoxia.

With DMSO perfusion of whole hearts and tissue incubation of myocardium in DMSO, Shlafer and Karow (1975) described functional effects, which include (1) a concentration-dependent heartbeat decrease, where the negative chronotropic effect is totally reversible with DMSO removal and (2) an effect on cardiac contractile strength—DMSO concentrations of 0.7 M and lower generally produce positive inotropy. These authors suggest that DMSO may provide relief of transient cardiac anoxia or ischemia and thus may be useful as a cardiac stimulant.

DMSO has been used as a carrier of many

drugs. In one study, DMSO was used in conjunction with certain antineoplastic compounds in the rat. Potentiation of antitumor activity was reported, such as the antiblastic action of cyclophosphamide (Warren et al., 1975).

Using 6 percent DMSO with isolated frog sciatic nerve, Sams (1967) demonstrated the reversible ability to lower velocity of nerve conduction. Pain relief, seen clinically, is further considered in the work of Shealy (1966), using feline peripheral small nerve fibers. Concentrations of 5 to 10 percent DMSO blocked C fiber conduction within one minute. Davis et al. (1967) found that DMSO served to block motor nerves in frog nerve-muscle preparations.

Peterson and Robertson (1967) studied the acute effects of intravenous DMSO in the dog. Incremental doses (5 to 10,000 mg/kg) produced remarkably few alterations in cardiopulmonary dynamics, selected autonomic reflex mechanisms, and arterial pH, pO_2, and pCO_2. These dosage levels bridge those used when DMSO was given intravenously to offset laboratory-induced CNS injury (de la Torre et al., 1975). De la Torre and associates concluded that DMSO was of significant benefit in treating acute extradural mass-forming lesions, middle cerebral artery occlusion, respiratory anoxia, and spinal cord injuries in rhesus and squirrel monkeys, dogs, and cats.

Use of DMSO for CNS trauma therapy is further supported. Cloned rat astrocytoma cells, in culture, are protected by DMSO when they are sonic stressed (Lim and Mullan, 1975).

DMSO (25 percent) completely inhibited *in vitro* growth of pleomorphic microorganisms (Seibert et al., 1967). DMSO was effective in overcoming streptomycin resistance in Escherichia coli. With DMSO at a noninhibitory concentration of 1.4 M, the minimum inhibitory concentration of streptomycin was lowered from over 5000 (control) to 7.5 micrograms/ml (Feldman et al., 1975).

DMSO increased the interferon titers (2- to 16-fold) in the mouse infected with Sindbis and Calova viruses (Kunze, 1975).

DMSO, at concentrations of 3 and 5 percent w/v in culture media, significantly and reversibly suppresses fibroblast proliferation (Berliner and Ruhmann, 1967). Using cortisol at 0.1 microgram/ml plus 1 percent DMSO, these investigators reported significant fibroblast growth depression, although neither agent alone was effective at these concentrations.

The interaction of DMSO and alcohol has been studied in animals and man (Mallach, 1967). Although concurrent DMSO failed to accelerate ethanol absorption, it caused a more rapid decline in blood level, potentiated psychomotor impairment and reduction of nerve conductivity, and achieved a reduction in alcohol mortality.

Clinical Findings and Considerations

Musculoskeletal Disorders

Historically, the first extensive clinical evaluation with DMSO in man concerned musculoskeletal disorders. Such disorders received special attention owing to the many clinical studies under the sponsorship of major U.S. pharmaceutical firms at the time of the November 1965 FDA ban. Millions of dollars in private and public funds had been expended in support of the program. These pharmaceutical firms, reflecting the opinion of their clinical investigators, were generally enthusiastic about the basic toxicologic and clinical DMSO findings. The ban hurt both the program and drug firm interest in the drug—despite a widely recognized need for a therapeutic entity such as DMSO.

An early publication of clinical findings concerned a study of seven patients with acute subdeltoid bursitis (Rosenbaum and Jacob, 1964). Therapy involved 6 to 8 ml of topically applied 90 percent aqueous DMSO. Pain relief was evident in all patients within 20 minutes, and improved shoulder joint range of motion was observed.

Topical application was practiced in thousands of subsequent patients. This topical mode of treatment actually plays a part in the controversy. Although topical administration is convenient, there is evidence that other routes of administration provide superior clinical improvement and totally circumvent the annoying skin reactions. In the treatment of genitourinary disorders described later, DMSO applied to the skin clearly gives results inferior to those shown with intravesical instillation. Unpublished findings indicate that injection yields superior results to topical application in inflammation of the olecranon bursa. There is a need for a comprehensive study of routes of administration that would better match route to disorder. Unfortunately, federal regulations suggest that each variation requires a separate IND/NDA filing, a prohibitively expensive procedure.

Before DMSO was introduced as a prescription drug in Europe, 308 patients were evaluated with topically applied 90 percent aqueous DMSO. This study included 100 patients with acute and chronic periarthritis, 88 patients with arthrosis of the knee, and 125 other patients with various acute and chronic musculoskeletal disorders. Dosage was between 5 and 10 ml, applied topically once daily in most cases. In this study, 27.6 percent became asymptomatic during therapy, 53.6 percent improved unequivocally, and 18.8 percent showed no improvement (John, 1965). John and Laudahn (1967) published findings of 4180 cases studied in Europe under the sponsorship of Schering. The 90 percent aqueous gel was again used, and in 1025 patients with acute musculoskeletal traumatic injuries, 86 percent demonstrated improvement. In 3155 cases of chronic calcified bursitis and localized arthritis, objective improvement (with some showing radiographic disappearance of calcifications) was reported; 49 percent demonstrated complete symptom remission, there was partial relief in 35 percent, and 16 percent did not improve.

Representative of clinical findings in the United States is a report of approximately 1900 patients with a variety of musculoskeletal disorders (Demos et al., 1967). The summary findings are in essential agreement with those of John and Laudahn.

Effectiveness was demonstrated in cases with Grades I and II rheumatoid arthritis in studies with 50 to 90 percent DMSO in Japan (Matsumoto, 1967). The 90 percent solution was judged most effective.

Several double blind-type studies were attempted with DMSO. In one design, 75 patients were treated with the 80 percent DMSO gel; a 10 percent DMSO solution served as a placebo. Both methods were compared with standard therapy (Brown, 1971). Analysis of coded findings indicated that 80 percent DMSO gel provided significantly greater and more rapid relief of pain and relief lasted for longer periods. Significantly greater improvement in active and passive motion was measured in patients presenting acute, severe sprains and strains, when treated with 80 percent DMSO gel.

Paul (1967) described a new and different approach to administering DMSO termed *interval therapy*. Treatment was but once or twice weekly by the topical route. Paul advised of the need to apply generous quantities of DMSO, not only to the involved site but to a large surrounding area. With the knee, it was recommended that application be made to the entire lower extremity from groin to toes. In 180 patients studied, results were in essential agreement with the data for patients treated daily.

The FDA approved DMSO for acute musculoskeletal injuries in animals first for horses in 1970, then for dogs in 1972. Of the clinical studies included with the submitted NDAs, the following are cited. These are referenced in the U.S. National Academy Report (1974). One involved the treatment of 13 horses with the counterirritant technique called *point firing* to relieve foreleg edema and tenderness. After firing, the right foreleg was treated with 90 percent DMSO topically twice daily for a total of seven applications. The left was used as a control (untreated). The circumference of each limb and the horse's response to digital pressure were determined daily. The DMSO-treated legs showed less edema, with disappearance of tenderness in half the time required for that in the control leg.

In racing greyhounds with acute traumatic arthritis of the phalanges, 90 percent DMSO applied topically was compared with standard corticoid therapy. A population of 46 dogs received standard corticoid therapy; 50 dogs received DMSO. Two racing season trials saw two dogs treated with DMSO demonstrate a recurrence of arthritis, whereas eleven dogs on standard therapy demonstrated a recurrence. Dogs on DMSO returned to racing in half the time required for those on standard therapy.

In a double blind study in racing greyhounds suffering with strain of the deltoideus or gracilis muscles, 10 dogs received 90 percent DMSO and 9 dogs received 10 percent (placebo) DMSO. Recovery time for the two groups was not statistically different, but none of those treated with DMSO had a recurrence of the musculoskeletal disorder, whereas 8 of 9 placebo-group dogs were seen to have a recurrence.

Urologic Disorders

The initial NDA approval for DMSO use in man was granted in 1978. A 50 percent aqueous solution is available for the treatment of interstitial cystitis, with administration by direct instillation into the bladder. This first approval is very specific and limiting. Since the product has demonstrated broader effectiveness, it may be possible to gain later approval for use in various other inflammatory urologic conditions such as radiation cystitis, urethritis, trigonitis, and abacterial prostatitis.

This use of DMSO in urology was first reported upon by Persky and Stewart (1967). Their clinical report considered DMSO in the treatment of Peyronie's disease, epididymitis, herpes of the genitalia, and other painful and inflammatory conditions of the genitourinary tract, including interstitial cystitis. This investigation saw significant improvement in a number of cases: 6 of 13 with Peyronie's disease and 7 of 12 with epididymitis.

Only 2 of 15 cases of interstitial cystitis were judged to have improved. Here, the route of administration proved critical. DMSO, in the first 15 cases, was applied topically over the suprapubic area on a twice daily basis using aqueous DMSO (50 to 90 percent concentrations). When the route of administration was changed to intravesicular instillation, marked improvement occurred in a majority of cases.

Stewart et al. (1972) describe additional studies with 21 patients. Follow-up after treatment ranged from six months to five years. Stewart and associates concluded that intravesicular instillation of 50 cc of 50 percent DMSO effectively controlled symptoms for as long as five years in about two thirds of the patients seen. It was judged that the treatment could be conducted safely as an office procedure.

Stewart and Shirley (1976) describe further experience with DMSO for interstitial cystitis in 46 patients. Of this series of patients, 80 percent were deemed to be objectively improved.

Collagen Metabolic Disorders

Frommhold and associates (1967) utilized a topically applied 90 percent gelled DMSO preparation in patients with subcutaneous fibrosis induced by telecobalt irradiation of deep-seated malignant tumors. DMSO was effective in softening and reducing the size of the plaque areas.

Systemic scleroderma (progressive systemic sclerosis) has been studied by numerous investigators after Scherbel et al. (1965) published the first preliminary report describing findings with ten patients. With this serious disease (and others), a double blind-type evaluation method is impossible, in the opinion of DMSO-experienced clinicians. The average dosage is greater than that required for a muscle strain. Treatment regimens may extend from several months to years. No attending physician, no patient, and no attendant would mistake topical 70 to 90 percent DMSO for any placebo. Identification requires only sight, smell, or touch.

Failure to gain approval to use DMSO for various disorders in man relates in part to the inability to employ the double blind method. The subject is broached in nearly every written criticism of the drug.

The National Academy of Sciences (1974) considered this matter and reached the following conclusion:

> The fact that, in most patients on whom it is used, topical application of DMSO produces an immediate skin reaction that in nearly all cases is soon followed by a characteristic breath odor complicates problems in designing and maintaining mechanisms for double-blind observations. In most instances, the control group, when one was used, actually received a low concentration of DMSO in an attempt to "blind" both the patient and the investigator with regard to the actual DMSO concentration used. Although this technique may help to preserve the double-blind features of a study, it is probably less than foolproof in most instances. The absence of mechanisms for ensuring double-blind observations is particularly serious because of the nature of the endpoints being observed in most DMSO studies.

A further report by Scherbel et al. (1967) describes findings with an additional 42 scleroderma cases. The eight criteria used in evaluating possible cutaneous improvement are described. They include softening of skin and subcutaneous tissues, healing of ulcers, increased finger movement and grip strength, and disappearance of collagen bundles. Of these 42 cases, 26 showed good to excellent improvement and 16 showed fair to poor response. Ischemic ulcers were present in 19 of the 42 patients. With topical DMSO, the ulcers generally healed in from one to six weeks of daily treatment. Evidence that DMSO therapy also has a beneficial effect in reducing interstitial calcinosis was presented.

Scherbel, at the DMSO Symposium sponsored by Schering (Austria, 1966), presented further encouraging findings with 61 patients; clinical improvement was confirmed histologically.

One early negative report is available concerning the use of DMSO in scleroderma (Tuffanelli, 1966). Duration of treatment was given as two to five months, but neither dose nor frequency of treatment is described.

Ehrlich and Joseph (1965) evaluated DMSO in 13 scleroderma patients, usually only treating the more severely disease-afflicted side. Duration of treatment varied up to five months. An increased range of motion was noted in nine patients, increased flexibility of the skin in nine, and increased grip strength in eight.

Engel (1972) supplemented a previous report describing "remarkable improvement in 5 patients with scleroderma treated with dimethyl sulfoxide." These findings concern 20 patients: three with linear scleroderma, nine with systemic sclerosis, one with morphea, two with coup de sabre, and five with generalized scleroderma. Topical, aqueous 90 percent DMSO was applied twice daily, and treatment continued for one year. Engel noted increase in skin mobility, rapid relief of pain, healing of persistent ulcers, regrowth of hair, and return of sensation and sweating.

DMSO was approved for general clinical use in the Soviet Union by 1972, and it is usually referenced as Demexide. Sergeyev and Zakhiyeu (1976) describe the use of 30 to 90 percent DMSO in a large population of patients presenting generalized, laminated, and linear manifestations of scleroderma. Applications of 10 to 15 ml "or more" were administered twice daily. The treatment course ran from 6 to 30 months. These investigators, employing objective methods of appraisal, reported clinical findings that closely match those of Scherbel, Engel, and others.

Ten patients with keloids received 50 to 80 percent DMSO applied topically two or three times daily over several months. After this time, a flattening of the scar was seen, with microscopic changes in the dermis characterized by a loosening of the collagen bundles (Engel, 1967).

Vehicle Usage

DMSO penetrates membranes, including the skin, and rapidly appears as a humoral constituent. The ability to penetrate such barriers without causing irreversible damage and to render the organ permeable to other drugs is one intriguing pharmacologic property not matched by other drugs and vehicles.

It was apparent from the earliest experiments that DMSO possessed unique drug vehicle value. It is expected that the utilization of DMSO as the solvent/vehicle for other important drug substances in the treatment of skin diseases will prove to be one of its more important medical uses. Many DMSO-drug combinations are in use in foreign countries.

In the United States, each combination made with DMSO, even a differing strength aqueous solution of DMSO alone, is deemed to be a new drug substance. This interpretation has stilled commercial interest in DMSO combinations.

Before the federal government enforced the "new combination as new drug" interpretation with DMSO, American studies that recognized special values of DMSO combinations, including lowered danger of toxic side reactions with concurrent improved drug efficacy, already existed.

To illustrate, one clinical study of a DMSO combination will be briefly described. Thiabendazole (TBZ) is an anthelmintic and broad spectrum fungicide. Its normal route of administration is oral. Side effects include dizziness, vomiting, and anorexia. One use of TBZ is for the control of larva migrans or creeping eruption (Katz and Hood, 1966; Smith, 1966). Katz described the oral TBZ problem for the patient thusly: "The primary disadvantage of thiabendazole is that the large dose required incurs bothersome side effects in a large proportion of patients."

Katz and associates carried out a double blind-type study, evaluating a 2 percent TBZ solution in 90 percent DMSO against placebo 90 percent DMSO alone. It was concluded: "Thiabendazole in dimethyl sulfoxide applied topically favorably alters the natural course of creeping eruption and is as effective as the drug (TBZ) administered orally." With this DMSO combination, the side effects were noted to be "local burning and erythema" in most patients, but it became severe in only one. No systemic symptoms of toxicity were observed.

Barriers now block United States approval of such a combination as DMSO-TBZ. One fundamental obstacle is economic—the enormous cost incurred in gaining an NDA approval, which is required since DMSO-TBZ is interpreted to be a new drug. This barrier alone will slow commercial development of DMSO combinations, whether with steroids, antibiotics, anesthetics, antivirals, or TBZ.

Perhaps there is a plausible way of resolving this dilemma that would not break new regulatory ground. It is the approach loosely practiced with other vehicles. Alcohols and various tars are now accepted vehicles for medical practice. The safety of DMSO, by any route of administration, compares favorably with that of any currently approved vehicle, and DMSO is a much better solvent. Would it therefore be feasible to file and gain one NDA approval as a dermatologic solvent/vehicle? Any pharmacy, on receipt of a prescription, could provide 2 percent TBZ formulated in Drug Grade DMSO with a label reading "DMSO for vehicle use only." The FDA could thus limit usage by label and package insert.

The value of DMSO as a vehicle for idoxuridine (IDU) in the treatment of zoster has been described (Juel-Jensen et al., 1970). IDU-DMSO combinations were studied in several double blind controlled-type studies. In one publication, the results were summarized as follows:

> The antiviral effect of 5 percent idoxuridine in dimethyl sulphoxide intermittently applied and of 40 percent idoxuridine in dimethyl sulphoxide continuously applied for four days to the lesions in patients with zoster of recent onset was studied in two double-blind controlled trials. Most, but not all, of the patients receiving intermittent active treatment had pain for a short period only. The effect of continuous treatment was striking; pain had disappeared within nine days in all the patients, and healing was accelerated. The results were statistically significant.

DMSO (20 percent) in a combination serves as the vehicle useful in the treatment of acute and chronic venous disorders. Formulation is as a convenient aerosol spray. Several clinical groups in Europe have evaluated the combination using the double blind technique, demonstrating effectiveness and safety (Kappert, 1975).

Conclusions

1. Historically, DMSO is an old chemical but a new drug substance. Synthesis is relatively simple and the various required materials are in abundant supply.
2. DMSO demonstrates a wide range of primary pharmacologic actions.
3. In subacute and chronic animal experiments, DMSO administered topically, subcutaneously, intravesically, intramuscularly, intraperitoneally, orally, into the eye, and into the mucous membrane is generally well tolerated.
4. Clinical studies were temporarily terminated in the United States in November of 1965, after it was reported that lenticular changes occurred in lower animals. This effect has not been seen in man.
5. DMSO has demonstrated clinical usefulness in treating musculoskeletal diseases, urologic inflammations, and microbial infections, serving as an adjunct.
6. In the United States, DMSO has been approved as a veterinary drug since 1970, and it was recently (1978) approved in humans for the treatment of interstitial cystitis.
7. The history of DMSO's trials and tribulations on the way to even limited FDA approval illustrates the tortuous route that such agents have to traverse under the current regulatory system.

References

Ashwood-Smith, M.J.: Radioprotective and cryoprotective properties of dimethyl sulfoxide in cellular systems. Ann. NY Acad. Sci. 141:45, 1967.

Berliner, D.L., and Ruhrman, A.G.: The influence of dimethyl sulfoxide on fibroblastic proliferation. Ann. NY Acad. Sci. 141:159, 1967.

Brobyn, R.B.: The human toxicology of dimethyl sulfoxide. Ann. NY Acad. Sci. 243:497, 1975.

Brown, J.H.: A double-blind clinical study–DMSO for acute injuries and inflammations compared to accepted therapy. Curr. Ther. Res. 13:536, 1971.

Brown, V.K., Robinson, J., and Stevenson, D.E.: A note on the toxicity and solvent properties of dimethyl sulfoxide. J. Pharm. Pharmacol. 15:688, 1963.

Demos, C.H., Beckloff, G.L., Donin, M.N., and Oliver, P.M.: Dimethyl sulfoxide in musculoskeletal disorders. Ann. NY Acad. Sci. 141:517, 1967.

Denko, C.W., Goodman, R.M., Miller, R., and Donavan, T.: Distribution of dimethylsulfoxide-35S in the rat. Ann. NY Acad. Sci. 141:77, 1967.

De la Torre, J.C., Kawanaga, H.M., Rowed, D.W., Johnson, C.M., Goode, D.J., Kajihara, K., and Mullan, S.: Dimethylsulfoxide in central nervous system trauma. Ann. NY Acad. Sci. 243:362, 1975.

Ehrlich, G.E., and Joseph, R.: Dimethyl sulfoxide in scleroderma. Penn. Med. J. 68:51, 1965.

Engel, M.F.: Indications and contraindications for the use of DMSO in clinical dermatology. Ann. NY Acad. Sci. 141:638, 1967.

Engel, M.F.: Dimethylsulfoxide in the treatment of scleroderma. South Med. J. 65 (1):71, 1972.

Feldman, W.E., Punch, J.D., and Holden, P.C.: In vivo and in vitro effects of dimethyl sulfoxide on streptomycin-sensitive and resistant Escherichia coli. Ann. NY Acad. Sci. 243:269, 1975.

Finney, J. W., Urschel, H.C., Bolla, G.A., Race, G.J., Jay, B.E., Pingree, H.P., Dorman, H.L., and Mallams, J.T.: Protection of the ischemic heart with DMSO alone or DMSO with hydrogen peroxide. Ann. NY Acad. Sci. 141:231, 1967.

Franz, T.J., and Van Bruggen, J.J.: A possible mechanism of action of DMSO. Ann. NY Acad. Sci. 141:302, 1967.

Frommhold, W., Bublitz, G., and Gries, G.: The use of DMSO for the treatment of postirradiation subcutaneous plaques. Ann. NY Acad. Sci. 141:603, 1967.

Gerhards, E., and Gibian, H.: The metabolism of dimethyl sulfoxide and its metabolic effects in man and animals. Ann. NY Acad. Sci. 141:65, 1967.

Görög, P., and Kovacs, I.B.: Effects of topically applied dimethyl sulfoxide. Ann. NY Acad. Sci. 243:91, 1975.

Hägglund, E.K.M., and Enkvist, T.U.E.: Method of improving the yield of methyl sulfide obtained by heating waste liquors from cellulose manufacture by adding inorganic sulfides. U.S. Patent Office No. 2,711,430, June 21, 1955.

Herschler, R.J., and Jacob, S.W.: A new drug from lignin. TAPPI 48:43, 1965.

Jacob, S.W., Bischel, M., and Herschler, R.J.: Dimethyl sulfoxide (DMSO): a new concept in pharmacotherapy. Curr. Ther. Res. 6:134, 1964.

Jacob, S.W., Bischel, M., and Herschler, R.J.: Dimethylsulfoxide: Effects on the permeability of biologic membranes (preliminary report). Curr. Ther. Res. 6:193, 1964.

Jacob, S.W., Bischel, M.G., Eberle, G.A., and Herschler, R.J.: The influence of dimethylsulfoxide on the transport of insulin across a biologic membrane. Fed. Proc. 23:410, 1964.

Jacob, S.W., Rosenbaum, E.R., and Wood, D.C.: *Dimethyl Sulfoxide, Basic concepts of DMSO* (Vol. 1). New York, Marcel Dekker, Inc., 1971.

John, H.: Therapautische Erfahrungen mit Dimethylsulfoxyd in der orthopadischen Praxis. Arzneim. Forsch. 15:1298, 1965.

John, H., and Laudahn, G.: Clinical experiences with the topical application of DMSO in orthopedic diseases: evaluation of 4180 cases. Ann. NY Acad. Sci. 141:506, 1967.

Juel-Jensen, B.E., MacCallum, F.O., Mackenzie, A.M.R., and Pike, M.C.: Treatment of zoster with idoxuridine in dimethyl sulphoxide. Br. Med. J. 4:776, 1970.

Kappert, A.: Experimental and clinical evaluation of topical dimethyl sulfoxide in venous disorders of the extremities. Ann. NY Acad. Sci. 243:403, 1975.

Katz, R., and Hood, R.W.: Topical thiabendazole for creeping eruption. Arch. Dermatol. 94:643, 1966.

Kocsis, J.J., Harkaway, S., and Snyder, R.: Biological effects of the metabolites of dimethyl sulfoxide. Ann. NY Acad. Sci. 243:104, 1975.

Kolb, K.H., Janicke, G., Kramer, M., and Schulze, P.E.: Absorption, distribution and elimination of labeled dimethyl sulfoxide in man and animals. Ann. NY Acad. Sci. 141:85, 1967.

Kunze, M.: Production of interferon in the white mouse by dimethyl sulfoxide. Ann. NY Acad. Sci. 243:308, 1975.

Lackey, H.B., Jacob, S.W., and Herschler, R.J.: Purification of dialkyl sulfoxides. Belgian Patent No. 656,879, June 9, 1965.

Lim, R., and Mullan, S.: Enhancement of resistance of glial cells by dimethyl sulfoxide against sonic disruption. Ann. NY Acad. Sci. 243:358, 1975.

Mallach, H.J.: Interaction of DMSO and alcohol. Ann. NY Acad. Sci. 141:457, 1967.

Matsumoto, J.: Clinical trials of dimethyl sulfoxide in rheumatoid arthritis patients in Japan. Ann. NY Acad. Sci. 141:560, 1967.

National Academy of Sciences-National Research Council, Contract FDA 70-22, Task Order No. 14: Dimethyl sulfoxide as a therapeutic agent. 1974.

Paul, M.M.: Interval therapy with dimethyl sulfoxide. Ann. NY Acad. Sci. 141:586, 1967.

Persky, L., and Stewart, B.H.: The use of dimethyl sulfoxide in the treatment of genitourinary disorders. Ann. NY Acad. Sci. 141:551, 1967.

Peterson, C.G., and Robertson, R.D.: A pharmacodynamic study of dimethyl sulfoxide. Ann. NY Acad. Sci. 141:273, 1967.

Rubin, L.F., and Mattis, F.A.: Dimethylsulfoxide: lens changes in dogs during oral administration. Science 153:83, 1966.

Sams, Jr., W.M.: The effects of dimethyl sulfoxide on nerve conduction. Ann. NY Acad. Sci. 141:242, 1967.

Scherbel, A.L., McCormack, L.J., and Poppo, M.J.: Alteration of collagen in generalized scleroderma after treatment with dimethylsulfoxide. Cleveland Clinic Quart. 32:47, 1965.

Scherbel, A.L.: Further observations on the effect of DMSO on patients with generalized scleroderma. *DMSO Symposium*. Vienna, Schering, 1966.

Scherbel, A.L., McCormack, L.J., and Layle, J.K.: Further observations on the effect of dimethyl sulfoxide in patients with generalized scleroderma. Ann. NY Acad. Sci. 141:613, 1967.

Seibert, F.B., Farrelly, F.K., and Shephard, C.C.: DMSO and other combatants against bacteria isolated from leukemia and cancer patients. Ann. NY Acad. Sci. 141:175, 1967.

Sergayev, V.P., and Zakiev, R.Z.: Treatment of scleroderma with dimethyl sulfoxide. Vestn. Dermatol. Venerol. 1976 (3):70, 1976.

Shealy, C.N.: The physiological substrate of pain. Headache 6:101, 1966.

Shlafer, M., and Karow, Jr., A.M.: Pharmacological effects of dimethyl sulfoxide on the mammalian myocardium. Ann. NY Acad. Sci. 243:110, 1975.

Smith, G.C.: Observations in treating cutaneous larva migrans. J. SC Med. Assoc. 62:265, 1966.

Sommer, S., and Tauberger, G.: Toxicologic investigations of dimethyl sulfoxide. Arzneim. Forsch. 14:1050, 1964.

Stewart, B.H., Branson, A.C., Hewitt, C.B., Kiser, W.S., and Straffon, R.A.: The treatment of patients with special reference to intravesical DMSO. J. Urol. 107:377, 1972.

Stewart, B.H., and Shirley, S.W.: Further experience with intravesical dimethyl sulfoxide in treatment of interstitial cystitis. J. Urol. 116 (1):36, 1976.

Tuffanelli, D.L.: A clinical trial with dimethylsulfoxide in scleroderma. Arch. Dermatol. 93:724, 1966.

Ward, J.R., Miller, M.L., and Marcus, S.: The effect of dimethyl sulfoxide on the local Shwartzman phenomena. Ann. NY Acad. Sci. 141:280, 1967.

Warren, J., Sackisteder, M.R., Jarosz, H., Wasserman, B., and Andreotti, P.E.: Potentiation of antineoplastic compounds by oral dimethyl sulfoxide in tumor-bearing rats. Ann. NY Acad. Sci. 243:194, 1975.

Weissman, G., Sessa, G., and Bevans, V.: Effect of DMSO on the stabilization of lysosomes by cortisone and chloroquine in vitro. Ann. NY Acad. Sci. 141:326, 1967.

Williams, K.I., Burstein, S.H., and Layne, D.S.: Dimethyl sulfone—isolated from human urine. Arch. Biochem. Biophys. 113:251, 1966.

Willson, J.E., Brown, D.E., and Timmens, E.K.: A toxicological study of dimethylsulfoxide. Toxicol. Appl. Pharmacol. 7:104, 1965.

Yorio, T., and Bentley, P.J.: The effects of hyperosmotic agents on the electrical properties of the amphibian lens in vitro. Exp. Eye Res. 22 (3):195, 1976.

25

Should Physician Prescribing Be Monitored and Controlled?

MONITORING AND CONTROL OF PHYSICIAN PRESCRIBING ARE NEEDED

Daniel L. Azarnoff, M.D.

NEW CONTROLS ON PHYSICIAN PRESCRIBING ARE NOT NEEDED

James H. Sammons, M.D.

Medicines are nothing in themselves if not properly used, but the very hands of the gods, if employed with reason and prudence.

Herophilus

You know that medicines when well used restore health to the sick . . .

Leonardo da Vinci, *Codice Atlantico*

Thou speak'st like a physician, Helicanus,
That ministers a potion unto me
That thou wouldst tremble to receive thyself.

Shakespeare, *Pericles*

Among the perils of disease we must not refuse to reckon the errors of physicians . . . .

Peter Mere Latham, *General Remarks on the Practice of Medicine*

Introduction

Physicians are often accused these days of improper prescribing. As a logical consequence, there has been a call, in some quarters, for systematic monitoring and control of prescribing behavior.

Azarnoff urges that the profession mend its own ways before nonprofessional controls are imposed. He sees no reason to assume that an M.D. degree provides an unlimited privilege to prescribe any and all drugs, and in support of this concern, he cites a series of studies that suggest deficiencies in the performance of doctors. One of the problems in evaluating these studies is that many of them are subject to a variety of interpretations.

Access of patients to hospitals in the United States and Scotland, for instance, is probably substantially different, and the available data do not allow one to judge whether the different rates of prescribing may be thus explained, at least in part. Nor is it possible to say anything with confidence about the overall therapeutic outcomes in the two countries. (Indeed, it is pathetic that no one can really say whether a country with tighter controls on drug usage fares any better than one with looser controls, or vice versa.)

The chloramphenicol story is also tricky. Except for aplastic anemia and the "gray baby" syndrome, chloramphenicol is almost a perfect antibiotic. It rarely produces gastrointestinal complaints or rashes, and it is not particularly expensive. Yet it has, for most academicians, a "toxic drug" image, whereas the same is not true for penicillin (which can cause death due to anaphylactic shock) or other broad spectrum antibiotics (which can be fatal by causing acute pseudomembranous enterocolitis). In evaluating the prescribing of a drug like chloramphenicol, one has to consider not only instances in which it should not be prescribed at all (because it would not produce any benefit) but also those in which other antibiotics would be equally advantageous. In the latter situation, we need a balance sheet to provide a view of the available alternatives and an unbiased look at the costs and risks of each, remembering that even experts disagree about "the drug of choice" in many instances.

It is important to keep in mind the goals of control programs. Some of these programs are aimed primarily at containing fiscal costs. This is not necessarily the same as optimizing quality of use, and we must be sure that the differences are kept clearly in mind.

I confess to a certain confusion when people put out lists of 100 or 200 "essential drugs." It is no doubt true that one can practice medicine with this number of drugs, but those of us who have spent considerable time in university hospitals, as well as those who are consultants to physicians in community outpatient programs, are often grateful for the availability of other, more rarely indicated drugs. As Azarnoff points out, it is important to insure that patients are not deprived of such drugs when they need them.

Sammons contends that doctors are overly maligned, and he reminds us that the use of drugs is not exactly uncontrolled at present. He also stresses the need for treating patients as individuals and not in "cookbook" style. The latter is surely one of the greatest fears of those who question either the practicality or the wisdom of any form of central bureaucratic control. The fear of imperilled confidentiality of patients' records is also real; no one can afford to feel complacent about electronic data processing that is available to the eyes of governmental (or other) snoopers.

Louis Lasagna, M.D.

Monitoring and Control of Physician Prescribing Are Needed

Daniel L. Azarnoff, M.D.
University of Kansas Medical Center, Kansas City

When physicians are licensed to practice medicine, they are granted certain privileges, including the authority to prescribe any and all marketed drugs for approved or unapproved indications in whatever doses they believe to be appropriate. Almost all physicians utilize this privilege; some do so quite extensively. The average practitioner writes approximately 8000 prescriptions per year. Two of every three patients entering a physician's office will receive at least one prescription (Stolley et al., 1972). On the other hand, there are very few other privileges the physician could or would undertake without further training and certification—e.g., surgery. Does a medical degree qualify a physician to prescribe drugs? Indeed, does an internship, residency, or fellowship in any medical speciality provide sufficient training to qualify physicians to prescribe any and all drugs? I believe not. Because this latitude has been granted to all physicians without regard to qualifications and ability, and without monitors and controls, significant problems in drug utilization, which are detrimental to the patient, have arisen.

The Task Force on Prescription Drugs (1969) concluded:

> . . . few practicing physicians seem inclined to voice any question on their competency in this field of therapeutic judgments. We also find, however, that the ability of an individual physician to make sound judgments under quite confusing conditions is a matter of serious concern to leading clinicians, scientists and medical educators.

These conclusions were based on the opinions of medical experts in drug usage. Unfortunately, facts were not provided to document their opinions, and I provide, therefore, evidence that I believe to be substantiating.

Inappropriate Prescribing

It has been estimated from pharmaceutical production figures that there has been a doubling of drug usage in the past decade (Department of Health, Education and Welfare, 1976). I doubt that anyone would state that patients have become twice as healthy. One must wonder if there has been even a 10 or 20 percent improvement in health or in the patients' feeling of well-being. We do know, however, that there has been a significant increase in the cost of drug usage.

Inappropriate prescribing may be divided into four major types: over-prescribing, under-prescribing, incorrect prescribing, and multiple prescribing (Council of Europe, European Public Health Community, 1976).

Over-Prescribing

American physicians prescribe four times as many drugs for hospitalized patients as do Scottish physicians (Lawson and Jick, 1976). Although the incidence of adverse reactions per dose of drugs was the same in both countries, total incidence of adverse reactions was significantly greater in the American patients because of the greater use of the drugs. Data on the outcomes of treatment are not available, but there is no reason to believe that the Scottish patients fare any worse than their American counterparts. In addition to prescribing an excessive number of drugs, American physicians may also prescribe an excessive amount of drug per prescription. Even if the latter is not detrimental to the patient *per se,* it certainly is costly (Maronde et al., 1971).

Incorrect Prescribing

Incorrect prescribing of drugs is probably the most common prescribing error. The authors of a study of the quality of general practice in North Carolina concluded that the quality of drug therapy was less than it should be (Peterson et al., 1956). It is also not easy to believe that physicians prescribe rationally when the drug efficacy study panels of the National Research Council (NRC) eliminated as "ineffective" some 400 drug products regularly used by physicians. Even today, many other drugs evaluated as only "possibly effective" are still being used by large numbers of physicians.

Antibiotics are the drugs whose use by physicians has been most frequently evaluated. Although criteria may be established for rational antibiotic use, at times even expert consultants cannot agree on proper drugs, indications, or length of treatment. Recently, however, an excellent set of guidelines was developed (Veterans Administration Ad Hoc Interdisciplinary Committee on Antimicrobial Drug Usage, 1977), and it can be used to evaluate appropriateness of antibiotic utilization.

As pointed out by the Committee on Drugs of the American Academy of Pediatrics, there are virtually no indications for the use of tetracyclines in children less than eight years old. Yet, in a recent survey of a two-year period (1973 to 1975) in a Tennessee Medicaid program, it was found that 7 percent of children in this age group received tetracycline, which was prescribed by 27 percent of the 1947 participating physicians. Over 50 percent of these inappropriate prescriptions were written by 5 percent of the physicians. The family practitioner was the most common offender; the pediatrician was the least common. In all medical specialties, a prescription for tetracycline was more likely to be written for the under-eight age group if the physician was in rural practice. Recent graduates from medical school were less likely than earlier graduates to prescribe tetracycline incorrectly (Ray, Federspiel, and Schaffner, 1977).

A study of 50 randomly selected charts from one week in June 1973, at a well known university medical center, showed that 56 courses of antibiotics were given (Castle et al., 1977). Of 17 courses of antibiotics given for infection to patients on medical services, 81 percent were considered appropriate, whereas only 7 percent of 39 courses given to 22 surgical patients for prophylaxis were considered appropriate. Of all the prescriptions for antibiotics, 63 percent were considered not indicated, inappropriately selected, or given in inappropriate doses.

Misuse of chloramphenicol has been particularly common, considering the educational efforts that have been made to curb irrational prescribing (Best, 1967; Becker et al., 1972; Stolley et al, 1972; Ray, Federspiel, and Schaffner, 1976). In a recent study made during a one-year period, 6 percent of 3409 physicians prescribed chloramphenicol for outpatients (Ray, Federspiel, and Schaffner, 1976). Twenty-one percent of the rural family practitioners prescribed the drug on this basis. These statistics alone do not support my contention that physicians prescribe inappropriately. Therefore, consider that it is generally agreed that chloramphenicol should be used almost exclusively in hospitalized patients with severe infections—and that of 992 ambulatory patients who received chloramphenicol, over half took it for treatment of upper respiratory infections, a disorder not considered an indication for the use of this potentially quite dangerous antibiotic. In addition, over half the patients receiving prescriptions for chloramphenicol received 6 gm or less, an amount inadequate for appropriate therapy of *any* indicated infection.

These physicians were not a random sample of all physicians. However, if the remaining 99 percent of physicians in this country prescribe in essentially the same way, approximately 100,000 patients per year would have been unnecessarily exposed to the hazards of chloramphenicol. It has been estimated that aplastic anemia occurs in 1 of 20,000 to 1 of 30,000 patients receiving chloramphenicol. Thus, three to five patients per year would have needlessly developed a potentially fatal disease.

Approximately 60 percent of patients with the "common cold" were observed to have received antibiotics in one study (National Disease and Therapeutic Index, 1967-1968). We are all aware that antibiotics are not indicated, nor are they of benefit, for a viral disease. In a review of these data, Stolley and Lasagna (1969) hedged on the appropriateness of this prescribing practice by stating that they did not know how many of the patients had bacterial complications. In a recent controlled trial, antibiotics did not alter the course of illness in patients with upper respiratory infections even when their cough was associated with purulent sputum (Stott and West, 1976). These data support the thesis that antibiotics are used inappropriately in patients with this illness. The authors of another survey reported that in 340 patients, antibiotic use was irrational in 66 percent and questionable in another 21 percent (Roberts and Visconti, 1972). Even more disturbing is that in another study, 62 percent of 1608 patients receiving antibiotics were considered to have no evidence of infection (Scheckler and Bennett, 1970).

Although other examples of inappropriate use of antibiotics are available (Kunin, 1973; Simon et al., 1975; Achong, Hauser, and Krusky, 1977), we should not believe that this is the only class of drugs that is misused. For example, I find it difficult to believe that the 3 percent of prescriptions written for amphetamines in one survey (Stolley et al., 1972) were all for acceptable indications. Diethylstilbestrol was used to prevent miscarriages for many years after it was shown to be ineffective for this indication (Dieckmann et al., 1953), and it would probably still be used today if its carcinogenic potential in the offspring of women receiving it had not been demonstrated (Herbst et al., 1975). Although there is controversy as to whether tolbutamide increases cardiovascular mortality in maturity onset diabetics, the evidence, in my opinion, is reasonably good that neither tolbutamide nor insulin reduces mortality (The University Group Diabetes Program, 1970). Similarly, these drugs do not reduce the morbidity associated with the eyes, the kidneys, or the nervous and cardiovascular systems (Miller et al., 1976) of patients with this disease. Yet physicians continue to prescribe sulfonylureas in ever increasing amounts.

The Coronary Drug Project Group (1975) has published results that make it clear that clofibrate has no effect in preventing further infarctions when given to males who have sustained one or more myocardial infarctions. In the same study, it was demonstrated that the use of this drug also increased the incidence of cholelithiasis, pulmonary emboli, and a variety of other adverse reactions. But do you doubt that clofibrate is still being prescribed for a number of males with previous myocardial infarctions?

The incidence of toxicity from phenylbutazone is greater in individuals above age 40 than in younger patients. In a recent survey (Crosby, 1977), over two thirds of patients receiving phenylbutazone or oxyphenbutazone were above this age. Indeed, one third of the use was in patients over the age of 60. In the latter group, therapy with these agents should be limited to a week in duration; yet the average use was for approximately two weeks. Thus, physicians use these drugs predominantly in the group most susceptible to the toxic effects, even though other effective, less toxic agents are available.

Multiple Prescribing

In a review of prescribing practices in a university medical service, it was noted that of 254 patients receiving spironolactone, 104 were also receiving oral potassium chloride (Simborg, 1976). This combination of drugs frequently has deleterious effects on the patient. The author then reviewed 25 charts and found that seven patients receiving both drugs had a serum potassium equal to or greater than 6.0 mEq/L, and another six had levels between 5 and 6 mEq/L. Two patients even required polystyrene sulfonate therapy for their hyperkalemia.

Physicians with any understanding at all of the pharmacologic action of spironolactone should realize that a potentially fatal drug-drug interaction can occur when these drugs are given concomitantly. It is even more disconcerting when one considers that the consequences of this interaction have been published in a journal widely read by many physicians (Greenblatt and Koch-Weser, 1973). If misuse of drugs occurs at teaching institutions that have strong peer review and supervision, what is happening in less well supervised situations, since the quality of hospital care is reported to be far superior to office-based (ambulatory) care (Brook, 1974)?

It is not necessary to continue the litany of examples of inappropriate prescribing. I do not deny that we cannot quantitate prescribing behavior totally satisfactorily, but it must at least be conceded that prescribing by most of us is in need of improvement. These observations do not mean that physicians are ignorant, unconcerned, or negligent about drug therapy. However, for a variety of reasons, physicians have not kept abreast of the latest knowledge in rational prescribing practices, and some have lagged considerably further behind the vast majority.

Since all effective drugs have inherent hazards, unnecessary or inappropriate use is unwarranted and must be eliminated.

Control of Prescribing

If the drug utilization of even a small proportion of physicians is inappropriate, how can we control their prescribing behavior? We can either regulate the prescribers (occasionally the dispensers) by fiat, or we can attempt to modify their behavior through teaching programs. The ideal system for control of irrational prescribing should be voluntary, based on changes brought about by education. Becker et al. (1972) have provided evidence supporting the concept that prescribing patterns are largely determined by educational experiences. Obviously, at this point it is only appropriate to underscore the importance of strong clinical pharmacology programs at all medical schools and the need for continuing postgraduate education in therapeutics. In general, one's own practice does not teach a great deal about therapeutics. In my experience, the poor prescriber is unaware of his deficiencies, or if aware, is reluctant to seek consultation. How then do we educate a poor prescriber?

Some information exists about the effectiveness of education in altering prescribing behavior. A successful program for the housestaff at a Montreal hospital reduced the incidence of digitalis toxicity from 21.4 to 12.3 percent over a two-year period by simply stressing the importance of body weight and renal function in prescribing a loading and maintenance dose of digoxin (Ogilvie and Ruedy, 1972). In general, however, educational programs designed to correct irrational drug use have not been particularly successful. Although one program on errors of prescribing antibiotics in a university-affiliated Veterans Hospital decreased the cost of unjustified antibiotic use, little noticeable effect on specific prescribing errors was observed as a result of the program (Jones et al., 1977). The knowledge of 4513 physicians about antibiotics was determined before and after a national television educational program (Nell and Howrey, 1975). Their overall score on a 50-question test was only 68 percent correct. Even though the score increased from 55 percent on the preteaching test to 71 percent on the postteaching test, important therapeutic information was not gained. For example, 26 percent selected oxacillin or cloxacillin in the posttest for treatment of a staphylococcal infection in a child allergic to penicillin, even after a discussion of the cross antigenicity of the various penicillins. As I pointed out, the continued unwarranted use of chloramphenicol after extensive educational efforts to improve prescribing patterns of this drug makes one wonder if education of the practicing physician is effective, particularly when counteracted by advertising and educational programs sponsored by pharmaceutical companies.

On the other hand, requiring an informal consultation with an infectious disease expert before prescribing antibiotics did substantially decrease unwarranted use of some drugs. This method has the advantage that it does not prevent the attending physician from making the decision and at least theoretically provides him with the most recent information (McGowan and Finland, 1974).

CURRENT CONTROLS

Voluntarily and otherwise, physician prescribing is already regulated in a variety of ways. These constraints include cost containment, restricted formularies, Food and Drug Administration (FDA) and Drug Enforcement Agency regulations, and, in some states, modification of antisubstitution statutes.

Cost Containment

Prescribing excessive amounts of any drug is also considered irrational prescribing (Maronde et al, 1971). The result is not only excessive cost but also increases in accidental and intentional overdosages as well as unsupervised use of the extra drug by the patient, a relative, or a friend for what may erroneously be considered the same disorder as that for which the drug was initially prescribed. The Task Force on Prescription Drugs (1969) estimated that this type of prescribing error increases our drug bills approximately 3 to 12 percent. For a several billion dollar drug bill, this is a great deal of money, even in a country with a one trillion dollar gross national product. Definitive data from computerized drug dispensing systems for ambulatory patient populations have corroborated this opinion (Maronde et al., 1971; Egdahl, 1973).

In some states, selection of the drug product by the pharmacist is now allowed, unless specifically prohibited by the physician. This control may provide a modicum of cost containment, but it certainly does not influence irrational prescribing.

Another type of control, present in 1975 in 33 states, specified maximum quantities that could be dispensed on drug prescriptions paid for by Medicaid. Thirty-one states and some federal agencies that sponsored programs, such as the Department of Defense and the Veterans Administration, specified the number of allowable refills. Morgan (1977) reviewed the methods of one drug utilization review group, PAID, and concluded that the purpose of the review is primarily to decrease costs rather than to determine if the selection was in patient's best interests. It has also been pointed out by Knoben (1976) that existing drug utilization review systems utilize quantity rather than quality standards and also are retrospective. If such reviews are retrospective, control of physicians' prescribing can only be attained by educational programs that are successful or by regulations that dictate how physicians are to prescribe. Any drug utilization review process should not concern itself only with quantity and cost. However, the task becomes exceedingly difficult with our current methods if quality of prescribing is also to be included.

Formularies

Another means of control depends on the use of a restricted formulary. For example, benefits for drugs are paid by the United Mine Workers of America Health and Retirement Fund (1977) only if the drug is on a list of basic drugs prepared by panels of experts assembled by the United States Pharmacopoeia (USP).

Hospitals are required to have pharmacy and therapeutics committees for accreditation. Many such committees have developed local formularies that are accepted by physicians. (Physicians abide by restricted formularies because they normally control the pharmacy and therapeutics committees and because most hospitals will obtain a drug not in the formulary if the physician demonstrates special need for it.) In general, a brand of a generically equivalent drug product is selected for use in the specific hospital. Committees seldom make decisions regarding the relative efficacy of therapeutically similar but not generically equivalent products. In their defense, it must be acknowledged that few studies are available on relative efficacy. Thus, such decisions become a matter of local preference and opinion rather than decisions based on facts. I believe enough data are available, however, to restrict formularies to reasonably rational selections. Criteria for such selections were published recently by an expert committee of the World Health Organization (WHO) (1977).

The number of drugs in such a formulary may vary from 100 to 1600. Several countries already have national formularies. Controls imposed by formularies do not guarantee that the physician will use the available drugs rationally, but at least they restrict his use of questionably useful drugs. If only local formularies are used, concern has been voiced about the development of widely differing standards among regions and the perpetuation of poor prescribing habits. If such concerns are legitimate, a national advisory council could be appointed to set national standards. If this mechanism were to be used for control, a Physicians Service Review Organization (PSRO) Council, the USP, or another group representing all medical specialities could be utilized. Regional PSRO groups could also carry out drug utilization reviews under national guidelines. The Joint Commission on Hospital Accreditation already requires hospitals to develop and undertake reviews of local antibiotic usage.

Agency Regulations

Some European countries limit the authority to prescribe or to administer unusually toxic drugs to physicians with specialized training. To my knowledge, an evaluation to determine whether this level of control alters drug utilization or efficacy has not been done. The FDA has tried similar controls on a voluntary basis. For example, at one time it recommended that tranylcypromine be used for depression only by psychiatrists and methotrexate for psoriasis only by dermatologists. The FDA currently does not have the statutory authority to force such restrictions on physicians. However, in the

FDA/HEW draft of the Drug Regulation Reform Act of 1978, the government is seeking legislation that would allow it to restrict the use of drugs to settings of its own selection for as long as it wishes. Under these proposed changes in the Food, Drug and Cosmetic laws, the FDA could direct where a drug could be used, indications for use, how many doses could be dispensed, and how often the prescription could be refilled. Severe criminal penalties would be imposed for noncompliance. At present, once a drug is marketed, physicians may use it for an individual patient however they deem best, regardless of what is stated on the official label.

Most drugs prescribed today were not available when many of us were in medical school. How have we learned to use these agents? Drug company literature (advertising and detail men) would be my first guess. To assure that at least the prescribers are cognizant of the important therapeutic facts about a drug, they could be required to pass an examination before being allowed to prescribe any new drug or drug for which they were not qualified, by specialty training, to prescribe. Knowledge, unfortunately, is not always translated into practice. Another obvious drawback to this proposal is that any type of prescribing restrictions could adversely affect the patient who needs a specific drug but does not live where there is a locally qualified prescriber. In this instance, emergency permission could be provided after telephone consultation with a regional or national expert. Several countries (Great Britain, Australia, New Zealand, Sweden, Norway) provide all physicians with prescribing guidelines (prepared by panels of independent medical experts) that are widely accepted by the medical profession. Physician prescribing in these countries is monitored, since all prescriptions are recorded in a regional or national computer. A government medical representative visits those physicians whose prescribing appears irrational to discuss the reasons and to suggest corrective measures. In Australia and Great Britain, visits are scheduled only when the cost of the drugs prescribed by a physician appears unusually high.

Although we live in a free society, we all submit to regulation of various types—presumably for the good of the public. However, regulation of any type of behavior carries risks. My major concerns would be that the regulator's decisions were incorrect and would perpetuate irrational therapy, such as leeching and purging did as the accepted therapeutic dogma of their day. In addition, restrictive regulations imposed improperly would stifle therapeutic innovation.

Conclusions

Evidence shows that the prescribing techniques of a significant number of physicians could be improved. As a result I recommend that:

1. Methods be developed that would initially evaluate the process of physician prescribing, but, in time, would also evaluate quality and outcome thereof.
2. The initial review be concerned primarily with drugs that have the greatest potential for misuse.
3. Physicians who prescribe these drugs most and least frequently (5 percent at each end, corrected for type of practice) be further evaluated by visiting physicians who are experts in therapeutics.
4. Those prescribers deemed inappropriate be required to participate in educational programs aimed at correcting their deficiencies. If these programs do not correct their deficiencies, these prescribers should be required to obtain consultation before prescribing the drug in question.
5. Pilot studies be undertaken to determine if restricted formularies alter outcome. If it can be demonstrated that the patient is benefited by their use, preparation of a national formulary should be given serious consideration.

I am well aware that these recommendations are fraught with difficulties, and that monitoring and remedial activities will add to the cost of drug utilization. However, the signs are quite clear. We as physicians must either regulate our own prescribing or it will be regulated for us, probably in an unpalatable manner. The privilege to prescribe may even be given to others, such as the clinical pharmacist. I prefer the regulation to be voluntary and to come from within our profession.

References

Achong, M.R., Hauser, B.A., and Krusky, J.L.: Rational and irrational use of antibiotics in a Canadian teaching hospital. Can. Med. Assoc. J. 116:256, 1977.

Becker, M.H., Stolley, P.D., Lasagna, L., McEvilla, J.D., and Sloane, L.M.: Characteristics and attitudes of physicians associated with the prescribing of chloramphenicol. HSMHA Health Rep. 86:993, 1971.

Becker, M.H., Stolley, P.D., Lasagna, L., McEvilla, J.D., and Sloane, L.M.: Differential education concerning therapeutics and resultant physician prescribing patterns. J. Med. Educ. 47:118, 1972.

Best, W.R.: Chloramphenicol-associated blood dyscrasias. JAMA 201:181, 1967.

Brook, R.H.: Quality of care assessment. A comparison of five methods of peer review. DHEW L-HRA-74-3100, Washington, D.C., U.S. Government Printing Office, 1974.

Castle, M., Wilfert, C.M., Cate, T.R., and Osterhout, S.: Antibiotic use at Duke University Medical Center. JAMA 237:2819, 1977.

Coronary Drug Project Research Group: Clofibrate and niacin in coronary heart disease. JAMA 231:360, 1975.

Council of Europe, European Public Health Community, Report by Working Party, 1975: Abuses of medicines. II, Prescription medicines. Drug Intel. Clin. Pharm. 10:94, 1976.

Crosby, D.L.: Personal Communication, 1977.

Department of Health, Education and Welfare: Health in the United States (1975). (HRA) 76-1233, Washington, D.C., U.S. Government Printing Office, 1976.

Dieckmann, W.J., Davis, M.E., Rynkiewicz, L.M., and Pottinger, R.E.: Does the administration of diethylstilbestrol during pregnancy have therapeutic value? Am. J. Obstet. Gynecol. 66:1062, 1953.

Egdahl, R.H.: Foundations for medical care. N. Engl. J. Med. 288:291, 1973.

Greenblatt, D.J., and Koch-Weser, J.: Adverse reactions to spironolactone. JAMA 225:40, 1973.

Herbst, A.L., Poskanzer, D.C., Stanley, J.R., Friedlander, L., and Scully, R.E.: Prenatal exposure to stilbestrol. A prospective comparison of exposed female offspring with unexposed controls. N. Engl. J. Med. 292:334, 1975.

Jones, S.R., Pannell, J., Barks, J., Uanchick, V.A., Bratton, T., Brown, R., McKee, E., and Smith, J.W.: The effect of an educational program upon hospital antibiotic use. Am. J. Med. Sci. 273:79, 1977.

Knoben, J.E.: Current status and relationship to assessing quality control. Drug Intel. Clin. Pharm. 10:222, 1976.

Kunin, C.M.: Use of antibiotics. A brief exposition of the problem and some tentative solutions. Ann. Intern. Med. 79:555, 1973.

Lawson, D.H., and Jick, H.: Drug prescribing in hospitals. An international comparison. Am. J. Public Health 66:644, 1976.

Maronde, R.F., Lee, P.V., McCarron, M.M., and Seibert, S.: A study of prescribing patterns. Med. Care 9:383, 1971.

McGowan, J.E., Jr., and Finland, M.: Usage of antibiotics in a general hospital. J. Infect. Dis. 30:164, 1974.

Miller, M., Knatterud, G.L., Hawkins, B.S., and Newberry, W.B., Jr.: A study of the effects of hypoglycemic agents on vascular complications in patients with adult-onset diabetes. VI, Supplementary report on non-fatal events in patients treated with tolbutamide. Diabetes 25:1129, 1976.

Morgan, J.P.: Drug utilization review: watching the monitors. N. Engl. J. Med. 296:251, 1977.

National Disease and Therapeutic Index, Reference file: Diagnosis-common cold. Ambler, Pa., Lea Assoc. Inc., Oct. 1967–Sept. 1968.

Ogilvie, R.I., and Ruedy, J.: An educational program in digitalis therapy. JAMA 222:50, 1972.

Peterson, O.L., Andrews, L.P., Spain, R.S., and Greenberg, B.G.: An analytical study of North Carolina general practice 1953–1954. J. Med. Educ. 31:part 2, 1956.

Ray, W.A., Federspiel, C.F., and Schaffner, W.: Prescribing of chloramphenicol in ambulatory practice. An epidemiologic study among Tennessee medicaid recipients. Ann. Intern. Med. 84:266, 1976.

Ray, W.A., Federspiel, C.F., and Schaffner, W.: Prescribing of tetracycline to children less than 8 years old. JAMA 237:2069, 1977.

Roberts, A.W., and Visconti, J.A.: The rational and irrational use of systemic antibiotics. Am. J. Hosp. Pharm. 29:828, 1972.

Scheckler, W.E., and Bennett, J.V.: Antibiotic usage of seven community hospitals. JAMA 213:264, 1970.

Simborg, D.W.: Medication prescribing on a university medical service. The incidence of drug combinations with potential adverse interactions. Johns Hopkins Med. J. 139:23, 1976.

Simon, W.A., Thompson, L., Campbell, S., and Lantos, R.L.: Drug usage review and inventory analysis in promoting rational parenteral cephalosporin therapy. Am. J. Hosp. Pharm. 32:1116, 1975.

Stolley, P.D., and Lasagna, L.: Prescribing patterns of physicians. J. Chronic Dis. 22:395, 1969.
Stolley, P.D., Becker, M.H., Lasagna, L., McEvilla, J.D., and Sloane, L.M.: The relationship between physician characteristics and prescribing appropriateness. Med. Care 10:17, 1972.
Stolley, P.D., Becker, M.H., McEvilla, J.D., Lasagna, L., Gainor, M., and Sloane, L.M.: Drug prescribing and use in an American community. Ann. Intern. Med. 76:537, 1972.
Stott, N.C.H., and West R.R.: Randomized controlled trial of antibiotics in patients with cough and purulent sputum. Br. Med. J. 2:55, 1976.
Task Force on Prescription Drugs: Approaches to drug insurance design. Washington, D.C., U.S. Government Printing Office, 1969.
Task Force on Prescription Drugs.: Final report. Washington, D.C., U.S. Government Printing Office, 1969.
The University Group Diabetes Program. II, Mortality results. Diabetes 19 (Suppl. 2):789, 1970.
United Mine Workers of America Health and Retirement Funds: Basic Drug List, 2nd ed. Washington, D.C., 1977.
Veterans Administration Ad Hoc Interdisciplinary Committee on Antimicrobial Drug Usage: Guideline for peer review. JAMA 237:1001, 1241, 1355, 1481, 1605, 1723, 1859 and 1967, 1977.
World Health Organization Expert Committee: The selection of essential drugs. WHO Technical Report Series 615, Geneva, 1977.

New Controls on Physician Prescribing Are Not Needed

James H. Sammons, M.D.
Executive Vice President, American Medical Association

The Demand for Regulation

More significant breakthroughs in medical science have occurred in the last two decades than in any previous period in history. Although more and better services are being provided to the American people, concomitant cynicism about the ability of the medical profession to deliver services competently has emerged. In the field of drug usage, this concern has been highlighted in the public mind because of the development of new, more powerful therapeutic agents—agents that produce greater benefits but also are substantially more hazardous than ones used in the past.

As a result of this change in attitude, representatives from government, academia, and consumer groups have demanded greater monitoring and control of medical practice. Nowhere is the call for greater regulation more prominent than in the area of prescription drug usage, where a massive regulatory apparatus is already in existence.

When considering the need to monitor and control prescribing practices, one must first determine why such constraints are thought to be desirable. It is assumed that no one would advocate the development of large-scale reporting and regulatory systems for prescription drugs without compelling justification. Reasons for the demand of such programs are alleged to be irresponsible prescribing by physicians, misprescribing leading to severe adverse reactions and even fatalities, excessive delays in data collection on adverse drug reactions (e.g., those caused by phenformin), and a general public concern that drugs are being overused and that physicians are not adequately informing patients about proper drug usage or alternative modes of therapy.

Although specific examples to justify all these reasons can be cited, the truth is that the vast majority of prescribing by physicians in the United States is based upon sound scientific principles and rational clinical judgment. Reported studies on drug-related injuries and deaths are based on small samples that should not be extrapolated to represent national prescribing practices (Ballin, 1974). Yet, such limited results are often thus presented, increasing the public's undue fear and concern and causing commensurate loss of confidence in physicians and still louder calls for more governmental intervention. This problem has been well summarized in an editorial that appeared in the British Medical Journal (1977):

> No matter how carefully the clinical course is reviewed, it is often difficult or impossible to decide whether a particular patient died solely as a consequence of his or her underlying disorder or in part from the effects of drug administration. Good quality studies of the prevalence of drug-related deaths are rare and have usually been confined to highly selected areas: most have concerned medical in-patients in university hospitals—a select group of severely ill patients. Extrapolation to the whole range of hospital treatment from information based on such narrow observations is clearly unjustified and has been strongly condemned.

Several recent studies of drug-related deaths have found that about 1 per 1,000 medical inpatients die at least in part as a consequence of drug treatment. One of these studies came from the Boston Drug Surveillance Program and is of particular interest since it reviewed data from selected hospitals in seven countries. The message of this study is clear: most of the patients who died from drug therapy (in part at least) were suffering from severe, terminal illness such as cancer, leukaemia, pulmonary embolism, and cirrhosis. Viewed retrospectively, only six out of 24 deaths occurring in 26,500 consecutive patients could have been prevented, and in only three cases did death result from treatment of patients who otherwise were only mildly unhealthy. The prevalence of preventable deaths in this group of medical inpatients was 1 per 10,000 and the drugs responsible were predominantly intravenous fluids and potassium chloride.

The picture that emerges is, then, less serious than has been alleged. Few patients appear to die as a result of our therapeutic endeavours, and most of those who do, have been treated with powerful drugs given to delay the progress of otherwise fatal disorders. While it is important to remain vigilant, the problem of drug-related deaths has yet to become a public health issue and should be viewed in the light of the mortality arising in other types of human endeavour.

Are Regulations Applicable to Prescribing Drugs?

Two points must be made before discussing whether control and monitoring of prescription drug use will be a cureall for some or all the perceived ills already described. First, the practice of medicine, although based upon scientific discovery, techniques, and technologies, is still very much an art. Contrary to common belief, all treatment cannot be based upon well controlled clinical studies. All patients do not respond in the manner cited in textbooks. Furthermore, the conscientious physician does not make a diagnosis and simply rely on some type of formulary or on the pharmacist to determine which drug will be best for his particular patient at the time of the diagnosis. He not only uses reference materials but makes a professional judgment based upon his education and clinical experience, the scientific literature, comments of peers (in settings such as hospital review meetings), product labeling, and the patient's drug history. Secondly, it must be noted that when monitoring drug use and adverse drug reactions, the mere fact that they exist cannot be equated with misprescribing, negligence, or poor medical practice. By the very nature of drug therapy, different patients may respond differently to the same drug. Even the same patient may respond differently at different times. Also, a physician may knowingly prescribe a drug that is capable of producing a serious adverse reaction after determining that the benefits to be derived from the drug might outweigh the consequences of the adverse reaction. Therefore, any system or program to monitor and control the prescription of drugs must reflect the variable nature of the practice of medicine in individual patients under very different circumstances. Such programs, if developed, should not be a modality that limits options in the treatment of the patient or that regiments the practice of medicine to meet some theoretical nationwide standards. Such constraints would constitute a disservice to the patient.

Monitoring Drug Usage

The organized medical profession has continued to support appropriate systems and programs for monitoring prescribing practices in order to determine the frequency of unexpected, severe reactions caused by drugs. Such programs have been voluntary, and although they do not have the force and effect of law, they have had the advantage of being flexible. In retrospect, the achievements of these voluntary programs have been notable. No reputable hospital in the nation operates without a continuing program of physician review and education concerning drug usage. Regular audits of charts and peer review of unusual cases, along with periodic staff meetings, provide a means of analyzing and developing information on the proper use of drugs. These routines, along with those conducted by Professional Standards Review Organizations (PSRO), are intended to insure that the care provided is necessary, appropriate, and carried out according to professionally developed standards. Furthermore, many physicians, on an ad hoc and voluntary basis, report significant adverse drug reactions to appropriate authorities for further analysis and dissemination. Also, a significant number of physicians regularly publish information on their experience with drugs in the scientific literature. Commercial ventures (e.g., the National Disease and Therapeutic Index) have also been developed to survey prescribing patterns and drug usage, and these fulfill a useful function.

Yet with all these existing mechanisms for

voluntary drug monitoring, there has still been a plethora of additional proposals for mandatory monitoring of drug use by the federal government. Members of Congress, medical and other health care professions, and the pharmaceutical industry have recognized the need to develop a rational, adequate monitoring system. To this end, they have joined together to form the Joint Commission on Prescription Drug Use, the primary mission of which is to determine the feasibility and design of a workable national system for collecting data on adverse drug reactions. This commission realizes that the scope of the adverse drug reaction problem has yet to be identified, and that until the problem can be defined, completely satisfactory systems cannot be developed to monitor drug usage.

The numerous proposals introduced into Congress for the mandatory reporting of all drug usage are objectionable for the following reasons:

1. There is a substantial risk that the confidentiality of patients' treatment records will be destroyed as more and more aspects of medical treatment, both of beneficiaries of federal health care programs and of private patients, undergo more and more scrutiny, reporting, and data collection. Electronic data processing increases the vulnerability of patients to unjustified intrusions and invasions of the privacy of their individual medical records.

2. The collection of such data creates the potential for abuse via misrepresentation of the conclusions from the information generated. Misuse of these data by private individuals in order to profit from the manipulation of the information also is possible. There are numerous examples of limited data being used to form erroneous conclusions on the incidence of adverse drug reactions and deaths (Jick, 1974).

3. Monitoring of this type would be onerous; it would require a large number of written reports to be filled out by physicians and other health professionals, as well as a large bureaucracy to receive, analyze, and store the data submitted.

4. Innovative uses of drugs by physicians would be stifled.

5. Such a monitoring system could be turned into a modality to enforce controls on drug usage if such controls are subsequently developed.

Monitoring systems are not objectionable *per se*. Such programs have great potential benefit. However, mandatory, large-scale reporting systems controlled by the federal government could lead to greater intervention into the practice of medicine with undesirable results.

Controls for Drug Usage

The organized medical profession has always accepted and supported the development of certain controls on drugs and drug usage. As far back as 1890, the American Medical Association (AMA) supported congressional action designed to limit the importation of adulterated drug products. In 1905 and again in 1937, the AMA endorsed the passage of major legislation designed to insure that drugs marketed in the United States would be safe, properly labeled, and unadulterated, including the requirement that a drug must be approved by the Food and Drug Administration (FDA) before it can be marketed. The AMA continues to support proposals that do not limit the availability of safe, efficacious drugs or impinge upon and interfere with the proper exercise of professional judgment by a physician.

Specific controls on drug use that the AMA has supported include (1) standards for the safety and purity of drugs, (2) limitations of prescribing privileges to physicians who are competent (judged by education and state licensure), (3) limitations upon the prescribing of controlled substances, (4) severely restricted use of investigational drugs, and (5) prohibited use of drugs that have not been approved for marketing in the United States.

The most prominent proposals to impose additional controls on physician prescribing are (1) limitations on the use of drugs to indications contained in approved labeling, (2) requirements that the use of certain drugs be limited to specified clinical settings or medical specialties, (3) mandatory patient package inserts for all drugs, and (4) more explicit labeling for physicians.

The AMA objects to imposing controls that would limit physician prescribing and the use of drugs to indications and dosages contained in FDA-approved labeling (often incorrectly called "approved uses") because:

1. Such controls would limit the innovative and serendipitous discovery of new uses of already approved drugs.

2. Such controls would place the potential new uses of drugs in the complete control of manufacturers who apply for and establish (usually at great expense and after long delay) the safety and efficacy of secondary uses. Man-

ufacturers may not be willing to assume such expensive projects if there is evidence that the cost of preparing an application and receiving approval would be excessive. It must be noted that the mere absence of an indication in the FDA-approved labeling does not mean that the drug is not, in fact, safe or effective for that use. It only means that the manufacturer has not requested that such an indication appear in the labeling or that the FDA has not approved the indication.

3. Such controls could expose the physician to criminal and civil liability if, in his professional judgment, the treatment of choice is not one approved by the FDA.

4. Such controls could be interpreted to include labeled dosage and, therefore, the physician would have to prescribe only the dosage contained in the labeling, even if, in his judgment, a higher or lower dosage would be more appropriate.

5. Such controls would limit the options available to the physician when usual therapeutic programs have been exhausted and the patient's condition has not improved.

6. Such controls would introduce direct federal intervention into the determination of how a physician is to treat the individual patient. This would lead to the development of strict federal criteria on practice and, ultimately, to cookbook medicine.

Another area of control could include limitations on which licensed physicians would be allowed to prescribe certain drugs and in what types of settings (e.g., hospital). This would be objectionable because (1) it would lead to the development of criteria on accreditation of medical specialties by the federal government; (2) it would limit patients' access to medical care by interfering with their freedom of choice of physician, increasing travel requirements for certain therapies, and fragmenting medical care; (3) it would establish a division of the medical market (antitrust in reverse) by limiting competition among specialists and nonspecialists in the use of certain therapy; (4) it could increase the cost of medical care by encouraging more hospital treatment and greater specialization; and (5) it could hamper treatment in remote, rural, and underserved areas where either the required facility or specialist would not be readily available.

The control exerted indirectly by the proposed requirement that patient package inserts be mandatory for all drugs is also of concern. The patient package inserts thus far developed by the FDA have tended to cause alarm because of the requirement that there be substantial evidence (controlled animal and clinical studies) before an indication and dosage may appear in the labeling and patient package insert, without the concomitant requirement that there be substantial evidence to verify proposed risks from use of the drug. Therefore, potential hazards appearing in a patient package insert are often based on sporadically reported or anecdotal data. Although, in certain circumstances, a patient package insert can improve medical treatment by informing the patient of certain hazards and precautions to be observed for proper drug usage, a long list of potential adverse effects could cause undue concern—so much so that a prescribed treatment regimen might not be carried out or completed. Furthermore, physician liability could increase if a drug was used for an indication not included in the patient package insert or if a contraindication listed therein was ignored, even if the prescription was based upon the physician's best judgment.

Finally, the labeling for a drug has an influence on the physician. For whatever reason, such labeling carries certain credibility. Although the labeling is appropriate to inform physicians of specific data on efficacy and safety of the drug, it was never intended that such labeling become a mini-treatise on the diagnosis and treatment of a disease. Yet the growing trend in FDA-approved labeling has been to specify the FDA's concept of proper medical practice, including admonitions about the criteria for selection, testing, diagnostic procedures, and even physical examination of the patient. Instructions on how to be a doctor do not belong in drug labeling!

The use of drugs by the medical profession since the passage of the original Food and Drug Act has been far from unfettered. Both formal and informal controls, including the physician's desire to treat patients properly, have prevented most effectively the improper prescribing of drug products. Further governmental controls in this area can only result in the denigration of medical practice and the corresponding lowering of the quality of medical care for patients.

Conclusion

The medical profession has never advocated uncontrolled and unfettered use of drug products. Therefore, organized medicine has been a long-time supporter of laws to insure the purity and safety of drugs available to the American people and has continually advocated increased funding so that the FDA can carry out its assigned functions more effectively. This does not, however, alter the conviction that physicians have been trained for, and are most capable of determining, the proper usage of drugs in their patients. A physician's extensive education and licensing requirements, along with his familiarity with the patient's medical history, indicate that he, and not a federal agency, should determine prescribing practices. Quality medical care would undeniably be threatened if treatment were dictated on a statistical basis for the average patient rather than for the individual one. Such generalized, cookbook medicine is totally unacceptable.

References

Ballin, J.C.: The ADR numbers game. JAMA 229:1097–1098, 1974.
Editorial: Deaths due to drug treatment. Br. Med. J. 1:1492–1493, 1977.
Jick, H.: Drugs—remarkably nontoxic. N. Engl. J. Med. 291:824–828, 1974.

26

How Can We Improve Patient Compliance?

Is There a Patient Compliance Problem? If So, What Do We Do About It?

D.L. Sackett, M.D.

Should We Improve Patient Compliance with Therapeutic Regimens, and, if so, How?

Carl C. Peck, M.D.

How to Improve Patient Compliance

Harold S. Solomon, M.D.

It is a distinct art to talk medicine in the language of the non-medical man.

Edward H. Goodman

Never believe what a patient tells you his doctor has said.

Sir William Jenner

It's no trifle at her time of life to part with a doctor who knows her constitution.

George Eliot, *Janet's Repentance*

A sick person who lies to his physician cheats only himself, wastes the physician's efforts and aggravates his sickness.

Bechya ben Joseph ibn Paauda,
Duties of the Heart

Introduction

Patient compliance is now an enormously popular term, despite its somewhat graceless character. Some have complained that it smacks of intimidation and the imposition of the physician's will on a reluctant and helpless patient-victim and have urged that medicine come up with a happier phrase.

Here, the term is used to denote a willingness on the part of a patient to adhere to a therapeutic regimen prescribed by a physician. As Sackett and Peck point out, compliance is not always in the patient's best interest, and Weintraub has coined the phrase *intelligent noncompliance* for the disregarding of doctors' orders when such uncooperativeness is wiser than a sheeplike compliance.

Nonetheless, most discussion on this topic assumes that physicians' directions are not only well intentioned but actually wise. If so, patients obviously stand to benefit from compliance and to be harmed by noncompliance. Study after study has shown that failure to follow directions is very common, although the literature is far less convincing if one seeks data on the deleterious consequences of such behavior.

Sackett proposes that strategies for improving compliance should be recommended only on the basis of proper randomized trials. He puts himself into the category of "snails" rather than that of "evangelists," who argue that to await scholarly proof is to adopt an iconoclasm that patients cannot afford.

Peck describes ways of estimating compliance by either subjective or objective techniques. None of these is perfect, but many such techniques give a reasonably accurate "ballpark" quantification of the problem. Attempts to identify important determinants of compliance have mostly failed; especially disquieting to academics and pedagogues is the repeated failure of educational efforts to improve patient compliance.

The impact of noncompliance on clinical trials can be substantial. Failure to take an active drug (or to take it properly) can obviously affect its therapeutic or toxic performance, and this factor should be considered in designing, executing, and analyzing clinical trials. Some would merely count noncompliants as "failures" or "dropouts," arguing that noncompliance may reflect either therapeutic failure or adverse effects, and thus constitute an assessment of the drug's likelihood of performing satisfactorily in practice. I would suggest at least an attempt to account for the compliance failures. We need to know not only how many people *can* take a given drug as directed, but how the drug works if it *is* used and taken in the best possible way. Peck also reminds us of the ethical implications of trying to force compliance on unwilling patients.

Solomon describes the "Health Belief Model," which has considerable *prima facie* appeal, arguing that what matter are (1) an expectation that treatment will yield benefit, (2) the attachment of importance to those benefits, and (3) cues to trigger appropriate behavior (symptoms, for instance). His essay provides a strategy not only for thinking about compliance but possibly for doing something about it.

I find his concluding bits of advice especially attractive.

LOUIS LASAGNA, M.D.

Is There a Patient Compliance Problem? If So, What Do We Do About It?*

D. L. Sackett, M.D.
McMaster University, Ontario, Canada

And I say that if a rhetorician and a physician were to go to any city, and had there to argue in the Ecclesia or any other assembly as to which of them should be elected state-physician, the physician would have no chance... (Plato)

Whether standing at the front or seated in the back of the hall, I don't enjoy debates, nor do I believe that they provide the shortest path to the truth. In a debate, the answer to the question is determined first, and one then constructs support from an assortment of famous men, straw men, incomplete observations, and quotes from Bartlett's Familiar Quotations (Bartlett, 1958). Accordingly, victory is more likely to attend duplicity than honesty; a good debator needs validity like a fish needs a bicycle.

The methodologist's search for truth invokes a fundamentally different strategy: the answer to the question remains unknown until the end of the journey. The first steps are devoted to establishing a hierarchy of rules of evidence and criteria against which all available evidence will be assessed. A detailed search for and evaluation of the available data follow (the latter often carried out by several independent reviewers) and the results are then synthesized, both for their conclusions and for the methodologic adequacy of the research that led to these conclusions. It is only at the end of this last step that the answer to the question becomes known, and the verdict frequently is "neither proven nor disproven," a conclusion unacceptable in debate.

As I understand the topic at hand, this debate is focused upon the basis for making recommendations to clinicians on how they can improve low compliance, and therefore boils down to a confrontation between the scientific method and that peculiar distillate of wisdom, anecdote, and prejudice called common sense. Since this dispute is fundamental to decision-making throughout clinical and health care, and is one I have joined elsewhere in another context (Sackett and Holland, 1975), a compromise is in order.

The compromise takes form in the two separate and contrasting portions of this essay. The first is an abbreviated methodologic review of all the true experiments upon compliance-improving strategies that my colleagues and I have uncovered in the last five years (Sackett and Haynes, 1976; Haynes, Taylor and Sackett, 1979), augmented by selected data on the magnitude of low compliance. It is intended to inform, but to persuade only by appeals to reason. The second section simply seeks to win the argument.

Three questions are to be considered:

1. Is there a compliance problem?
2. Should low compliance be attacked?

* Support for the collation and review of compliance articles has come from a number of sources, including the Medical Research Council of Canada, the National Health Research and Development Program, the Ontario Heart Foundation, the Sun Life Assurance Company, and several pharmaceutical manufacturers.

3. Upon what basis should compliance-improving strategies be recommended?

The Facts

In collecting, evaluating, and collating the 598 original articles we have gathered in our five-year search, each has been assessed and scored with respect to the rigor with which it recognized and dealt with six methodologic issues of central importance to the investigation of compliance: study design, sample selection and specification, description of the illness, description of the regimen, completeness of the definition of compliance, and adequacy of the measurement of compliance (Haynes et al., 1976a). As a result it becomes possible to insert appropriate "filters" of methodologic adequacy when selecting articles on a specific topic, restricting the final set to those that have properly dealt with key issues. Thus, the following section on the magnitude of compliance is based upon that subset of investigations that successfully handled sampling problems, and the section on compliance-improving strategies is restricted to randomized trials.

Is There a Compliance Problem?

The results of investigations upon carefully selected inception cohorts can be summarized as follows (Sackett, 1976; Sackett 1979):

1. Patients keep 80 percent of appointments that they make, and 50 percent of appointments made by providers.

2. Compliance with short-term preventive regimens (e.g., immunizations) is cyclic and now stands at 75 percent. For long-term preventive regimens (e.g., rheumatic fever prophylaxis) about 50 percent of prescribed doses are taken.

3. Compliance with therapeutic medication regimens averages 50 percent and falls dramatically with the passage of time.

4. Compliance with life-style regimens is generally lower than that for therapeutic regimens; the majority of inception cohorts in voluntary weight-reduction and exercise programs drop out without reaching their goals, and only about 20 percent of those who join smoking cessation groups become long-term abstainers.

These data show that low compliance is common. For compliance to constitute a problem, however, two additional criteria must be met. First, the associated regimens must be efficacious (that is, they must do more good than harm to those who comply). This criterion is tested by the randomized trial and has been met by a number of regimens, most prominently those for tuberculosis, some psychoses and endocrine deficiences, epilepsy, moderate and severe hypertension, active immunizations, and rheumatic fever prophylaxis. The second criterion is the demonstration that the low levels of compliance that have been observed clinically actually impede the achievement of treatment goals. Again, this has been met by several regimens. For example, the achievement of goal blood pressure by hypertensives is closely linked to their compliance (Lowenthal et al., 1976), and the risk of rheumatic fever recurrence is also proportional to compliance with prophylactic penicillin (Feinstein et al., 1968).

In summary, low compliance with efficacious regimens is widespread, and it leads to failure to achieve the goals of prevention and cure. In terms of these three criteria (magnitude, efficacy, and relation to treatment goals), there indeed is a compliance problem.

Should Low Compliance Be Attacked?

The reader may be surprised to find this question posed in a section on facts, since it is, on the surface, a matter of ethics. However, the fact is that a set of criteria for answering this question has been identified at compliance symposia (Sackett, 1976b; Jonsen, 1979). Moreover, it is possible to specify certain circumstances in which an attack upon low compliance is demonstrably unethical.

The following criteria have been identified as requiring satisfaction before launching an attack on low compliance:

1. The diagnosis must be correct.*

2. The therapy must be efficacious.*

3. Low compliance must be suspected or documented.

4. A compliance-improving strategy of established effectiveness must be available.

5. The patient must provide free, informed consent to receive this strategy.

---

* If either of these criteria is breeched, the patient whose compliance is increased has been needlessly exposed to an increased risk of side-effects and toxicity from an unnecessary or useless regimen. Of course, it is theoretically possible (though improbable) that the right drug is given for the wrong diagnosis, but this constitutes luck, not judgment.

Ethical issues in compliance have been discussed in detail elsewhere (Jonsen, 1979). Just as the acceptance of specific methodologic standards led to a "yes" answer to the first question in this series, the acceptance of the foregoing ethical standards leads to an affirmative answer to the second.

Upon What Basis Should Compliance-improving Strategies Be Recommended?

The bases for recommending strategies to improve compliance can form two groups: those derived from subexperimental observations or experiences and those derived from true experiments (i.e., randomized trials). Recommendations of the first sort are far more common and are less expensive to generate, since they tend to arise from everyday experience. Thus, if they could be shown to meet a criterion of validity, they would constitute a preferable source of strategies.

Recommendations of the second sort arise from experiments that parallel those used to establish the efficacy and safety of new drugs. In this case, the randomized trial has become the standard index of validity because subexperimental observations have repeatedly been shown to produce erroneous conclusions. It is appropriate, therefore, to apply this same criterion to the assessment of compliance-improving strategies: if strategies that have previously been recommended on the basis of prior experience and other subexperimental observations can be shown to be valid in randomized trials, the subexperimental basis for making these recommendations would be vindicated.

By late 1977, we had gathered 27 published randomized clinical trials of compliance-improving strategies (mostly for therapeutic regimens) in which the strategy being tested had been proposed as sensible and reasonable on the basis of subexperimental observations. These trials are summarized in Table 26–1. Although several useful strategies—especially those with a large behavioral component—have been identified, there are two major areas in which common sense approaches failed to produce the anticipated changes in compliance.

For example, teaching patients about their diseases and about the need for specific long-term health behaviors, although it may substantially increase their knowledge, does not improve their compliance. Furthermore, the provision of comprehensive care through largely organizational approaches—a shift of traditional care to the worksite (Sackett et al., 1975) or care for all complaints at all hours by the same clinician (Gordis and Markowitz, 1971)—does not improve medication compliance.* Thus, two of the common sense approaches to improving compliance that have been repeatedly recommended in clinical journals have been shown to be invalid when tested in randomized trials. If one accepts the foregoing criterion, failure to achieve validation in randomized trials renders the recommendations of compliance-improving strategies on the basis of subexperimental evidence inappropriate.

The Polemic: Evangelists Versus Snails

The evangelists, usually for impeccable motives, hold that the burden of preventable disability and untimely death is great, and that compliance-improving strategies based on common sense and experience must be applied now, even in the absence of experimental evidence on their validity.** On this and similar issues, dissent is not well tolerated. "Can we afford iconoclasm while awaiting proof?" In "keeping the faith," evangelists find themselves forced to accept or reject evidence not on the basis of its scientific merit but on the extent to which it supports or refutes their public stand. Cognitive dissonance abounds.

The snails of Table 26–1, on the other hand, are wed not to a conclusion about whether this or that strategy works, but to the experimental method—which, if rigorously applied, will maximize the likelihood that the compliance-improving strategies ultimately put into general use will do more good than harm. The snails insist that compliance-improving strategies are therapeutic maneuvers: they are prescribed for specific health problems, are instituted to produce specific changes in patients, and may produce unwanted side effects (such as preoccupation with illness and infirmity) as well as benefits. Accordingly, before their general use, strategies for improving compliance with therapy should undergo the same valida-

* A third trial (Becker et al., 1974) demonstrated a 10 percent improvement in attendance when continuous care by the same team was provided; medication compliance was not studied.

** See Editorial, American Journal of Public Health, 1971; Finnerty, 1973; Stokes et al., 1973.

Table 26-1. *Randomized Trials of Compliance-Improving Strategies*

Reference	Situation	Strategy	Result (Compared with the control group)
Shepard & Moseley, 1976	Appointment-Keeping at a Pediatric Clinic	Mailed or telephone reminders shortly before the appointment date.	Mailed reminders led to a 17% improvement, and telephone calls a 22% improvement in appointment-keeping.
Levy & Claravall, 1977	Appointment-Keeping at a Pediatric Clinic	Telephone reminders shortly before the appointment date.	No effect on short interval (<14 days) appointments, but longer interval appointment-keeping rose by 31%.
Glogow, 1970	Appointment-Keeping after Glaucoma Screening	Health messages with "in-depth", "minimal" and "no" information content.	Appointment-keeping rose by the same amount in all 3 experimental groups.
Haefner & Kirscht, 1970	Appointment-Keeping for a Health Check-Up	Instruction about disease.	No effect.
Radelfinger, 1965	Appointment-Keeping for a Tetanus Immunization	High and low fear messages about the need for immunization.	No effect.
Barnes et al., 1971	Appointment-Keeping after a Dental Check-Up	High and low fear messages about the need for dental care.	Appointment-keeping rose by the same amount in both experimental groups.
Steckel & Swain, 1977	Appointment-Keeping at a Hypertension Clinic	Education plus counselling.	Fourfold rise in drop-outs.
		Contingency contracting.	No drop-outs and improved attendance.
Becker et al., 1974	Appointment-Keeping in a Pediatric Clinic	Continuous care by the same team.	Appointment-keeping rose 10%.
Colcher & Bass, 1972	Short-Term (10 day) Medication Compliance	Instruction by therapist or intramuscular injection.	Equally effective in increasing, by 25%, the proportion of patients with drug in their urine 9 days later.
Linkewich et al., 1974	Short-Term Medication Compliance	Calendar plus instruction.	Progressive improvements in compliance.
		Unit doses plus instruction.	
		Reminder package of medications.	
Fink et al. 1969	Short-Term Pediatric Regimens	Care from a specially trained "Family Health Management Specialist"	Compliance rose by 51%.
Sackett et al., 1975	Hypertension	Programmed instruction.	No effect from either strategy.
		Care at the work site.	
Tagliacozzo et al., 1974	Diabetes or Hypertension	Lectures.	No effect.
Eshelman & Fitzloff, 1976	Hypertension	Calendar medication pack.	No effect.
Steckel & Swain, 1977	Hypertension	Contingency contracting.	Better blood pressure control and weight loss.
Haynes et al., 1976b	Hypertension	Self home blood pressures, tailoring doses to daily rituals and positive reinforcement.	22% improvement in medication compliance.
Blackwell, 1976	Hypertension	Counselling and/or mechanical calendar dispenser.	Dispenser increased proportion of patients taking >95% of medication, but blood pressure fell only when this was coupled with counselling.
Meyer & Henderson, 1974	Coronary Risk Factors	Counselling.	No effect.
		Behavior modification.	Substantial changes in diet, cholesterol, exercise and cigarette consumption.
Porter and McCullough, 1972	Cigarette Smoking	Counselling.	No effect.
Mann & Janis, 1968	Cigarette Smoking	Role-playing.	Smoking reduced.
Evans et al., 1970	Dental Hygiene	Instructions with varying information, appeal and fear-arousal.	No difference in dental hygiene 6 weeks later.
Starfield & Sharp, 1968	Enuresis	Instruction plus assistance in implementing exercises.	Decrease in enuresis.
Lund et al., 1964	Epilepsy	Blood drug levels and feedback.	38% improvement in compliance.
Feinstein et al., 1968, 1959	Rheumatic Fever Prophylaxis	Intramuscular injection.	Statistically significantly fewer relapses.

Table 26-1. *(Continued) Randomized Trials of Compliance-Improving Strategies*

Reference	Situation	Strategy	Result (Compared with the control group)
Cody & Robinson, 1977	Schizophrenia	Lowered cost of medications.	Relapses increased.
Gordis & Markowitz, 1971	Well-Child Care	Continuous, comprehensive care.	No effect.
	Rheumatic Fever Prophylaxis		

tion procedures as are undergone by new drugs, the most important of which is the controlled experiment in man (Sackett et al., 1976).

Why not simply forge ahead on the basis of "it is generally acknowledged that . . ." (Ingelfinger, 1966)? First, both the time and the money spent applying useless strategies are wasted. Second, although even an effective strategy cannot be expected to help every patient, any compliance-improving strategy carries the potential to harm all patients.* Third, the loss of credibility when experiments show the touted "common sense" strategies to be worthless will reinforce public skepticism toward other advice such as the need for polio immunization or the use of seat belts. Finally, the general acceptance of common sense compliance-improving strategies will retard experimental research into alternative maneuvers that really work.

* For example, our programmed instruction strategy (Sackett et al., 1975) not only failed to improve the compliance of hypertensive steelworkers but it was accompanied by striking deteriorations in measures of psychosocial function and dramatic increases in absenteeism among those who learned how yet failed to take their medicine.

The issue is simple. In establishing the basis from which to recommend compliance-improving strategies, should we insist upon validation by the randomized experiment or should we retreat to the idolatry of that same common sense expedient that brought us the internal mammary ligation for angina pectoris, mass screening for sickle-cell trait, and the gastric freeze for peptic ulcer?

Conclusion

Is there a compliance problem? Yes. *Should low compliance be attacked?* Yes, but only if the diagnosis is correct, the regimen is efficacious, the patient freely consents, and the compliance-improving strategy selected has been experimentally validated. *Upon what basis should compliance-improving strategies be recommended?* As with any other therapeutic maneuver, only on the basis of proper randomized trials.

References

Barnes, K.E., Gunther, D., Jordan, I., and Gray, A.S.: The effects of various persuasive communications on community health: a pilot study. Can. J. Public Health 62:105, 1971.

Bartlett, J., ed.: *Familiar Quotations.* New York, Philos Lab, 1958.

Becker, M.H., Drachman, R.H., and Kirscht, J.P.: A field experiment to evaluate various outcomes of continuity of care. Am. J. Public Health 64:1062, 1974.

Blackwell, B.: Treatment adherence in hypertension. Am. J. Pharm. 148:75, 1976.

Cody, J., and Robinson, A.: The effect of low-cost maintenance medication on the rehospitalization of schizophrenic outpatients. Am. J. Psychiatry 134:73, 1977.

Colcher, I.S., and Bass, J.W.: Penicillin treatment of streptococcal pharyngitis: A comparison of schedules and the role of specific counselling. JAMA 222:657, 1972.

Editorial: The need for patient education. Am. J. Public Health 61:1277, 1971.

Eshelman, F.N., and Fitzloff, J.: Effect of packaging on patient compliance with an antihypertensive medication. Curr. Ther. Res. 20:215, 1976.

Evans, R.I., Rozelle, R.M., Lasater, T.M., Dembroski, T.M., and Allen, B.P.: Fear arousal, persuasion, and actual versus implied behavioral change. J. Pers. Soc. Psychol. 16:220, 1970.

Feinstein, A.R., Wood, H.F., Epstein, J.A., Taranta, A., Simpson, R., and Tursky, E.: A controlled study of three methods of prophylaxis against streptococcal infection in a population of rheumatic children. II, Results of the first three years of the study, including methods for evaluating the maintenance of oral prophylaxis. N. Engl. J. Med. 260:697, 1959.

Feinstein, A.R., Spagnjolo, M., Jonas, S., Kloth, H., Tursky, E., and Levitt, M.: Prophylaxis of recurrent rheumatic fever. JAMA 206:565, 1968.

Fink, D., Malloy, M.J., Cohen, M., Greycloud, M.A., and Martin, F.: Effective patient care in the pediatric ambulatory setting: a study of the acute care clinic. Pediatrics 43:927, 1969.

Finnerty, F.A., Jr.: The hypertension problem: what we can do about it. Circulation 48:681, 1973.

Glogow, E.: Effects of health education methods on appointment breaking. Public Health Rep. 85:441, 1970.

Gordis, L., and Markowitz, M.: Evaluation of the effectiveness of comprehensive and continuous pediatric care. II, Effectiveness of continuous care in influencing patient compliance. Pediatrics 48:766, 1971.

Haefner, D.P., and Kirscht, J.P.: Motivational and behavioral effects of modifying health beliefs. Public Health Rep. 85:478, 1970.

Haynes, R.B., Sackett, D.L., Taylor, D.W., Hackett, B.C., Luterbach, E., and Cloak, J.R.: An annotated bibliography including notes on methodologic standards for compliance research. In Sackett, D.L., and Haynes, R.B., *Compliance with Therapeutic Regimens,* Baltimore, Johns Hopkins University Press, 1976a.

Haynes, R.B., Sackett, D.L., Gibson, E.S., Taylor, D.W., Hackett, B.C., Roberts, R.S., and Johnson, A.L.: Improvement of medication compliance in uncontrolled hypertension. Lancet 1:1265, 1976b.

Haynes, R.B., Taylor, D.W., and Sackett, D.L., *Compliance in Health Care,* Baltimore, Johns Hopkins University Press, 1979.

Ingelfinger, F.J.: Introduction. In Ingelfinger, F.J., *Controversies in Internal Medicine,* Philadelphia, W.B. Saunders Co., 1966.

Jonsen, A.R.: Ethical issues in compliance. In Haynes, R.B., Taylor, D.W., and Sackett, D.L., *Compliance in Health Care,* Baltimore, Johns Hopkins University Press, 1979.

Levy, R., and Claravall, V.: Different effects of a phone reminder on appointment keeping for patients with long and short between-visit intervals. Med. Care 15:435, 1977.

Linkewich, J.A., Catalano, R.B., and Flack, H.L.: The effect of packaging and instruction on outpatient compliance with medication regimens. Drug Intell. Clin. Pharmacy 8:10, 1974.

Lowenthal, D.T., Briggs, W.A., Mutterperl, R., Aldeman, B., and Creditor, M.A.: Patient compliance for antihypertensive medication: the usefulness of urine assays. Curr. Ther. Res. 19:405, 1976.

Lund, M., Jorgenson, R.S., and Kuhl, V.: Serum diphenylhydantoin (phenytoin) in ambulant patients with epilepsy. Epilepsia 5:51, 1964.

Mann, L., and Janis, I.L.: A follow-up on the long-term effects of emotional role-playing. J. Pers. Soc. Psychol. 8:339, 1968.

Meyer, A.J., and Henderson, J.B.: Multiple risk factor reduction in the prevention of cardiovascular disease. Prev. Med. 3:225, 1974.

Plato: Gorgias. 456 B.C. (translated by B. Jowett).

Porter, A.M., and McCullough, D.M.: Counselling against cigarette smoking. Practitioner 209:686, 1972.

Radelfinger, S.: Some effects of fear-arousing communications on preventive health behavior. Health Educ. Monogr. 19:2, 1965.

Sackett, D.L.: The magnitude of compliance and noncompliance. In Sackett, D.L., and Haynes, R.B., *Compliance with Therapeutic Regimens,* Baltimore, Johns Hopkins University Press, 1976a.

Sackett, D.L.: Introduction. In Sackett, D.L., and Haynes, R.B., *Compliance with Therapeutic Regimens,* Baltimore, Johns Hopkins University Press, 1976b.
Sackett, D.L.: The magnitude of compliance and noncompliance. In Haynes, R.B., Taylor D.W., and Sackett, D.L., *Compliance in Health Care,* Baltimore, Johns Hopkins University Press, 1979.
Sackett, D.L., and Holland, W.W.: Controversy in the detection of disease. Lancet 2:357, 1975.
Sackett, D.L., Haynes, R.B., Gibson, E.S., Hackett, B.C., Taylor, D.W., Roberts, R.S., and Johnson, A.L.: Randomized clinical trial of strategies for improving medication compliance in primary hypertension. Lancet 1:1205, 1975.
Sackett, D.L., Haynes, R.B., Gibson, E.S., Taylor, D.W., Roberts, R.S., Johnson, A.L., Hackett, B.C., Turford, C., and Mossey, J.: Randomized trials of compliance-improving strategies in hypertension. In Lasagna, L., *Patient Compliance,* Mt. Kisco, Futura Publishing Company. 1976.
Shepard, D.S., and Moseley, T.A.: Mailed versus telephoned appointment reminders to reduce broken appointments in a hospital outpatient department. Med. Care 14:268, 1976.
Starfield, B., and Sharp, E.: Ambulatory pediatric care: the role of the nurse. Med. Care 6:507, 1968.
Steckel, S.B., and Swain, M.A.: Contracting with patients to improve compliance. Hospitals 51:81, 1977.
Stokes, J.B., III, Payne, G.H., and Cooper, T.: Hypertension control: the challenge of patient education. N. Engl. J. Med. 289:1369, 1973.
Tagliacozzo, D.M., Luskin, D.B., Lashof, J.C., and Ima, K.: Nurse intervention and patient behavior. Am. J. Public Health 64:596, 1974.

Should We Improve Patient Compliance with Therapeutic Regimens, and, if so, How?

Carl C. Peck, M.D.
Letterman Army Institute of Research, San Francisco

Many physicians suppose that the patient who voluntarily seeks medical attention will faithfully accept and execute medical directives. Those practitioners aware that some patients deviate from prescribed recommendations are reluctant to admit that their patients would do so. The most deceived of all are doctors who believe they know which of their patients are not following their sage advice (Berkowitz, 1963; Preston and Miller, 1964).

Reflection on the nature and complexity of medical counsel is revealing. Medical recommendations range from suggestions to consult with other health professionals and instructions for a wide variety of diagnostic procedures to specific advice on surgical, physical, psychologic, dietary, and pharmacologic therapies. Details of drug prescription are typically complex: a specific drug or family of drugs is to be taken, in precise dosage, at particular times of the day, for a defined length of time. Consider the hypertensive patient for whom hydrochlorothiazide 50 mg b.i.d., propranolol 10 mg ii q.i.d., and hydralazine 10 mg ii q.i.d. are prescribed, who is seen in consultation every three months and who is subjected to a chest X-ray, electrocardiogram, and multiphasic blood testing annually. This patient is responsible for complying with an enormous number of instructions in one year. Only the most naive physician would think that perfection in compliance with this medical advice is even possible!

Extent of Compliance with Therapeutic Regimens

Little is known about the true extent of patient compliance with medical advice, because the tools currently available are limited in their ability to measure this complex phenomenon objectively. Biased opinions of physicians or their patients are practically worthless; both groups tend to overestimate the degree of patient compliance (Bergman and Werner, 1963 ; Berkowitz, 1963). However, patients who admit to noncompliance usually do so truthfully (Park and Lipman, 1964; Sackett, 1977). Although it is theoretically a "global" measure, direct observation of patients medicating themselves invites behavior that is unrepresentative of their usual routine. Nevertheless, this method was used to study the self-management of 60 diabetics in their homes. "Best effort" results indicated that 31 patients made quantitative errors in insulin dosage—20 injected greater than 115 percent of the prescribed dose, 46 used unsterile equipment, only 15 followed the recommended diet, 40 incorrectly tested their urine for glucose, and 27 used the results of urine testing in a manner that was detrimental to their health (Watkins, 1967).

More objective measures aimed at specific aspects of medical compliance behavior provide spotty, although important, insights into patient compliance with prescribed drug regimens. Counting by medical personnel to ascertain if the correct number of pills or ounces of medication had been removed from the prescription bottle has been used to study compliance in numerous therapeutic situations, including the use of antacids for peptic ulcer, penicillin for streptococcal pharyngitis, imipramine for depression, and penicillin for prophylaxis of rheumatic fever (Bergman and Werner, 1963; Park and Lipman, 1964; Caron and Roth, 1968; Gordis et al., 1969). These studies revealed that the average "nonremoval" rates ranged from 25 to 50 percent of the medication prescribed. More recently, portable medication dispensers that document drug removal by continuous photographic or electronic surveillance have been devised to study this aspect of patient compliance (Moulding, 1971; Yee et al., 1974). Such devices have shown wide variations in medication removal patterns despite medical advice to take the doses on a regular basis.

Documentation of medication missing from its storage container does not mean necessarily that the patient actually administered it or that the correct dose was taken. Although comparisons of pill counting with other objective measures of compliance have generally revealed a high correlation (Berkowitz, 1963; Roth et al., 1970), techniques that validate actual drug intake have been developed to remedy the limitations in medication counting. These methods assay drugs, drug metabolites, or concurrently administered inert markers in biologic fluids or tissues. Urine and blood have been extensively investigated in this way. Although drugs or their metabolites also enter saliva, sweat, and hair, these easily accessible body constituents have not been exploited for this purpose (Inaba and Kalow, 1975; Peck et al., 1977; Chaput de Saintonge, 1977).

Tests for the presence of urinary metabolites of paraaminosalicylic acid and isoniazid have been used to study compliance among tuberculous outpatients. One such study revealed that 24 of 25 patients claimed faithfulness in self-medication, whereas only 18 showed evidence of drug intake (as measured by urine tests) during the 24 to 28 hours prior to the clinic visit (Preston and Miller, 1964).

Riboflavin and phenol red have been used as inert markers in studies of compliance with therapy for tuberculosis and hypertension. Over 50 percent of candidates for the Veterans Administration Cooperative Hypertension Study were denied entrance to the study because of absence of both urinary fluorescence (riboflavin) and reasonably correct pill counts at each of two pretrial observation visits (Veterans Administration, 1967; Feinstein, 1974). Riboflavin, 25 mg once a day for up to three months, was found to be a safe, simple, and reliable measure of compliance in a trial of anorectic agents in the treatment of obesity (Smith et al., 1973). Its presence can be detected for 12 to 24 hours after a dose (25 mg) simply by holding a Wood's lamp (fluorescent light) up to a urine sample in a darkened room and looking for a bright yellow-orange fluorescence.

Although detection of drugs or drug metabolites in urine can be used to validate qualitatively whether any drug is being taken (in the absence of false positives), exact dosage is not quantitated. However, pharmacokinetic analyses of many drugs have revealed a direct proportional relationship between dosage intake and concentration in blood at steady state (Wagner, 1971). This knowledge has been used to assess dose, dosing frequency, and duration of intake in peptic ulcer disease patients taking antacid containing a bromide "tracer" (Roth et al., 1970) and in cardiac patients treated with digoxin. Sheiner et al. (1974) reported a study comparing general hospital cardiology clinic outpatients with university hospital inpatients. Concentrations of digoxin in the serum of outpatients averaged 72 percent of those achieved by inpatients after individual pharmacokinetic differences were taken into account. Based on this observation, it was argued that compliance of outpatients might be lower than that of inpatients. Individual concentrations of digoxin in outpatients ranged from 40 percent to 104 percent of the expected concentrations. However, a second study of elderly outpatients from the same clinic on a prospective basis revealed contrary results (Peck et al., 1975). Patients taking digoxin were enrolled at random when they presented at the pharmacy for refills and agreed to allow serial blood samplings upon return clinic visits. The patients were not aware that concentrations of digoxin were being measured in their blood samples for the purpose of studying compliance. The mean concentration of digoxin was 1.04 ± 0.76 ng/ml (160 levels measured in 42 patients). This average value is suggestive of acceptable compliance, although there is considerable variability in the individual values. Less than 25 percent of values were less than 0.4 ng/ml. Later, pharmacokinetic parameters established for each patient during a supervised dosing phase enabled a retrospective evaluation of the measured concentrations in terms of concentrations predicted on the basis of individual kinetics. The group as a whole evidenced no significant shift from expected concentrations under the assumption of 100 percent compliance by the patients. One probable poor complier was identified, and only a few patients appeared to be "borderline." These results were surprising when one considers the complexity of the medical regimen for which many patients were responsible. Patients took an average of five other drugs and were responsible for 13 administrations each day. One patient (not the poor complier) was taking 21 different drugs and had to remember to take a pill 62 times each day. The apparent "better than average" compliance (relative to results in most other studies) found in this study has been reported elsewhere for cardiac drugs and antidiabetic agents (Hulka et al., 1975).

Determinants of Compliance

Studies have been undertaken to assess a possible correlation between the tendency to comply poorly with the physician's instructions and personal characteristics of the patient (e.g., sex, age, race, education, demographic factors). Sackett and Haynes (1976) catalogued studies of over 200 proposed candidate factors for determinants of compliance. However, these studies have failed to identify factors that would be helpful in predicting which individuals are likely to display poor compliance (Davis, 1968; Marston, 1970; Hulka et al., 1975; Haynes, 1976). Certain subgroups of patients have special circumstances that contribute to difficulties in self-medication. For example, elderly patients may have problems with eyesight, memory, or ability to follow complex instructions (Schwartz et al., 1962; Hall, 1975). Faithfulness in following prescriptions among pediatric patients may be dependent upon the parents' perception of the illness (Mattar and Yaffe, 1974).

Only a few factors have been identified as determinants of good compliance. Minimizing the complexity of the regimen is important (Malahy, 1966; Hulka et al., 1975). Even nurses working on a hospital ward make more errors in administration of drugs as the number of drug orders increases, especially when a patient receives more than six different drugs concurrently (Vere, 1965). Ayd (1973) has published a convincing review of evidence that supports the thesis that simplifying the self-medication regimen to once-a-day dosages will result in better compliance.

Education of the patient with regard to his disease(s) and the rationale for the prescribed drug regimen is another important factor in effecting optimal compliance. Although some studies have not shown benefit from educating the patient, several recent reports have strongly argued the efficacy of this procedure (Malahy, 1966; Colcher and Bass, 1972; Marsh and Perlman, 1971; Boyd et al., 1974; Hecht, 1974; Neufeld, 1976). However, in those reports in which patient education appeared efficacious, it was necessary to exert extraordinary effort. Best results occurred when in-hospital, clinic, in-home, and follow-up training sessions were all used. For example, a 17 percent "serious error" rate in self-medication in intensely educated patients was significantly less than the 45 percent rate found in a comparable group who received no instruction beyond the usual (Hecht, 1974).

Uncomfortable side effects of drugs may discourage compliance (Bulpitt and Dollery, 1973). They may be particularly important in a setting in which the disease being treated produces minimal or no symptoms—e.g., mild essential hypertension. In such cases, the treatment indeed may be worse than the disease, at least from the patient's point of view.

Consequences of Inadequate Compliance

Because standards for compliance and noncompliance vary, it is difficult to interpret the literature on the consequences of noncompliance. Each study either proposes its own criteria or merely reports intake relative to the theoretical 100 percent compliance. If it is assumed that a prescribed drug regimen will result in some observable clinical effects if adhered to by the patient, an operational definition may be based on measurable consequences of compliance. *Adequate compliance* is established from objective evidence of (1) drug-intake and (2) drug-related benefit or toxicity. *Inadequate compliance* is established by failure to meet these criteria. Such operational criteria suggest several consequences of inadequate compliance.

In clinical practice, inadequate compliance may be obstructive to therapeutic management and may increase the risk of hospitalization (Peck, 1978). On the other hand, minor departures of compliance may be inconsequential, either because the therapy is not efficacious even when taken faithfully, or because 100 percent compliance is unnecessary for efficacy. Noncompliance may even be beneficial at times; for example, when the drug actually produces more harm than benefit. Such a situation can arise when the diagnosis is incorrect, the therapy is inappropriate for a correct diagnosis, excessive dosage is employed, or an adverse reaction occurs.

At times, poor compliance may be obstructive to effective clinical management because the physician may erroneously conclude that his initial therapy is ineffective or that his diagnosis is in error if he is unable to recognize inadequate compliance as a cause of therapeutic failure. Changing to an incorrect diagnosis or prescribing a more toxic therapy may subject a patient to unnecessary risk. On the contrary, the patient who takes only 50 to 75 percent of the stated dose of a drug that has a narrow therapeutic index may be at risk when hospitalized. For instance, a poorly complying outpatient may develop digitalis toxicity several days after admission to the hospital as a result of being given his "usual dose" in a setting in which compliance can be enforced.

From a research point of view, the effect of inadequate compliance among test subjects is particularly important in planning and interpreting results of clinical trials. Joyce (1962) reported that in his crossover comparison of phenylbutazone with a second experimental drug and a placebo in 72 arthritic patients, initial results did not show a statistically significant effect of phenylbutazone. However, when he reanalyzed the data after eliminating those judged to be noncompliant by both pill counts and a urinary inert marker technique, phenylbutazone emerged as statistically superior to both other drugs. This phenomenon of diminishing the sensitivity of a comparative trial by effectively diluting all treatment groups with inadequate compliers has been seen in other studies (Bonnar et al., 1969). Feinstein (1976) has suggested that one major methodologic defect in the University Group Diabetes Project (UGDP) lies in the fact that only 26 percent of all UGDP patients faithfully maintained their initially assigned treatments. Recall that in the VA Cooperative Hypertension Study (1967), over 50 percent of candidates were denied entry into the trial because of demonstration of poor reliability in the pretrial period (Feinstein, 1974). The results of the VA trial would have been considerably less convincing if the poor compliers had been retained in the treated group. For example, if 50 percent of the group of trial subjects with diastolic blood pressure averaging 90 to 114 mm Hg being treated with antihypertensive agents had been inadequate compliers, the difference in percentage of deaths attributable to hypertension would have been reduced from 5.5 percent (control-treated group) to 2.8 percent (analysis of data from Veterans Administration, 1970).

Ethical Considerations

The physician who discovers that his patient is an inadequate complier may entertain the question "How can I induce my patient to follow my instructions?" This question presupposes that the physician has the right to induce improvement in compliance, and thus raises a serious ethical issue.

Although a patient may present himself voluntarily for diagnostic and therapeutic advice, this does not constitute implied acceptance of all prescribed maneuvers. On the contrary, the patient often (and rightly) feels free to accept or reject any aspect of medical advice. Whereas the physician may feel compelled to inform the patient of the probable consequences of inadequate compliance (if the doctor indeed knows them), it seems imperative to respect the patient's right to determine the extent to which he complies *as long as it does not affect others.* Protecting the patient from himself by forced compliance is seen by many to be an infringement on the patient's right of self-determination.

As long as it does not affect others as an operational criterion may not always provide a clear-cut basis for deciding whether to employ measures designed to improve compliance. Most would agree that protection of others from infectious diseases such as syphilis, gonorrhea, and tuberculosis, or homicidal psychosis, justifies the use of parenteral therapy or hospitalization as measures to insure compliance. However, when inadequate compliance may adversely affect a patient's ability to interact with or support his family, the ethics of physician intervention aimed at induction of improved compliance become problematic.

Another instance in which the justification for encouraging compliance is enigmatic is the planning and execution of clinical drug trials. There is no doubt that information derived from trials in which participants have been selected who are highly compliant with the drug regimens under study affords the most sensitive and efficient means of discerning relative efficacy and toxicity. However, such information may not be applicable to the patient group that will actually receive the drug therapy in practice (Feinstein, 1974). In fact, studying drug performance only in compliant patients may preclude the discovery of important features of the regimen that adversely influence compliance.

Strategies for Improving Compliance

Occasionally, a patient with good intentions may request or agree to accept assistance in improving his compliance with the therapeutic regimen. Of special interest is the recent observation that self-admitted noncompliers have shown greater improvement when offered help with taking medication than those poor compliers who claim good compliance (Haynes et al., 1976). Although many strategies for improving compliance have been proposed, few have been put to objective test and even fewer have been proven effective (Sackett, 1978). Sackett and Haynes (1976) list 44 reports on six educational and nine behavioral approaches that claim variable success in improving compliance. Patient education has not been as effective as might be expected. This approach appears to be useful only when applied in a high intensity, repetitive program involving multiple health personnel located in strategic points of the health care system or when combined with behavioral techniques.

Behavioral strategies aim at the logistics, cueing, and reinforcement of compliant behavior. Simplification of the drug regimen by replacing multiple doses with single, longer-acting formulations, especially when supervised or parenteral administration can be employed, has been one of the most consistently successful methods of effecting improved compliance. Use of medication containers containing signal alarm devices, consensual regimens,* telephone reminders, and home visits by nursing personnel have been successful in research settings, but they do not lend themselves to widespread use. More practical behavioral approaches include serum drug monitoring coupled with feedback, encouragement or praise, convenient packaging of medications, and hospitalization when necessary (Sackett, 1978).

Monitoring Compliance in Clinical Practice

A consideration of whether and how to improve compliance in a patient presupposes that inadequate compliance can be detected in the practice setting. Likewise, documenting response to an attempt at improving compliance requires an objective and practical method of assessing compliance. Although a variety of compliance measurement techniques are available, each of which exhibits certain assets and limitations, most techniques are impractical in clinical practice. Whereas nonthreatening interview techniques may be useful in eliciting admissions of noncompliance, patient reporting of improvement in compliance must be viewed with skepticism (Peck, 1976).

There are three techniques, however, that are convenient to use and may assist in detecting inadequate compliance as well as in documenting improvement. Medication counts are simple for office personnel to perform and yield information that generally correlates well with serum drug levels. Drug levels in serum are now widely available and can assist in the assessment of adequacy of drug intake. Knowledge of the contributions of individual differences in body size (distribution space), drug elimination rate (clearance), and effects of disease states on serum levels is essential for their proper interpretation (Sheiner and Tozer, 1978). Finally, ingestion of some drugs that are excreted in the urine may be documented by the fluorescence created by holding a postingestion urine sample near a Wood's light. Two such drugs are riboflavin, which may be used as an inert marker, and triamterene (Smith et al., 1973). The latter is not uncommonly used in the treatment of hypertension, a condition in which inadequate compliance may have profound consequences.

Conclusion

Compliance with the prescribed therapeutic regimen often is ignored or underplayed by physicians as a determinant of therapeutic outcome. Detecting inadequate compliance and

* A consensual regimen is a product of negotiation between patient and physician and represents a consensus or mutual contract (Fink, 1976).

assessing its improvement in the clinical setting can be done by using pill counts, serum drug levels, or the Wood's light technique. There is considerable evidence that patient compliance is less than perfect, but less certain is knowledge of the extent and consequences of inadequate compliance.

Inadequate compliance may or may not adversely affect the patient, his family, or society. Forced improvement in compliance appears justified only in the case of diseases that are of considerable nuisance or danger to others. Otherwise, the patient's right to accept or reject his physician's recommendations must be respected. Few methods for improving compliance have been shown to be efficacious, although simplification of the drug regimen, intensive patient education, parenteral therapy administered by medical personnel, and hospitalization have proven effective. Physicians are well advised to educate themselves as to the extent and implications of patient compliance and to integrate this knowledge into clinical practice.

References

Ayd, F.J.: Rational pharmacotherapy: once-a-day drug dosage. Dis. Nerv. Syst. 34:371, 1973.

Bergman, A.B., and Werner, R.J.: Failure of children to receive penicillin by mouth. N. Engl. J. Med. 268:1334, 1963.

Berkowitz, N.H.: Patient follow-through in the out-patient department. Nurs. Res. 12:16, 1963.

Bonnar, J., Goldberg, A., and Smith, J.A.: Do pregnant women take their iron? Lancet 1:457, 1969.

Boyd, J.R., Covington, T.R., Stanaszek, W.R., et al.: Drug defaulting. II, Analysis of noncompliance patterns. Am. J. Hosp. Pharm. 31:485, 1974.

Bulpitt, C.J., and Dollery, C.T.: Side effects of hypotensive agents evaluated by a self-administered questionnaire. Lancet 3:485, 1973.

Caron, H.S., and Roth, H.P.: Patients' cooperation with a medical regimen. JAMA 203:922, 1968.

Chaput de Saintonge, D.M.: A new method for measuring compliance from samples of hair (abstract). Workshop Manual, Workshop/Symposium on Compliance, McMaster University, Hamilton, Ontario, Canada, 1977.

Colcher, I.S., and Bass, J.W.: Penicillin treatment of streptococcal pharyngitis. JAMA 222:657, 1972.

Davis, M.S.: Physiologic, psychological and demographic factors in patient compliance with doctors' orders. Med. Care 6:115, 1968.

Feinstein, A.R.: Clinical Biostatistics. XXX, Biostatistical problems in 'compliance bias'. Clin. Pharmacol. Ther. 16:846, 1974.

Feinstein, A.R.: Clinical biostatistics. XXXV, The persistent clinical failures and fallacies of the UGDP study. Clin. Pharmacol. Ther. 19:78, 1976.

Fink, D.L.: Tailoring the consensual regimen. In Sackett, D.L., and Haynes, R.B., *Compliance with Therapeutic Regimens*, Baltimore, Johns Hopkins University Press, 1976.

Gordis, L., Markowitz, M., and Lilienfeld, A.M.: Studies in the epidemiology and preventability of rheumatic fever. IV. A quantitative determination of compliance in children on oral penicillin prophylaxis. Pediatrics 43:173, 1969.

Hall, M.R.: Use of drugs in elderly patients. NY State J. Med. 75:67, 1975.

Haynes, R.B.: A critical review of the "determinants" of patient compliance with therapeutic regimens. In Sackett, D.L., and Haynes, R.B., *Compliance with Therapeutic Regimens*, Baltimore, Johns Hopkins University Press, 1976.

Haynes, R.B., Sackett, D.L., Gibson, E.S. et al.: Improvement of medication compliance in uncontrolled hypertension. Lancet 1:1265, 1976.

Hecht, A.B.: Improving medication compliance by teaching outpatients. Nurs. Forum 13:112, 1974.

Hulka, B.S., Kupper, L.L., Cassel, S.C., and Efird, R.L.: Medication use and misuse: physician-patient discrepancies. J. Chronic Dis. 28:7, 1975.

Inaba, T., and Kalow, W.: Salivary excretion of amobarbital in man. Clin. Pharm. Ther. 18:558, 1975.

Joyce, C.R.B.: Patient cooperation and the sensitivity of clinical trials. J. Chronic Dis. 15:1025, 1962.

Malahy, B: The effect of instruction and labeling on a number of medication errors made by patients at home. Am. J. Hosp. Pharm. 23:283, 1966.

Marsh, W., and Perlman L.V.: Patient understanding of congestive heart failure and self-administration of digoxin. Clin. Notes Respir. Dis. 19:662, 1971.

Marston, M.V.: Compliance with medical regimens: a review of the literature. Nurs. Res. 19:312, 1970.

Mattar, M., and Yaffe, S.J.: Compliance of pediatric patients with therapeutic regimens. Postgrad. Med. 56:181, 1974.

Moulding, T.: The medication monitor for studying the self-administration of oral contraceptives. Am. J. Obstet. Gynecol. 110:1143, 1971.

Neufeld, V.R.: Patient education: a critique. In Sackett, D.L., and Haynes, R.B., *Compliance with Therapeutic Regimens*, Baltimore, Johns Hopkins University Press, 1976.

Park, L.C., and Lipman, R.S.: A comparison of patient dosage deviation reports with pill counts. Psychopharmacologia 6:299, 1964.

Peck, C.C.: Outpatient compliance with prescriptions for self-medication. In *Present Concepts in Internal Medicine,* Internal Medicine Symposium, 1976.

Peck, C.C.: Qualitative aspects of therapeutic decision making. In Melmon, K.L., and Morrelli, H.F., *Clinical Pharmacology, Basic Principles in Therapeutics,* New York, Macmillan Publishing Company, 1978.

Peck, C.C., Egan, J., and Sheiner, L.B.: Compliance among digoxin-taking patients. Unpublished data, Letterman Army Medical Center, 1975.

Peck, C.C., Phillips, M., and Becker, C.: Drug measurement in sweat: a new technique for estimating patient compliance (abstract). Workshop/Symposium on Compliance, McMaster University, Hamilton, Ontario, Canada, 1977.

Preston, D.F., and Miller, F.L.: The tuberculosis outpatient's defection from therapy. Am. J. Med. Sci. 247:55, 1964.

Roth, H.P., Caron, H.S., and Bartholomeau, P.: Measuring intake of a prescribed drug, a bottle count and a tracer technique compared. Clin. Pharmacol. Ther. 11:228, 1970.

Sackett, D.L.: Patients and therapies: getting the two together. N.Engl. J. Med. 298:278, 1978.

Sackett, D.L.: Why won't patients take their medicine? Can. Fam. Physician 23:462, 1977.

Sackett, D.L., and Haynes, R.B., eds.: *Compliance with Therapeutic Regimens.* Baltimore, Johns Hopkins University Press, 1976.

Schwartz, D., Wong, M., Zeitz, L., et al.: Medication errors made by elderly chronically ill patients. Am. J. Public Health 12:2018, 1962.

Sheiner, L.B., Rosenberg, B.; Marathe, M.A., and Peck, C.C.: Differences in serum digoxin concentrations between outpatients and inpatients: an effect of compliance? Clin. Pharmacol. Ther. 15:239, 1974.

Sheiner, L.B., and Tozer, T.N.: Clinical pharmacokinetics: the use of plasma concentrations of drugs. In Melmon, K.L., and Morrelli, H.F., *Clinical Pharmacology, Basic Principles in Therapeutics,* New York, Macmillan Publishing Company, 1978.

Smith, D., Peck C.C., Egan, J., and Deller, J.J.: A prospective comparison of three anorectic agents, a tranquilizer and a placebo in the short term treatment of exogenous obesity. Unpublished data, Letterman, Army Medical Center, 1973.

Vere, D.W.: Errors of complex prescribing. Lancet 1:370, 1965.

Veterans Administration Cooperative Study Group on Antihypertensive Agents: Effects of treatment on morbidity in hypertension: results in patients with diastolic blood pressure averaging 115–129 mm Hg. JAMA 202:1028, 1967.

Veterans Administration Cooperative Study Group on Antihypertensive Agents: Effects of treatment on morbidity in hypertension. II, Results in patients with diastolic blood pressure averaging 90 through 114 mm Hg. JAMA 213:1143, 1970.

Wagner, J.G.: *Biopharmaceutics and Relevant Pharmacokinetics.* Hamilton, Ill., Drug Intelligence Publications, 1971.

Watkins, J.C.: A study of diabetic patients at home. Am. J. Public Health 57:452, 1967.

Yee, R.D., Hahn, P.M., and Christensen, R.E.: Medication monitor for ophthalmology. Am. J. Ophthalmol. 78:774, 1974.

How to Improve Patient Compliance

Harold S. Solomon, M.D.
Peter Bent Brigham Hospital, Boston

The title of this chapter infers that there is room for improvement in health-related behavior and that we as physicians can contribute to that improved behavior. There are large gaps in our understanding of the causes of noncompliance with medical instructions. The opinions offered are syntheses from available data and from personal clinical experience, and they are still largely unsubstantiated by scientific evidence.

Compliance with medical advice is not a single entity. The act of following a physician's instructions requires a variety of behaviors that depend upon the instructions given. Brushing one's teeth, for example, necessitates different kinds of motivators and cues than does taking one's pills, and taking pills for contraception differs from taking antibiotics to prevent rheumatic fever. In recalling the care given to renal transplant recipients over a two-year period, never once was there a suspicion that a patient failed to comply with his azathiaprine or prednisone, medications used to suppress and prevent transplant rejection. On the other hand, among dialysis patients, there is often suspicion that patients do not take their antacid-phosphate binders consistently. The transplant patient is willing to tolerate disfiguring side effects to prevent transplant rejection. The dialysis patient perhaps is less willing to tolerate the side effects of antacids when the consequences of noncompliance are not so dire and not easily conceptualized (secondary hyperparathyroidism). Rates of compliance vary according to the condition being treated, although data are available for only a few conditions. Measures of compliance are so poorly standardized that comparisons are very difficult to make. The number and type of instructions given, the way patients are instructed by the physician or other health professionals, and the characteristics of the patients who receive those instructions all are determinants of compliance.

Ample documentation exists in the literature of failure of patients to comply consistently with antihypertensive regimens, as well as of the consistent overestimation by physicians of their patients' compliance (Mushlin and Appel, 1977). Recently reported reductions in death rates in the United States due to cardiovascular disease—stroke in particular—suggest that many patients are controlling their blood pressure by complying with antihypertensives, but it is estimated that two thirds of the hypertensives are still not adequately controlled. It is reasonable to assume that poor compliance with antihypertensive treatment is the major reason for lack of blood pressure control, although inadequate dosages or inappropriate selection of medication by physicians contributes to poor blood pressure control as well. For a given individual, failure to comply might be the fault of the patient, the physician, or even the health care system as a whole.

Synopsis of Compliance Research

Compliance research can be divided roughly into three general categories: (1) observational studies of determinants of patient compliance behavior (patient characteristics), (2) observational studies of physician behavior and interventions directed toward the physician (physician characteristics), and (3) intervention studies directed toward the patient.

Patient Characteristics

Early research in patient compliance with medical recommendations assumed that noncompliance was some sort of deviant behavior. Many studies of personality traits—such as intelligence, personality type, authoritarianism, and other parameters of adjustment—have been made without consistently identifying factors related to noncompliance. The noncomplier is not characteristically different from the complier in any specific personality trait. Various demographic and sociologic measurements have been made (Becker and Maiman, 1975) in relation to the type of instructions studied (psychotropic drugs, antihypertensives, parental compliance with pediatric treatments); again, consistency is hard to find. Additionally, even if a patient's race, age, or sex predicts compliance with a certain treatment, we are still left unable to explain the relationship between the demographic factor and the behavior. Another characteristic of compliance studies in adult populations is that most of the studies have been done in urban teaching hospitals where the poor and racial minorities are overrepresented. This population is clearly a special one; in a Louis Harris Poll conducted in 1973, only 15 percent of a sample of the American public reported that they obtained their health care in an urban clinic setting, whereas the other 85 percent received their care predominantly from private practitioners. The private sector is poorly studied. At the National Conference on High Blood Pressure Control in 1977, only one of 123 abstracts represented research done in the private sector.

From a demographic standpoint, and specifically for compliance with antihypertensive medications, the elderly comply better than the young, females better than males, and whites better than blacks. Patients in medical care for a longer time are more apt to stay in care than those in care for a short time. Most physicians are surprised to find that knowledge of the adverse consequences of hypertension, the nature of treatment, and other information about the disease do *not* contribute to compliance. Imparting this information to the American public may result in more patients being screened and detected, but at least two studies show that knowledge *per se* does not result in long-term compliance (McKenney et al., 1973; Haynes et al., 1976). According to the *Health Belief Model* (Rosenstock, 1966; Becker and Maiman, 1975), compliance depends not upon knowledge of the disease process and its consequences but upon (1) the value placed by an individual on a particular outcome (benefits), (2) the patient's expectation that the treatment will result in that benefit, and (3) cues that trigger appropriate health behavior (symptoms, mass media, and interpersonal communication).

It is thought that the information alone does not serve as a strong motivator, but belief in efficacy of treatment and severity of the disease does. The nature of the condition treated and of the medical treatments are clearly related to compliance. If a condition causes pain or loss of a bodily function, and the treatment results in immediate benefit, likelihood of compliance is great. Because hypertension is relatively asymptomatic and noncompliance rarely results in immediate adverse consequences, patients comply less well with treatment for this disease than for other ailments. Medication side effects interfere with drug compliance as do the complexity and dosage interval of treatment.

Physician Characteristics

Doctor-patient interaction is critical to patient compliance. This encounter is one of the most anxiety-laden of all professional consultations. The amount of information transmitted from physician to patient is great, and the patients may be asked to remember too much within too short a period. The manner of the physician, his choice of technical terms, and the sincerity that the patients sense all probably play a role in subsequent compliance behavior. One study (Svarstad, 1974) found that short-term patient compliance was much better when physicians employed compliance-promoting strategies than when they did not. The nature of the instructions and the efforts made by the physician had a measurable outcome on short-term patient medication compliance. Another study (Inui et al., 1976) showed that a tutorial given to physicians in training at a teaching hospital, focusing on compliance skills, resulted in measurable increases in patient compliance with antihypertensive regimens. Together, these two studies reinforce my belief that noncompliance is often the consequence of physicians' lack of skills in the interactive process.

Intervention Studies

When one looks at successful compliance intervention studies (Finnerty et al., 1973a; Finnerty et al., 1973b; McKenney, 1973; Alderman and Schoenbaum, 1975; Haynes et al., 1976), one finds that improving the organization of the practice (appointment reminders, shortened waiting times, consistent care-giver), increasing the amount of time spent by professionals with patients, and increasing efforts designed to establish rapport between physicians and patients all contribute to increased compliance by patients. These studies demonstrate that paraprofessionals can apply compliance-improving strategies with successful outcomes; yet it also seems that physicians should already be using these strategies. For example, the results of one study (McKenney, 1973) showed that a pharmacist, meeting with a patient following the doctor-patient encounter, was able to improve compliance by spelling out medication instructions clearly, reducing the number of medication errors, and explaining side effects. it should not require a pharmacist or other paraprofessional to give instructions clearly or to explain side effects carefully!

Patients make decisions to comply with medical instructions when the benefits from treatment are perceived to exceed the costs, as listed in Figure 26-1. In our hypothetical model (derived from the literature and personal experience), positive numbers represent contributors to compliance and negative numbers represent detractors; zero makes no contribution. For a given patient, the magnitude of the positive or negative number determines the level of importance of a given category in enhancing or preventing compliance. The higher the total positive number, the more likely the patient would be to comply. Data from our Hypertension Education Project show that the current "cost" of being hypertensive in treatment is far greater than most physicians would estimate. We asked our patients, "*In addition to* taking your hypertension medication, what other things has your doctor asked you to do for hypertension?" Then, "How successful have you been at. . . ?" The number of patients reporting that they were requested to make lifestyle changes, and the number of those changes per patient, are shown in Table 26-2. The type of behavioral changes

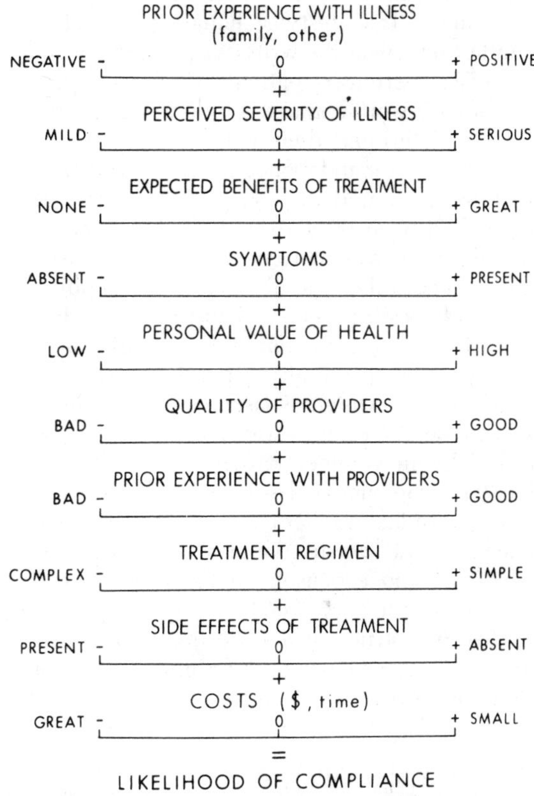

Table 26-2. *Number of Health Behavioral Changes Asked of 300 Hypertensive Patients*

Number of Changes Asked	Number of Patients Reporting	Percent of Patients
0	20	7
1	35	12
2	50	17
3	80	27
4 or more	115	38

From: Hypertension Education Project, Peter Bent Brigham Hospital.

requested and the perceived success that the patients achieved are shown in Table 26–3. Only 7 percent of our patients were told only to take medication; thirty-eight percent of our patients reported they were asked to make at least four changes. From these data, it is clear that treatment for hypertension is "expensive" in terms of the lifestyle changes required. In another review of the writer's office experience, 23 of 52 hypertensive patients who had dropped out of care were contacted by a research assistant to determine their reasons for dropping out. The writer independently reviewed those records and found that 30 percent of the patients had been treated for their hypertension initially with weight reduction diets and were all unsuccessful. None of the patients reported that unsuccessful dietary changes caused them to drop out of care, but it is not difficult to imagine that possibility. It seems that with hypertension—which is usually asymptomatic and not perceived as a serious immediate threat, especially in younger patients who are more likely to drop out of care—initial treatment with a weight reduction diet may establish an imbalance of "cost" versus "benefit" and render the treatment too expensive in terms of lifestyle changes for the perceived benefits. The question of dietary instructions interfering with compliance with other parts of the regimen is important and clearly needs further study.

Table 26–3. *Types of Health Behavioral Changes Asked of 300 Hypertensive Patients*

	Number Asked	Percent Asked	Percent Asked Achieving Some Success
Use less salt	224	75	87
Stop smoking	61	20	57
Avoid fatty-fried Foods	177	59	90
Lose weight	201	67	52
Relax	114	38	68
Other instructions	58	19	67
None	20	7	N.A.

From: Hypertension Education Project, Peter Bent Brigham Hospital.

Conclusion

Compliance with a physician's instructions seems to be enhanced when patients sense that their doctor (or health facility) cares that they comply. The decision to stay in treatment, at least with antihypertensives, seems to be made within the first few encounters with the care process. Compliance is unlikely when side effects of medication are prominent. If the intrusion of a treatment into a patient's lifestyle is perceived by the patient to be too great, the patient is more likely to drop out of care. Individuals make decisions about compliance for many reasons, and for each patient these reasons may be multiple, difficult to identify, and even more difficult to substantiate. To the physician, reasons for noncompliance may seem illogical or irrational; to the patient, the reasons may make good sense. If a patient thinks that a medication is causing a side effect and the physician does not feel this to be true, unless that physician can explain to the patient's satisfaction the lack of relationship of medication to the symptom, the patient will continue to adhere to his belief and eventually stop the treatment.

How, then, can a physician maximize, or at least improve, patient compliance?

Minimize the number of dietary and other life style instructions given, especially during the early phases of treatment. Start with the easier instructions, such as pill taking, and add the more difficult changes later on. A 35-year-old moderately obese patient who is referred because of mild asymptomatic hypertension may perceive hypertension to be a small problem. The obesity may have been dealt with in the past unsuccessfully, and may be considered an insurmountable problem to the patient. If the doctor initiates therapy for hypertension by prescribing weight reduction, and the patient fails to achieve that weight reduction (a likely outcome in seven of eight patients given dietary instruction for weight loss), the patient may drop out of care. The patient may perceive his relationship with the physician as contingent upon a positive outcome (weight loss); failure to lose weight jeopardizes the relationship. In such a patient, I would first institute simple pharmacotherapy appropriate for the hypertension. The patient is more likely to take once- or twice-daily medication than adhere to an 800-calorie diet. Once the blood pressure is brought under control (success) and the person is transformed into a compliant patient, the patient can be offered the opportunity to lose weight. If the patient loses weight, an additional positive reward is that the medication might be discontinued or reduced in dosage. On the other hand, if the patient fails to lose weight, he is still under treatment for hypertension and is still compliant overall. Many casual instructions for which the physician has little expectation of success create negative feelings of failure and guilt on the part of patients. Thus, suggestions to "knock off a few pounds," "add a few bananas a day to your diet," or "relax" are easy to suggest but may be difficult goals to reach. It is essential if a patient is to be "compliant" that success be experienced by the patient, especially in the first six months of treatment. Failures early on lead to dropping out.

Simplify the drug regimen and teach compliance cues. Tell the patient that you are simplifying the drug regimen so as to reinforce the feeling that the physician cares that he complies. No antihypertensive drugs need be given more than twice daily. A twice-a-day dosage regimen is fairly easy for the patient to maintain. The patient can take the medication with breakfast and dinner, at which time there are environmental cues to take medication that the physician can help the patient to identify. Drugs that need to be taken more than twice daily often require patients to remember to take medication to work with them, a potentially embarrassing situation. Home blood pressure devices may also serve as a reinforcer or cue to remember to take medications. Three fourths of my patients have their own devices.

Tell the patient exactly what is expected of him, and exactly what he can expect from the doctor-patient relationship. Eliminate all extraneous instructions. Give patients written instructions wherever possible. It has been useful for me to make the following statement to the hypertensive patient: "A successful outcome requires that you do three things and that I do three things. I expect you to take your medication as prescribed, keep your next appointment, and telephone if you have any questions or if you decide to stop the medication for any reason. In return, I will see you within 30 minutes of your scheduled appointment, return your phone calls promptly, and provide you with the most up-to-date treatment for your condition." The patient gets a sense of mutuality of involvement in the treatment process. In addition, when the patient has left the often anxiety-provoking atmosphere of the doctor's office, there are only three instructions to remember. Other health instruction, including dietary changes, can be dealt with in exactly the same way, but in subsequent visits. Another useful tool to increase the feeling of the mutual nature of the relationship between doctor and patient is to define clear treatment goals. For the hypertensive patient, knowing that a diastolic blood pressure less than 90 mm Hg is a treatment goal gives the patient an idea of how serious the condition is and how well he is doing.

Build upon successes. Patients seem to comply better if their physicians care that they comply, and they are more likely to remain in care if they are successful at being a "patient," especially in the first few months of treatment. The easiest health changes—usually taking medication—should be suggested first. The more difficult health changes, such as weight loss, smoking, and exercise, should be dealt with in such a way as not to overwhelm the patient.

Audit patient behavior. Physicians overestimate compliance, and quickly forget patients who drop out of care. A review of your patient population will identify patients who have dropped out of care, many of whom will return to care following a call from the office.

More research is needed, especially on compliance in the noninstitutional primary care setting. Although the purpose of this textbook is to air controversy, there are still not enough scientific data in this area to warrant more than strong opinions.

References

Alderman, M.H., and Schoenbaum, E.E.: Detection and treatment of hypertension at the work site. N. Engl. J. Med. 293:65, 1975.

Becker, M.H., and Maiman, L.A.: Sociobehavioral determinants of compliance with health and medical care recommendations. Med. Care 13:10, 1975.

Finnerty, F.A., Jr., Mattie, E.C., et al.: Hypertension in the inner city. I, Analysis of clinic dropouts. Circulation 47:73, 1973.

Finnerty, F.A., Jr., Shaw, L.W., et al.: Hypertension in the inner city. II, Detection and followup. Circulation 47:76, 1973.

Haynes, R.B., Sackett, D.L., et al.: Improvement of medication compliance in uncontrolled hypertension. Lancet 1:1265, 1976.

Inui, T.S., et al.: Improved outcomes in hypertension after physician tutorials. Ann. Int. Med. 84:646, 1976.

McKenney, J.D., Slining, J.M., et al.: The effect of clinical pharmacy services on patients with essential hypertension. Circulation 48:1104, 1973.

Mushlin, A.I., and Appel, F.A.: Diagnosing potential noncompliance. Arch. Int. Med. 137:318, 1977.

Rosenstock, I.M.: Why people use health services. Milbank Memorial Fund Q. 44:94, 1966.

Svarstad, B.L.: The doctor-patient encounter: an observational study of communication and outcome. Doctoral Dissertation, University of Wisconsin, 1974.

27

Should Saccharin Be Banned?

An article of food or drink which is slightly worse, but more palatable, is to be preferred to such as are better but less palatable.

Hippocrates, *Aphorisms*

Tell me what you eat, and I will tell you what you are.

A. Brillat-Savarin, *La Physiologie du Goût*

What is worse than keeping a diet! It can make your whole life miserable.

August Bier

Introduction

At the moment, the American public is down to its last artificial sweetener. A decade ago, cyclamates were banned as carcinogens. Although the Canadians reversed their stand on these agents (it had been similar to that of our FDA) in 1978 and concluded that there is not a shred of evidence that cyclamates are carcinogenic, these products are still disapproved by the U.S. regulatory agency.

In 1977, saccharin came under attack on the basis of controversial animal and human data. If the U.S. Congress had not forced a delay, there is little doubt that the FDA would have banned saccharin as a food additive.

Aaron believes that saccharin is a weak carcinogen—which is an opinion shared by many experts—and he believes that the latest epidemiologic study will be crucial in deciding the fate of "the last sweetener."

Kessler, in contrast, finds the case for saccharin's dangers to be unconvincing, especially since the bulk of the epidemiologic data argues for its safety. His critique of the animal and human data makes interesting reading, and his closing section on "the regulatory dilemma" posed by a Delaney Amendment philosophy is must reading for those who feel any degree of complacency about this general problem.

As a clinical pharmacologist, I hope that our society does not have to do without artificial sweeteners. Regardless of the merits of such additives for dieters or diabetics, sweeteners are very important in the preparation of drug formulations. The world has enough bitter pills as it is.

LOUIS LASAGNA, M.D.

Saccharin: The Evidence of Carcinogenicity

Harold Aaron, M.D.
The Medical Letter, Inc., New Rochelle, N.Y.

Many chemicals added to or found in food, water, and workplaces turn out to have unsuspected injurious properties when tested with new chemical and biologic techniques. Such has been the fate of saccharin: it was used for more than 80 years as a sweetening agent, believed to be harmless, and known to have toxic effects only when given to animals in heroic doses, far larger than would ever be likely in human experience. Today, saccharin is under a cloud of suspected carcinogenicity, becoming one more chemical to be added to the long list of harmful agents in our environment (National Academy of Sciences, 1974; National Institutes of Health: National Institute of Environmental Health Sciences, 1977; Select Committee on Small Business, United States Senate, 1977).

Human exposure to the carcinogenic and genetic effects of ionizing radiation and fallout by the use of nuclear weapons led to international agreements restricting such tests to the underground. Acute lymphoblastic and chronic myelogenous leukemia, lymphosarcoma, and tumors of the thyroid, respiratory tract, breast, and intestinal tract have resulted from whole body irradiation among survivors of the atomic bomb explosions in Japan during World War II. Concern has also been voiced about excessive exposure of patients and healthy subjects to radiation and radionuclides for diagnosis, screening programs, and therapy. Accordingly, any increment of a carcinogen, no matter how small, added to the already substantial exposure of the population to carcinogens during a lifetime, must be taken very seriously and its risks must be carefully balanced against its benefits. Against this background, interest in saccharin has shifted from its toxic to its potential carcinogenic effects.*

Power to regulate carcinogenic chemicals in the environment resides mainly in two federal statutes—The Food, Drug and Cosmetic Act of 1938 (and its amendments) and The Toxic Substances Control Act of 1976. Both contain provisions for regulating carcinogens that are distinct from those regulating toxic agents. The 1938 statute generally takes precedence over other federal and state laws for regulating carcinogenic substances in foods, drugs and cosmetics.

Of all the federal laws regulating hazardous substances in the environment, only the Food, Drug and Cosmetic Act contains provisions such as the Delaney clause, which permits little discretion in banning carcinogens in foods and beverages. The Delaney clause, at the core of the controversy over the safety of saccharin, is found in the 195th Amendment to the Act dealing with food additives and states "No addi-

* Protection of the general public from hazardous chemicals including carcinogens is entrusted to several federal agencies: The Occupational Safety and Health Administration, which has regulatory authority over the workplace; the Food and Drug Administration (FDA), which regulates foods, drugs, and cosmetics; the Consumer Product Safety Commission, whose mandate is to protect the public against unreasonable risks of injury associated with consumer products; and the Environmental Protection Agency (EPA), which regulates air and water pollution and the manufacture and use of pesticides, and administers the Toxic Substance Control Act.

tive shall be deemed to be safe if it is found to induce cancer when ingested by man or animal, or if it is found, after tests which are appropriate for the evaluation of the safety of food additives, to induce cancer in man or animal." The clause is always interpreted as meaning zero tolerance for additives that induce cancer, regardless of any health or economic benefits provided by the additives.

Food Additives

GRAS is an acronym for food additives "generally recognized as safe" by the FDA. In 1958, the FDA solicited opinions from the scientific community about the usefulness and safety of all substances added to foods, and in 1959 and 1960, it published GRAS lists in the Federal Register. No further testing of the safety of these initial GRAS compounds was required (the "grandfather" clause), but any additions to the list were expected to be adequately tested by the manufacturer for usefulness and safety. Currently, there are probably over 700 GRAS compounds. There are also approximately 1200 natural and synthetic flavoring agents added to foods that are generally recognized as safe but listed separately in the Code of Federal Regulations.

The presumed safety of so many chemicals added to foods or migrating into foods during packaging has been based on common experience and the lack of adverse information, rather than on extensive toxicologic testing and knowledge of the biologic effects of such chemicals (LaDu, 1977). Although the burden of proof of safety remains with the original manufacturer, the task of providing new evidence of possible harm shifts to the FDA. Under the Delaney clause, the FDA's responsibility is met as soon as it finds that a food additive is carcinogenic (Federal Register Part III, April 15, 1977).

The most troublesome aspect of the review process has been the lack of adequate biologic and toxicologic information from the world literature on most of these food additives. Relatively few GRAS substances have been sufficiently studied in man to determine their metabolic fate, disposition, and acute and chronic toxicity. Furthermore, although most of any GRAS compound added to foods or migrating into foods from packaging material is consumed in extremely small quantities (a few milligrams or less per day), there is no generally regarded safe dose or tolerance for a carcinogen. In other words, there is no threshold below which carcinogens are inactive; lowering the dose decreases the risk but does not abolish it.

Prior to 1972, saccharin was classified by the FDA as GRAS, and thus it was considered by the public to be a safe substitute for sugar in (or on) foods and in drinks. Most of the studies on the metabolism, excretion, and toxicity of saccharin were made in the earlier part of the century. Large amounts of it were used during wartime periods of sugar shortages, and no adverse effects were reported. Since 1969, when cyclamates were banned by the FDA as sweetening agents as a result of animal tests showing them to be carcinogens, saccharin has been the only synthetic sweetener used in the United States.

Saccharin crosses the placenta in primates and tends to accumulate in fetal tissues. In 1972, after bladder tumors were discovered in rats fed saccharin *in utero* and also throughout life, the FDA removed it from the list of GRAS food additives (National Academy of Sciences, Subcommittee on Nonnutritive Sweeteners, 1974). Its continued use was allowed, however, while a National Academy of Sciences (NAS) Committee reviewed the evidence of carcinogenicity. The Subcommittee reported that existing evidence was insufficient to determine whether saccharin is carcinogenic in animals.

On March 18, 1977, the Subcommittee on Health and Scientific Research of the Senate Committee on Human Resources requested that the Office of Technology Assessment (OTA) of the U.S. Congress convene a panel of scientists to study the technologic basis for the FDA ruling.*

Methods for Detecting Carcinogens

The OTA report (1977) discussed four methods available for identifying substances in

* The panel consisted of John Burns, Vice President for Research, Hoffman-La-Roche, Inc.; Emilio Daddario, Former Director, Office of Technology Assessment; Cyrus Levinthal, Professor of Biology, Columbia University; Matthew Meselson, Chairman of the Department of Biochemistry and Molecular Biology, Harvard University; David Rall, Director of the National Institute of Environmental Health Sciences; Frank Rauscher, Former Director, National Cancer Institute and Vice President for Research, American Cancer Society; Frederick Robbins, Dean, Case Western Reserve Medical School and Chairman, Health Advisory Committee, Office of Technology Assessment.

the environment that are potential carcinogens: analysis of the substance's molecular structure, animal tests, short-term (mutagenic and other) tests, and epidemiologic studies. Although analysis of molecular structure provides some information concerning the likelihood that a substance will cause cancer, in most instances, prediction on this basis alone is not helpful, since the substance may be metabolized and the metabolite may be a carcinogen.

Animal Tests

Animal tests are known valuable methods for predicting carcinogenicity. All substances demonstrated to be carcinogenic in animals can be regarded as potential human carcinogens; no clear distinctions exist between substances that cause cancer in laboratory animals and those that cause it in humans. A large number of animal tests performed with chemicals overwhelmingly supports this hypothesis (Office of Technology Assessment, 1977).

The best animals for such tests (apart from testing suspected carcinogens directly in humans) are primates, but in order to detect carcinogens of low incidence and long incubation periods, experiments require that hundreds of primates be exposed to the suspected carcinogen at the same dose and by the same route of administration as in humans. Guidelines set up by the National Cancer Institute (NCI) also require that animals be followed for at least two generations in order to detect a carcinogenic effect. The best practical model, therefore, is to use small animals that have lifetimes of two to three years. Several agents now recognized as being carcinogenic in humans—bischloromethyl ether, diethylstilbestrol, and vinyl chloride—were first recognized as carcinogens on the basis of animal tests.

Standard procedure in animal cancer tests is to feed the suspected substances at the "maximum tolerated dose." In the case of saccharin, this is 5 percent of the diet, even though humans are exposed to much lower doses. Contrary to popular opinion, all chemicals do not cause cancer at high dose levels. Many food additives and other chemicals have been tested in animals at very high levels without causing cancer.

Feeding large doses of a substance in animal tests is generally acknowledged to be a valid experimental procedure. As the dose of a carcinogen is increased, the number of exposed animals that develop cancer also increases. To conduct a sound experiment at high dose levels, only a small number of animals (perhaps several hundred) is required. However, to conduct a valid experiment at low dose levels, a very large number of animals is required. The smallest incidence rate detectable with 10 animals is 10 percent (or one animal). To detect a 1 percent incidence rate, several hundred animals would be required. Another important variable is the strength of the carcinogen—the stronger the carcinogen, the greater the number of animals getting cancer at a particular dose. Thus, there are three important variables to be considered in any animal experiment: the strength of the carcinogen, the exposure level or dose, and the number of animals exposed.

Genetic variation among humans and their exposure to other carcinogenic substances in the environment affect susceptibility to carcinogenic agents. This causes difficulties in making quantitative estimates of human risk based on data even from genetically similar animals. In general, if the substance produces cancer in test animals and the route of administration is equivalent to that in humans, the agent is likely to have a carcinogenic effect in humans.

Extrapolation to humans. Evidence that the potency of carcinogens in rodents is a rough indicator of their potency in people is not conclusive. To compare the strength of carcinogens in animals with that in people requires more data. Because controlled oral dosage experiments cannot be conducted in humans, available information is limited to animal, mutagenic, and epidemiologic population studies. Although some extrapolations to humans have been validated, others are more complex. In the case of diethylstilbestrol (DES), for example, the chemical caused cancer of the liver in animals but affected the female reproductive organs in humans. Nevertheless, although the animal experiments did not predict the organ site, they did show that exposure to the chemical involved a risk.

Early Animal Studies

Preliminary results of a long-term feeding study of saccharin by the Food and Drug Administration (FDA) indicated the formation of bladder tumors. In February 1977, the FDA removed saccharin from the GRAS list and issued an interim food additive regulation limiting the use of saccharin in foods. The FDA extended the interim regulation while awaiting a review of the experimental data by the National Academy of Sciences (NAS), including the two long-term feeding studies by the FDA at the Wisconsin Alumni Research Foundation that showed bladder tumors developing in rats fed on diets containing 5 and 7.5 percent saccharin (Federal Register Part III, April 15, 1977). The 1974 NAS report stated that saccharin itself could not be positively identified as the cause of the tumors because of the presence of impurities, as well as because of problems in experimental design and procedures. The FDA therefore continued interim regulations while awaiting results of new tests.

A Canadian study was designed to answer the objections raised in the NAS report, principally that an impurity in the saccharin, orthotoluenesulfonamide (OTS), might have been the carcinogen. The Canadian study separated rats into control, saccharin, and OTS populations. The results showed that the saccharin group had an increased incidence of bladder tumors, whereas the OTS group did not (Health Protection Branch, National Health and Welfare Department, Canada, 1976).

On the basis of animal tests alone, the FDA was required to ban the use of saccharin as a sweetening agent and to hold hearings that would permit consumers and manufacturers of saccharin and dietetic foods and drinks containing it to state their objections to or support for the proposed ban. However, manufacturers and distributors of the chemical and of products containing it raised such a clamor about the Delaney clause and the relevance of animal experiments showing that saccharin caused cancer in mice and rats that the FDA was compelled to postpone enforcing prohibitive regulations. Congress went a step further; in November 1977, the House of Representatives and the Senate passed and sent to the President the "Saccharin Study and Labeling Act" (SSLA), which the President signed. The SSLA prohibited the FDA from banning the use of saccharin as a food additive or in drugs and cosmetics solely on the basis of scientific evidence about the cancer-causing properties of saccharin available to FDA on the day the SSLA was enacted (November 23, 1977). It also directed the FDA to arrange for various studies to be conducted on "carcinogenic and other toxic substances in food and concerning the toxicity of saccharin and the health benefits, if any, resulting from the use of nonnutritive sweeteners."

In the meantime, the SSLA required that after February 21, 1978, the labeling of food containing saccharin bear the following warning in a conspicuous place: "Use of this product may be hazardous to your health. This product contains saccharin which has been determined to cause cancer in laboratory animals." Food containing saccharin that does not bear this warning would be misbranded under a new section of the Food, Drug and Cosmetic Act.

Short-Term Tests

About 20 short-term studies of saccharin have been reported (reviewed by OTA), and they can be divided into three general types: tests using Drosophila; *in vitro* (Ames salmonella/microsome test) and *in vivo* tests (in mammals) for induction of chromosome abnormalities; and tests for the induction of dominant lethal mutations in mice. The OTA commissioned a battery of 12 such tests on saccharin, designed to determine whether highly purified saccharin is mutagenic or if it causes other genetic alterations. Saccharin had been tested previously by only 2 of 12 methods. All participating laboratories received a sample of saccharin that had been specially purified.

Results from three tests—"sister chromatid exchange," "mouse lymphoma," and "chromosome aberration"—were positive. Although highly purified samples of saccharin were weakly active in these tests, the results are clearly suggestive that saccharin itself has mutagenic properties. According to the OTA, the results should be regarded with some caution, since the responses were weak in the three tests, even at the high dose levels tested.

The negative results do not invalidate the positive results. In animal studies, saccharin is detected to be carcinogenic in rats only at high doses and is therefore called a "weak carcinogen." Mutagenic effects were also detected only at very high dosages. Thus, positive mutagenicity may not be detected in many short-term tests. According to the OTA, each of the short-term tests has its own set of limitations, both in sensitivity and in the range of chemical classes it can detect. Although it would be surprising if a potent carcinogen were negative in many different kinds of short-term tests, it is not surprising that a carcinogen such as saccharin might be detected in only a few systems. Uncertainties regarding impurities are characteristic of the published short-term data on saccharin. Samples of saccharin used in the

Canadian cancer tests contained far lower levels of impurities than commercial saccharin (to which humans are exposed), and it is possible that carcinogenic impurities in commercial saccharin pose a greater human health hazard than saccharin itself.

Epidemiologic Studies

Epidemiologic studies attempt to determine if there is a positive association between a particular exposure and the occurrence of disease in the population, and, if there is, whether the association is causal. Humans are usually exposed to carcinogens in far smaller doses than those used in animals. Effects in humans are consequently less frequent, and it is necessary to examine large numbers of people in order to detect them.

The usual sensitivity limits of even a properly conducted study make detecting a carcinogen with a low incidence unlikely. A long induction time also makes detection difficult. Thus, positive or negative epidemiologic evidence could make a strong case for or against the existence of a carcinogen with a high incidence and a short induction time. Negative evidence alone would not provide the basis for a case against a carcinogen with an expected low incidence or a long induction time.

Three kinds of epidemiologic evidence have been examined. In Great Britain, where a large increase in saccharin consumption occurred during World War II, time trends in per capita use of saccharin and of cigarettes have been compared with trends in death rates from cancer of the bladder (Armstrong and Doll, 1974). Increased cigarette smoking can account for the steady increase in bladder cancer mortality among males born after 1870. These data, although revealing no association between saccharin and cancer, cover only two or three decades of increased saccharin use.

In a series of patients with cancer of the bladder, using a control group of normal subjects, information was obtained on patient use of saccharin (or beverages containing saccharin) and their medical histories with respect to diabetes. In none of several studies of this type—in the United States, Canada, and Britain (Morgan and Jain, 1974; Kessler, 1978; Armstrong and Doll, 1975)—were statistically significant differences found between the cancer subjects and the controls. Data on saccharin use were in many instances incomplete and were not available for those patients who had died of bladder cancer, making valid comparison impossible.

A series of patients with diabetes who were known to use more saccharin than the general population was followed for many years to determine the cause of their deaths. The observed number of deaths from cancer was compared with the number expected on the basis of cancer mortality rates in the general population of the same age and sex. This method permits assessment not only of bladder cancer risk, but of risk of all cancers that are likely to cause death. In two studies conducted to date (Kessler, 1978; Armstrong and Doll, 1975), no significant excess of bladder cancer mortality was observed.

The Positive Canadian Experiment

A total of 821 newly diagnosed cases of primary bladder cancer were identified (Howe et al., 1977) in three Canadian provinces between April 1974 and June 1977. Of these, 632 (480 males and 152 females) were personally interviewed in their homes and asked questions about their use of artificial sweeteners. Information from these interviews was compared with that obtained from interviewing an equal number of controls. Each case was matched with a control of the same sex and same age (within 5 years) and who lived in the same neighborhood.

The conclusions drawn from these data are that artificial sweetener use increases the risk of bladder cancer in males by a factor of 1.6 but there is no association between sweetener use and bladder cancer in females. However, too few cases of female bladder cancer were found to conclude with any assurance that sweeteners had no effect on bladder cancer incidence in women.

The inconclusive findings of the various epidemiologic studies led to a decision to carry out a well controlled investigation of a large group of the population. On January 25, 1978, the FDA and the National Cancer Institute (NCI) announced plans to conduct a nationwide study on the role of saccharin in bladder cancer in humans. The epidemiologic study will cost $1.375 million and will require about 18 months to complete. The study will include about 3000 people with bladder cancer diagnosed during 1978 and 6000 randomly chosen healthy individuals living in the same areas. All 9000 people will be interviewed. The NCI will analyze the data and compare the saccharin consumption patterns of the cancer patients with those of the healthy individuals to determine whether there is a causal association between the sweetener and bladder cancer.

The study also will develop information on other factors that may play a role in bladder cancer, including cyclamates, drinking water, cigarettes, and occupational exposures.

Benefit Versus Risk

Some scientists, while acknowledging that saccharin may be a carcinogen, urge that it remain on the market since it is helpful in weight reducing regimens and in the control of diabetes. In other words, they feel that the benefits outweigh the risks.

The benefits of a sweetener such as saccharin are difficult to assess, in part because it has become an integral item in the diet of many Americans and in part because of the scarcity or absence of controlled studies on its effectiveness. The OTA concluded that no scientific data were found to prove or to disprove that use of the nonnutritive sweetener leads to any health benefits.

Weight control. Only two studies employing controls were found in the literature with respect to the value of saccharin in a weight control regimen. In a study of the effectiveness of noncaloric sweeteners among 247 obese and 100 diabetic people (McCann et al., 1956), the authors found "No significant difference ... when the weight loss of users and non-users of these products was compared. No correlation was found between the length of time these products were used and weight loss ...."

A study was undertaken to investigate the effects of substituting an artificially sweetened solution for a sucrose solution on spontaneous food consumption and weight gain in mice (Friedhoff et al., 1971). It was concluded that mice offered a normal diet and a sucrose solution do not gain weight faster than animals eating the same diet plus either artificially sweetened solution or plain water. Whereas these findings are not necessarily applicable to human use of sugar-containing or noncaloric beverages, they question the value of simple substitution of noncaloric beverages for sucrose-containing beverages as a weight control measure.

Noncaloric beverages may be useful when total caloric intake is closely regulated, but if this is not the case, the loss of calories in drink may be compensated for by ingestion of caloric solids. Conversely, the ingestion of sugar-containing beverages may not increase body weight, because spontaneous reduction of solid food intake may occur, perhaps by an appetite-depressing effect of sugar solutions (Mellinkoff and Frankland, 1956).

Diabetes. The view of a select committee on sugar substitutes of the American Diabetes Association probably represents the prevailing judgement of physicians who manage diabetic patients. The committee concludes "... that much more research of broader scope and greater detail is needed before the saccharin controversy can be resolved.... Surveillance of new information by the Association will continue. However, based on evidence now available, there appears to be little justification for placing further governmental restrictions on the use of saccharin by the American public at the present time." (June 10, 1978).

The committee took no position on the usefulness of saccharin in the management of diabetes.

Conclusion

There is evidence from animal lifetime studies and from short-term tests that saccharin is a carcinogen, albeit a weak one. Epidemiologic studies are less convincing, but they have many weaknesses in design. An epidemiologic study has been started by the National Cancer Institute and the Food and Drug Administration, employing an adequate number of subjects, a proper design, and appropriate controls. The results of this study will soon be known and should have a crucial effect on the evaluation of saccharin as a carcinogen.

References

Armstrong, B., and Doll, R.: Cancer mortality and saccharin consumption in diabetics. Br. J. Prev. Soc. Med. 30:151, 1974.

Armstrong, B., and Doll, R.: Bladder cancer mortality diabetics in relation to saccharin consumption and smoking habits. Br. J. Prev. Soc. Med. 29:73, 1975.

Department of Health, Education, and Welfare: Saccharin and its salts. Federal Register Part III, April 15, 1977.

Friedhoff, R., et al.: Sucrose solution vs no-calorie sweetener vs water in weight gain. J. Am. Diet. Assoc. 59:485, 1971.

Howe, G.R., et al.: Artificial sweeteners and human bladder cancer. Lancet 2:578, 1977.

Kessler, I.I.: Saccharin, cyclamate and human bladder cancer. JAMA 240:349, 1978. J. Urol.

LaDu, B.N.: Effects of GRAS substances on pharmacologic effects of drugs. Clin Pharm. Ther. 22:743, 1977.

McCann, M.F., et al.: Non-caloric sweeteners and weight reduction. J. Am. Diet. Assoc. 32:327, 1956.

Mellinkoff, S.M., and Frankland, M.: Effect of amino acid and glucose on arteriovenous blood sugar and appetite. J. Appl. Physiol. 9:85, 1956.

Morgan, R.W., and Jain, M.G.: Bladder cancer; smoking, beverages and artificial sweeteners. Can. Med. Assoc. J. 111:1067, 1974.

National Academy of Sciences: How safe is safe? The design of policy on drugs and food additives. Washington, D.C., 1974.

National Academy of Sciences (Subcommittee on Nonnutritive Sweeteners): Report on safety of saccharin and sodium saccharin in the human diet. Washington, D.C., 1974.

National Institutes of Health: National Institute of Environmental Health Sciences: Human health and the environment: some research needs. Washington, D.C., 1977.

Office of Technology Assessment (OTA): Cancer testing technology and saccharin. Washington, D.C., 1977.

Select Committee on Small Business, United States Senate Hearings: Food additives: competitive, regulatory, and safety problems. Washington, D.C., 1977.

Saccharin Should Not Be Banned

Irving I. Kessler, M.D., Dr.P.H.
University of Maryland School of Medicine

Saccharin, Son of Cyclamate

My interest in the saccharin controversy stems from the earlier debates on cyclamates. Abbott Laboratories began to market cyclamates in 1950. The principal use of this hexylsulfamate, usually in combination with smaller amounts of saccharin, was to sweeten soft drinks and canned foods. During the succeeding decade, cyclamate production increased more than 300 percent; diet drinks alone came to account for some 15 percent of the total soft drink market.

The appearance of studies linking sugar consumption with obesity and chronic disease, the rising diet-consciousness of Americans, and the encroachment of nonnutritive sweeteners on sugar sales may all have encouraged the interest of the Sugar Research Foundation in contracting with the University of Wisconsin Alumni Research Foundation (WARF) for studies on the toxicologic effects of cyclamate ingestion in rats. At about the same time and perhaps in response to these efforts, Abbott Laboratories, the leading cyclamate producer, arranged for Food & Drug Research Laboratories of New York to conduct additional studies on the safety of cyclamates.

The results of these "defensively motivated" investigations were ironic. The WARF studies sponsored by the sugar industry failed to demonstrate serious adverse effects of cyclamate feeding. On the other hand, the studies supported by the cyclamate manufacturers revealed tumors in some laboratory rats fed this substance, leading to its removal from the GRAS (generally recognized as safe) list in October 1969 and an outright ban a few months later.

Several aspects of the cyclamate saga paved the way for the saccharin dilemma. Firstly, there was the question of how food additives are selected for study of possible health hazards. With millions of distinct chemical entities in our environment, and with more than 60,000 chemicals in common use, what rational means are there for society to decide which substances require the expenditure of limited fiscal resources for carcinogenic or toxicologic testing? (Competing commercial interests played crucial roles in the generation of evidence against cyclamates.)

The cyclamate saga is impressive because it represents a rare instance in which the Delaney clause of the Food Additives Amendment of 1958 has been invoked as the principal basis for health hazard regulation of food additives. It is pertinent to consider why this well intentioned law has been applied so infrequently—perhaps only 9 or 10 times since its passage by the Congress more than 20 years ago.

The alacrity with which the Abbott study findings were accepted by the Food and Drug Administration (FDA) and then adopted as the basis for a Delaney clause action less than two weeks later suggests a third issue: whether a single study—however well designed and executed—can or should be regarded as "definitive" with respect to important scientific questions and serve as the basis for regulatory action by government. How is truth approached in science? More particularly, what kinds of data should serve as the basis for scientific inference?

A fourth issue raised by the cyclamate ban was the novel spectacle of scientific pronouncements and regulatory decisions made under the glare of klieg lights—of scientists interacting with the press and political figures rather than with professional colleagues. A perhaps inevitable consequence of this intrusion of politics into science was an increasing polarization of opinion among scientists, industry representatives, consumer advocates, and government officials, with a predictable rise in the level of the public's anxiety.

The poor quality of the scientific evidence invoked for the regulatory decision on cyclamates was also striking. The Abbott study involved feedings of cyclamate-saccharin mixtures, rather than of pure cyclamate; therefore, saccharin was as likely as cyclamate to have been the hypothesized carcinogenic agent. Years later, when the shortcomings of the study were finally acknowledged, subsequent rat feeding studies employing pure cyclamates yielded negative results. *Yet, no reversal of the regulatory decision was forthcoming,* although a law suit toward this end is still pending.

The difficulties in extrapolating experimental findings from animals to man are well recognized. It is thus all the more surprising that until last year, the need for human epidemiologic evidence on the presumed carcinogenicity of cyclamates or saccharin had never been publicly supported by the FDA despite the fact that both artificial sweeteners had been in use for many years and that substantial observational data on the outcomes of such use could readily be derived from epidemiologic investigation.

These considerations, most particularly the absence of any studies on human subjects, impelled me to design a case-control investigation on the role of artificial sweeteners in human bladder cancer. The study was conducted during a quiescent period of the early 1970s, after the cyclamate ban but before the government's action against saccharin. It is crucial that scientifically and socially acceptable means for resolving the issue be forthcoming. Otherwise, saccharin will become not only a bitter sweet but a Pandora's box as well.

The Epidemiologic Evidence

At the height of the cyclamate controversy in 1969, an impressive number of toxicologic studies on artificial sweeteners were either underway or being planned. However, there were no studies on human subjects, nor was there any apparent interest on the part of the government in initiating any.

Some indirect evidence of toxicity was available from the results of our prospective study of 20,000 diabetic patients who could be presumed more likely to use artificial sweeteners than the general population. At about the same time, Burbank and Fraumeni (1970) published their correlational analysis of time trends in artificial sweetener use and bladder cancer mortality. No suggestion of a carcinogenic risk from artificial sweeteners emerged from either of these studies, although neither was designed expressly to provide a substantial test of this hypothesis.

In late 1972, a three-year grant of $115,000 from the National Bladder Cancer Project enabled us to undertake the first full-scale epidemiologic investigation of the possible carcinogenicity of artificial sweeteners in man. The level of financial support may be compared, for whatever it is worth, with the 18-month $1.4 million study recently commissioned by the government. Even taking into account its larger patient sample, the yield of subjects per dollars expended is less than half that achieved in the university-sponsored study.

Our initial findings were presented in 1974 at the International Cancer Congress in Florence, Italy. Publications in the scientific literature appeared in 1976 and, most recently, in July 1978. The significance of these dates lies in their demonstration that substantial evidence bearing on the saccharin controversy was available to the FDA long before the appearance of the controversial Canadian study, to be discussed later.

With the following detailed description of our study, my hope is that readers who are unfamiliar with the epidemiologic method will have an opportunity to judge for themselves the contributions that this relatively new approach may make in the assessment of human health hazards.

Controlled Studies on the Effects of Artificial Sweeteners in Man

All metropolitan Baltimore residents discharged from any hospital in the area between 1972 and 1975 with a diagnosis of bladder cancer were identified. Senile, dying, or other uninterviewable patients, as well as a few refusers, were excluded. Five hundred and nine subjects died before they could be contacted, and 157 cases identified too late were unprocessed. Out of a total of 634 surviving patients with histopathologically confirmed malignancies of the bladder, 519 (82 percent) agreed to participate in the study. Because patients from all the local hospitals were included, the study subjects were probably representative of the community as a whole rather than of any given institution. Their selectivity was further reduced by including most newly diagnosed cases and matching them to demographically similar controls.

For each bladder cancer case, a control subject was randomly selected from hospital registration lists of cancer-free patients without bladder conditions who were hospitalized in the institution at the same time as the bladder cancer case and who were of the same sex, race, age, and current marital status. The last condition was imposed in order to control for variations in the validity of responses concerning dietary habits. A patient living alone might, for example, have more difficulty recalling precise details of sweetener ingestion as compared with a married individual.

All patients and controls were then personally interviewed with respect to their use of artificial sweeteners in any and all forms. They were probed about the frequency, quantity, and duration of exposure to table sweeteners, diet beverages, diet foods, and other artificially sweetened products by type and brand name. The nonnutritive sweetener constituents were verified from industrial sources and by direct examination of product labels. In order to reduce the likelihood of including cancers unrelated to sweetener use, ingestion of saccharin or cyclamates from one year prior to the date of cancer diagnosis and thereafter was ignored in the analysis.

Study subjects were also investigated in detail with respect to smoking habits, occupational exposures, diabetic conditions, and other factors that might have influenced their risk of developing bladder cancer. Such information lessened the possibility that the observed sweetener effects were distorted by "confounding" factors.

Two other, somewhat related, essential study conditions were also satisfied by our investigational protocol: the interviewers were not aware of the case or control status of their subjects at the time of interview, and, as previously noted, the study was conducted at a time when public attention on the artificial sweetener issue was slight. Thus, neither the interviewers nor the interviewees were likely to have been sensitized—and therefore potentially biased—at the moment of their encounter. Analysis was in terms of relative frequencies, quantities, and duration of artificial sweetener use among bladder cancer cases and controls, with appropriate computations of the statistical significance of differences. Comparisons were also made in terms of relative risk after simultaneous adjustment for the potential confounding factors already mentioned. Finally, the data were carefully examined for evidence of dose-response relatonships that might shed further light on the nature of the association, if any, between artificial sweetener use and bladder cancer in man.

Our bladder cancer patents and controls were remarkably similar in artificial sweetener exposure, however measured. Since several hundred different comparisons on sweetener use in one form or another were made, we expected to find between 10 and 20 statistically significant case-control differences on the basis of chance alone. In fact, considerably fewer were noted, and these had no consistent direction, either positive or negative. The data are notable for the unexceptionable similarity between cases and controls in their patterns of table-top, diet beverage, diet food, and other artificial sweetener exposure.

These findings suggest to us that ingestion of artificial sweeteners, at least at the moderate dietary levels reported by the patients sampled, is unlikely to be associated with an increased risk of bladder cancer. This conclusion is strengthened by the consistency of the normal findings for nearly all possible artificially sweetened substances, even after considering frequency, quantity, and duration of use. It is further substantiated by the persistence of the findings after adjusting for the effects of smoking, occupation, age, diabetes mellitus, and several other potential confounding factors. Most importantly, the relative risk of bladder cancer does not increase with increasing exposure to artificial sweeteners. This absence of a dose-response effect is inconsistent with an etiologic relationship.

During the three years prior to the FDA's recent action, several other epidemiologic analyses of the saccharin issue appeared. These included a cohort analysis of bladder cancer mortality trends, another analysis of bladder cancer mortality among diabetics, and three retrospective studies designed for other purposes but incorporating information relevant to the artificial sweetener issue. The results of all these studies were unequivocally negative.

Among epidemiologic studies, only one has yielded findings that might be interpreted as suggesting the possible carcinogenicity of saccharin in human beings. An intriguing feature of this study (Howe, Burch, et al., 1977) is that it found its way to the FDA several months before its publication and very shortly after the FDA proposal to ban saccharin except as an over-the-counter drug. On June 27, 1977—a time when his agency was subjected to widespread criticism for its proposal—Commissioner Kennedy discussed the Canadian study and its possible relevance to the proposed saccharin ban in considerable detail before the Subcommittee on Health and the Environment of the Committee on Interstate and Foreign Commerce of the House of Representatives. No mention whatever was made of our findings, which were then available to the FDA in both published and prepublished forms.

The Canadian study used the classical case-control method. Bladder cancer cases were identified through provincial cancer registries and cooperating pathologists and neurologists. Controls were selected from residential neighborhoods among individuals matching the cases on sex and age. The subjects were questioned at length on occupation, use of water supplies, and medical histories, as well as artificial sweetener exposure.

With respect to saccharin, only three questions were asked, though the answers were recorded in detail. An anomaly in this study was that the subjects were questioned on their use of tablets and drops but not powders, which represent a significant proportion of artificial sweetener use. Furthermore, the calendar period during which sweeteners were used was not ascertained at the interview. Thus, patients who began using saccharin *after* the onset of cancer might well have been included in the analysis.

Several findings in the Canadian study are unexpected, biologically inconsistent, or otherwise in need of explanation. The data suggest a 60 percent increased risk of bladder cancer among male saccharin users as well as a statistically significant 40 percent *decrease* in such risk among females. If regulation of food additives were to be made—as some appear to recommend—on the basis of statistical considerations alone, one might exploit Canadian findings to recommend saccharin use to women in order to reduce their cancer risk!

Another serious inconsistency is that Canadian users of saccharin-containing beverages or foods, as contrasted with table-top drops or tablets, experienced no increase in cancer risk. The issue is a crucial one because diet beverages contribute far more to artificial sweetener exposure (perhaps 80 percent of the total) than do saccharin tablets or drops alone. These inconsistencies suggest that selective biases rather than true case-control differences might account for some of the findings in the Canadian study.

I agree with several comments made in a Lancet editorial (1977) that concluded that "most readers will find the case against saccharin unimpressive." The editor surmised:

> No non-hormonal carcinogen in man is known to affect only one sex, and the case made by the Canadian workers that saccharin is the first such example is less than convincing . . . . The methods of analysis do little to clarify whether the apparent effect of artificial sweeteners is real or whether it is merely due to cigarette smoking and/or coffee consumption . . . . It is not reassuring that the investigators failed to report any respect in which the cases and controls were similar and substantial differences were detected in education, occupation, history of urinary infection, and source of water supply, besides tobacco and coffee consumption.

Thus, it is fair to conclude that the epidemiologic evidence on saccharin is largely and consistently negative, with the Canadian study findings representing only a partial exception. Anamnestic evidence of the epidemiologic kind is certainly not adequate *per se* to resolve this important health issue.

Statistical inferences. One can argue, for example, that the sample sizes of even the largest of saccharin studies were insufficient to rule out a weak carcinogenic effect. However, although this limitation of individual epidemiologic studies may be conceded, no one seems to have estimated the statistical power of *all* the epidemiologic studies combined to rule out a carcinogenic effect of saccharin. Since each of the studies was conducted under somewhat different circumstances and among different population groups, I should think that a small but consistent carcinogenic risk attributable to artificial sweeteners would not easily remain undetected for long.

Minuscule or demographically insignificant risks might continue to elude statistical detection, but this involves the question of the risk level at which governmental regulation should be invoked.

Assessments of low level carcinogenic hazards can be mischievous in settings like our own. The secret is to multiply the risk factor (1 percent or 0.1 percent or 0.01 percent, etc.) by the population of 215,000,000. Thus, instead of describing a potential cancer risk attributable, for example, to saccharin as 0.01 percent, define it in terms of a risk that potentially affects 21,500 people. Such statistical manipulations may have enormous public impact but they are demagogic because society presently lacks the means to detect such low risks—if they do indeed exist—against the variety of background noises involved.

Epidemiologic studies are viewed skeptically by some because of their presumed lack of specificity. They are certainly less specific than laboratory studies conducted on inbred animal strains under highly controlled conditions. On the other hand, the naturally occurring cancers in human society probably arise from a complex of interactions between environmental agents (e.g., saccharin) and host factors such as genotype, constitution, hormone profile, and immune status. Thus, one may argue that epidemiologic studies conducted in their natural milieu are eminently appropriate and realistic. They would, by this definition, contrast favorably with what might be regarded as the rather abstract setting of the typical laboratory experiment.

Sex differences in susceptibility. There is one more somewhat perplexing but persistent epidemiologic finding related to artificial sweetener effects that requires elucidation. In several of the studies, including our own, the relative risks of bladder cancer are greater among male sweetener users than female. This may be important if only because of the relatively greater ease of induction of bladder tumors in male rats with such substances as diethyleneglycol. On the other hand, the higher relative risks among males was obtained for both saccharin and cyclamate usage. This suggests the operation of an artifact because the two sweeteners are chemically distinct and would not be expected to produce the same effect. One possible explanation may stem from the fact that our male subjects drank significantly more coffee than did the controls, whereas there were no differences in this regard between female cases and controls. Coffee is often taken with artificial sweeteners and may itself be a weak bladder carcinogen.

A Dilemma

Epidemiologists interested in the saccharin controversy today face a peculiar dilemma. Epidemiologic and other evidence on saccharin carcinogenicity is so unimpressive that under ordinary circumstances, few if any additional studies would be undertaken. However, the massive intervention of the regulatory agencies into this arena, and their proposed ban on saccharin, clearly dictates that additional epidemiologic evidence be compiled. Unfortunately, because of the publicity and apprehension engendered, epidemiologic studies conducted at this time are unlikely to yield unbiased responses concerning the saccharin exposure of human subjects.

Curiously, the government has nevertheless embarked on a congressionally mandated $1.4 million epidemiologic study on saccharin! Nine thousand patients with and without cancer from five states and four metropolitan areas from coast to coast are to be investigated over an 18-month period. Some, though not all, controls will be selected by random digit dialing, thus excluding people who do not have telephones. Furthermore, the study protocol makes it appear likely that blind interviews will not be routinely conducted; i.e., interviewers will tend to know whether they are dealing with a bladder cancer case or a control. The potentially serious biasing effects of this situation have already been noted.

Such major investigational initiatives as the nine-area saccharin study should be undertaken by university-based epidemiologists following competitive peer review of their grant or contract proposals. No methodologic, inferential, or administrative advantages are apparent in the ongoing government study as compared with the traditional grant-supported research mechanism. If 9000 subjects were deemed necessary for a study, a collaborative effort among experts from several academic institutions could easily have been arranged. There are many precedents for this in conjoint studies of diabetes, cardiovascular disease, and cancer. Not the least of the advantages of this approach would have been a cleaner separation of the information gathering effort from the regulatory function of the federal government.

Laboratory-Based Studies

Since its discovery in 1879, saccharin has been subjected to a wide variety of toxicologic studies, both here and abroad. The literature of the late Victorian era is replete with conflicting reports on the use of this substance for diabetes as well as for the treatment of various gastrointestinal and other conditions. In 1912, a Board of Scientific Advisors to the Secretary of Agriculture appointed by President Theodore Roosevelt concluded that 0.3 grams per day of saccharin was safe, but that intake of more than one gram per day caused digestive disturbances.

Saccharin consumption was greatly increased in Europe during World Wars I and II without any apparent adverse effects, although no systematic epidemiologic studies on the consuming public were undertaken at the time. Between the wars, numerous toxicologic studies on experimental animals were conducted. These raised no serious questions about the sweetener's safety.

However, by 1954, as saccharin became more prevalent in the American diet, the Committee on Food Protection of the National Academy of Sciences (NAS) was requested to review the toxicologic literature on the subject. It was concluded that the maximum probable tolerance level for saccharin in the human diet was at least as high as 1.0 gram per day. Another NAS Committee on Food Protection report, issued in 1968, came to similar conclusions but recommended that new studies be undertaken utilizing the current, higher standards of testing.

Still another NAS committee reviewed the existing data in 1970, shortly after the cyclamate ban, and it concluded that saccharin was safe. Like its predecessor, the committee also suggested further toxicologic investigations as well as comparative studies on the metabolic processes of animals and man.

In early 1972, saccharin was removed from the GRAS list on the basis of preliminary reports from a Wisconsin Alumni Research Foundation (WARF) study in which bladder tumors were found in four rats fed a 5 percent saccharin diet over their lifetimes. The comparable human dosage would be in excess of 1200 bottles of diet soda per day for life. Rats in the WARF study that were fed a saccharin-containing diet more comparable to that in human populations showed no adverse effects.

During the ensuing two years, the WARF and FDA conducted studies in which rats were fed maximum tolerable doses of saccharin over two successive generations. The results were inconsistent. At a 5 percent dietary intake level, the incidence of bladder cancer in the treated F_1 generation male rats was significantly increased over that in the control rats of the WARF series but not of the FDA series. However, at a 7.5 percent dietary level, the differences between the treated and untreated male rats of the FDA study became statistically significant.

These results were apparently sufficiently equivocal to deter further FDA action until early 1977, when the results of a new two-generation feeding study were reported by the Canadian National Health and Welfare Ministry. This study had been designed primarily to evaluate the separate effects of saccharin and its major contaminant ortho-toluenesulfonamide (OTS), which was not possible in the WARF and FDA studies. Seven of 38 F_0 generation male rats on the saccharin diet developed bladder tumors (3 malignant, 4 benign), a significantly higher proportion than in the control group (0 malignant, 1 benign). Twelve of 45 F_1 generation male rats on the saccharin diet developed bladder tumors (8 malignant, 4 benign), as compared with none among the control animals. Since the experiment was conducted with 50 rats per group, it is apparent that 12 treated and 14 control F_0 generations rats and 5 treated and 8 control F_1 generation rats were unaccounted for.

On March 9, 1977, the FDA announced the results of the Canadian study and stated that the law required the removal of saccharin from the food supply, citing the Delaney clause of the Food, Drug and Cosmetic Act. On April 14, 1977, FDA Commissioner Kennedy announced the intention to propose a ban on saccharin, which was published in the Federal Register on the following day. Essentially, this would ban the use of saccharin from foods, beverages, cosmetics, drugs, and animal feeds, but would permit its marketing as a single ingredient over-the-counter drug.

The Canadian study results pose difficult inferential problems. None of the first generation female rats—even those fed the 5 percent saccharin diet over a lifetime—developed bladder cancer. In fact, out of the 300 female rats in the several treatment groups, only one developed even a benign bladder tumor—and this was an animal fed the lowest of all the saccharin diets. Among the second generation female rats, only two—again those on the lowest saccharin diet—developed benign bladder tumors, and only two at the 5 percent dosage level manifested bladder cancer. The curious fact that bladder cancer incidence was identical among the treated (5 percent saccharin) and control F_1 generation rats in the FDA study has already been noted.

A serious problem is posed by the observation that in many of the earlier toxicologic studies, several types of tumors were reported to be associated with saccharin feeding. These included lesions of the reproductive and hematopoietic systems, the lungs, and the cardiovascular organs, as well as of the squamous epithelium. Unless one is willing to entertain a theory of universal carcinogens, it is difficult to accept such evidence as supporting a specific carcinogenic effect of saccharin.

The issue is an important one because it provides much of the rationale for the Delaney-type approach to cancer regulation. Those who support this view are impressed by the fact that with the possible exception of arsenic, every substance proven to cause cancer in man has also been shown to cause cancer in animals. Therefore, it is argued, extrapolation from mouse to man makes eminent good sense. Those of us on the other side of this judgmental fence believe that specific host-agent interactions produce site-specific neoplasms. Uncritical extrapolation from animal studies to man is unjustified. Thus, the fact that saccharin feeding studies were associated with ovarian, lymphatic, or respiratory tumors in rats does not substantiate the carcinogenicity of saccharin to the human bladder.

The Canadian Study

The Canadian study that precipitated the most recent FDA action was, as already mentioned, not designed to evaluate the carcinogenicity of saccharin but rather to differentiate between the effects of saccharin and OTS. Accordingly, only one dose level of saccharin was employed, thus making it impossible to generate any information on the presence of a dose-related response to the sweetener.

In contrast with other carcinogenicity experiments, the animals were not sacrificed for necropsy at scheduled intervals during the trials; instead, they were merely examined each day for clinical signs of tumors. This apparent weakness in the study protocol may be responsible for the confusion that persisted with respect to the precise number of bladder tumors developing in the different trial groups. At various times, it was suggested that 14 or 12 or 8 of the second generation male rats had developed histopathologically confirmed bladder cancer. Another cause of concern is that the second generation tumors that developed among the Canadian study rats, and possibly among those in the WARF and FDA studies as well, appeared to be unlike human bladder carcinomas in their low degree of invasiveness and complete absence of metastases.

Some anomalies in the FDA and WARF studies also require resolution. For example, in the FDA study, more bladder cancers occurred among the control male rats than among those fed saccharin, except at the 7.5 percent dose level. In fact, rats fed moderate dosages of saccharin actually had a lower incidence of bladder hyperplasia than the controls. In the WARF study, very small numbers of animals were employed, and bladder tumors were found only among male rats at the highest saccharin dose levels. To aggravate the confusion, the incidence of adrenal, pancreatic, uterine, thyroid, pituitary, and other tumors was considerably higher among the control rats than among rats exposed to saccharin.

There is also some evidence that rats clear high doses of saccharin differently than they clear low doses, as the mechanism for renal tubular secretion becomes overloaded. This alone would make it difficult to justify extrapolation from high dose to low dose animal experiments, let alone to low dose human exposures.

In recent years, a number of short-term *in vitro* tests have been developed for use in predicting whether substances are likely to cause cancer. Most commonly, these evaluate the extent to which suspect substances (such as saccharin) are mutagenic or interactive with DNA. The large majority of short-term tests for genetic effects of saccharin and some of its impurities have been negative. Thus, the substance may not even be mutagenic, although more research on this question is certainly necessary.

The Committee for Study on Saccharin and Food Safety Policy of the National Academy of Sciences-National Research Council recently concluded that "either saccharin is unusual in that its carcinogenic effects are due to the unmetabolized parent compound or the effects are due to small quantities of undetected metabolites" (NAS-NRC, 1978). The Committee was led to this conclusion because little biotransformation of saccharin has been detected in laboratory animals and none at all has been observed in humans. The fact that people do not metabolize saccharin but excrete essentially all of it unchanged in the urine poses a formidable problem to those who support its carcinogenicity.

Confounding factors. Certain technical problems have added to the difficulties in interpreting the toxicologic studies. For example, the tumors observed in the *in utero* studies were often associated with altered urine composition and crystalluria. In addition, such animals often demonstrated body weight losses in excess of 10 percent, suggesting that the experiments might have been conducted at saccharin levels exceeding the maximum tolerable dose.

One might also ask whether it is appropriate to employ saccharin dosages that kill perhaps 50 percent of the rats because of toxicity long before the anticipated development of cancer among the survivors. The other effect of these high dosages—i.e., saturation of the renal tubular secretion mechanism—becomes manifest at approximately the 5 percent dietary level of saccharin. Therefore, at feeding dosages exceeding 5 percent, the excretion of other, possibly carcinogenic, metabolites may be impeded, thus producing bladder cancers that are fundamentally unrelated to the saccharin.

The Regulatory Dilemma

Not too many years ago, a president of the United States declared war on heart disease, cancer, and stroke. Many millions of dollars later, with expenditures unmatched by achievements, this moonshot-type endeavor was allowed to die. That initiative was succeeded almost immediately by the National Cancer Program of another president, an effort characterized by organ-site cancer task forces dispensing cornucopias of research ideas, money, and advice to the academic community.

Spanning most of the years between these presidential initiatives was the Era of Viral Carcinogenesis, an epoch based upon the conviction that oncogenic viruses were an important, if not *the* important, factor in human cancer. For historical reasons among others, research on cancers associated with RNA viruses was supported as never before. The carcinogenic potential of the DNA viruses (e.g., genital herpes virus) received marginal funding, whereas chemical and environmental carcinogens were out of fashion.

The Era of Viral Carcinogenesis came to an abrupt end when (1) essentially no evidence on the role of RNA viruses in any human cancer was convincingly developed, (2) the Special Virus Cancer Program was dissolved, and (3) two recent winners of the Nobel Prize in Medicine specifically discounted the relevance of their work to the viral etiology of cancer in man.

Almost predictably, the Era of Viral Carcinogenesis was succeeded by the Era of Environmental Carcinogenesis. The government now cited such statements as "Reasonable estimates are that not more than 5 percent of human cancer is due to viruses and less than 5 percent to radiations. Some 90 percent of cancer in man is therefore due to chemicals." Most recently, the public has been reading regulatory agency statements suggesting that 20 or 40 or 60 percent of all cancers are due to occupational exposures of one sort or another.

As a clinical epidemiologist, I find myself wondering what has happened to the classical triad in disease etiology of agent, host, and environment. In the highly contrived setting of the animal laboratory, tumor induction may sometimes be produced by straightforward exposure of test animals to known carcinogens. In the real and complex world of human beings, however, the situation is far different.

Although heavy cigarette smokers incur an eight- or tenfold greater risk of lung cancer than do nonsmokers, most heavy smokers will never develop lung cancer at all. The same is probably true for all the known human carcinogens. The enormous variability of tumor inductibility in man is related in part to the genetic, immunologic, hormonal, and other constitutional differences among individuals; in part to the degree and duration of carcinogenic exposure; and in part to other factors as yet unknown.

The multifactorial nature of human cancer etiology presents serious problems to the investigator, to the regulator, and to the general public. The investigator is obliged to conduct his experiments in such fashion as to take account of, or control, as many of the host and environmental factors that might affect the agent's potency as possible. For all its shortcomings, the epidemiologic method of studying the development of cancer in human subjects in their natural habitat under controlled conditions represents a rational and effective approach to this challenge. For all its evident simplicity, the classic toxicologic testing situation—although it may contribute greatly to our knowledge of carcinogenic mechanisms—is in fact quite an artificial setting, particularly if one wishes to extrapolate findings from animals to man.

To the health regulator, the epidemiologic triad poses an especially vexing problem because the government, having embarked on a well publicized crusade to protect its citizens against the menace of cancer, must make good its promise. Impatient as the government is with the complexity of the situation and with our rather humbling ignorance concerning cancer, bureaucratically simple mechanisms for decision making on the carcinogenicity of suspected substances have earned highest priority.

Whereas those of us in academia may be perfectly content to advance knowledge deliberately and circumspectly, government regulators are under enormous public pressure to make decisions and to make them rapidly. This explains their oft expressed disenchantment with epidemiologic studies that usually require three or four years for completion and that are basically unsuited for randomized testing of suspected carcinogens to which human populations have not been spontaneously exposed. This also explains their reliance upon laboratory animal studies in which potential confounding factors such as species specificity, strain specificity, experimental conditions, and extrapolation problems are unresolved. In good measure, this also explains the enthusiasm with which the short-term *in vitro* tests for mutagenicity were supported and highly publicized, despite their obvious limitations.

The conflict is obvious. Bombarded on all sides by the daily media warnings of new threats to life, the public reads of cancer risks in articles written by scientifically uneducated reporters and is confronted by warning labels on products readily available in the neighborhood supermarket.

Our regulatory dilemma today is due, in part, to the very real fact that the prevalence of cancer is increasing. This in turn stems from our increasing longevity and possibly from the increasing number and variety of chemical substances in the environment. Because of the relatively sudden appearance of these agents, our normal evolutionary adaptive mechanisms may be proving inadequate. The regulatory dilemma also arises from the increasingly consumer-oriented society in which we live. Disease is no longer regarded as an act of God but rather as a challenge to government, which is responsible for protecting us therefrom, regardless of whether the means are at hand.

Many thousands of citizens and scientists now owe their livelihood to the existence of regulatory agencies and research laboratories concerned with the human cancer problem. These individuals constitute what may be termed a *cancer constituency*, because they benefit personally from the belief, for example, that saccharin causes human bladder cancer. Were saccharin and a number of other suspected substances finally deemed safe for human consumption, this would contract the activities of the regulatory agencies and research laboratories, thereby reducing employment or promotion possibilities for many individuals therein.

I have the impression that the regulatory agencies are considerably more interested in positive (i.e., cancer-associated) results than in negative findings among studies that are equally well designed and executed. In fact, a number of high-level regulatory officials have publicly supported the notion that positive epidemiologic findings should be taken seriously by the government, but that negative findings may be ignored because of the inherent weaknesses of the epidemiologic method.

A crucial factor in the regulatory situation is introduced by the Delaney Amendment to the Food, Drug and Cosmetic Act. The effect of the Delaney clause is to make the regulatory process more perfunctory, automatic, and bureaucratic, and to influence it by statistical rather than by biologic considerations. Should the question of saccharin's safety be resolved on the basis of the statistical significance of differences between case and control groups or in terms of the power of the statistical test at given α and β levels?

The saccharin question is a biologic issue that must be resolved primarily by the application of scientific reasoning to the biomedical data at hand. Thus, instead of focusing upon the statistical significance of the increased bladder cancer among the Canadian males, one should be assessing the biologic significance of the findings, including the remarkable sex disparity, the absence of a relationship with diet drinks or foods, and the absence of a substantial dose-response association. The fact that man does not metabolize saccharin is another biologic reality that cannot be simply dismissed on statistical grounds or otherwise ignored. Coherence of one's observations with previously established facts is an essential element in the process of imputing cancer to saccharin or to any other suspect agent.

Epidemiologic evidence on saccharin should be taken seriously. The purported weakness of the epidemiologic approach is contradicted by the specious argument often used—i.e., that the studies are not based upon large enough samples of individuals to permit a definitive test of the hypothesis. The argument is specious, in my opinion, because it is made by the same critics who defend the use of 40 or 50 animals per experiment in the toxicologic setting as representing a reasonable approach. This limitation in turn necessitates the feeding of nonphysiologic doses of saccharin or other test substances, with all the inferential consequences that this entails.

We should not have it both ways. If epidemiologic studies are defective because of inadequate sample size—generally 500 or 600 subjects—this should also apply to the classical rat feeding study involving 50 or so rats per treatment group. If it is difficult and expensive to investigate 10,000 people, it would certainly be less difficult and less expensive to investigate 10,000 rats. Yet, with very few exceptions, this is not being done. If the saccharin issue is sufficiently important to justify Congressional hearings, numerous NAS evaluations, and other costly activities, the use of 100,000 rats exposed to varying doses of saccharin down to physiologic levels is also justified. At the very least, such a study would go far to answer the question of whether thresholds exist for cancer induction by such substances as saccharin.

The threshold question is a crucial one if only because it evokes the question of absolute safety. Some have argued that the food and drug laws should be applied so as to assure the public of the absolute safety—i.e., the total absence of a carcinogenic risk—of all foods and food additives. Absolute safety could be assured for substances in which there is a dose threshold. Without it, the only other option would be a total ban of the suspected substance.

In the light of the complexity of the human carcinogenetic process, however, the concept of absolute safety is difficult to defend. For example, how should one regulate saccharin if it were proven to be weakly carcinogenic only in immunodeficient people? Would it be more rational to banish the substance from the general marketplace or to make special provision for protecting the susceptible few?

I regret that little or no consideration is being given these days to host factors in human cancer. Government regulators appear to be taking a simplistic course in which they seek to characterize saccharin as a carcinogen without in any way determining the conditions under which it may or may not be carcinogenic. Elucidation of host factors that protect most of us but predispose some of us to cancer would represent an extremely rational approach to cancer control at the public level.

The Delaney-based orientation of our current regulatory system is well intentioned but unduly susceptible to bureaucratic whim. It singles out cancer to the exclusion of cardiovascular and other chronic diseases that kill and disable most of us. It calls for judgments on the basis of *appropriate tests* without providing any definition of the term. Does one positive test override three negatives? Should seven well designed negative studies refute one positive study?

The Delaney approach permits no balancing of the presumed risks against the benefits to the obese, the carious, or the diabetic. It does not represent a bending over backwards to protect the public against carcinogenic risk because these risks are generally species-specific. Under the Delaney clause, a negative saccharin feeding study might be regarded as implying the safety of the substance, when in fact other species, including man, might actually test positive. Thus, the injudicious application of the Delaney clause could confer a false sense of security with respect to many substances to which we are exposed and that happen to prove negative in the particular animal species tested.

Conclusion

Well controlled epidemiologic studies, conducted on relatively large numbers of people in their natural habitat, are in accord on the safety of saccharin in moderate doses. A Canadian study suggests that saccharin feeding may actually protect women from bladder cancer while increasing the risk among men who ingest the substance in the form of tablets or drops, rather than in powders, diet beverages, or diet foods.

A host of toxicologic studies on saccharin, including two two-generation trials, were considered essentially negative for carcinogenicity in a succession of evaluative reviews by such elite bodies as the National Academy of Sciences. However, when 8 Canadian F_1 generation male rats on a lifetime 5 percent saccharin diet developed malignant tumors—a yield far exceeding expectation—some of the earlier studies were reinterpreted as being confirmatory of these findings, and a saccharin ban was proposed by the Food and Drug Administration.

However, the evidence against saccharin is weak, inconsistent, and lacking coherence with existing knowledge on the physiologic, metabolic, and dose-response relationships of the carcinogenic process. In view of the two-generation findings among male rats, it would be prudent for pregnant or lactating women and their offspring to avoid saccharin, at least until adequate epidemiologic studies on second generation effects in humans have been completed. Otherwise, I recommend against the banning of saccharin.

References

Armstrong, B., and Doll, R.: Bladder cancer mortality in England and Wales in relation to cigarette smoking and saccharin consumption. Br. J. Prev. Soc. Med. 28:233–240, 1974.

Armstrong, B., and Doll, R.: Bladder cancer mortality in diabetics in relation to saccharin consumption and smoking habits. Br. J. Prev. Soc. Med. 29:73–81, 1975.

Armstrong, B., et al.: Cancer mortality and saccharin consumption in diabetics. Br. J. Prev. Soc. Med. 30:151–157, 1976.

Arnold, D.L., Moodie, C.A., Grice, H.D., Charbonneau, S.M., Stavrice, B., Collins, B.T., McGuire, P.F., and Munroe, I.C.: Long term toxicity of ortho-toluenesulfonamide and sodium saccharin in the rat: an interim report. Ottawa, Canada, Toxicology Research Division, Health Protection Branch, National Health and Welfare Ministry, 1977.

Burbank, F., and Fraumeni, J.F., Jr.: Synthetic sweetener consumption and bladder cancer trends in the U.S. Nature 227:296–297, 1970.

Department of Health, Education and Welfare: Saccharin and its salts: proposed rules and hearings. Federal Register Part III, April 15, 1977.

Department of Health, Education and Welfare (Division of Pathology): Sub-acute and chronic toxicity and carcinogenicity of various dose levels of sodium saccharin, P-169-170. Final Report, 1973a.

Editorial: Bladder cancer and saccharin. Lancet II:592–593, 1977.

Howe, G.R., Burch, J.D., Miller, A.B., et al.: Artificial sweeteners and human bladder cancer. Lancet II:578–581, 1977.

Kessler, I.I.: Cancer mortality among diabetics. J. Natl. Cancer Inst. 44:673–686, 1970.

Kessler, I.I.: Non-nutritive sweeteners and human bladder cancer: preliminary findings. J. Urol. 115:143–146,1976.

Kessler, I.I., and Clark, J.P.: Saccharin, cyclamate and human bladder cancer; No evidence of an association. JAMA 240:349–355, 1978.

National Academy of Science-National Research Council (Committee for a Study on Saccharin and Food Safety): Saccharin: technical assessment of risks and benefits. Washington, D.C., 1978.

Office of Technology Assessment, Congress of the United States: Cancer testing technology and saccharin. Washington, D.C., October, 1977 (Lib. of Congress Card #77-600051).

Renwick, A.G.: The metabolism, distribution and elimination of non-nutritive sweeteners. In Guggenheim, B., ed., Health and Sugar Substitutes (Proceedings of ERGOB Conference on Sugar Substitutes), Geneva, S. Karger Basel, 1978.

Thomas, D.L.: Bitter and sweet. Barron's, September 29, 1975.

Thomas, H., and Maugh I.I.: Chemicals: how many are there? Science 199:162, 1978.

Wisconsin Alumni Research Foundation: Long-term saccharin feeding in rats. Final Report, WARF, Madison, Wisconsin, 1973.

Index

Page numbers in *italic* type refer to illustrations; (t) denotes tabular material.

B

C

M

N

O

P

Q

R

S